C0-ATK-185

Medical Radiology

Diagnostic Imaging

For further volumes:
http://www.springer.com/series/4354

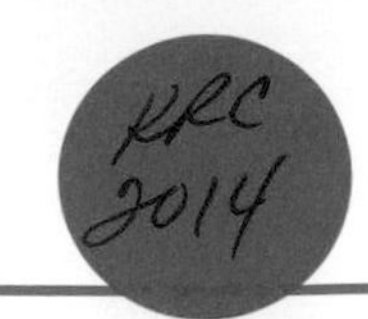

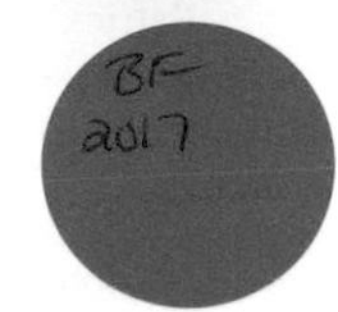

Patrick Peller • Rathan Subramaniam
Ali Guermazi
Editors

PET-CT and PET-MRI in Oncology

A Practical Guide

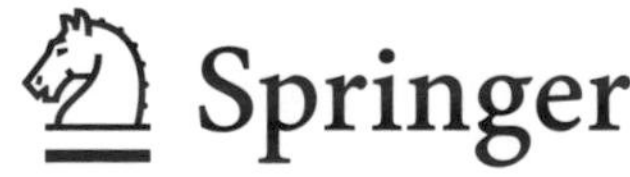

Editors
Patrick Peller
Rochester, MN
USA

Ali Guermazi
Boston University Medical Center
Boston, MA
USA

Rathan Subramaniam
Boston University School of Medicine
Boston, MA
USA

ISBN 978-3-642-01138-2 ISBN 978-3-642-01139-9 (eBook)
DOI 10.1007/978-3-642-01139-9
Springer Heidelberg New York Dordrecht London

Library of Congress Control Number: 2012949365

Printed on acid-free paper

Springer is part of Springer Science+Business Media (www.springer.com)

"We should not be ashamed to acknowledge truth from whatever source it comes to us, even if it is brought to us by former generations and foreign people. For him who seeks the truth there is nothing of higher value than truth itself"

Abu Yusuf Yaqub ibn Ishaq as-Sabbah al-Kindi (Alkindus) 801–873

"The scientists of today think deeply instead of clearly. One must be sane to think clearly, but one can think deeply and be quite insane"

Nikola Tesla 1856–1943

"Chance favors only those who know how to court her"

Charles Nicolle 1866–1936

Foreword

PET-CT is growing faster than any other imaging modality, and oncology is still by far the most frequent application of this modality. PET-CT has sometimes been termed a "no brainer" examination, insinuating that it does not require deep knowledge and extensive experience. Evidently, this is not true by any means. In order to fully exploit the diagnostic information provided by PET-CT and PET-MRI, deep knowledge of both PET and the corresponding method—CT or MRI—is indispensable.

The editors of this book, Patrick Peller, Rathan Subramaniam, and Ali Guermazi, have been able to gather distinguished experts in the field who, in part I of the book, have contributed most informative chapters on physics and technology, radiochemistry, and the basics of interpreting PET-CT and PET-MRI results. These important chapters provide the reader with the knowledge required in order to interpret adequately the results of hybrid examinations.

Biology, staging, and therapy monitoring of different tumor entities vary widely, and diagnosticians should also be aware of current treatment strategies in order to provide the best possible advice to clinicians. In part II of the book, the results of PET-CT and PET-MRI in common cancer entities are described in a series of informative chapters organized according to different organ systems and clinical disciplines: central nervous system, head and neck, chest, breast, gastrointestinal, genitourinary, gynecologic, musculoskeletal and soft tissue sarcoma, hematology, dermatologic, and pediatric.

Further important topics addressed in the book include radiotherapy planning and assessment of therapeutic response and metastatic disease.

PET-CT has become an important and most valuable modality in planning radiotherapy since it permits more accurate definition of the target volume and allows the biology and response of the tumor tissue to the radiation therapy to be taken into account, thus enabling "dose painting".

Owing to the increasingly effective means of cancer treatment, including drugs for targeted therapy, various cancer entities have become chronic diseases. Therefore, assessment of therapy response and metastatic disease is key to the selection of personalized therapy that is most appropriate for a particular patient.

The editors of *Medical Radiology—Diagnostic Imaging* would like to express their gratitude and appreciation to the editors and authors of *PET-CT and PET-MRI in Oncology* for this outstanding book. We are confident that readers and ultimately our patients will benefit greatly.

Maximilian F. Reiser

Foreword

The field of oncology remains a formidable challenge for the entire medical field. We have made so much progress and yet we have such a long way to go. Many advances are still needed to truly help individuals who have yet to be diagnosed with cancer as well as those already diagnosed. Positron emission tomography (PET) has emerged as a key imaging technology that has helped to radically change how we stage and manage cancer. The field has grown so rapidly over the last decade that a book such as this is critical to help both new and seasoned physicians.

This is a very well-written and organized book to help introduce the reader to rigorous interpretation of PET-CT oncological images. The book also addresses the important emerging area of PET-MRI that is likely to play an increasing role in the upcoming decade. The image examples are numerous and will clearly benefit physicians at all levels. Detailed coverage of the basic physics and radiochemistry is followed by the basics of image interpretation. Details of oncological applications (e.g., head & neck cancer) allow one to quickly synthesize important issues for each cancer type. Three chapters in this book are unique and make this book a standout—HIV disease, Therapy Response, and PET/CT interpretation. The final chapter on PET pitfalls and artifacts is also unique and an excellent way to stay up-to-date on key image interpretation issues.

This book will be an important resource for years to come and is a welcome addition to the growing knowledge base behind PET-CT and PET-MRI. Although the field of oncology and the use of imaging in cancer will continue to rapidly evolve, the fundamentals covered in this book should remain timeless.

Sanjiv Sam Gambhir

Preface

This book deals with various aspects of PET/CT and PET/MRI in oncology. When we began to plan the book, we aimed to give the reader a clear understanding of the physics that underlie these very complex technologies, before describing how the scanners are applied in clinical oncology. We begin with a chapter explaining in some detail how PET/CT and PET/MRI scanners work and how to maximize their inherent qualities for optimum results. The next chapter gives a fairly detailed overview of PET radiochemistry and radiotracers. The third chapter introduces, step by step, the basics of interpreting PET/CT and PET/MRI results. We think these three introductory chapters will provide readers with a strong basis for understanding the technology behind these imaging modalities. This understanding is absolutely necessary to interpret images that can be very complicated indeed, and it provides a foundation for the center of the book, 14 chapters on PET/CT and PET/MRI as applied to the most commonly encountered cancers including HIV issues. The significant role of PET/CT in planning radiotherapy is also included. These chapters are generously illustrated. In the final chapter, the theoretical understanding of the first three chapters and the practical aspects of various oncological situations are brought together with a detailed and thorough chapter on common errors associated with the use of PET/CT and PET/MRI. These are powerful but very complex technologies, and the path to diagnosis is strewn with pitfalls and artifacts that can easily lead the reader to the wrong diagnosis. Foreknowledge of these potential problems will save time and money, and will improve patient care.

All of the authors who participated in this work are renowned experts in their fields, from North America, Europe, Asia and Australia. We are indebted to them for their work and dedication and we hope the book will meet their best expectations.

We would like to dedicate this book to our wives Maribeth, Sakila and Noura and children Cynthia, Katrina, John, Meera, Anjana, Santhiya, Dorra, Elias and Manel. Without their patience and love, this book will certainly will not be public today.

Rochester	Patrick Peller
Baltimore	Rathan Subramaniam
Boston	Ali Guermazi

Contents

Contributors

M. Abou-Zied Department of Nuclear Medicine, State University of New York at Buffalo, 105 Parker Hall South Campus, 3435 Main Street, Buffalo, NY 14214, USA

A. Agarwal Boston University School of Medicine, Boston, MA 02118, USA

Bruce Barron Department of Radiology, Emory University School of Medicine, Atlanta, GA 30322, USA

François Bénard Department of Radiology, BC Cancer Agency, Functional Cancer Imaging, Centre of Excellence for Functional Cancer Imaging, University of British Columbia, Vancouver BC V5Z 4E3, Canada

David Brandon Department of Radiology, Emory University School of Medicine, Atlanta, GA 30322, USA

Jacqueline Brunetti Department of Radiology, Holy Name Medical Center, 718 Teaneck Road, Teaneck, NJ 07666, USA

Alin Chirindel Russell H Morgan Department of Radiology and Radiological Science, Johns Hopkins Medical Institutions, Baltimore, MD 21205, USA

T. Cooley Department of Oncology, Boston University School of Medicine, Boston, MA 02118, USA

J. M. Davison Department of Radiology, Boston Medical Center, Boston University School of Medicine, 820 Harrison Ave., FGH Building 3rd Floor, Boston, MA 02118, USA

Frederic H. Fahey Division of Nuclear Medicine, Harvard Medical School, Children's Hospital Boston, Boston, MA 02115, USA

Ali Gholamrezanezhad Russell H Morgan Department of Radiology and Radiological Science, Johns Hopkins Medical Institutions, Baltimore, MD 21205, USA

Ali Guermazi Department of Radiology, Boston Medical Center, Boston University School of Medicine, 820 Harrison Avenue, Boston, MA 02118, USA

Christopher Harker Hunt Department of Radiology, Mayo Clinic, Rochester, MN 55905, USA

Roland Hustinx Division of Nuclear Medicine, University Hospital of Liège, Domaine Universitaire du Sart Tilman B35, 4000, Liège 1, Belgium

T. Jackson Department of Radiology, Stanford University School of Medicine, Stanford, CA 94305-5105, USA; Department of Radiology, Boston Medical Center, Boston University School of Medicine, Boston, MA 02118, USA

Mark S. Jacobson Department of Radiology, Mayo Clinic, 200 1st Street SW, Rochester, MN 55905, USA

Hossein Jadvar Division of Nuclear Medicine, Keck School of Medicine, University of Southern California, 2250 Alcazar Street, Los Angeles, CA 90033, USA

Geoffrey Bates Johnson Department of Radiology, Mayo Clinic, Rochester, MN 55905, USA

Brad Kemp Department of Radiology, Mayo Clinic, 200 1st Street SW, Rochester, MN 55905, USA

Gustavo A. Mercier Department of Radiology, Boston University School of Medicine, Boston, MA 02118, USA

Jeffrey A. Miller Division of Nuclear Medicine, Department of Radiology, Duke University Medical Center, Box 3949, Durham, NC 27710, USA

Felix M. Mottaghy Department of Nuclear Medicine, Maastricht University Medical Center, P. Debeylaan 25, 6229 HX, Maastricht, The Netherlands; Clinic for Nuclear Medicine, University Hospital RWTH Aachen University, Pauwelsstr. 30, 52074, Aachen, Germany

Ujas Parikh, Boston University School of Medicine, Boston, MA 02118, USA

Patrick J. Peller Division of Nuclear Medicine, Department of Radiology, Mayo Clinic, 200, 1st Street SW, Rochester, MN 55905, USA

Jeffrey J. Peterson Department of Radiology, Mayo Clinic, 4500 San Pablo Road, Jacksonville, FL 32224-3899, USA

Leonne Prompers Department of Nuclear Medicine, Maastricht University Medical Center, P. Debeylaan 25, 6229 HX, Maastricht, The Netherlands

Felix-Nicolas Roy Department of Radiology, Centre Hospitalier de l'Université de Montréal (CHUM), 3840 Saint Urbain Street, Montreal, QC H2W 1T8, Canada

Gregory Russo Department of Radiation Oncology, Boston University School of Medicine, 3rd Floor, Boston, MA 02118, USA

Barry L. Shulkin Division of Diagnostic Imaging, St. Jude's Children's Research Hospital, Memphis, TN 38105, USA

Raymond A. Steichen Section of Equipment Services, Mayo Clinic, 200 1st Street SW, Rochester, MN 55905, USA

Rathan M. Subramaniam Russell H Morgan Departments of Radiology and Radiological Sciences, Johns Hopkins School of Medicine, Baltimore, MD 21205, USA

Devaki S. Surasi Department of Radiology, Boston Medical Center, Boston University School of Medicine, 820 Harrison Ave., FGH Building 3rd Floor, Boston, MA 02118, USA

Minh Tam Truong Department of Radiation Oncology, Boston Medical center, Boston, MA 02118, USA; Harvard Medical School, Boston, MA 02115, USA

Terence Z. Wong Division of Nuclear Medicine, Department of Radiology, Duke University Medical Center, Box 3949, Durham, NC 27710, USA

Part I

Basics

PET Physics and Instrumentation

Brad Kemp

Contents

B. Kemp (✉)
Department of Radiology, Mayo Clinic,
Rochester, MN, USA
e-mail: kemp.brad@mayo.edu

Abstract

In this chapter the basic principles of positron emission tomography (PET) imaging will be introduced. The physics of coincidence detection and the instrumentation used to acquire PET data will be presented. Finally, the factors that degrade PET image quality and the correction techniques employed to compensate for these factors will be reviewed.

1 Key Points

Biologically important radionuclides (C-11, N-13, O-15 and F-18) undergo positron decay. The annihilation of this emitted positron results in two 511 keV photons, which travel 180° from each other. Coincident detection of these two photons allows precise localization by the tomographic scanner in positron emission tomography (PET). Attenuation correction is crucial in the reconstruction of PET images. CT images provide a rapid and relatively noise-free means to obtain attenuation correction with the integration of PET and CT into a single scanner. Adapting the MR signal to provide attenuation correction for PET images is one of the largest hurdles in creating a successful PET and MR instrument.

2 Physics of Positron Emission Imaging

2.1 Positron Decay

In positron decay a radionuclide with an excess number of protons may decay through the emission of a positron, whereby a proton is converted into a

P. Peller et al. (eds.), *PET-CT and PET-MRI in Oncology*, Medical Radiology. Diagnostic Imaging,
DOI: 10.1007/174_2011_526, © Springer-Verlag Berlin Heidelberg 2012

Table 1 Physical properties of radionuclides commonly used in PET

Radionuclide	Half-life (min)	Maximum positron energy (MeV)	Positron range in water (mm)	β^+ Branching fraction
^{11}C	20.4	0.96	3.9	1.00
^{13}N	10.0	1.19	5.1	1.00
^{15}O	2.1	1.7	8.0	1.00
^{18}F	109.8	0.64	2.3	0.97
^{64}Cu	762	0.65	2.3	0.29
^{68}Ga	67.8	1.89	9.0	0.89
^{82}Rb	1.3	3.15	18.0	0.96
^{124}I	5,904	1.53, 2.14	7.4/10	0.23

neutron and a positron. A positron has the same mass as an electron but has a positive electric charge. Positron decay is denoted as

$$^{A}_{Z}X \rightarrow ^{A}_{Z-1} Y + \beta^{+} + v \tag{1}$$

where X is the original radionuclide of mass number A and atomic number Z, Y is the daughter nuclide, β^+ is the positron and v is a neutrino. Y has the same mass number as X but the atomic number has decreased by 1. The neutrino has no electric charge and has very little mass.

The positron and the neutrino share the energy released during positron decay, and, as a result, the positron can have a spectrum of kinetic energies from zero up to a maximum value (E_{max}) characteristic of the original nuclide. The energy will determine the distance the positron travels in matter; the direction of the positron emission is isotropic. Table 1 lists properties of radionuclides that are commonly used in positron emission tomography (PET). Radionuclides that decay primarily by positron emission and not by electron capture (i.e. that have a high positron branching fraction) are preferred for PET imaging.

2.2 Positron Annihilation

The positron travels a certain distance or range in matter, losing its kinetic energy through inelastic interactions with atomic electrons. When the positron has lost its kinetic energy and comes to rest (with thermal energy $E \sim 0.025$ eV) it will combine with a free electron in the process of annihilation. This annihilation interaction results in the creation of two 511 keV photons traveling in opposite directions from the annihilation site. The conservation of energy is obeyed, in that the masses of the positron and electron are converted into a total energy release of 1.022 MeV that is shared equally between the two photons. In addition, the conservation of momentum is obeyed such that the two photons travel away from the annihilation site at 180° from each other. If the positron had not lost its kinetic energy prior to annihilation the photons would not travel in exactly opposite directions; they would be noncolinear. Positron decay and annihilation are shown in Fig. 1.

2.3 Coincidence Detection

Positron imaging, in which detectors are placed on opposite sides of a patient, has been developed to exploit the directional relationship of the two simultaneously emitted 511 keV photons. Positron imaging uses coincidence detection circuitry to determine whether two photons are detected simultaneously or within a short ($\sim$5–10 ns) coincidence timing window. When two opposing detectors detect a pair of photons in coincidence the system assumes that the point of annihilation occurred within the volume between the two detectors. The detected event is recorded and a line joining the two detectors passes through the point of annihilation; this line is called a line of response (LOR). See Fig. 2.

The process of coincidence detection intrinsically provides positional information about the location of the annihilation event (and positron decay). This is referred to as electronic collimation and, unlike a gamma camera, it does not require absorptive or mechanical collimation to obtain positional information. As a result the sensitivity of a system employing electronic collimation is an order of magnitude greater than a system employing physical collimation.

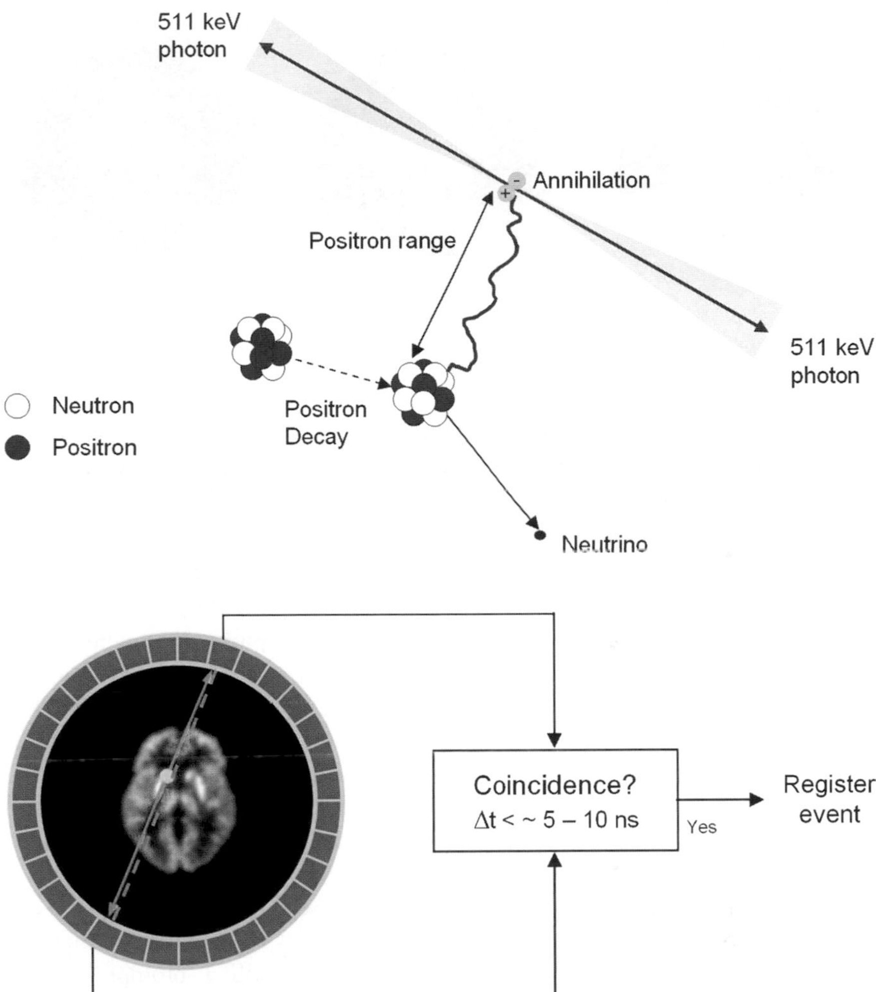

Fig. 1 Positron decay and annihilation. A nucleus with excess protons undergoes positron decay whereby a proton is transformed into a neutron and a positron and neutrino are emitted. The positron undergoes multiple inelastic interactions with electrons before annihilating with an electron in the surrounding tissue. Two 511 keV photons are emitted $180 \pm 0.25°$ from each other. The *shaded areas* represent the uncertainty in the direction of the annihilation photons

Fig. 2 Diagram showing coincidence detection of two annihilation photons. Coincidence detection circuitry measures the time of detection to determine whether two photons (*green lines*) were detected simultaneously or within a short time interval (typically 5–10 ns). If the coincidence detection criterion is met the annihilation event occurred within the volume between the two detectors. This volume is referred to as a line of response (LOR, *dashed orange line*)

The position of annihilation can be further localized by using time-of-flight (TOF) information. Basically, if the detection time of both coincidence photons can be measured accurately then the time difference in the detection times can provide information about where along the LOR the annihilation occurred. Simply stated, the location of the positron decay is closer to the detector that records the earlier detection time.

A PET scanner or tomograph is comprised of multiple cylindrical rings of detectors that surround the patient, with each detector in coincidence with a group of detectors on the opposite side of the ring. That is, each detector acquires a fanbeam of LORs. A detected event is considered valid if the following criteria are satisfied: the two annihilation photons are detected within the coincidence timing window; the LOR formed by the two photons subtends the trans-axial FOV and is within the ring difference of the system (explained below); and both photons have an energy within a predefined energy window.

2.4 Types of Coincidence Events

There are several types of coincidence events in PET imaging: true, scatter, randoms (or accidental) and multiple coincidence events. See Fig. 3 for an illustration of the various coincidence events. In PET a singles event is an individual photon that falls within the energy window of the system and is considered a valid photon. The singles rate increases linearly with the amount of radioactivity in the FOV. A true

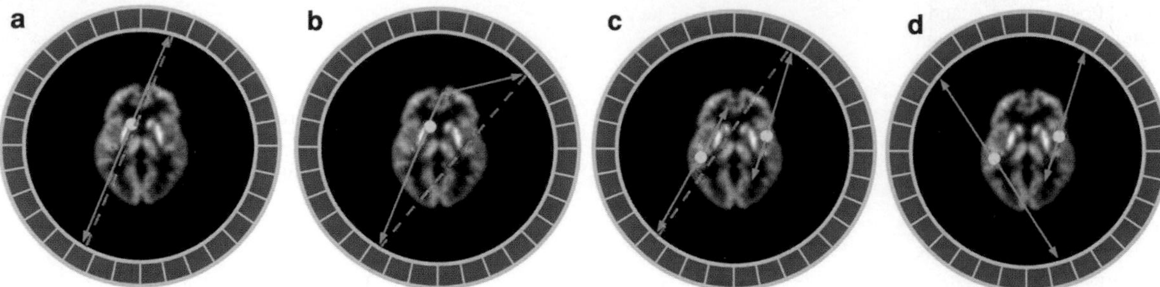

Fig. 3 Diagram showing (**a**) true, (**b**) scatter, (**c**) random and (**d**) multiple coincidence events. A detected annihilation photon is referred to as a single. The *solid lines* represent the singles while the *dashed orange line* represents the assigned line of response. The prompts coincidence events are composed of the true, scatter and random coincidence events

coincidence event occurs when both annihilation photons that are detected have not undergone any interactions within the patient.

In a scatter coincidence event one or both of the photons from the same annihilation undergo a Compton scatter interaction prior to detection. Compton scatter results in a photon with change in direction and a loss of energy, and since the scanner has a finite energy resolution, not all the scattered photons can be discriminated. Therefore, the photons are considered valid singles and the system assumes that the point of annihilation for the photon pair occurred on a line joining the two detectors. Consequently, scatter results in mispositioned events that result in a background noise within reconstructed PET images.

In random coincidence events, photons from two unrelated positron annihilations are detected within the coincidence timing window. The system assumes the photon pair were produced from the same annihilation and an LOR that does not pass through either point of annihilation is assigned. This LOR is not correlated to the location of the annihilations and image quality and quantitative accuracy are reduced. The random coincidence event rate between a pair of detectors is given as

$$R_{12} = 2\tau S_1 S_2 \tag{2}$$

where 2τ is the coincidence timing window and S_1 and S_2 are the singles rates for detector 1 and 2, respectively. Typically S_1 is approximately equal to S_2 so that the random coincidence event rate is proportional to S^2 or to the square of the activity in the scanner.

Multiple coincidence events occur when three or more singles are detected within the coincidence timing window. In this situation the system cannot determine which two singles, if any, belong to the same annihilation pair. As a result the singles are discarded and no LOR is assigned. Another type of coincidence event occurs for radionuclides that do not have a high positron branching ratio; they emit prompt gamma rays that may be in cascade with each other or with the positron decay. These spurious coincidence events are not spatially correlated to the site of the positron decay and, as such, they degrade image quality and quantitative accuracy of the PET images. Spurious coincidence events are detected when imaging ^{64}Cu or ^{124}I.

During a PET acquisition all the true, scatter, randoms and coincidence events are detected and are called prompt coincidence events (or ‘prompts’). Only true coincidence events represent the true signal from the patient; the scatter and random coincidence events represent unwanted events (noise) with incorrect positional information and must be removed from the reconstructed image. Methods to correct for random coincidence events are discussed below.

3 PET Performance

A reconstructed PET image should represent the true distribution of the radiopharmaceutical within the body. However, representation of the true radiopharmaceutical distribution in the reconstructed image will be degraded by the spatial resolution of the scanner, by noise due to limited sensitivity and by the inclusion of random and scatter events. Spatial resolution, sensitivity and the effect of random and scatter events are discussed below.

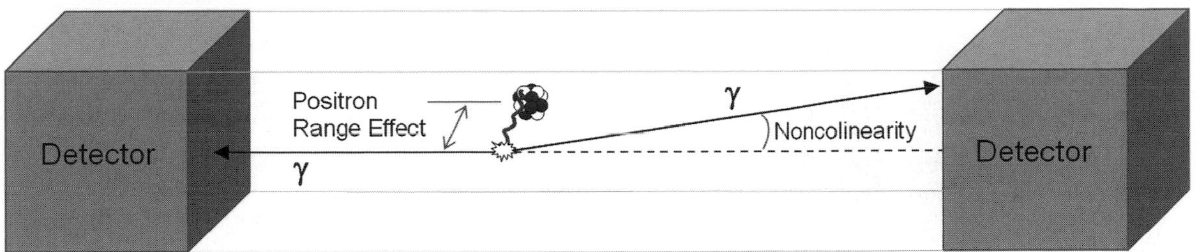

Fig. 4 Detection of annihilation photons within a volume defined by two detectors operating in coincidence. The degradation in spatial resolution due to the positron range effect is determined by the perpendicular distance the positron travels before annihilation. The degradation in spatial resolution due to noncolinearity is also shown. Because of these two effects the assigned line of response will not pass through the site of positron decay

3.1 Spatial Resolution

The spatial resolution of a PET scanner is fundamentally limited by the range of the positron and by the noncolinearity of the annihilation photons. These two effects determine the error in defining the LOR for a true coincidence event and whether it passes through the location of the radionuclide. As shown in Fig. 4 (and in Fig. 1), the positron will travel a finite distance before annihilation with an electron. As a result, the assigned LOR passes through the site of annihilation and not the location of the radionuclide (i.e. the site of positron emission). However, the effective range is much smaller than the maximum range since the positron takes a tortuous path through matter. As a result, the perpendicular distance from the site of emission to annihilation is shorter than the path length traveled. This effect, combined with the isotropic emission of the positron and the spectrum of possible positron energies suggests that the degradation of spatial resolution due to the positron range is small for clinical scanners (Levin and Hoffman 1999).

The noncolinearity of the annihilation photons arises when the positron does not come to rest before annihilation with an electron. As a result the annihilation photons will not be emitted at exactly 180° to each other but with a distribution of angles about 180°; the distribution of angles is approximately 180 ± 0.25° (Beneditti and Cowan 1950). This results in an error in the positioning of the LOR as the PET scanner defines an LOR assuming the photons were emitted at exactly 180° to each other. The effect of noncolinearity is illustrated in Fig. 4. The degradation of the spatial resolution expressed as a full-width at half maximum (FWHM) due to noncolinearity is defined as

$$\mathrm{FWHM}_{\mathrm{nc}} = \Delta\theta \times D = 0.0022 \times D \quad (3)$$

where D is the ring diameter of the PET scanner in millimeters. From this equation, the blurring caused by noncolinearity increases as the diameter of the ring increases; it will be about 2 mm for a clinical whole-body PET scanner.

There are two instrumentation factors that also limit the spatial resolution of a PET scanner. Firstly, for discrete detectors of width w in a ring, the intrinsic resolution along an LOR varies from $w/2$ at the center of the ring to w adjacent to either detector. The second factor limiting spatial resolution is referred to as parallax error or radial elongation, and the depth of an interaction within discrete detectors causes it. See Fig. 5. For increasing radial offsets from the center of the scanner, annihilation photons impinge on detectors at oblique angles and may pass through the first detector before being detected in a neighboring detector. As such the LOR that passes through the point of detection is shifted from the point of entry. As a result the effective width of a detector increases and resolution will degrade in the radial direction. Both the intrinsic resolution and parallax error are spatially variant and together with the positron range and photon noncolinearity define the resolution of PET scanners.

3.2 Sensitivity

The PET system should possess a high sensitivity for detecting the 511 keV photons that impinge on their surface. Sensitivity is defined as the number of detected true coincidence events per unit activity of

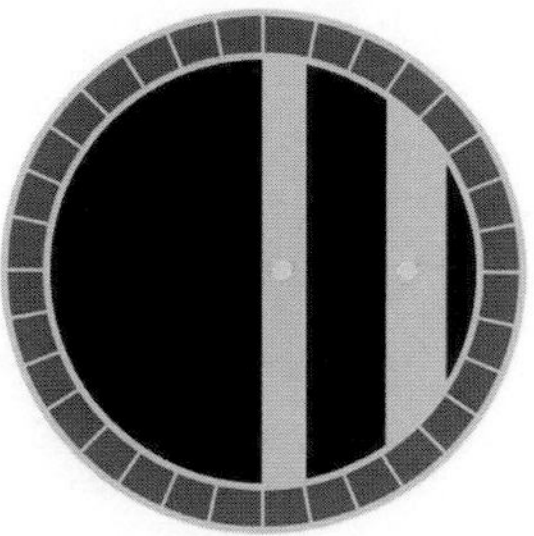

Fig. 5 Parallax error in PET systems. Annihilation photons emitted from a location off-center can penetrate more than one detector before being stopped, which results in a degradation of the spatial resolution in the radial direction. The width of the *gray bands* represents this radial elongation; this effect becomes more pronounced as the source is moved away from the center of the ring

radionuclide. A system with high sensitivity means that more true coincidence events will be detected and the resultant images will have an improved signal-to-noise ratio (SNR).

Sensitivity is determined by the geometric and intrinsic efficiencies of the system. The geometric efficiency is the fraction of emitted radiations that strike a detector and it is dependent on the overall solid angle coverage at the source subtended by the detectors. The geometric efficiency can be increased by increasing the axial coverage of the source (i.e. adding more rings), removing axial collimation, reducing the diameter of the rings and by increasing the packing fraction of the block detectors (block detectors will be discussed later).

The intrinsic efficiency is the probability that a photon striking a detector will be stopped and counted by the detector. It is defined as

$$\varepsilon = 1 - e^{-\mu d} \tag{4}$$

where μ is the attenuation coefficient of the detector and d is the thickness of the detector. Using a detector material with high stopping power for the 511 keV photons can increase the intrinsic efficiency of a PET scanner. For PET imaging the coincidence intrinsic efficiency is ε^2 since *both* photons must be stopped in a detector. The sensitivity of the scanner will also depend on the coincidence timing and energy windows used and the location of the radioactivity within the scanner.

3.3 Noise Equivalent Count Rate

Random and scatter coincidence events represent noise and can reduce the contrast and quantitative accuracy of PET images. Detecting more true coincidence events and detecting less random and scatter coincidence events increases the SNR of PET images. In addition, the number of true events is increased by scanning longer (at the expense of patient motion) or injecting more activity (at the expense of increased radiation dose to the patient). An increase in activity will proportionally increase the number of true coincidence events, assuming negligible deadtime effects. However, the randoms event rate is proportional to the square of the activity, so that an increase in activity will increase the randoms events to a greater degree than the true events. This is shown in the count rate curves in Fig. 6a.

Depending on the activity level in the scanner an increase in activity can have a deleterious effect on image quality. The statistical quality of PET raw data is measured by the noise equivalent count rate (NECR); the NECR is a measure of the SNR of the PET raw data. NECR is defined as

$$\mathrm{NECR} = \frac{T^2}{T + S + kR} \tag{5}$$

where T, S and R are the true, scatter and random coincidence count rates, respectively (Strother et al. 1990). The scalar k is equal to 1 or 2 for noiseless or noisy estimates of random events, respectively. A typical noise equivalent count rate curve is shown in Fig. 6b. The maximum NECR is less that the maximum trues rate and occurs at a lower activity concentration because of the detrimental effects of random and scatter events.

The SNR in the raw data is defined as

$$\mathrm{SNR}^2 = \mathrm{NECR} \times \Delta t \tag{6}$$

where Δt is the acquisition duration. This equation shows that the SNR in the raw data can be increased by increasing the NECR (and activity, assuming the scanner is not saturated) or the scan duration. For the activity levels of clinical 2D imaging the randoms events are a small fraction of the prompts and the NECR is similar to the true coincidence event rate. However, for 3D imaging the randoms events

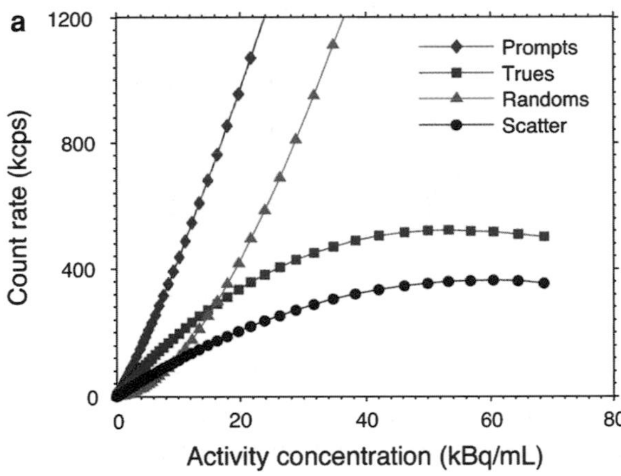

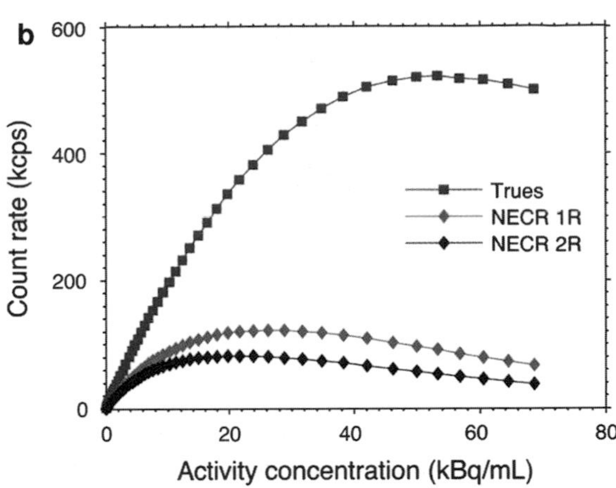

Fig. 6 Count rate curves for a typical PET scanner, measured using methodology prescribed by National Manufacturer's Association NU 2-2007 performance standard. **a** At low activity the true count rate increases linearly with activity whereas the randoms count rate increases as the square of the activity. Increasing the activity beyond the level where the true and randoms count rates are equal provides no further gain in effective count rate. **b** Noise equivalent count rates for noiseless and noisy estimates of random events (denoted as 1R and 2R, respectively). The peak NECR is lower than the peak trues rate due to the inclusion of scatter and randoms events in the prompts

represent the majority of the prompts so there is an optimum activity level.

The NECR represents the SNR of the raw data and not the SNR of the reconstructed images. NECR does not consider the reconstruction algorithm and the resolution and noise correlations in reconstructed images (Badawi and Dahlbom 2005). In addition, NECR does not consider TOF information. As such, NECR is not a metric of lesion detection. Nevertheless, NECR has been employed to demonstrate that increasing the acquisition duration is more effective in improving image quality than increasing the administered dose in 3D imaging.

4 PET Instrumentation

4.1 Detectors

The most commonly used detector in PET imaging is an inorganic scintillation detector. The scintillation crystals used in PET must have a high probability of stopping the 511 keV photons that impinge on it: they must have a high linear attenuation coefficient as shown in Eq. 4. A high linear attenuation coefficient will also reduce the parallax error due to reduced depth of interaction effects. Moreover, the scintillators must have a high photoelectric fraction and low Compton scatter so that all the energy of the annihilation photon is deposited locally within the scintillator (Humm et al. 2003). Finally, differences in linear attenuation coefficient are accentuated since the coincidence intrinsic efficiency is given as ε^2 (from Eq. 4). Table 2 lists the properties of common scintillators used in commercial PET systems.

A scintillator must produce a large number of light photons for each MeV of energy stopped; this property is referred to as the light output or brightness of a scintillator. A bright scintillator reduces statistical uncertainty in the light signal from each scintillation, which improves energy resolution and scatter rejection. Greater light output from a scintillator also allows for more precise localization of the annihilation photon in the detector block. The decay time of a scintillator is also important as it defines the deadtime and maximum count rate capability of the system. A scintillator with a short decay time, called a fast scintillator, will also improve the accuracy of the time measurement of a detected event. Therefore, a faster crystal will permit the use of a shorter coincidence timing window, thereby reducing the random coincidences. In addition, time-of-flight PET scanners require scintillators with very short decay times and good timing resolutions. Unfortunately no single scintillator possesses all these ideal properties. NaI(Tl) has high light output but does not have high stopping power. Bismuth gemanate (BGO) possesses a high stopping power but it has low light output and

Table 2 Physical properties of PET scintillators

Material	Density (g/cm^3)	Effective atomic number Zeff	Linear attenuation coefficient (cm^{-1})	Total light yield (photons/MeV)	Scintillation decay time (nsec)
NaI(Tl)	3.67	51	0.34	37,700	230
$Bi_4Ge_3O_{12}$	7.13	76	0.95	8,200	300
$GdSiO_5(Ce)$	6.71	59	0.70	~10,000	~60
$Lu_2SiO_5(Ce)$	7.40	65	0.88	~30,000	~40

$Bi_4Ge_3O_{12}$, $GdSiO_5(Ce)$, $Lu_2SiO_5(Ce)$ are commonly referred to as BGO, GSO and LSO, respectively. LYSO has properties similar to LSO

long scintillation decay times. Lutetium oxyorthosilicate (LSO) and lutetium yttrium oxyorthosilicate (LYSO) have good stopping power and fast scintillation decay which lead to high count rate capability.

The light photons created from a scintillation event in a crystal are converted to an electrical signal by photomultiplier tubes (PMT) or solid state photodetectors. PMTs have been used exclusively in commercial PET scanners because of their high amplification of the light signal into an electrical signal. However, avalanche photodiodes have been used in small animal scanners and in areas of high magnetic fields, such as PET/MR systems.

4.2 Block Detectors

The detectors in early PET scanners consisted of a single scintillation crystal coupled to a single PMT. However, to improve spatial resolution the detectors must be made smaller, but to achieve a 4–5 mm spatial resolution is difficult as the PMT cannot be made concomitantly smaller with the crystal. Because of this limitation and the high cost of many PMTs the block detector was developed (Casey and Nutt 1986). The block detector consists of a piece of scintillator that has been divided into a rectangular array of detector elements and coupled to four PMTs. In some systems the large scintillator is segmented using saw cuts of different lengths, and the cut lines are filled with reflective material to isolate each detector element. Alternatively, small crystals of the same size and length are etched or wrapped in reflective tape and assembled into a scintillator block. Regardless of the approach each individual detector element creates a unique distribution of light into the PMTs.

The position at which the annihilation photon deposited its energy in the crystal is determined by Anger logic using the output signals from the four PMTs. The position of this event is then assigned to an individual crystal by using a two-dimensional lookup table (called a crystal or position map) that has been created during system calibration. In this manner the block detector permits an array of many crystals to be spatially encoded using four PMTs.

A modification of the block design is the quadrant sharing block design, in which each block of crystals is coupled to four PMTs, but these four PMTs are shared by four blocks (Wong et al. 1995). This reduces the number of PMTs required to decode a given number of crystals but it results in a system with higher dead time than the standard block approach. An interaction in a block in the quadrant sharing design will deaden the adjacent eight blocks whereas in the standard block only the block involved with the interaction will deaden.

A number of block detectors are assembled together into an array called a module or bucket. Each row of crystals in a block detector is part of a detector ring, and the number of rows of crystals in the module defines the number of rings. For example, a PET scanner may have an 8 × 8 array of crystals in a detector block with a 4 × 2 array of blocks in a module (4 blocks in axial direction and 2 blocks in the transaxial direction) and 36 modules in the system. Therefore, there are 32 (i.e. 8 × 4) rings in the scanner, 576 (i.e. 8 × 28 × 36) crystals in a ring and 18,432 crystals (i.e. 8 × 8 × 4 × 28 × 36) in the system.

4.3 Data Collection

PET acquisitions can be performed in two-dimensional (2D) or three-dimensional (3D) modes. Regardless of acquisition mode, a 3D volumetric dataset with $2N-1$ images (or slices) is reconstructed, where N is the

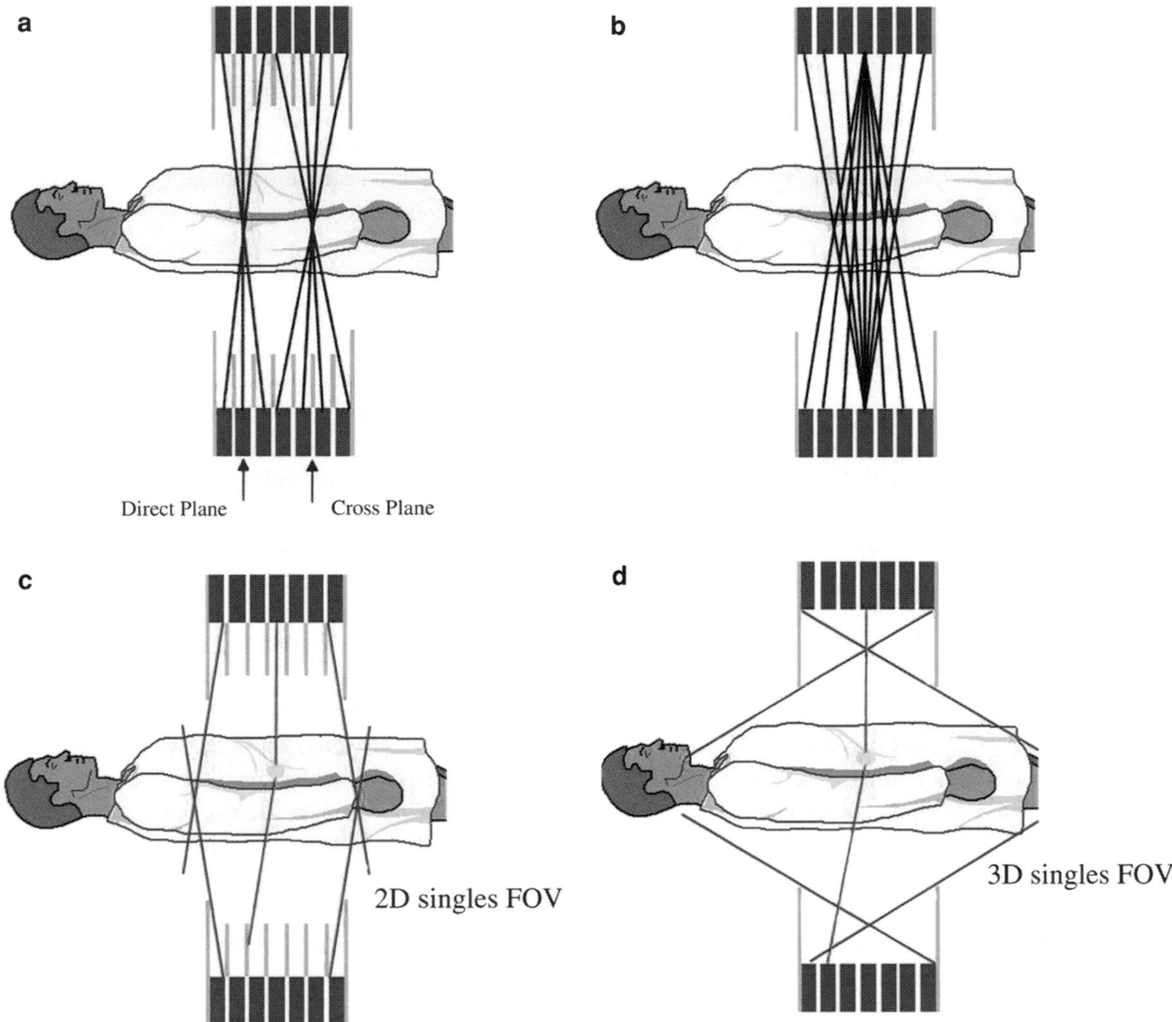

Fig. 7 2D and 3D acquisition geometries. **a** In 2D PET septa are positioned between rings. In high sensitivity 2D PET imaging LORs span adjacent rings; a detector in one ring can have a fanbeam of LORs that extends into adjacent rings. Direct planes are defined at axial positions mid-ring, cross planes are defined at axial positions between rings and each ring has an index. In this example the LORs assigned to direct planes can have a ring difference of 0 or $\pm$ 2 (*red lines*) while the LORs assigned to cross planes can have a ring difference of $\pm$ 1 or $\pm$ 3 (*blue lines*). **b** In 3D PET the septa are removed and a detector in one ring can have a fanbeam of LORs that extends to all rings. **c** The axial FOV in 2D PET is defined by the end shielding and the septa of the first ring (*green lines*). The septa reduce the amount of detected scatter (orange lines). **d** The axial FOV in 3D PET is much larger than for 2D PET. Single events emitted from outside the gantry can increase the random events. The amount of scatter also increases for 3D acquisitions (*orange lines*)

number of rings. For example, the system described above has $N = 32$ rings and it will create 63 transaxial images.

For a 2D acquisition mode axial collimation is employed by positioning annular tungsten septa between the detector rings, as shown in Fig. 7a. The septa are approximately 1–2 mm thick and extend approximately 8–12 cm radially from the detector face into the gantry bore. The septa define slice-by-slice LORs and eliminate out-of-slice annihilation photons. Hence the septa reduce the detection of out-of-slice scatter and random coincidence events (see Fig. 7c), which serves to improve image quality, but the septa also reduce sensitivity as most true coincidence events are also reduced. In the simplest 2D acquisition mode the tomograph operates as a series of separate rings with only those events in which both annihilation photons are detected in the same ring

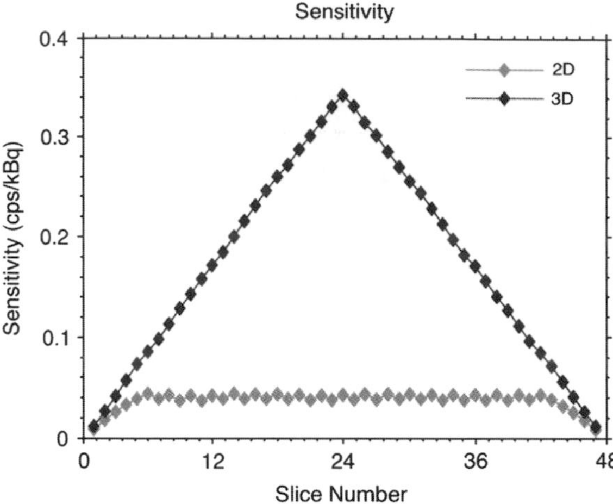

Fig. 8 Axial sensitivity profile for a PET scanner operating in 2D and 3D acquisition modes. The scanner has greater sensitivity in 3D than 2D but there is greater variation in sensitivity across slices when operating in 3D. The oscillation in sensitivity in 2D is due to alternating direct and cross planes. The cross planes have greater sensitivity as they include more lines of response, as shown in Fig. 7a

(ring difference = 0) considered as valid events. To increase the sensitivity of the scanner additional LORs are included in a given slice if the annihilation photons are detected in adjacent rings (ring difference ± 2 or ± 3, as shown in Fig. 7a).

To maximize the sensitivity of a PET scanner the septa are removed and all possible LORs from all detectors can be acquired (see Fig. 7b). This is known as 3D PET (Cherry et al. 1991; Townsend et al. 1991). In 3D PET the system sensitivity increases five fold over the 2D system sensitivity, with the sensitivity greatest at the axial center of the system. The axial sensitivity of a scanner in 2D and 3D is shown in Fig. 8. Typically the sensitivity of a PET scanner is 1–2 cps/kBq in 2D and 5–15 cps/kBq in 3D. The drawback of 3D PET is increased deadtime, an increased acceptance of scattered photons and increased singles rates from activity outside the FOV. The latter effect leads to increased random coincidence events. To minimize the increased random events and deadtime losses a shorter coincidence timing window and faster scintillator and system electronics are required. Typically the scatter fraction (defined as Scatter/(Trues + Scatter)*100) of a PET scanner is 11% in 2D and 32–40% in 3D. To minimize the effects of increased scatter, detectors with better energy resolution and model-based scatter correction algorithms are required.

4.4 PET Scanners of Today

The state-of-the art PET scanner is actually a PET/CT scanner with the PET scanner located behind a CT scanner; a common bed moves the patient sequentially from the CT acquisition to the PET acquisition. The CT images are used for attenuation correction of the PET data and they assist in the localization of lesions visualized in the PET images. In current systems the ring diameter is 80–90 cm and the transaxial field of view (FOV) is 70 cm. The axial FOV depends on the size of the detectors and the number of rings stacked together; the axial field of view is 15–20 cm. Tungsten septa can be positioned between the rings or the system can have no septa.

5 Data Corrections

5.1 Randoms Corrections

As mentioned above, only the true coincidence events represent the true signal from the patient. Random and scatter events give erroneous information about the position of the positron decay and their detection, and if not corrected for, results in reconstructed images with reduced contrast and quantitative accuracy. Therefore, estimates of the randoms and scatter events are subtracted from the prompts events to provide a measure of the true coincidence events. Randoms corrections are described below; scatter corrections are outside the scope of this book chapter.

There are two methods for estimating the amount of random events included in the prompts events rate. The first method uses an additional, delayed coincidence window to directly measure the random events. This delayed coincidence window is of the same temporal width as the standard coincidence window. In this technique the timing pulse from one of the detectors in a detector pair is delayed in time by greater than 50 ns. As a result the probability of detecting a true event in the delayed coincidence window is zero, while the probability of detecting a random event is the same as in the standard coincidence window. Therefore, these delayed events provide an estimate of the number of random events in the standard coincidence timing window. This estimate can be subtracted from the prompts events during the acquisition or a separate sinogram can be

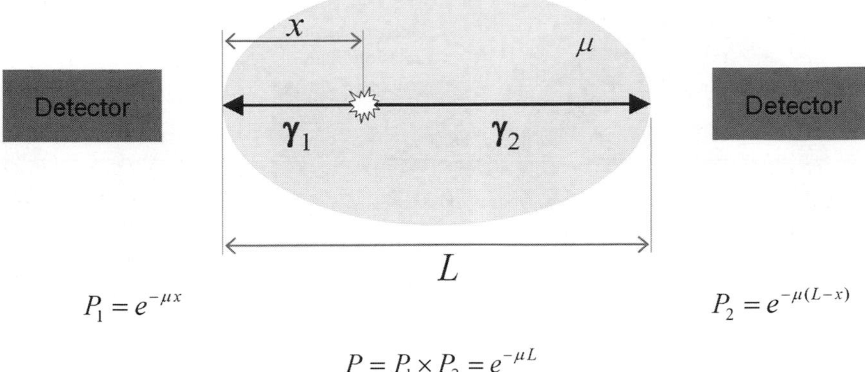

Fig. 9 Attenuation in PET imaging. Attenuation of the annihilation photons depends on the total path length (L) through the object and is independent of the position of the source within the object

saved and subtracted from the prompts sinogram during image reconstruction. Generally the delayed events random correction is considered a noisy correction and the scalar k in Eq. 5 is equal to 2.

The second method estimates the number of random events in each LOR using Eq. 2. This singles-based randoms correction requires that the tomograph can accurately measure the singles rate for each crystal and it requires accurate knowledge of the coincidence timing window for each detector pair. The singles-based randoms correction produces a lower noise estimate of the number of randoms events because the singles rate is much greater than the delayed event rate. This randoms correction is considered a noiseless correction and the scalar k in Eq. 5 is set to 1. However, singles-based randoms corrections may generate a biased estimate of the number of random events if the acquisition duration is long with respect to the half-life of the radionuclide. It should be mentioned that both delayed event and singles-based randoms corrections estimate the number of random events detected by each detector pair during an entire acquisition, and they do not determine whether each individual coincidence event is a random event.

5.2 Attenuation Correction

Attenuation is the physical factor that produces the greatest effect on the reconstructed images. Attenuation is the reduction of the number of detected photons due to photoelectric absorption and Compton scatter in the patient. At 511 keV the predominant interaction is Compton scatter. Mathematically attenuation in a uniform medium is defined as

$$N = N_o e^{-\mu x} \qquad (7)$$

where N_o is the number of emitted photons, N is the number of photons that escape the attenuating medium without interaction, x is the path length the photon travels in the medium and μ is the linear attenuation coefficient and the probability per unit distance that an interaction will occur. Attenuation is manifested as a progressive underestimation in the radioactivity from the edge to the center of the body and an artifactual increase in radioactivity in the skin and the lungs. The amount of attenuation depends on the body size and the composition of the attenuating medium. Attenuation in PET depends on the total thickness of the attenuating medium as both annihilation photons must escape to be detected.

Consider a point source located at depth x in a uniformly attenuating medium with a linear attenuation coefficient μ. The thickness of the attenuating medium is L along the LOR. See Fig. 9. The probability that annihilation photon 1 will escape the object is given as

$$P_1 = e^{-\mu x} \qquad (8)$$

The probability that annihilation photon 2 will escape is given as

$$P_2 = e^{-\mu(L-x)} \qquad (9)$$

The probability that both annihilation photons escape the object is the product of the two probabilities P_1 and P_2:

$$P = P_1 \times P_2 = e^{-\mu L} \qquad (10)$$

Therefore, the probability of both photons escaping the object without being attenuated is independent

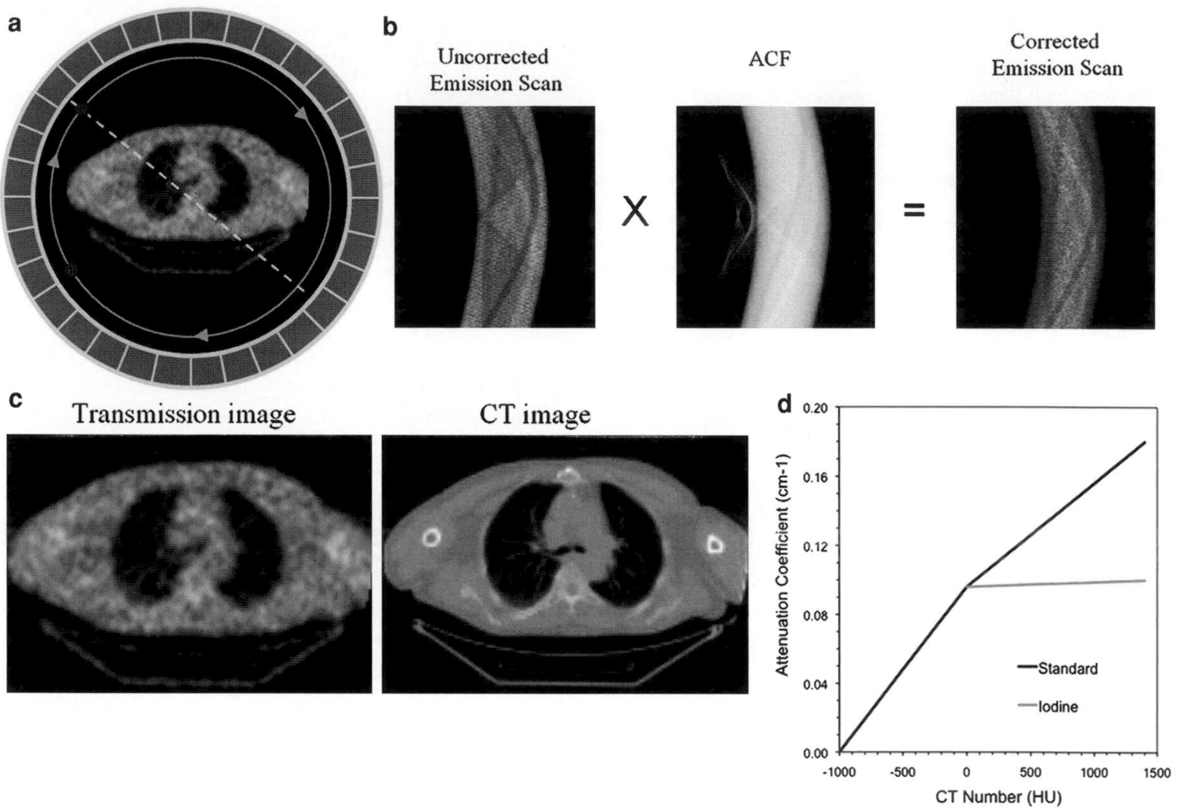

Fig. 10 **a** A transmission acquisition using two positron emitting sources (*red circles*). The transmission sources rotate around the patient for several minutes as depicted by the green trace. **b** Utilization of the measured attenuation correction factors (ACFs) in the attenuation correction of the PET scan data. **c** A transmission image and a CT image from the same patient. The CT image has been blurred to match the PET resolution and the CT numbers scaled to represent attenuation coefficients; this scaling of the CT numbers utilized the bilinear curve shown in (**d**)

of the depth of the source in the object and only dependent on the total thickness of the object along the LOR and the attenuation coefficient of the object. Probability P represents the reduction in the photon flux along a given LOR due to attenuation and to correct for attenuation requires applying attenuation correction factors (ACFs) to the emission data. These ACFs are the reciprocal of P:

$$\mathrm{ACF} = e^{\mu L} \tag{11}$$

The ACFs can be measured by acquiring transmission scans. PET-only tomographs acquire transmission scans by using external sources—either positron emitting sources (Ge-68) or single photon sources (Cs-137). These sources rotate around the patient and produce low-quality CT images in several minutes.

Transmission scanning utilizing positron emitting sources provide ACFs that are directly measured at the same 511 keV energy as the emission study. For transmission imaging the coincidence detection criteria also requires that the LOR pass through the location of the source so contamination from emission activity is reduced. In transmission imaging with a positron source the detector near the source can experience high deadtime as it is exposed to the full flux of photons without attenuation. Therefore, to minimize detector deadtime the source strength is low, two to three sources are used simultaneously and the acquisition is several minutes. Figure 10a shows transmission imaging with two sources, and Fig. 10b shows the application of the ACF to correct emission data for attenuation.

The duration of the transmission scan is almost the same duration as the PET scan. Shortening the transmission scan duration results in noisier ACFs, which create noisier attenuation corrected PET images. Segmented attenuation correction algorithms have been developed to reduce the noise and acquisition duration of transmission scans. Single photon sources generate images that contain less noise than the positron emitting sources, but the attenuation coefficients must be adjusted to the 511 keV energy prior to use in the ACFs. Alternatively, uniform attenuation correction can be applied in which a constant attenuation coefficient is applied to all pixels within a predefined contour around the object.

One benefit of PET/CT is the ability to use the CT images for attenuation correction of the PET images. The rapid acquisition of the CT images significantly reduces the scan time compared to the duration of a transmission scan using rotating pin sources for PET. Moreover, the high X-ray flux provides a low-noise map of the attenuation coefficients and therefore improves the precision of the attenuation correction factors and reduces the propagation of noise from the transmission scans into the attenuation corrected emission images. Finally, the use of an X-ray tube eliminates the reduction of transmission scan quality as the transmission source decays.

Prior to their use in attenuation correction, the CT images are resampled to match the spatial resolution of the emission data. Since attenuation is dependent on the energy of the X-rays, the CT numbers (in Hounsfield units, HU) must be converted to linear attenuation coefficients at 511 keV. The conversion of CT numbers to attenuation coefficients requires an assumed effective energy of the polychromatic X-ray beam.

This conversion can be facilitated by segmentation or scaling techniques (see Kinahan et al. (2003) for more details). The most common method uses a bilinear curve to multiplicatively scale the CT numbers; in this method, tissue with a HU of $-1{,}000$ to 0 is modeled as a mixture of soft tissue and air, and tissue with an HU greater than 0 is modeled as a mixture of soft tissue and bone. See Fig. 10c for an example of a transmission image and CT image acquired for the same patient. An example of a bilinear curve used to convert CT number to attenuation coefficient is shown in Fig. 10d. The bilinear curve can be modified to have a different soft tissue-bone mixture when iodinated contrast agents are used. Iodinated contrast agents possess a high iodine concentration that increases the CT number but not the density of the tissue or the attenuation; this leads to an overcorrection of attenuation and an increase in the activity concentration in the PET images.

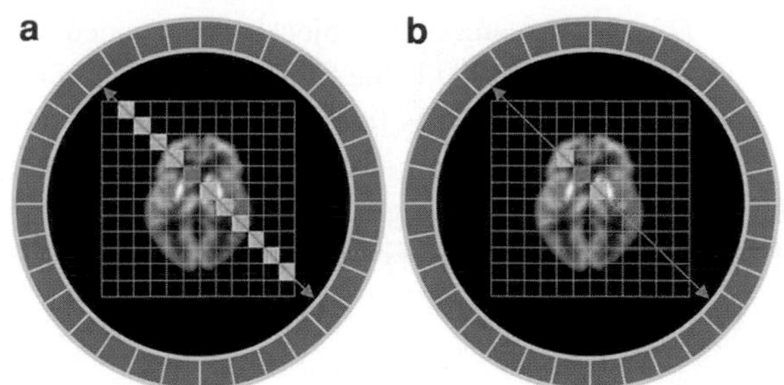

Fig. 11 Illustration of the reconstruction process of assigning count values to pixels in an image matrix for a given line of response for (**a**) conventional, non-TOF PET and (**b**) TOF PET. For conventional PET each pixel along the line of response is given uniform weight or probability of being the annihilation site. For TOF PET the timing information is used to adjust the pixel weighting by the probability that the annihilation site is at that pixel. As such the TOF information constrains the location of annihilation site

Other corrections that must be applied to the PET raw data include: normalization corrections that remove the variations in efficiency in each LOR; sensitivity correction to remove the axial variation in sensitivity; deadtime and decay corrections and a system calibration correction that converts counts per pixel in the reconstructed image to activity concentration.

6 Time-of-Flight

As mentioned previously, in TOF PET imaging the actual difference in detection times of the two photons is measured and used to deduce the approximate location of the annihilation site along the LOR (Ter Pogossian et al. 1981). This TOF information constrains the reconstruction algorithm as it localizes the annihilation site to a region, with the extent of the region dependent upon the timing resolution of the system (See Fig. 11). As a result, the TOF images will have a higher SNR over similar conventional, non-TOF images. For a uniform object the improvement in SNR over that obtained with a non-TOF PET scanner is given by

$$\mathrm{SNR_{TOF}} = \sqrt{\frac{2D}{c\Delta t}} \times \mathrm{SNR_{non-TOF}} \qquad (12)$$

where D is the diameter of the object being scanned, c is the speed of light and Δt is the timing resolution of the system. Empirically it was found that, for the filtered-backprojection (FBP) reconstruction algorithm, the improvement in SNR over that obtained with a non-TOF PET scanner is given by (Tomitani 1981):

$$\mathrm{SNR}_{\mathrm{TOF}} = \sqrt{\frac{2D}{1.6c\Delta t}} \times \mathrm{SNR}_{\mathrm{non-TOF}} \qquad (13)$$

The relative improvement in $\mathrm{SNR}_{\mathrm{TOF}}$ may be smaller than the magnitude predicted in Eq. 13 when using iterative reconstruction (IR) algorithms, as IR algorithms have been shown to provide images with lower noise and hence greater SNR over the FBP algorithm. Nevertheless, from these equations it can be seen that the improvement in TOF SNR increases as the size of the object increases. Karp has shown that the TOF images provide images of better contrast to noise than non-TOF images, especially for small lesions (Karp et al. 2008). In addition, the TOF images converged to a solution faster than the non-TOF images. This suggests a greater improvement in SNR for larger patients and it permits the use of a lower injected dose and/or shorter acquisition duration.

The benefits of TOF on image quality have been known since PET was first developed. Several research systems were designed in the 1980s (Lewellen 1998) but at that time the scintillator materials did not possess proper time resolution, stopping power and light output to produce images of acceptable image quality. In addition, the detector electronics were not stable and could not provide accurate timing measurements. For these reasons TOF PET technology research drastically decreased in the 1990s. Recently there has been renewed interest in TOF using lutetium-based scintillators to achieve reasonable timing accuracy while maintaining other desirable properties for PET such as good stopping power and high light output. Currently Philips Healthcare, GE Healthcare and Siemens Medical all offer TOF capability on their PET/CT systems. These systems employ lutetium-based scintillators and possess a coincidence timing resolution of 500–650 ps.

7 PET/MR

While current PET/CT systems are fully integrated devices, the acquisition of the PET and CT data is sequential; typically the CT data is acquired first. However, the simultaneous acquisition of multimodality data would permit accurate spatial and temporal registration of the data without motion artifacts. With PET/MR systems the emphasis has been on the simultaneous collection of PET and MR data. One benefit of simultaneous PET/MR scanning is improved spatial resolution of the PET images as the magnetic field will reduce the range of the positron. However, this improvement in resolution will only be realized at high magnetic fields and for radionuclides with a large positron range. Another benefit of simultaneous PET/MR would be real-time motion correction of PET data using anatomic MR data.

The integration of PET and MR systems faces technical challenges: space is limited and the fundamental principles of their design conflict (Cherry 2006). The operation of PMTs is sensitive to both the static and dynamic magnetic field of an MR scanner. Hence PMTs are not suitable for use in an MR system, as even weak magnetic fields will adversely affect their performance. In addition, the presence of the PET detectors can degrade the field homogeneity and imaging performance of the MR system. In early design concepts the PMTs of a single-slice PET scanner were located outside the main magnetic field using long light fibers to transport the signals. The disadvantages of this approach are the low PET sensitivity, the degradation of the energy and coincidence timing resolutions and the space required for the PMTs.

Therefore two alternative magnet designs have been suggested. In one approach the magnet is split and a PET detector array placed in the magnet structure. The gap in the magnet allows light fibers to couple the scintillation crystals to conventional PMTs in a region with low magnetic field but close enough to insure a proper signal. The second approach uses a field-cycled MR scanner, making it possible to bring the magnetic field close to zero during PET scanning. Finally, another MR/PET system design utilizes a PET detector, comprised of avalanche photodiodes (APD), inserted directly into the MR bore (Pichler et al. 2006). Semiconductor APDs are light sensitive detectors that can be operated inside a strong magnetic field without any performance degradation and they are compact and occupy less space than PMTs.

A major issue with PET/MR imaging is attenuation correction. The generation of an attenuation map from an MR image is not straightforward since the MR image represents proton density and tissue relaxation properties while attenuation is related to electron density. In MR images both air and cortical bone present with no signal yet obviously air and cortical bone have markedly different attenuation properties. There are several approaches in obtaining attenuation information based on MR images. These techniques use segmentation to assign attenuation coefficients or co-registration to an atlas to infer the attenuation coefficients. Alternatively, pulse sequences that image bone could be used in the conversion of MR images to attenuation factors. PET/MR systems will be an active area of development in the next several years.

References

Badawi RD, Dahlbom M (2005) NEC: some coincidences are more equivalent than others. J Nucl Med 46:1767–1768

Beneditti SD, Cowan CE, Konneker WR et al (1950) On the angular distribution of two photon annihilation radiation. Phys Rev 77:205–212

Casey ME, Nutt R (1986) A multi-slice two-dimensional BGO detector system for PET. IEEE Trans Nucl Sci 33:760–763

Cherry SR (2006) The 2006 Henry N. Wagner lecture: of mice and men (and positrons)—advances in PET imaging technology. J Nucl Med 47:1735–1745

Cherry SR, Dahlbom M, Hoffman EJ (1991) 3D PET using a conventional multislice tomograph without septa. J Comput Assis Tomogr 15:655–668

Humm JL, Rozenfeld A, Del Guerra A (2003) From PET detectors to PET scanners. Eur J Nucl Med Mol Imaging 30:1574–1594

Karp JS, Surti S, Daube-Witherspoon ME, Muehllehner G (2008) Benefit of time-of-flight in PET: experimental and clinical results. J Nucl Med 49:462–470

Kinahan PE, Hasegawa BH, Beyer T (2003) X-ray-based attenuation correction for positron emission tomography/computed tomography scanners. Semin Nucl Med 33:166–179

Levin CS, Hoffman EJ (1999) Calculation of positron range and its effect on the fundamental limit of positron emission tomography system spatial resolution. Phys Med Biol 44:781–799

Lewellen TK (1998) Time-of-flight PET. Semin Nucl Med 28:268–275

Pichler BJ, Judenhofer MS, Catana C, Walton JH et al (2006) Performance test of an LSO-APD detector in a 7-T MRI scanner for simultaneous PET/MRI. J Nucl Med 47:639–647

Strother SC, Casey ME, Hoffman EJ (1990) Measuring PET sensitivity: relating count rates to image-signal-to-noise ratio using noise equivalent counts. IEEE Trans Nucl Sci 37:783–788

Ter Pogossian MM, Mullani NA, Ficke DC (1981) Photon time-of-flight assisted positron emission tomography. J Comput Assist Tomogr 5:227–239

Tomitani T (1981) Image-reconstruction and noise evaluation in photon time-of-flight assisted positron emission tomography. IEEE Trans Nucl Sci 28:4582–4589

Townsend DW, Geissbuhler A, Defrise M et al (1991) Fully 3-dimensional reconstruction for a PET camera with retractable septa. IEEE Trans Med Imag 10:505–512

Wong W-H, Uribe J, Hicks K, Hu G (1995) An analog decoding BGO block detector using circular photomultipliers. IEEE Trans Nucl Sci 42:1095–1101

Further Reading

Bendriem B, Townsend DW (1998) The theory and practice of 3D PET. Kluwer, Dordrecht

Cherry SR, Sorenson JA, Phelps ME (2003) Physics in nuclear medicine, 3rd edn. W.B. Saunders, New York

Knoll GF (2010) Radiation detection and measurement, 4th edn. Wiley, New York

PET Radiochemistry and Radiopharmacy

Mark S. Jacobson, Raymond A. Steichen, and Patrick J. Peller

Contents

M. S. Jacobson (✉) · P. J. Peller
Department of Radiology, Mayo Clinic,
200 1st Street SW, Rochester, MN 55905, USA
e-mail: jacobson.mark17@mayo.edu

R. A. Steichen
Section of Equipment Services, Mayo Clinic,
200 1st Street SW, Rochester, MN 55905, USA

Abstract

The vast majority of PET radiopharmaceuticals today are cyclotron produced. Carbon-11 (^{11}C), Nitrogen-13 (^{13}N), Oxygen-15 (^{15}O) products are created for in-house use only due to their short half-lives. The longer half-life of Fluorine-18 means that ^{18}F-labeled PET radiotracers can be widely distributed. Production of radiopharmaceuticals is computer-controlled and automated. Automation increases both reliability and efficiency of PET operations while decreasing the radiation dose to the staff. For today, FDG remains the workhorse of oncologic PET imaging. Additional ^{18}F PET radiotracers directed at a range of molecular processes are being studied and should become available in the future.

1 Introduction

Positron emission tomography (PET) has become a powerful research and clinical imaging tool for evaluating complex biochemical processes in cancer patients. PET has developed rapidly as radiochemistry and radiopharmacy have advanced. The oncologic clinical applications of PET have increased dramatically over the past decade because of the synthesis and widespread distribution of one molecule, ^{18}Fluorine-2-Fluoro-2-Deoxy-glucose (FDG). FDG PET/CT has become essential in evaluating cancer patients in major medical centers throughout the world. Measurement of normal and altered biochemical pathways noninvasively is routinely performed with PET radiopharmaceuticals. The continued

P. Peller et al. (eds.), *PET-CT and PET-MRI in Oncology*, Medical Radiology. Diagnostic Imaging,
DOI: 10.1007/174_2012_703,

Table 1 PET radionuclides

Radionuclide	Half-life (min)
Carbon-11	20.4
Nitrogen-13	9.98
Oxygen-15	2.03
Fluorine-18	109.8
Copper-62	9.74
Gallium-68	68.3
Rubidium-82	1.25
Iodine-122	3.62
Iodine-124	6019.2

growth of PET will require the expansion of clinically available positron emitting radiopharmaceuticals (Vallabhajosula et al. 2011, Rice et al. 2011).

2 Positron Emitting Radionuclides

Of the more than 3,000 known neutron and proton configurations, approximately 250 are stable and more than 2,500 are radioactive. The majority of the radioactive nuclides are artificially produced in cyclotrons or reactors. Of these radioactive nuclides, ten are major positron emitters (Table 1). PET imaging makes use of these positron-emitting radionuclides for clinical and research applications (McCarthy and Welch 1998). There are three primary methods to produce radioactive atoms for nuclear imaging. Radioisotopes are either reactor produced from fission by-products by chemical separation, or by neutron irradiation of a specific target; or they are produced in a cyclotron from bombardment of a target material with charged particles.

2.1 Cyclotron Produced

Carbon-11 (^{11}C), Nitrogen-13 (^{13}N), Oxygen-15 (^{15}O) and Fluorine-18 (^{18}F) are low-molecular-weight radioisotopes produced in a cyclotron. One of the great advantages of positron emission tomography is the use of positron emitting radioisotopes that can be easily added to biomolecules, especially ^{11}C, ^{13}N, ^{15}O and ^{18}F. All 4 also possess simple decay schemes with each emitting a single positron. Substituting ^{11}C, ^{13}N and ^{15}O for stable ^{12}C, ^{14}N and ^{16}O does not alter the function or configuration of the compound. ^{18}F often replaces a hydroxyl group, which only mildly affects the biologic behavior of the molecule.

The disadvantage of ^{11}C, ^{13}N and ^{15}O labeled compounds is that their half-life is very short. The 2-minute half-life of ^{15}O requires a tube direct from the cyclotron and pumping the ^{15}O labeled compounds immediately into the scan room. The complicated chemistry of ^{13}N and its 10-min half-life leaves too little time for radiopharmaceutical synthesis and imaging. ^{11}C with its 20-min half-life has labeled a vast array of biological radiotracers in the research realm to measure molecular kinetics and function. ^{11}C radiopharmaceuticals require rapid synthesis and scanning, which make an on-site cyclotron mandatory. Only ^{18}F with its nearly 2-h half-life allows time for complex syntheses or delayed imaging and it can be transported significant distances (Schlyer 2004).

2.1.1 Cyclotron

A medical cyclotron (Fig. 1) is a particle accelerator that can produce PET radionuclides. It is composed of two flat D-shaped hollow metal electrodes in the vacuum chamber between the two poles of a large electromagnet. In the center hydrogen (H_2) or deuterium (D_2) gas is introduced to yield the particles to be accelerated (H^- or D^-). Under the effect of a strong magnetic field, these anions gain energy from high-frequency alternating voltage applied between the electrodes. The magnetic field and the increasing energy of the particles force the anions to travel in a spiral path. The radius of the anion's path increases until the particles hit a stripping foil at the perimeter of the vacuum chamber. The stripping foil removes the electrons from the anions forming positively charged particles, H^+ or D^+. The change in charge deflects the particles out of the acceleration chamber to collide with the contents of the target. The high-energy particle smashes into a stable isotope target, yielding positron-emitting radionuclides (Shaiju et al. 2009).

2.1.2 Cyclotron Created Radionuclides

The synthesis of positron emitting biomolecules begins from small precursor compounds that are generated from a cyclotron target. There a limited number of small precursors that can originate in a cyclotron. The energy of the particle and density of the beam particle as well as the nuclear reaction determines the quantity

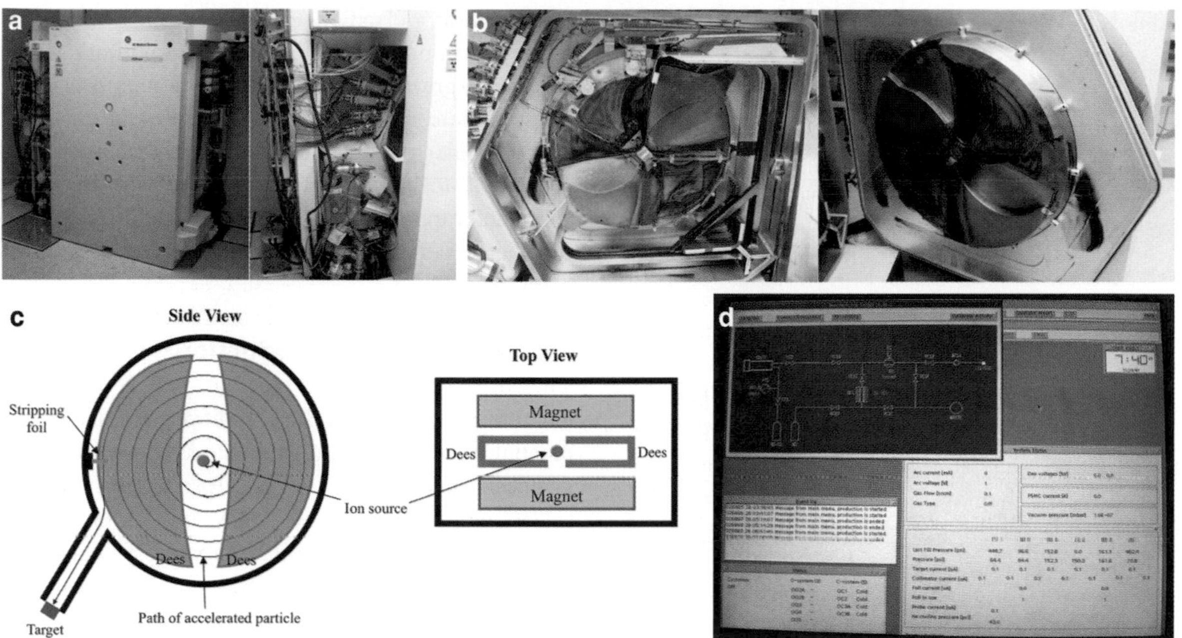

Fig. 1 This is the outside (**a**) and inside (**b**) of an upright PET cyclotron with dual particle capability. Six target ports on the left side of the cyclotron can be used for dual target irradiation. The cyclotron (**c**) contains two major parts: a large electromagnet and two semicircular, hollow electrodes called "dees" because of their D-shape. The ions are injected into the center of the cyclotron and come under the affect of the alternating current applied to the dees and the magnetic field supplied by the electromagnet. The current is carefully timed so that the polarization of the dees changes as the particles dart from side to side. This accelerates the ions propelling them in a spiral faster and faster. At the maximum radius of the spiral, the ions hit the stripping foil and exit the cyclotron. The charged particles exiting the cyclotron impact the target to produce PET radionuclides. The cyclotron is computer controlled (**d**), allowing easy and efficient production of PET radiopharmaceuticals

and type of radionuclide produced. The specific activity of the radionuclide produced is equal to the activity per unit of material, often given in terms of the activity per gram. The radionuclide purity is the percentage of the radioactive species that is the desired isotope (Sharma et al. 2006).

Four major positron emitters are produced within a medical cyclotron: Carbon-11 (^{11}C), Nitrogen-13 (^{13}N), Oxygen-15 (^{15}O) and Fluorine-18 (^{18}F). ^{11}C is produced by proton bombardment of natural nitrogen. The proton interacts with stable ^{14}N and produces a neutron and ^{11}C. The target typically contains 2 % oxygen in the nitrogen and yields ^{11}C-carbon dioxide. ^{13}N is produced by proton bombardment of distilled water. The proton interacts with stable ^{16}O and produces an alpha particle and ^{13}N. ^{15}O is produced by deuteron bombardment of natural nitrogen. The deuteron interacts with stable ^{14}N and produces ^{15}O. Oxygen-15 is produced as either ^{15}O-molecular oxygen, ^{15}O-water or ^{15}O-carbon dioxide. Fluorine-18 (^{18}F) is produced by proton bombardment of Oxygen-18 enriched water. The proton interacts with the ^{18}O and produces a neutron and ^{18}F (Schlyer 2004).

2.2 Generator Derived Radionuclides

The Molybdenum-99/Technetium-99m generator is the major source for radionuclides in general nuclear medicine practice. The Tc-99m used to label a wide variety of compounds is eluted from the molybdenum-99 generator. Similar generator systems exist for positron emitting radionuclides (Table 2). Radionuclide generator systems consist of a parent radionuclide, which is a relatively long-lived radionuclide that decays into a much shorter-lived and chemically different daughter radionuclide. The system typically has the parent nuclide in a column from which the daughter is eluted when needed. The advantage of generator-produced positron emitting radionuclides is

Table 2 Generator produced positron emitting radionuclides

Parent	Daughter
Strontium-82 (half-life 25 days)	Rubidium-82 (half-life 1.25 min)
Germanium-68 (half-life 275 days)	Gallium-68 (half-life 68.3 min)
Zinc-62 (half-life 9.13 h)	Copper-62 (half-life 9.74 min)

the increased availability of short-lived radionuclides without an on-site cyclotron (Breeman and Verbruggen 2007; Williams et al. 2005; Zhernosekov et al. 2007; Zweit et al. 1992). The Rubidium-82 from a Strontium-82 generator is FDA approved for myocardial perfusion imaging. Gallium-68 and Copper-62 are not available for clinical use in the US. These metal radionuclides can label peptides and proteins coupled by a chelating agent. A number of ^{68}Ga-somatostatin analogs are being studied for tumor imaging (Rufini et al. 2007).

3 PET Radiotracer Production

3.1 Synthesis

Within the radiochemistry lab, quality assurance and quality control are of paramount importance. Quality control includes chemical and radiochemical purity determination and radiopharmaceutical validation. Time dominates all aspects of a PET study, particularly in the production of PET radionuclides. PET tracers must be synthesized and imaged rapidly taking into account the half-life of the radioisotope. For Carbon-11 labeled tracers with a 20-min half-life, this typically means 10 min for isotope production, 40 min for synthesis and 60–90 min for PET imaging. Since radiotracers are typically administered intravenously, procedures must be developed to produce high yield radiotracers that are chemically, radiochemically and biologically pure (Schlyer 2004).

3.2 Quality Control

Each radiolabeling procedure is validated by testing batches for sterility, presence of endotoxins, heavy metal contamination, pH, chemical purity, radionuclide identification, and radionuclide purity. Since time is vital for a PET radiopharmaceuticals, only initial validation is performed prior to release of the radiopharmaceutical. Subsequent testing on each batch ensures the continued safety of the manufacturing process. PET radiopharmaceutical testing is often automated with thin layer chromatography, high performance liquid chromatography or gas chromatography (Sharma et al. 2006).

3.3 Automated Production

Routine production of PET radiopharmaceuticals is computer controlled and automated. These automated synthesis units allow regular production of PET tracers with speed and efficiency, but without significant radiation exposure to laboratory personnel. These modules allow a series of reactions to occur under computer control. The operator guides the computer software to perform the complex synthetic procedures required to make PET tracers. Automated synthesis units can produce different radiotracers with the same or similar equipment. Indeed, the modular approach has been extended to the point that sterile disposable cartridges are now available to produce pure and pyrogen-free PET radiotracers for clinical use. High-yield production of FDG has been validated and cartridges for other PET radiopharmaceuticals are now available (Gatley 2003; Schlyer 2004).

3.4 Dispensing

Originally, PET radiopharmaceuticals were dispensed and administered as unit doses by hand. As with so much else in busy PET practices, FDG dosing is now automated. An FDG-filled tungsten-shielded multidose vial is placed inside the shielded cart and each dose is automatically measured and calibrated (Fig. 2). The FDG dose measured by an ionization chamber is automatically delivered directly to the patient. An easy-to-use touch screen initiates the injection and clearly shows prescribed and actual activity. The touch screen interface controls delivery of a specific dose for each patient that is consistently within 2 % of the prescribed dose. The equipment cart is mobile allowing easy movement to patient location. By eliminating manual unit dose preparation and

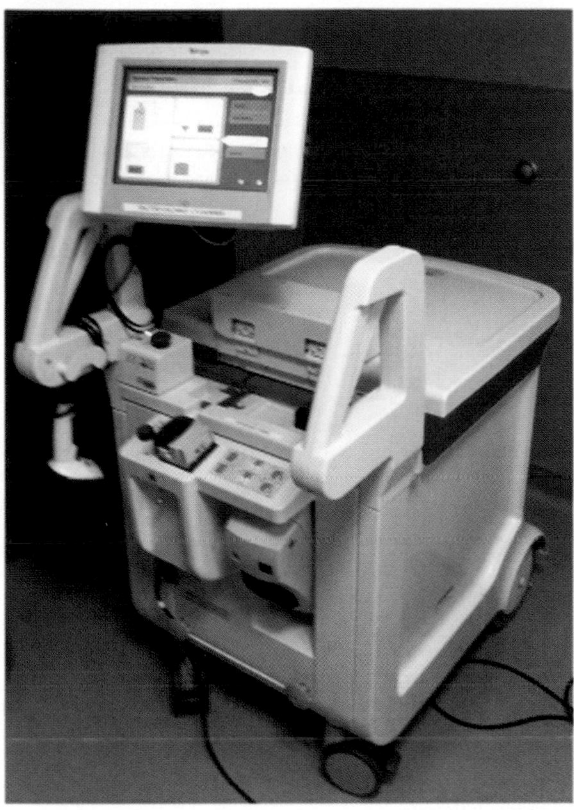

Fig. 2 This is an example of a mobile FDG administration device. From the shielded multidose vial within the machine, the individual patient's FDG activity is measured and administered. FDG dosing is controlled via computer to provide efficient delivery consistently within 2 % of the requested amount

injection, radiation exposure to both radiopharmacy and imaging personnel decreases more than 20 % (Carolan et al. 2012).

4 Oncologic PET Radiopharmaceuticals

In the last 30 years, several thousand PET radiotracers for oncologic imaging have been developed in more than 600 PET radiopharmacies worldwide. Despite the availability of so many PET radiopharmaceuticals for oncologic imaging, FDG remains the primary agent. Approximately 95 % of all PET studies for patients with cancer are performed with FDG.

4.1 FDA Approved

4.1.1 ^{18}F-2-Fluoro-2-Deoxy-Glucose

Warburg first reported increased glucose consumption by cancer cells compared to normal cells (Warburg 1956). In 1960 2-Deoxy-D-glucose was developed as a chemotherapeutic agent but it blocked glucose use by both normal and cancer cells (Laszlo et al. 1960). In 1976, ^{18}F-2-fluoro-2-deoxy-glucose (FDG) was first synthesized at Brookhaven National Laboratory (Ido et al. 1978; Pacák and Cerny 2002) (Fig. 3). Initially FDG PET was used to image cerebral glucose metabolism. Oncologic imaging began with brain tumors in part because of the small aperture in the early PET scanners. FDG was investigated in animal models with a wide range of malignancies. Clinical oncologic imaging was limited to the brain until PET body scanners became available (Nutt 2002).

Energy-dependent transmembrane transport proteins (GLUT) pump glucose into cells (Fig. 3). These GLUT receptors are over-expressed on the surface of malignant cells in proportion to the rate of increased glucose metabolism. GLUT-1 is hypoxia responsive, insulin independent and the most common on cancer cells. FDG uptake in tumor cells requires a sufficient blood supply for nutrients to reach the cell. The number of viable tumor cells within a lesion determines the intensity of FDG uptake. Hypoxia-inducible factor-1-alfa up-regulates GLUT-1 by increasing tumoral FDG uptake. Rapid cell proliferation in tumors, evident by the high mitotic rate, also increases glucose utilization (Avril et al. 2001; Mochizuki et al. 2001; Bos et al. 2002).

Tumor cells have increased intracellular hexokinase levels, which phosphorylate glucose and FDG, trapping them within the cell (Smith 2000). FDG is phosphorylated by hexokinase into FDG-6-phosphate. Phosphorylated glucose rapidly undergoes glycolysis but the presence of ^{18}F on FDG-6-phosphate blocks binding of enzymes leading to glycolytic pathways. Unlike normal cells, Tumor cells show reduced levels of glucose-6-phosphatase, the enzyme that dephosphorylates D-glucose or FDG-6-phosphate, aiding accumulation of intracellular FDG. FDG accumulation in malignant cells is generally proportional to the glycolytic rate of malignant cells, which allows their detection with PET FDG imaging (Coleman 1999; Delbeke 1999; Ak et al. 2000).

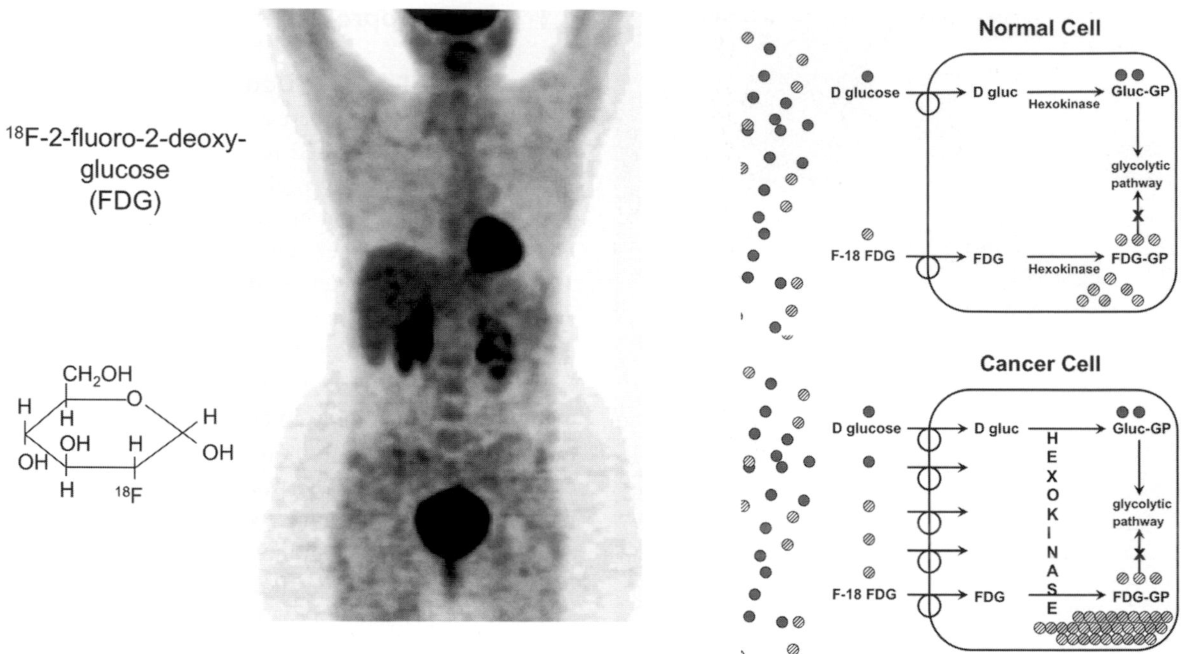

Fig. 3 ^{18}F-2-fluoro-2-deoxy-glucose (FDG) is a glucose analogue, which differs from D-glucose by the ^{18}F on the 2-carbon. Glucose and FDG are pumped into cells via the GLUT transporters on the plasma membranes. Once inside the cell, both glucose and FDG are immediately phosphorylated under the control of hexokinase. Glucose-6-phosphate can enter glycolytic pathways but the FDG-6-phosphate does not degrade because the enzyme-binding site is blocked by the ^{18}F. FDG accumulates within cancer cells in proportion to their accelerated glycolytic rate

Unfortunately, FDG is not a cancer-specific agent and accumulates avidly in inflammatory and infectious diseases, especially sarcoidosis, tuberculosis, fungal infection, and pneumonia. The increased FDG uptake is due to a marked increase in the glycolytic rate when leukocytes are activated. The increased expression of GLUT receptors and elevated hexokinase activity in activated leukocytes is very similar to tumor cells (Zhao et al. 2001; Higashi et al. 2002).

Glucose and FDG are freely filtered by the glomerulus. Glucose is then reabsorbed in the proximal convoluted tubule. The glucose transporters in the proximal convoluted tubule (SGLT1 and 2) have a limited affinity for FDG because of the ^{18}F on the 2-carbon. Only about half of the filtered FDG undergoes reuptake in the nephron. The FDG excreted in the urine leads to intense activity within the urinary system, which is normal. This normal urinary excretion of FDG clears the background activity and is beneficial for imaging. Rapid urinary excretion allows earlier imaging and lower plasma levels of FDG diminish the radiation dose to the patient (Gatley 2003).

4.1.2 ^{18}F-Sodium Fluoride

^{18}F-Sodium Fluoride (NaF) is a bone-imaging agent first introduced in 1962 and used with early gamma cameras (Blau et al.1962). NaF was the first FDA approved radiopharmaceutical. ^{18}F-NaF has a biodistribution similar to ^{99m}Tc-polyphosphonates, but with less protein binding. Following intravenous administration, NaF is rapidly removed from the plasma and either bound to bone or excreted by the kidneys. At 60 min only 10 % of the injected dose remains in the plasma. The fluoride ion is exchanged for a hydroxyl group on the hydroxyapatite crystal to form fluorapatite and is incorporated into the bone matrix. Fluoride is firmly attached at sites of osteoblastic activity and remains in the bone. NaF uptake has twice the target-to-background ratio of Tc-99m-MDP and accumulation is higher at sites of new bone formation due to the greater availability of binding

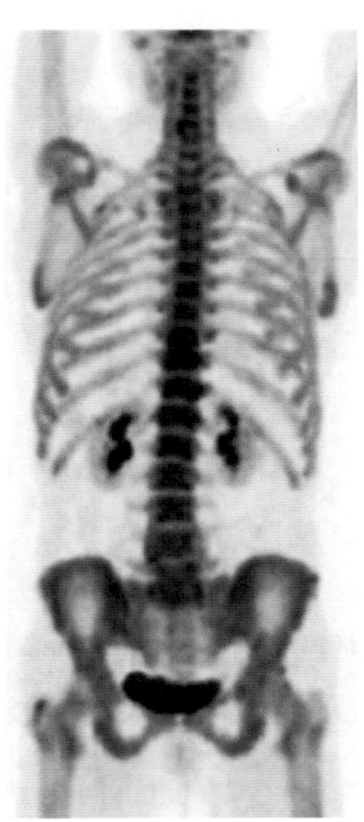

Fig. 4 ^{18}F-Sodium Fluoride (NaF) is a PET bone tracer used for evaluating osseous metastasis. NaF PET/CT is an extremely sensitive method for detecting bony metastases in patients with known malignancy. NaF normally accumulates in the bones and areas of active soft tissue calcification with renal excretion into the bladder

^{18}F-fluoroethylcholine (FECH)

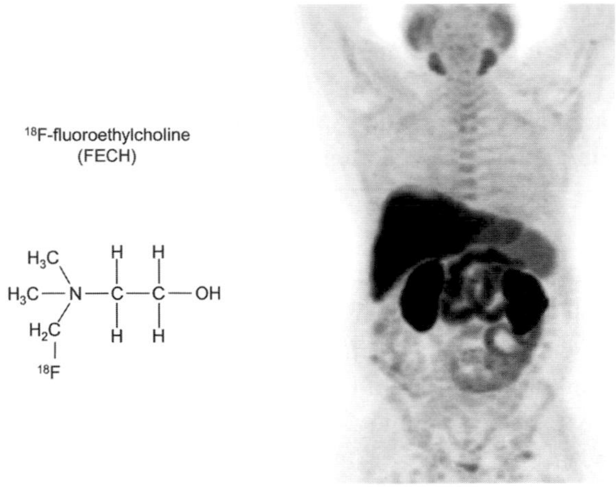

Fig. 5 ^{18}F-fluoroethylcholine (FECH) is a hypoxia tracer used for evaluating rapidly growing tumors. FECH PET/CT is extremely useful in restaging prostate cancer patients with biochemical recurrence. FECH normally accumulates in the salivary glands, pancreas, liver and intestines with renal excretion into the bladder

sites and regional hyperemia (Schiepers et al. 1997; Blake et al. 2001; Even-Sapir et al. 2004, 2006; Even-Sapir 2005) (Fig. 4).

NaF PET is very sensitive for the detection of both lytic and sclerotic bone lesions and combining it with CT increases specificity. NaF PET has a spatial resolution of 4–6 mm versus 10–15 mm for Tc-MDP imaging. NaF PET/CT has been shown to be more sensitive for detecting skeletal metastases than planar or SPECT Tc-99m-MDP skeletal imaging. Benign bone lesions like fractures, Paget disease, enchondroma, and osteoid osteomas also demonstrate increased NaF uptake. NaF PET/CT detects skeletal metastases from tumors that are typically sclerotic or have low FDG activity. FDG PET/CT is more likely to detect bone marrow metastases or small osteolytic lesions (Schirrmeister et al. 2001; Hetzel et al. 2003; Even-Sapir et al. 2004, 2006; Even-Sapir 2005).

4.2 Non-FDA Approved

The sensitivity and specificity of FDG are not optimal in all cancer types. FDG PET/CT images can not adequately differentiate between post-therapy inflammation and residual tumor, poor uptake in slow-growing tumors, and high uptake in normal cells such as the brain, which obscure tumor deposits. In the last decade, research has focused on new PET radiopharmaceuticals directed at a wide range of molecular targets including membrane synthesis, hypoxia, protein synthesis and DNA replication.

4.2.1 Membrane Synthesis

Phosphatidylcholine is an essential element of phospholipids of the cell membrane. Choline is its precursor. Choline enters most cells using specific energy-independent cell membrane transporters. Upon entering the cell, choline is phosphorylated in a reaction catalyzed by the enzyme choline kinase. The malignant transformation of cells elevates levels of choline kinase activity and phosphatidylcholine production (Howard and Howard 1975; Jackowski 1994). PET imaging with ^{11}C-choline was first evaluated in brain tumors because the normal brain has no significant phospholipid metabolism. (Hara et al. 1997) In prostate cancer ^{11}C-choline PET/CT is superior to FDG PET and conventional imaging for identifying nodal and bony metastases in patients with increasing PSA levels. (Roivainen et al. 2000; Picchio et al. 2003) The advantages of ^{11}C-choline PET imaging were apparent after initial studies, but ^{11}C-compunds have a significant logistical limitation–their half-life is only 20.4 min. Methods to label choline with fluorine-18 have been established: ^{18}F-fluoroethylcholine (FECH) is phosphorylated in vivo by choline kinase. (DeGrado et al. 2001; Hara et al. 2002) FECH (Fig. 5) is now distributed widely for PET/CT imaging in Europe where it is used primarily for imaging prostate cancer. FECH is also useful in PET imaging of hepatocellular carcinoma and primary and metastatic brain tumors (Hara et al. 1997; Mertens et al. 2010).

4.2.2 Hypoxia

^{18}F-Fluoromisonidazole (FMISO) is a tracer used for evaluating tumor hypoxia. Hypoxia occurs in rapidly growing tumors as their need for oxygen exceeds the supply available from blood and tissue diffusion. The anoxic center of tumors typically undergoes cell death and necrosis (Fig. 6). In the borderline zones of the tumor, hypoxia inhibits cell growth and division but often leads to adaptive changes as the tumor cells struggle to survive in the harsh environment (Vaupel et al. 1992). Tumor hypoxia is a key factor in tumor progression and therapy resistance (Lee and Scott 2007). FMISO (Fig. 6) enters cells by passive diffusion and under hypoxic conditions forms a charged molecule, which binds to cellular macromolecules. FMISO is not retained in necrosis (Rasey et al. 1987; Foo et al. 2004). PET/CT with FMISO is able to assess the evolving hypoxia level in tumors during radiotherapy. Hypoxic cells are less sensitive to the cytotoxic effects of ionizing radiation than well-oxygenated cells (Koh et al. 1995). Studies in sarcoma and head and neck cancer have demonstrated a correlation of FMISO uptake with poor outcomes for radiation and chemotherapy. (Hicks et al. 2005; Rajendran et al. 2006) Other hypoxia agents include: ^{18}F-fluoroerythronitroimidazole, ^{18}F-fluoroetanidazole, and ^{62}Cu-diacetyl-bis(N (4)-methylthiosemicarbazone (^{62}-Cu-ATSM) (Beck et al. 2007; Mees et al. 2009).

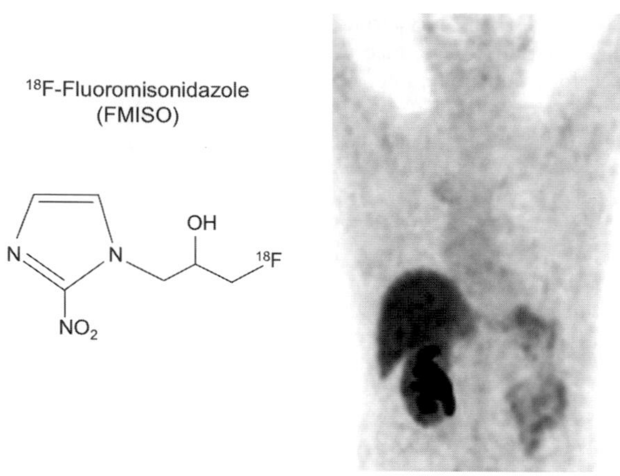

Fig. 6 ^{18}F-Fluoromisonidazole (FMISO) is a hypoxia tracer used for evaluating rapidly growing tumors. FMISO PET/CT is extremely useful in head and neck cancer patients treated with radiotherapy. FMISO normally accumulates in the liver with renal excretion into the bladder

4.2.3 Protein Synthesis

^{11}C-methionine is an amino acid that has been widely studied as a substrate for protein synthesis. Amino acids can freely diffuse into the cells, but the bulk of their transport depends on membrane glycoprotein transport. These transport systems in tumor cells can be energy-dependent, like glucose, or energy-independent. Amino acids are pumped into tumor cells in proportion to their metabolic activity. Malignant transformation drives the use of amino acids for protein synthesis as well as energy production.

Protein synthesis accelerates in proportion to the tumor mass and growth. C-methionone does not accumulate in normal brain tissue but over expressed amino acid transporters in gliomas allow visualization PET/CT. ^{11}C-methionine brain PET is useful for detection of primary tumors, evaluating suspected recurrence, predicting histopathologic grade, radiosensitivity and prognosis, guiding stereotactic brain biopsy, planning radiotherapy and assessing treatment response. (Kaschten et al. 1998; Nuutinen et al. 2000; Ribom et al. 2002; Jacobs et al. 2005; Ceyssens et al. 2006; Galldiks et al. 2006) ^{11}C-methionine PET/CT can also be used to measure increased protein synthesis in lung cancer and breast cancer (Buck et al. 2003).

3,4-Dihydroxy-^{18}F-6-fluoro-L-phenylalanine (FDOPA) was initially developed to examine the transport of a dopamine precursor in Parkinson's disease (Luxen et al. 1992). FDOPA Fig. 7 which enters the brain via a neutral amino acid carrier, is similar structurally to tyrosine but cannot be used in protein synthesis (Fig. 7). These amino acid carriers are commonly over-expressed on the plasma membranes of melanoma cells. FDOPA is extremely useful in staging and restaging of medullary thyroid carcinoma, gastrointestinal cancers, pheochromocytomas and other neuroendocrine tumors (Hoegerle et al. 1999, 2001a, b, 2002; Becherer et al. 2004). FDOPA PET/CT has greater diagnostic accuracy for detecting serotonin-expressing tumors than 111In-Octreotide SPECT or FDG PET/CT (Hoegerle et al. 2001a, b; Ilias et al. 2008). Other radiolabeled amino

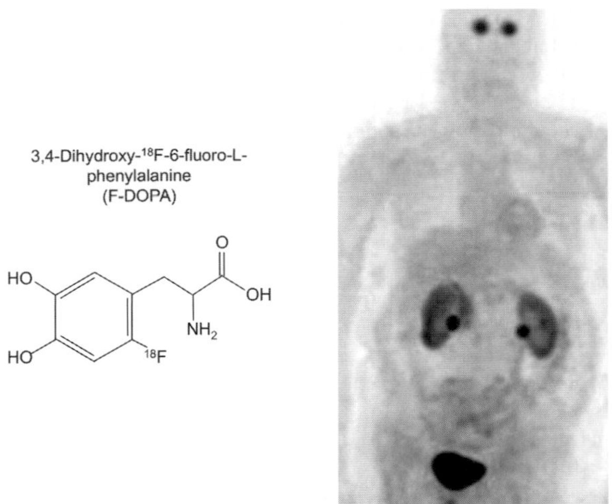

Fig. 7 3,4-Dihydroxy-^{18}F-6-fluoro-L-phenylalanine (FDOPA) is similar structurally to tyrosine and is pumped into cells by the neutral amino acid carrier FDOPA PET/CT is extremely useful in staging and restaging of neuroendocrine tumors. F-DOPA normally accumulates in the basal ganglia and liver with renal excretion into the bladder

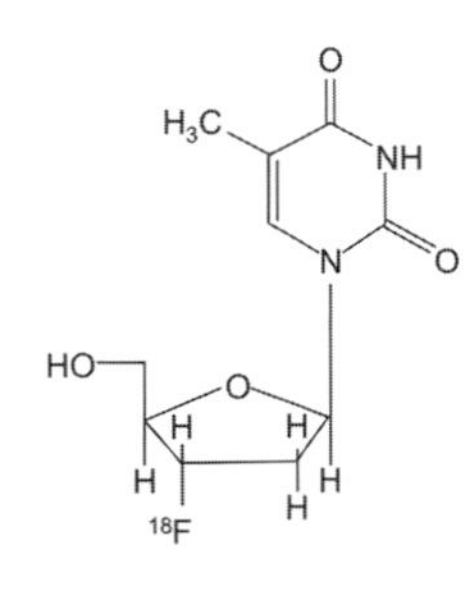

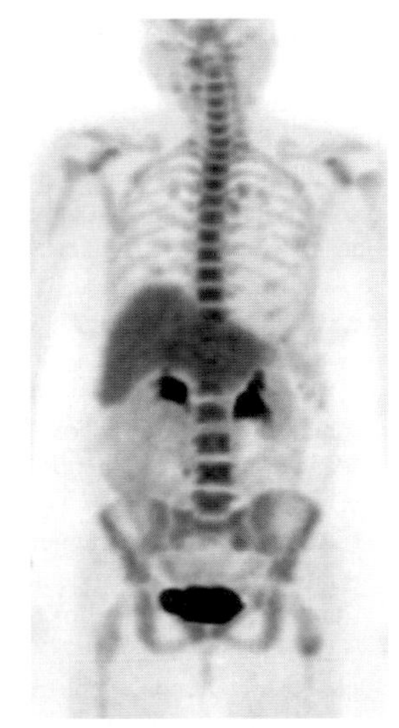

Fig. 8 ^{18}F-3-fluoro-3-deoxy-thymidine (FLT) is a radiolabeled thymidine analog, which is an indirect measure of DNA proliferation. FLT PET/CT is an imaging biomarker for early therapy assessment. FLT normally accumulates in the liver and bone marrow with renal excretion into the bladder

acid analogs include ^{18}F-L-tyrosine and ^{18}F-fluoro-cyclo-butane-1-carboxylic acid (FACBC) (Vallabhajosula 2007; Schuster et al. 2007).

4.2.4 DNA Replication

^{18}F-3-fluoro-3-deoxy-thymidine (FLT) is a pyrimidine analogue used to measure tumor cell proliferation (Fig. 8). Increased mitotic rate, cell multiplication and lack of differentiation are characteristics of the tumors. The accelerated growth of malignant tissue is the best measure of DNA replication. FLT is actively transported into the cell and phosphorylated similarly to thymidine (Sherley and Kelly 1988). FLT is trapped in the cell in proportion to the amount of DNA and RNA synthesis (Shields et al. 1996, 1998). There is a strong correlation between FLT uptake and the proliferation rate as determined by the Ki-67 index in lung, colorectal and breast cancer, melanoma, soft tissue sarcoma and brain tumors. (Vesselle et al. 2002; Francis et al. 2003; Cobben et al. 2003, 2004; Smyczek-Gargya et al. 2004; Chen et al. 2005) FLT uptake can differentiate between benign and malignant tissues and helps with tumor grading. PET/CT with FLT is useful for assessing tumor aggressiveness and early prediction of treatment response. FLT uptake does not increase with infection or inflammation like FDG. FLT, as a proliferative marker, is less affected by radiation inflammation and can detect response as early as 1 week after treatment. FLT PET/CT has a higher specificity for early therapy assessment than FDG PET/CT (Shields 2003). FLT offers more in vivo utility than FDG for evaluating patient response to novel therapies and to predict patient outcomes. Other proliferative tracers include ^{18}F-fluorouridine and ^{18}F-FMAU (Vallabhasojula 2007; Bading et al. 2008).

References

Ak I, Stokkel MP, Pauwels EK (2000) Positron emission tomography with 2-[18F]fluoro-2-deoxy-D-glucose in oncology. Part II. The clinical value in detecting and staging primary tumors. J Cancer Res Clin Oncol 126:560–574

Avril N, Menzel M, Dose J, Schelling M, Weber W, Jänicke F, Nathrath W, Schwaiger M (2001) Glucose metabolism of breast cancer assessed by 18F-FDG PET: histologic and immunohistochemical tissue analysis. J Nucl Med 42(1):9–16

Bading JR, Shields AF (2008) Imaging of cell proliferation: status and prospects. J Nucl Med 49(2):648-805

Becherer A, Szabo M, Karanikas G et al (2004) Imaging of advanced neuroendocrine tumors with ^{18}F-FDOPA PET. J Nucl Med 45:1161–1167

Beck R, Roper B, Carlsen JM et al (2007) Pretreatment 18F-FAZA PET predicts success of hypoxia-directed radiochemotherapy using tirapazamine. J Nucl Med 48:973–980

Blake GM, Park-Holohan SJ, Cook GJ et al (2001) Quantitative studies of bone with the use of ^{18}F-fluoride and ^{99m}Tc-methylene diphosphonate. Semin Nucl Med 31:28–49

Blau M, Nagler W, Bender MA (1962) A new isotope for bone scanning. J Nucl Med 3:332–334

Bos R, van Der Hoeven JJ, van Der Wall E, van Der Groep P, van Diest PJ, Comans EF, Joshi U, Semenza GL, Hoekstra OS, Lammertsma AA, Molthoff CF (2002) Biologic correlates of (18)fluorodeoxyglucose uptake in human breast cancer measured by positron emission tomography. J Clin Oncol 20(2):379–387

Breeman WAP, Verbruggen AM (2007) The 68 Ge/68 Ga generator has high potential, but when can we use 68 Ga-labeled tracers in clinical routine? Eur J Nucl Med Mol Imaging 34:978–981

Buck AK, Halter G, Schirrmeister H et al (2003) Imaging of proliferation in lung tumors with PET: 18FLT versus 18FDG. J Nucl Med 44:1426–1431

Carolan P, Hunt C, McConnell D et al (2012) Radiation exposure reduction to PET technologists with the use of an automated dosage delivery system. J Nucl Med 53:2185

Ceyssens S, Van Laere K, de Groot T et al (2006) [11C]methionine PET, histopathology, and survival in primary brain tumors and recurrence. AJNR 27:1432–1437

Chen W, Cloughesy T, Kamdar N et al (2005) Imaging proliferation in brain tumors with 18-FLT PET: comparison with 18F-FDG. J Nucl Med 46:945–952

Cobben DC, Elsinga PH, Suurmeijer AJ et al (2004) Detection and grading of soft tissue sarcomas of the extremities with 18F–3-fluoro-3-deoxy-l-thymidine. Clin Cancer Res 10:1685–1690

Cobben DC, Jager PL, Elsinga PH et al (2003) 18F–3-fluoro-3-deoxy-l-thymidine: a new tracer or staging of metastatic melanoma? J Nucl Med 44:1927–1932

Coleman RE (1999) PET in lung cancer. J Nucl Med 40(5):814–820

DeGrado TR, Coleman RE, Wang S et al (2001) Synthesis and evaluation of 18F labeled choline as an oncologic tracer for positron emission tomography: initial findings in prostate cancer. Cancer Res 61:110–117

Delbeke D (1999) Oncological applications of FDG PET imaging. J Nucl Med 40(10):1706–1715

Even-Sapir E, Metser U, Flusser G et al (2004) Assessment of malignant skeletal disease: initial experience with 18F–fluoride PET/CT and comparison between 18F–fluoride PET and 18F–fluoride PET/CT. J Nucl Med 45:272–278

Even-Sapir E, Metser U, Mishani E et al (2006) The detection of bone metastases in patient with high-risk prostate cancer: 99mTc-MDP planar bone scintigraphy, single- and -field-of view SPECT, 18F–fluoride PET, and 18F–fluoride PET/CT. J Nucl Med 47:287–297

Even-Sapir E (2005) Imaging of malignant bone involvement by morphologic, scintigraphic, and hybrid modalities. J Nucl Med 46:1356–1367

Foo SS, Abbott DF, Lawrentschuk N et al (2004) Functional imaging of intra-tumoral hypoxia. Mol Imaging Biol 6:291–305

Francis DL, Visvikis D, Costa DC et al (2003) Potential impact of [18F]-3-fluoro-3-deoxy-thymidine versus [18F]-fluoro-2-deoxy-D-glucose in positron emission tomography for colorectal cancer. Eur J Nucl Med Mol Imaging 30:988–994

Galldiks N, Kracht LW, Burghaus L et al (2006) Use of 11Cmethionine PET to monitor the effects of temozolomide chemotherapy in malignant gliomas. Eur J Nucl Med Mol Imaging 33:516–524

Gatley SJ (2003) Labeled glucose analogs in the genomic era. J Nucl Med 44(7):1082–1086

Hara T, Kosaka N, Kishi H (2002) Development of [18F]-Fluoroethylcholine for cancer imaging with PET: synthesis, biochemistry, and prostate cancer imaging. J Nucl Med 43:187–199

Hara T, Kosaka N, Shinoura N et al (1997) PET imaging of brain tumor with [methyl-11C] choline. J Nucl Med 38:842–847

Hetzel M, Arslandemir C, Konig HH et al (2003) F-18 NaF PET for detection of bone metastases in lung cancer: accuracy, cost-effectiveness and impact on patient management. J Bone Miner Res 18:2206–2214

Hicks RJ, Rischin D, Fisher R et al (2005) Utility of FMISO PET in advanced head and neck cancer treated with chemoradiation incorporating a hypoxia-targeting chemotherapy agent. Eur J Nucl Med Mol Imaging 32:1384–1391

Higashi T, Saga T, Nakamoto Y, Ishimori T, Mamede MH, Wada M, Doi R, Hosotani R, Imamura M, Konishi J (2002) Relationship between retention index in dual-phase (18)F-FDG PET, and hexokinase-II and glucose transporter-1 expression in pancreatic cancer. J Nucl Med 43(2):173–180

Hoegerle S, Altehoefer C, Ghanem N et al (2001a) 18F-DOPA positron emission tomography for tumor detection in patients with medullary thyroid carcinoma and elevated calcitonin levels. Eur J Nucl Med 28:64–71

Hoegerle S, Altehoefer C, Ghanem N, Koehler G, Waller CF, Scheruebl H, Moser E, Nitzsche E (2001b) Whole-body 18F dopa PET for detection of gastrointestinal carcinoid tumors. Radiology 220(2):373–380

Hoegerle S, Nitzsche E, Altehoefer C et al (2002) Pheochromocytomas: detection with 18F DOPA whole body PET—initial results. Radiology 222:507–512

Hoegerle S, Schneider B, Kraft A, Moser E, Nitzsche EU (1999) Imaging of a metastatic gastrointestinal carcinoid by F-18-DOPA positron emission tomography. Nuklearmedizin 38:127–130

Howard BV, Howard WJ (1975) Lipids in normal and tumor cells in culture. Prog Biochem Pharmacol 10:135–166

Ido T, Wan CN, Casella JS et al (1978) Labeled 2-deoxy-D-glucose analogs: 18F labeled 2-deoxy-2-fluoro-D-glucose, 2-deoxy-2-fluoro-D-mannose and 14C–2-deoxy-2-fluoro-D-glucose. J Label Compd Radiopharmacol 14:175–183

Ilias I, Chen CC, Carrasquillo JA et al (2008) Comparison of 6-[18F]-fluorodopamine positron emission tomography to [123I]-metaiodobenzylguanidine and [111In]-pentetreotide scintigraphy in the localization of non-metastatic and metastatic pheochromocytoma. J Nucl Med 49:1613–1619

Jackowski S (1994) Coordination of membrane phospholipid synthesis with the cell cycle. J Biol Chem 269: 3858–3867

Jacobs AH, Thomas A, Kracht LW et al (2005) 18F-fluoro-l-thymidine and 11C-Methylmetionine as markers of increased transport and proliferation in brain tumors. J Nucl Med 46:1948–1958

Kaschten B, Stevenaert A, Sadzot B et al (1998) Preoperative evaluation of 54 gliomas by PET with fluorine-18-fluoro-deoxyglucose and/or carbon-11-methionine. J Nucl Med 39:778–785

Koh WJ, Bergman KS, Rasey JS et al (1995) Evaluation of oxygenation status during fractionated radiotherapy in human non-small cell lung cancers using [F-18]fluoromisonidazole positron emission tomography. Int J Radiat Oncol Biol Phys 33:391–398

Laszlo J, Humphreys SR, Goldin A (1960) Effects of glucose analogues (2-deoxy-D-glucose, 2-deoxy-D-galactose) on experimental tumors. J Natl Cancer Inst 24:267–281

Lee ST, Scott AM (2007) Hypoxia positron emission tomography imaging with 18F-fluoromisonidazole. Semin Nucl Med 37:451–461

Luxen A, Guillaume M, Melega WP et al (1992) Production of 6-[18F]fluoro-L-dopa and its metabolism in vivo—a critical review. Int J Radiat Appl Instrum B 19:149–158

McCarthy TJ, Welch MJ (1998) The state of positron emitting radionuclide production in 1997. Semin Nucl Med 28(3): 235–46

Mees G, Dierckx R, Vangestel C et al (2009) Molecular imaging of hypoxia with radiolabeled agents. Eur J Nucl Med Mol Imaging 36:1674–1686

Mertens K, Slaets D, Lambert B, Acou M, De Vos F, Goethals I (2010) PET with (18)F-labeled choline-based tracers for tumor imaging: a review of the literature. Eur J Nucl Med Mol Imaging 37(11):2188–2193

Mochizuki T, Tsukamoto E, Kuge Y, Kanegae K, Zhao S, Hikosaka K, Hosokawa M, Kohanawa M, Tamaki N (2001) FDG uptake and glucose transporter subtype expressions in experimental tumor and inflammation models. J Nucl Med 42(10):1551–1555

Nutt R (2002) The history of positron emission tomography (PET). Mol Imaging Biol 4:11–26

Nuutinen J, Sonninen P, Lehikoinen P et al (2000) Radiotherapy treatment planning and long-term follow-up with [(11)C] methionine PET in patients with low-grade astrocytoma. Int J Radiat Oncol Biol Phys 48:43–52

Pacák J, Cerny M (2002) History of the First Synthesis of 2-Deoxy-2-Fluoro-D-Glucose the Unlabeled Forerunner of 2-Deoxy-2-[18F]Fluoro-D-Glucose. Mol Imaging Biol 4:353–354

Picchio M, Messa C, Landoni C et al (2003) Value of [11C]choline positron emission tomography for re-staging prostate cancer: a comparison with [18F] fluorodeoxyglucose-positron emission tomography. J Urol 169:1337–1340

Rajendran JG, Schwartz DL, O'Sullivan J et al (2006) Tumor hypoxia imaging with [F-18] fluoromisonidazole positron emission tomography in head and neck cancer. Clin Cancer Res 12:5435–5441

Rasey JS, Grunbaum Z, Magee S et al (1987) Characterization of radiolabeled fluoromisonidazole as a probe for hypoxic cells. Radiat Res 111:292–304

Ribom D, Engler H, Blomquist E, Smits A (2002) Potential significance of (11)C-methionine PET as marker for the radiosensitivity of low-grade gliomas. Eur J Nucl Med Mol Imaging 29:632–640

Rice SL, Roney CA, Daumar P, Lewis JS (2011) The next generation of positron emission tomography radiopharmaceuticals in oncology. Semin Nucl Med 41(4):265–282

Roivainen A, Forsback S, Grönroos T et al (2000) Blood metabolism of [methyl-11C]choline; implications for in vivo imaging with positron emission tomography. Eur J Nucl Med 27:25–32

Rufini V, Calcagni ML, Baum RP (2007) Imaging of neuroendocrine tumors. Semin Nucl Med 36:228–247

Schiepers C, Nuytes J, Bormans G et al (1997) Fluoride kinetics of the axial skeleton measured in vivo with fluorine-18-fluoride PET. J Nucl Med 38:1970–1976

Schirrmeister H, Glatting G, Hetzel J et al (2001) Prospective evaluation of clinical value of planar bone scans, SPECT, and18F-labeled NaF PET in newly diagnosed lung cancer. J Nucl Med 42:1800–1804

Schlyer DJ (2004) PET tracers and radiochemistry. Ann Acad Med Singapore 33:146–154

Schuster DM, John R, Votaw JR et al (2007) Initial experience with the radiotracer anti-1-amino-3-18F-fluorocyclobutane-1-carboxylic acid with PET/CT in prostate carcinoma. J Nucl Med 48:56–63

Shaiju VS, Sharma SD, Kumar R, Sarin B (2009) Target foil rupture scenario and provision for handling different models of medical cyclotrons used in India. J Med Phys 34(3):161–166

Sharma S, Krause G, Ebadi M (2006) Radiation safety and quality control in the cyclotron laboratory. Radiat Prot Dosimetry 118:431–439

Sherley JL, Kelly TJ (1988) Regulation of human thymidine kinase during the cell cycle. J Biol Chem 263:8350–8358

Shields AF (2003) PET imaging with 18F-FLT and thymidine analogs: promise and pitfalls. J Nucl Med 44:1432–1434

Shields AF, Grierson JR, Kozawa SM et al (1996) Development of labeled thymidine analogs for imaging tumor proliferation. Nucl Med Biol 23:17–22

Shields AF, Grierson JR, Dohmen BM et al (1998) Imaging proliferation in vivo with [F-18]FLT and positron emission tomography. Nat Med 4:1334–1336

Smith TA (2000) Mammalian hexokinases and their abnormal expression in cancer. Br J Biomed Sci 57:170–178

Smyczek-Gargya B, Fersis N, Dittmann H et al (2004) PET with [18F]fluorothymidine for imaging of primary breast cancer: a pilot study. Eur J Nucl Med Mol Imaging 31:720–724

Vallabhajosula S, Solnes L, Vallabhajosula B (2011) A broad overview of positron emission tomography radiopharmaceuticals and clinical applications: what is new? Semin Nucl Med 41(4):246–264

Vallabhajosula S (2007) (18)F-labeled positron emission tomographic radiopharmaceuticals in oncology: an overview of radiochemistry and mechanisms of tumor localization. Semin Nucl Med 37(6):400–419

Vaupel P, Schlenger K, Hoeckel M (1992) Blood flow and tissue oxygenation of human tumors: an update. Adv Exp Med Biol 317:139–151

Vesselle H, Grierson J, Muzi M et al (2002) In vivo validation of 3′deoxy-3′-[(18)F]fluorothymidine ([(18)F]FLT) as a proliferation imaging tracer in humans: correlation of [(18)F]FLT uptake by positron emission tomography with

Ki-67 immunohistochemistry and flow cytometry in human lung tumors. Clin Cancer Res 8:3315–3323

Warburg O (1956) On the origin of cancer cells. Science 123:309–314

Williams HA, Robinson S, Julyan P et al (2005) A comparison of PET imaging characteristics of various copper radioisotopes. Eur J Nucl Med Mol Imaging 32:1473–1480

Zhao S, Kuge Y, Tsukamoto E, Mochizuki T, Kato T, Hikosaka K, Hosokawa M, Kohanawa M, Tamaki N (2001) Effects of insulin and glucose loading on FDG uptake in experimental malignant tumors and inflammatory lesions. Eur J Nucl Med 28(6):730–735

Zhernosekov KP, Filosofov DV, Baum RP et al (2007) Processing of generator-produced 68 Ga for medical application. J Nucl Med 48:1741–1748

Zweit J, Goodall R, Cox M, Babich JW, Potter GA, Sharma HL, Ott RJ (1992) Development of a high performance zinc-62/copper-62 radionuclide generator for positron emission tomography. Eur J Nucl Med 19(6):418–425

PET/CT Interpretation

Patrick J. Peller

Contents

P. J. Peller (✉)
Division of Nuclear Medicine,
Department of Radiology, Mayo Clinic, 200,
1st Street SW, Rochester, MN 55905, USA
e-mail: Peller.patrick@mayo.edu

Abstract

PET/SPECT interpretation is a challenging task, which is aided by a systematic approach to image review. The PET/SPECT report is the final product of interpretation and needs to be crafted carefully. The impression should answer the referring physician's clinical question and delineate all diagnoses requiring his action. A thorough knowledge of the normal distribution of FDG is very important for PET/CT interpretation.

1 Key Points

Optimal PET/CT interpretation requires attention to details throughout the process from scheduling to reporting. FDG PET/CT should be performed at basal insulin and fasting-glucose levels, with minimal physical activity. A systematic approach to PET/image review is highly recommended. For each PET/CT scan set your images at the same intensity and use the cerebellum, blood pool, and liver as internal references while interpreting. Craft the PET/CT report to optimize communication with the referring physician and always answer the clinical question posed. Accurate PET/CT interpretation requires the reader to understand the variation of normal FDG uptake throughout the body.

2 Introduction

Integrated positron emission tomography and computed tomography (PET/CT) utilizing Fluorine-18 2-Fluoro-2-deoxyglucose (FDG) is now a well-established oncologic

P. Peller et al. (eds.), *PET-CT and PET-MRI in Oncology*, Medical Radiology. Diagnostic Imaging,
DOI: 10.1007/174_2012_602,

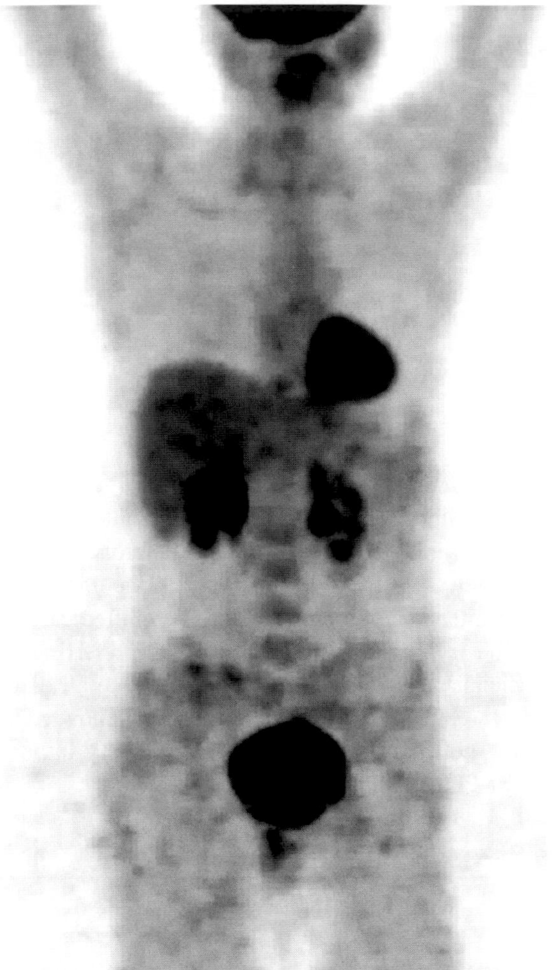

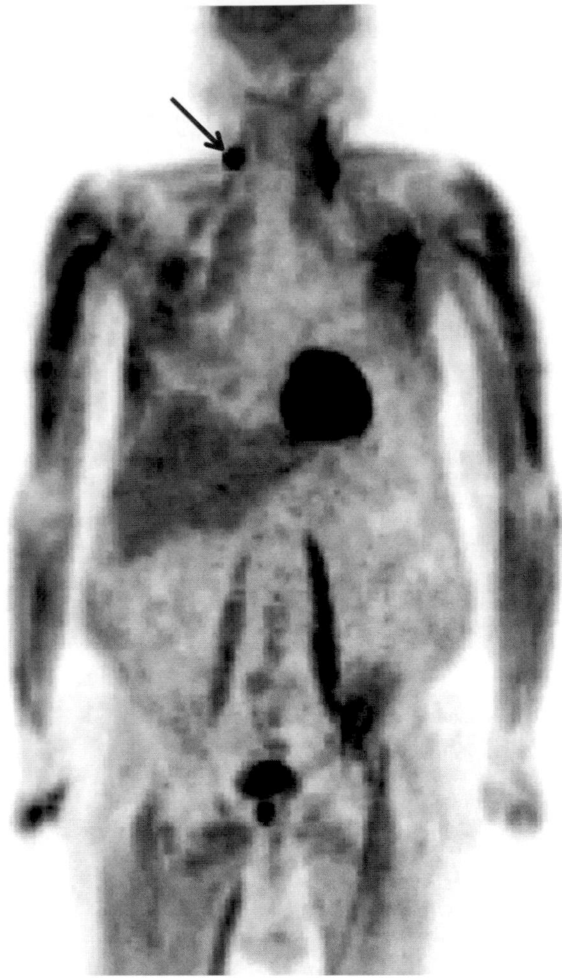

Fig. 1 Spinning the MIP FDG PET image is a useful first step to control the quality of the PET/CT scan. The interpreter is looking for the normal distribution of FDG. There is customarily intense activity in the brain and excreted urine in the kidneys and bladder. Variable activity is seen in the myocardium, predominantly the *left* ventricle, and moderate activity in the liver. In the resting fasting patient the remainder of the tissues have very low activity. Patient preparation is key to most imaging studies. To the *right* is an example of a patient who was fasting except for two cough drops. Minimal oral carbohydrate intake will produce no elevation in blood sugar, but high insulin levels drive the FDG into skeletal and cardiac muscles. The patient's *right* neck nodal metastasis is still visible (*arrow*)

imaging technique. The goal in combining PET and CT into a single scanner is to leverage the strengths of both modalities (Townsend 2008). The high FDG uptake of many malignancies results in lesion conspicuity on the PET portion yielding high sensitivity. The high spatial resolution of the multidetector CT portion provides localization clarity resulting in high specificity. Careful systematic review of PET, CT, and fused images should lead to a high degree of interpretive certainty. When optimally applied FDG PET/CT can detect, stage, and restage cancer patients with accuracy and can be reported with confidence.

3 PET/CT Image Evaluation

Optimal interpretation requires supervision and attention to details throughout the entire process from scheduling the PET/CT scan, to patient preparation, to the actual imaging, and ultimately to

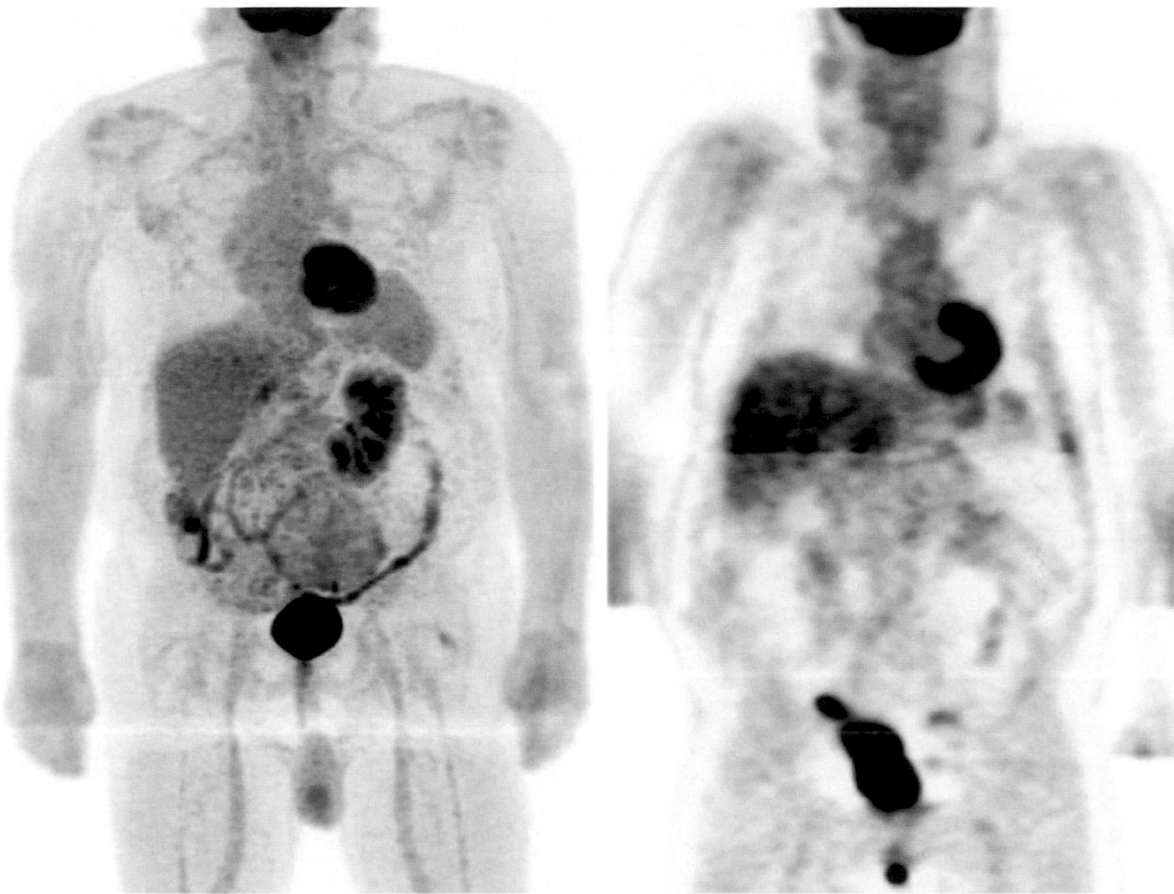

Fig. 2 The MIP images are useful to detect common artifacts such as patient motion. Patients most frequently move their head or hands. Linear motion artifacts can be produced by simple hand motion (*left*). Torso motion is uncommon but severely degrades the PET/CT (*right*)

reporting. For all imaging tests, proper patient preparation prior to and during the study is vitally important for maximal diagnostic yield. FDG PET patients are ideally imaged in the resting state with basal insulin and glucose levels to minimize physiologic activity. A careful, systematic approach to both imaging and interpretation is highly recommended (Agress et al. 2008).

3.1 Image Quality Control

Prior to initiating image interpretation, the interpreting physician should take a critical look at the images to ensure high quality and identify flaws that might create artifacts. The first step is to spin the FDG maximum intensity projection (MIP) image (Fig. 1). This image created from the transaxial images is a very good way to evaluate the integrity of the PET data. Patient motion is a common artifact and is frequently observed on this initial image quality control step (Fig. 2). The FDG MIP image allows the interpreter to review to FDG distribution globally. Tracer infiltration or extravasation can often be readily identified.

The CT and PET scans are performed sequentially on the same pallet, ideally without patient movement between scans. The alignment of CT and PET data is crucial for PET attenuation correction and image fusion. The rapid review of the transaxial fused images set can confirm that the PET and CT data are correctly registered (Fig. 3). Motion in head and neck is not uncommon. One should identify the FDG brain

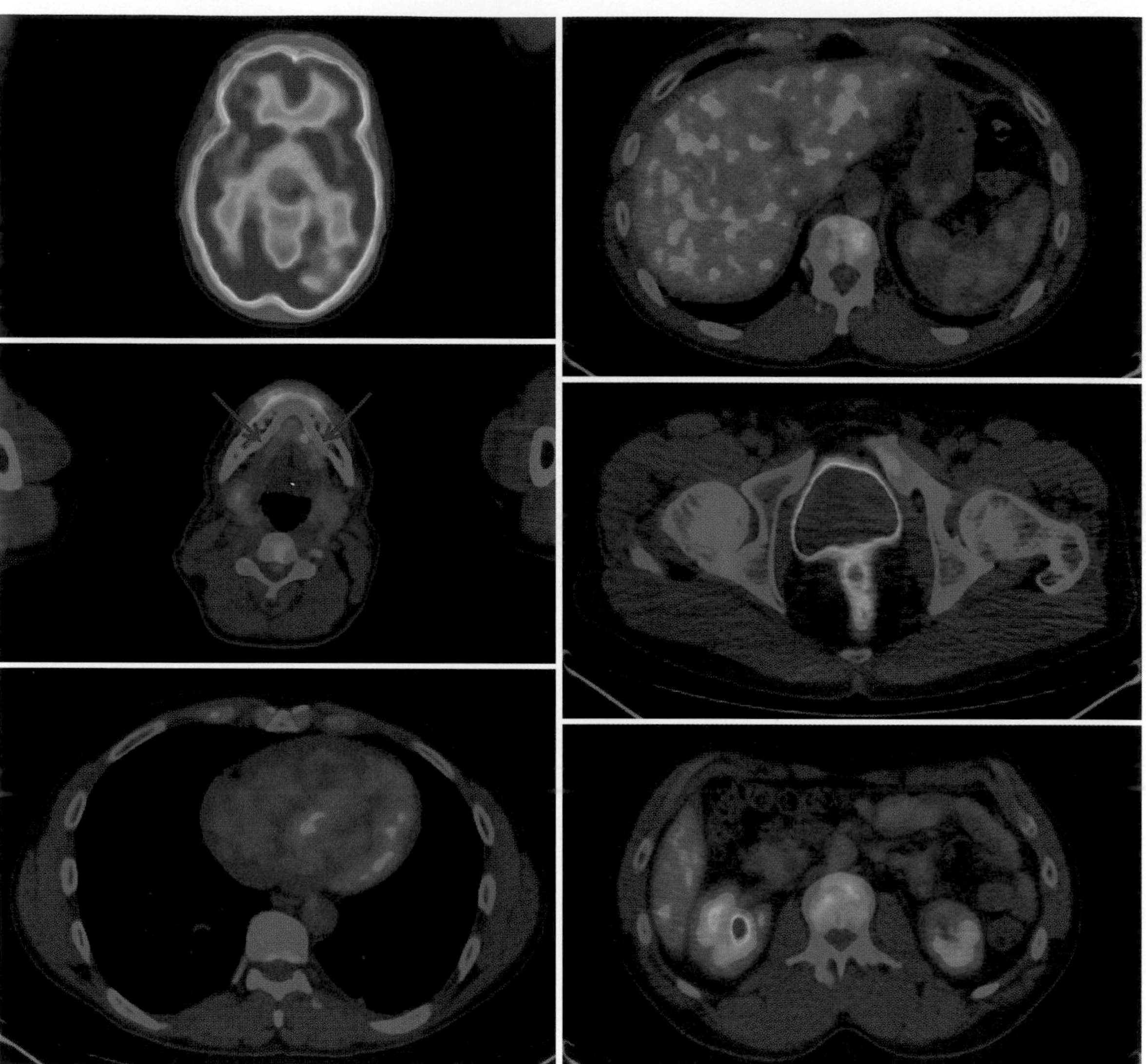

Fig. 3 It is extremely important that the CT and PET images are obtained without patient motion between the image sets. As part of PET/CT quality control, one should check for coregistration. It is important to see that the brain is within the skull, the liver and spleen correspond both in uptake and structure, and the urine activity in the kidneys and bladder are in appropriate locations. Head motion is common and to confirm neck registration the mylohyoid muscle—an upside down V in the floor of the mouth—should lie just within the mandible (*arrows*)

within the CT skull when progressing from head to toe. The inverted "V" of the mylohyoid muscle in the floor of the mouth should lie as just inside the mandible. If the brain and mylohyoid muscle are correctly registered it is likely that no significant patient head and neck motion was present. The FDG accumulation in the left ventricle, liver, kidneys, and bladder activity on PET images should also match the corresponding structures on CT.

3.2 Image Setup

The overlay or fusion of PET images on to the CT scan requires the conversion of the PET images to color. Many color scales are available on commercial PET/CT reading stations. Rainbow and hot iron are the most common color scales employed (Fig. 4). The operator should set the color intensity identically for every PET/CT scan. Setting the color intensity too high or too low

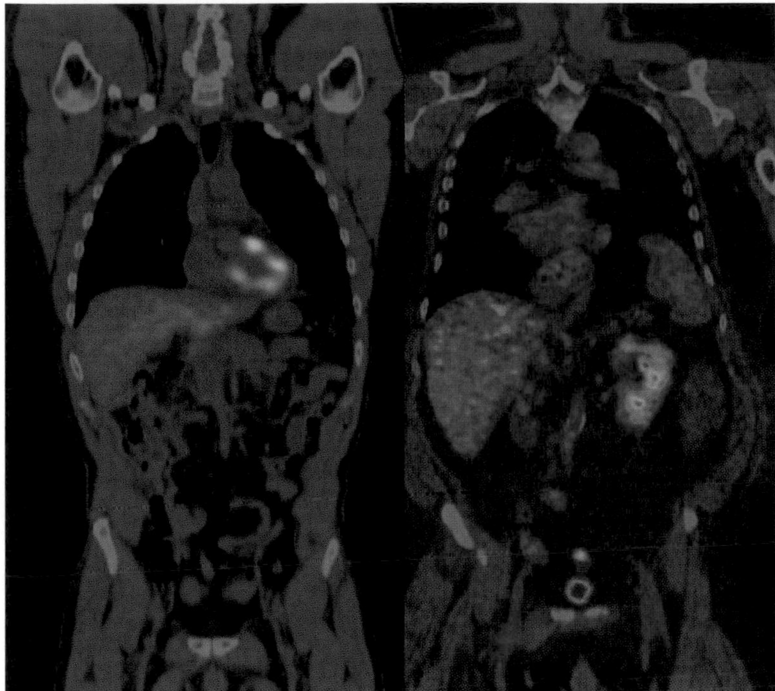

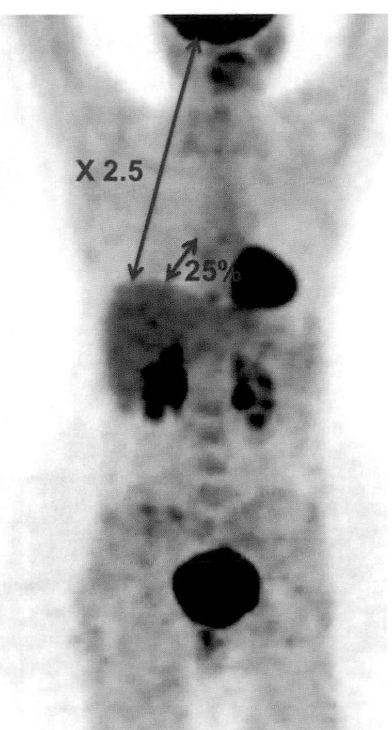

Fig. 4 A standard color scan should be used to display the PET data overlaid on the CT. The most common choices are hot iron (*left*) and rainbow (*right*). The intensity of these color images are set similarly for each PET/CT reading using the liver as the reference organ. Interpretation of PET images is aided by establishing visual standards: mediastinal blood pool, liver, and cerebellum. Typically the liver is 25 % more active than the mediastinal blood pool and the cerebellum is at least 2.5 times the activity in the liver

can lead to interpretive errors. Most commonly the color scale is adjusted to normal liver activity selecting a color in the middle of the color scale range. When two PET/CT scans are being compared, it is very helpful to set the liver activity in both scans the same.

Simplistically a CT image is a map of differential densities: air, fat, water, and bone. CT lesion characterization is aided by comparison of lesion density to adjacent structures of known density. PET is a map of differential FDG uptake throughout the body. It is useful during interpretation to compare and contrast FDG uptake in a potential lesion to normal structures, which have predictable, stable relative uptake. Interpreters frequently use the residual blood pool activity within the mediastinal great vessels, liver uptake, and cerebellar accumulation for this comparison. In normal patients liver uptake is approximately 25 % higher than mediastinal blood pool activity (Fig. 5). The cerebellum has more than 2.5 times the FDG accumulation of the liver. Creating a standard initial image color setup consistently and using the mediastinal blood pool, liver, and cerebellum activity as points of reference can significantly improve PET/CT interpretation and reproducibility.

1. Spin FDG PET MIP
2. PET + CT soft tissue window head to thigh/toe
3. PET + CT bone window thigh/toe to head
4. PET + CT lung windows apex to base
5. Review coronal and sagittals windowing CT as needed
6. Re-window PET to interpret brain

Fig. 5 Systematic PET/CT image review

3.3 Systematic Image Review

Oncologic PET/CT scans are some of the most complex, time-consuming, and difficult sets of images to interpret. The sheer number of CT, PET, and fused images to review is the initial challenge. Using a

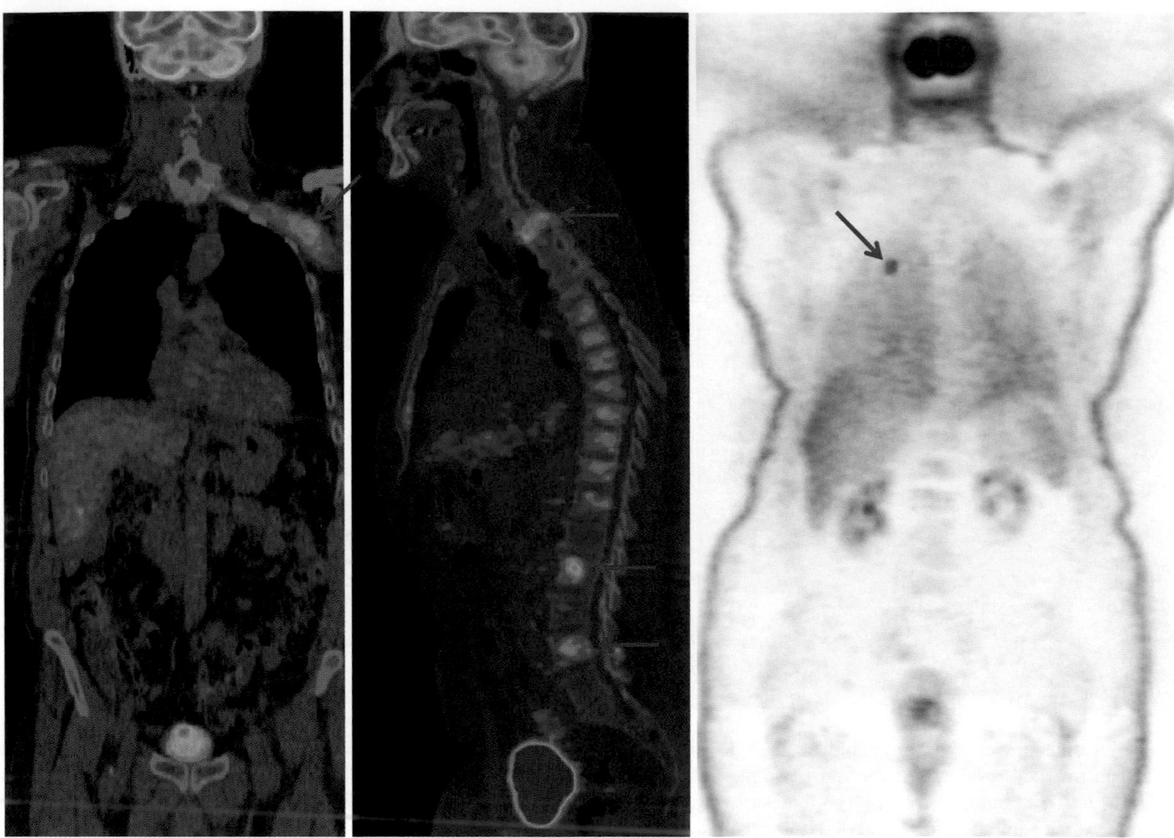

Fig. 6 This coronal fused image demonstrates a hypermetabolic neurogenic tumor infiltrating the *left* brachial plexus (*arrow*). The sagittal fused PET/CT image demonstrates recurrent bone metastases within two areas of bone marrow ablation from previous irradiation to the spine (*arrows*). The nonattenuation corrected coronal image demonstrates typical high activity in the skin and lung accentuating a mildly FDG-avid right upper lobe lung nodule (*arrow*)

systematic approach of image review for every PET/CT scan leads to complete study evaluation and avoids interpretive error (Fig. 5). The FDG PET MIP image can provide a general overview of disease distribution and extent. PET and CT transaxial images should be read side-by-side using the fusion images for correlation of potential abnormalities. One systematic approach is to start at the head on transaxial PET and CT soft tissue window and continue to mid thigh, returning cephalad viewing the PET and CT bone windows and covering the lungs from apex to base with CT lung windows. Typically review of coronal, sagittal, and nonattenuation corrected (NAC) PET images can increase diagnostic yield and confidence (Fig. 6). When setting the liver to the center on the color scale, the brain should be the maximum color. Prior to completing image review often the FDG PET color scale must be manipulated downward to interpret the brain.

Coronal, sagittal, and NAC images should be available for review on all PET/CT scans. Coronal images are particularly helpful in evaluating and measuring cephalad to caudal lesion extent and tracing the normal path of muscle, nerves, and vessels. Adding a small degree of obliquity to coronal images on the PET/CT review work station places the brachial plexus in one or two coronal slides matching those often acquired on MRI. Sagittal images readily evaluate spine structure, marrow activity and aid precise lesion localization. Comparison of bone marrow activity before and after treatment is often best performed with sagittal images. The NAC PET images amplifies skin and lung lesions. The NAC images are often crucial for identification of artifacts induced by CT attenuation correction.

Non FDG-avid CT findings are very important to identify. Pulmonary nodules smaller than 8 mm can be readily detected by CT, but can be poorly seen and

Clinical history: Reason for study, type, site and stage of cancer, therapy
Procedure: tracer dose and route, incubation time, scan coverage, type of CT, contrast, and blood glucose
Findings: Comparison or prior studies, abnormalities described and measured, differential diagnosis, incidental CT findings
Impression: Interpretation of findings, answer clinical question, next step if needed

Fig. 7 Essential PET/CT report elements

characterized with FDG PET. Cystic soft tissue lesions and sclerotic bone abnormalities are manifestations of malignancy that often have poor FDG uptake but are visible on CT. The presence of small pleural effusions or ascites will be detected only on CT. Significant vascular disease can be identified on the CT component primarily.

4 PET/CT Reporting

The PET/CT report remains the major source of communication between the interpreting and referring physicians. The PET/CT report is often the only permanent record of test performance and results. Coding and billing personnel typically use the report to support request for payment (Coleman et al. 2010). The report is ultimately the final product of PET/CT interpretation. Standardized and structured reporting are definitely useful and are recommended by many professional organizations (ACR; SNM). The report should contain four basic components: clinical history, procedure information, PET/CT findings, and impression (SNM PET Pros) (Fig. 7).

The clinical history should be a concise restatement of relevant patient information and the clinical question posed by the physician ordering the PET/CT scan. When possible the original pathologic diagnosis and stage plus recent treatments especially surgery and radiation therapy should be stated. Potential interfering inflammatory conditions, e.g., sarcoidosis should be included. Relevant laboratory markers, especially serum tumor markers, should be recorded. The new CMS billing requirements of initial or subsequent treatment strategy should be added here (CMS 2009).

The procedure section of the report should include concise technical details of both the PET and CT portion of the examination. Medications used including radiopharmaceutical, IV and oral contrast, and sedation should be recorded. The axial coverage of the scan should be noted in terms of the major body parts, which are included in the procedure. Additional images or special patient preparation should be documented, for example high-resolution neck images or a Foley catheter placed in the urinary bladder. The time of the scan relative to FDG injection and the fasting serum glucose at the time of FDG administration should be provided. Additional data such as injection site, specific PET/CT reconstruction parameters, CT settings, and a rate of IV contrast administration are typically recorded in a separate patient data sheet.

The findings section should provide a full description of abnormalities identified in both FDG PET and CT scans. Prior imaging should be correlated and integrated with current images. Both metabolic and morphologic findings should be measured and described completely. Standard measurement schemes such as RECIST and PERCIST should be employed, especially for patients enrolled in clinical studies. The PET/CT results should be recorded to aid communication of disease extent taking into account disease-specific staging, e.g., TNM or FIGO. Incidental clinically relevant CT or PET only findings should be recorded. Prominent variants and potential pitfalls should be clearly delineated.

In a patient with a prior PET/CT scan available for comparison the findings section should reflect both the metabolic and anatomic response to therapy. Changes in tumor uptake of FDG are frequently reported as change in maximum SUV (SUV_{max}). SUV_{max} is the easiest and most reproducible measurement reflecting tumor metabolism and corresponds to the strongest medical literature support. The relative FDG uptake, uptake pattern, and configuration are as important as the SUV number. When comparing two PET/CT scans reporting the SUV_{max} is numerically helpful to describe the magnitude of change. Progression of oncologic disease can be seen with increasing activity, size of lesions, or number of abnormalities, but newly visualized lesions represent the strongest evidence for progression.

The impression is the critical portion of the report. It is here that the interpreting physician should synthesize all of the data in the rest of the report and come to a clear, concise conclusion if possible. The clinical question of the referring physician must be answered. The impression should take into account all PET and

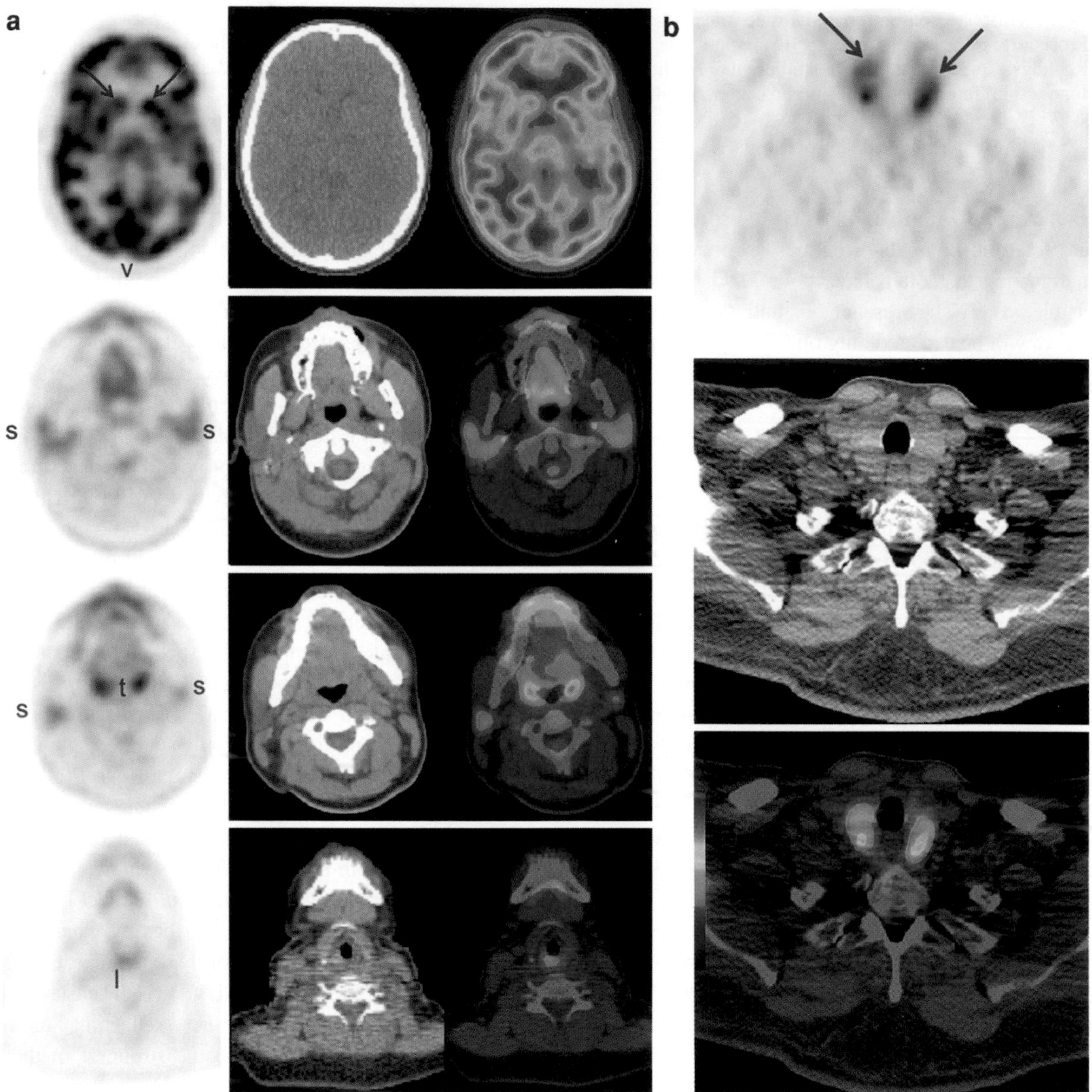

Fig. 8 **a** Normal head and neck. The basal ganglia (*arrows*) and visual cortex (v) are 10–15 % more FDG-avid than the remaining cerebral cortex. The cerebellum (not shown) is 30–40 % less active than the visual cortex. Mild FDG uptake is typically seen in the oral pharynx, and salivary glands (s). The lymphoid tissue in the tonsils varies greatly in intensity. Moderate symmetric activity in the young adult shown here is normal. In the resting state laryngeal activity is minimal to none (l). **b** Mild diffuse thyroid uptake and enlargement is typical of autoimmune thyroid disease, usually Hashimoto's thyroiditis (*arrows*)

CT findings as a whole and are best presented as bullet points. Single focused phrases are helpful as opposed to a paragraph or long differential. Typically only actionable items are listed in the impression. A concise, short differential, and suggested next step are especially helpful when a precise diagnosis is not possible. If urgent or emergent findings are present direct communication and documentation of contact is required (Reiner et al. 2007; Agress et al. 2008).

In the current environment PET/CT reports are also read by consulting and referring physicians, payers, regulators, and often the patients. Well-focused reports avoid vague descriptive phrases and communicate clearly whether the interpreter thinks that an imaging

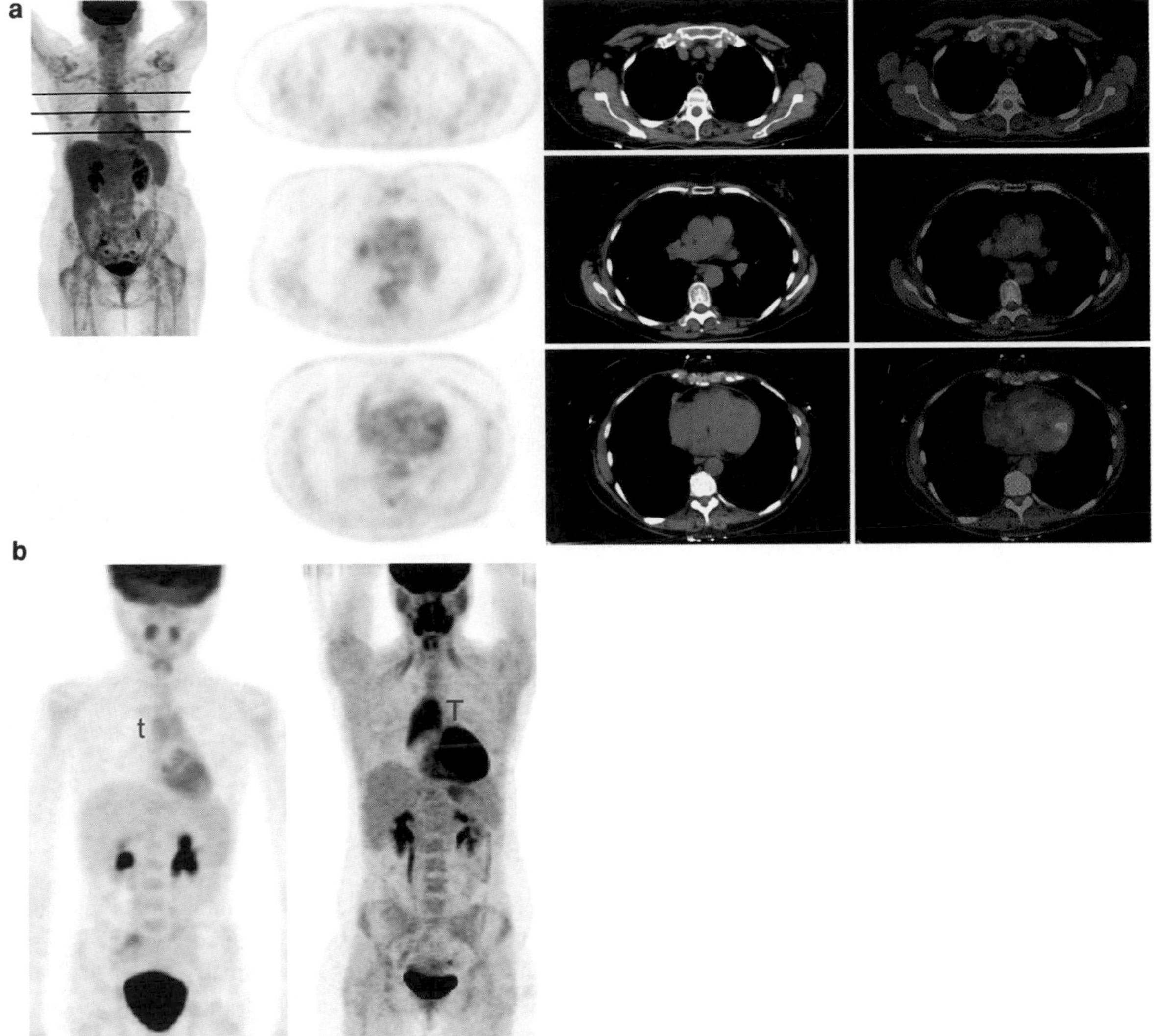

Fig. 9 **a** Normal chest. There is typically minimal activity in the lungs with mild FDG uptake in both hila. Mild residual activity is seen within the circulating blood at 60 min. *Left* ventricular uptake varies greatly from mild to intense activity. **b** Normal thymic uptake in an 8-year-old boy is mild (t) versus intense thymic rebound observed in this 27-year-old man (T). **c** FDG uptake within the breasts depends on the density of glandular tissue and the presence of estrogen stimulation. There is typically mild uptake in the breasts of a premenopausal (*left*) versus minimal uptake in a postmenopausal woman (*center*). Intense FDG uptake is observed in the breastfeeding women (*right*)

finding is likely benign or malignant. To the referring physician the most important part of a PET/CT report is the answer to the clinical question that prompted the referral for scanning. The interpretation and reporting of PET/CT scans in cancer patients requires careful integration of both clinical information and imaging findings to render a comprehensive evaluation that ends in a concise, focused impression (Coleman et al. 2010).

5 Normal FDG Distribution

The biodistribution of FDG reflects the utilization of glucose by the tissues and organs throughout the body. Identifying abnormal FDG tracer uptake requires a thorough knowledge of the normal and physiologic variant activity seen on PET/CT scans.

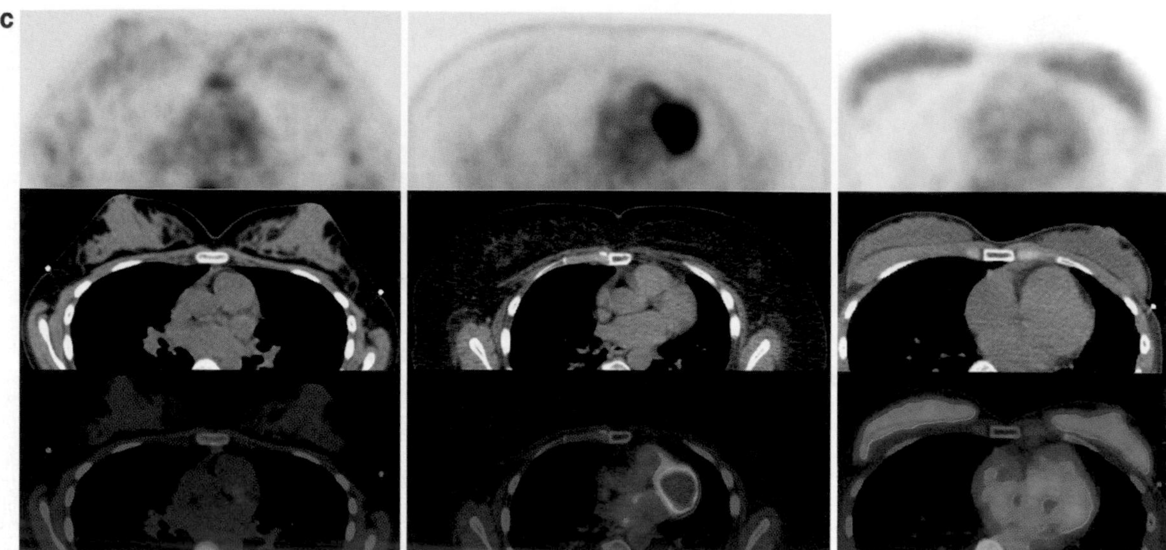

Fig. 9 (Continued)

Determining whether the level of FDG accumulation in a focal lesion, tissue, or organ is abnormally increased is aided by comparison with activity seen in normal reference sites, usually the mediastinal blood pool, liver, and cerebellum. When not diseased these reference sites provide reliable sources of intra-subject comparison and interval scan variation.

5.1 Head and Neck

The brain is an obligate user of glucose regardless of substrate availability and the total uptake in the brain is approximately 6 % of the injected dose (Ak et al. 2000). The cerebral cortex and basal ganglia exhibit the highest activity. The ocular muscles often have intense uptake due to active eye movements during the incubation period. Mild to moderate FDG uptake occurs in the lingual and palatine tonsils and at the base of the tongue because of the lymphatic tissue in Waldeyer's ring (Goerres et al. 2002). Tonsillar uptake can be intense in children and adolescents. The salivary glands commonly show mild FDG activity. Muscles in the oropharynx and hypopharynx may demonstrate symmetrical physiological FDG uptake, especially the muscles of the floor of the mouth (Nakamoto et al. 2005) (Fig. 8a). Normally, FDG uptake in the thyroid gland is low or absent, but diffuse uptake occurs in autoimmune thyroid disease, Hashimoto's thyroiditis, or less commonly Graves' disease (Karantanis et al. 2007) (Fig. 8b).

5.2 Chest

There is negligible activity within normal lung parenchyma. At 60 min only low-grade activity is seen within the blood of the mediastinal vascular structures. This mild uptake is usually accepted as a background reference level for characterizing abnormal FDG uptake elsewhere in the thorax. There can be normal mild FDG activity in the esophagus possibly due to swallowed saliva or smooth muscle activity. Esophagitis in the distal esophagus is also a common cause of tracer accumulation (Skehan et al. 2000).

Left ventricular myocardial uptake is highly variable even with appropriate fasting prior to FDG injection. In the fasting state the myocardium preferentially utilizes fatty acids for energy, but glucose still accounts for 30–40 % of the metabolic substrate. The left ventricle FDG uptake ranges from minimal to intense (Dilsizian et al. 2001) (Fig. 9a).

Moderate thymic uptake in a bat-winged configuration is commonly seen in children. This physiologic uptake of FDG in the thymus typically disappears in

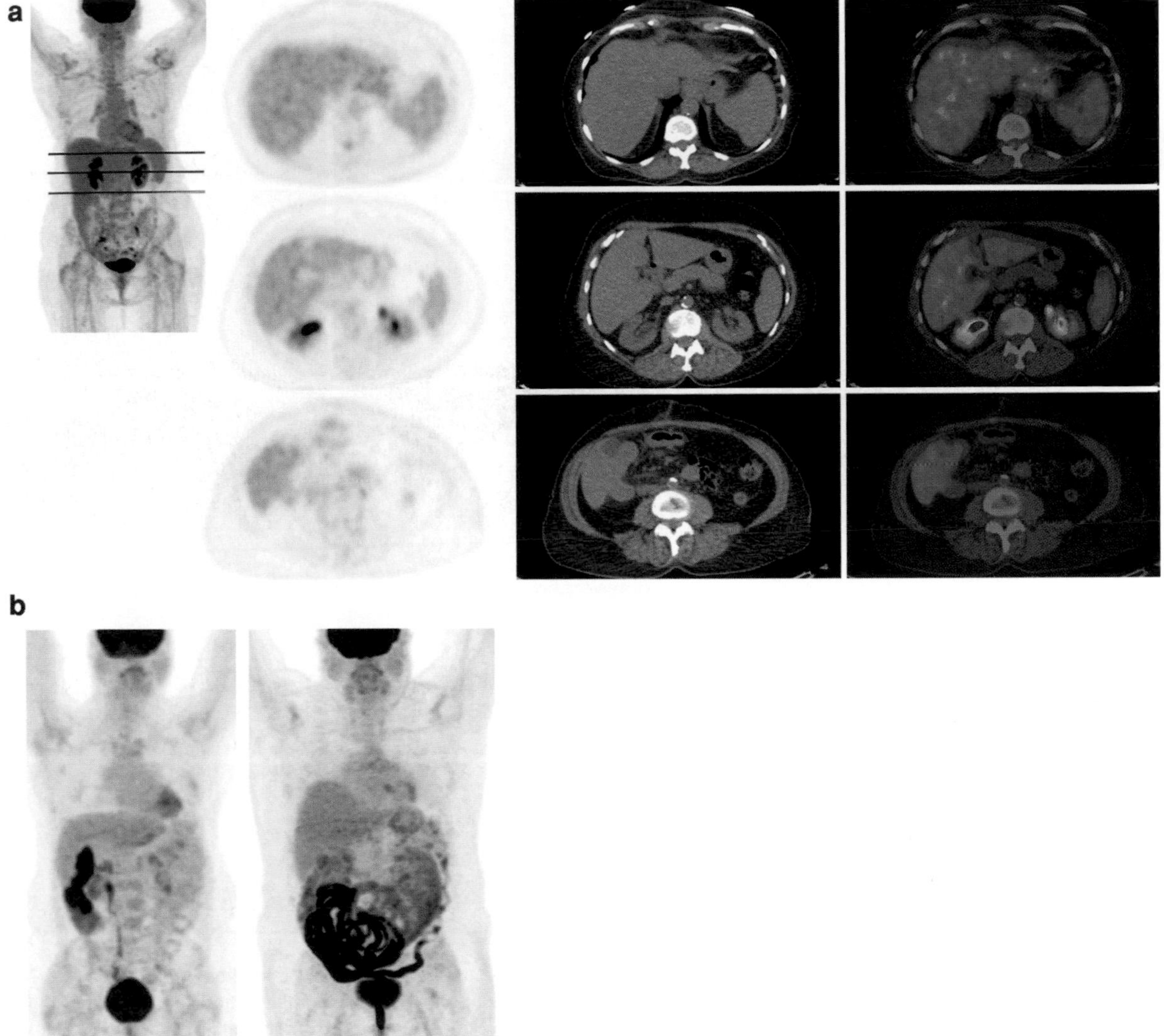

Fig. 10 **a** Normal abdomen. The liver has moderate heterogeneous FDG uptake, which is 10 % higher than normal splenic activity. FDG is rapidly extracted and excreted by normal renal parenchyma; with supine imaging the ureters may be visualized. **b** Normal gastrointestinal activity is minimal to mild. The *right* colon tends to have the greatest bowel uptake (*left*). Metformin significantly increases the FDG uptake of the colon and to lesser extent the small intestine. This increase is typically intense, diffuse, and continuous along the bowel (*right*)

adolescence with the involution of the thymus. However, a small focus of residual thymic tissue with FDG accumulation has been reported in adult patients. Following chemotherapy, reactivation of thymic FDG uptake is common in children and adolescents, often called "thymic rebound." In some adults after chemotherapy small thymic remnants in the anterior mediastinum can have moderate activity (Ferdinand et al. 2004; Brink et al. 2001) (Fig. 9b).

Variable uptake can be seen within glandular tissue of the breasts. Higher FDG uptake is seen in premenopausal women and those with dense breasts and on hormone replacement (Vranjesevic et al. 2003). The areolar complex also normally demonstrates FDG activity (El-Haddad et al. 2004). Very high uptake of FDG can be seen in the lactating breast due to intracellular trapping within the activated glandular tissue, which results in minimal FDG excretion into breast milk (Hicks et al. 2001) (Fig. 9c).

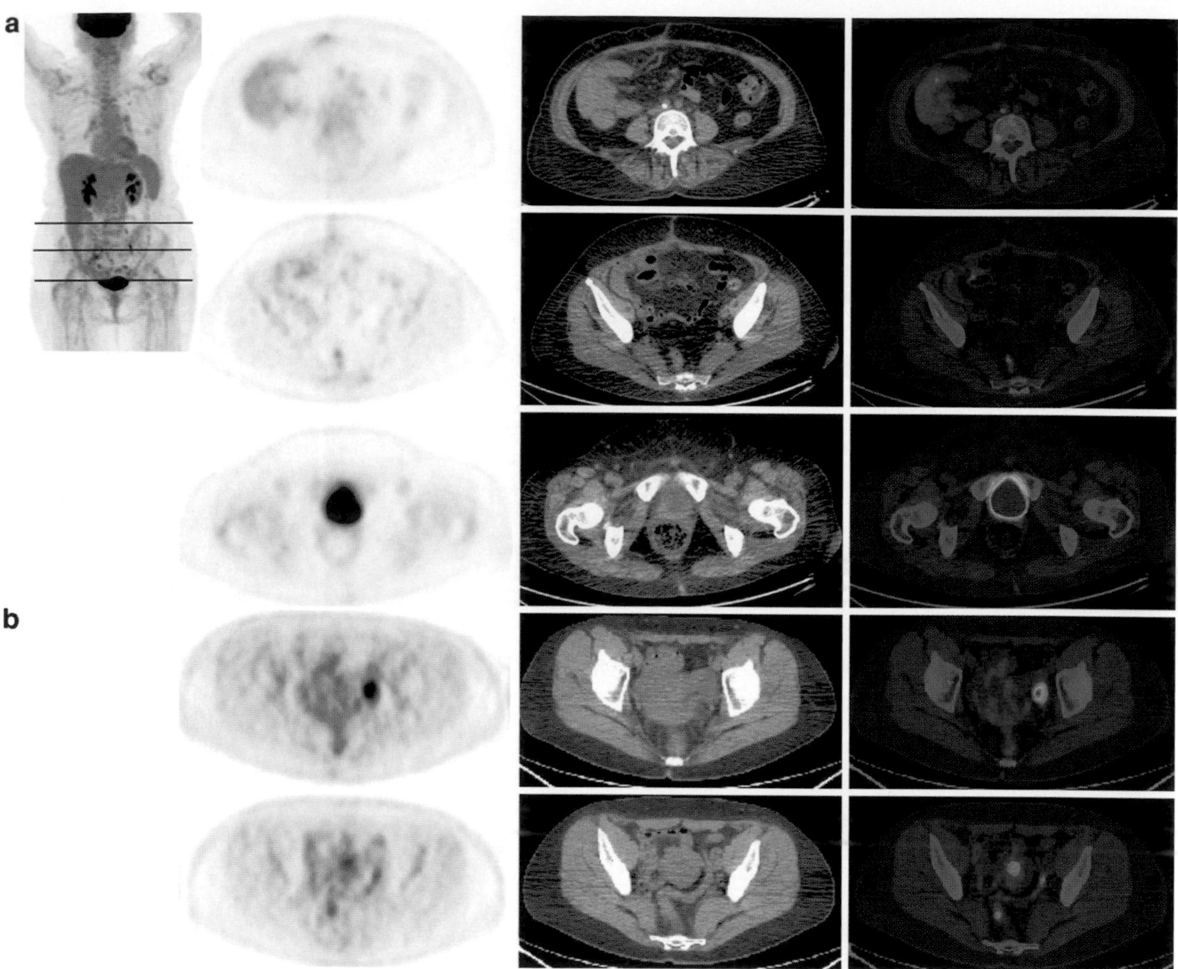

Fig. 11 **a** Normal pelvis. Mild increased activity is typically seen in the rectum. The intense increased activity in the ureters and bladder dominate the pelvis. **b** During mid-menstrual cycle, premenopausal woman will demonstrate intense FDG uptake in an ovary unilaterally. From mid-cycle through menses the endometrial lining will have mild to moderate FDG uptake. It is common to see both ovarian and endometrial activity synchronously

5.3 Abdomen/Gastrointestinal

The liver has moderate heterogeneous activity and is about 10 % more intense than normal splenic uptake. Bone marrow activity is similar to liver in patients in their teens and twenties declining slowly with age (Culverwell et al. 2011). Variable activity can be seen throughout the intestinal tract. The exact etiology of uptake is still unclear and is partly due to smooth muscle activity associated with peristalsis, bacterial uptake, gastrointestinal lymphoid tissue, and metabolically active mucosa (Kostakoglu et al. 2003). The stomach wall activity is usually faintly seen but normal uptake can also be intense. Small bowel activity is usually mild and heterogeneous, whereas large bowel activity is more commonly moderate in a multifocal, segmental, or diffuse distribution (Tatlidil et al. 2002; Israel et al. 2005) (Fig. 10a). Diffuse intense FDG uptake throughout the colon is frequently seen in diabetic patients treated with metformin (Gontier et al. 2008; Ozülker et al. 2010) (Fig. 10b).

5.4 Pelvis/Genitourinary

FDG undergoes glomerular filtration similar to glucose, but cannot be reabsorbed by the proximal tubular cells due the Fluorine-18 replacing the hydroxyl group.

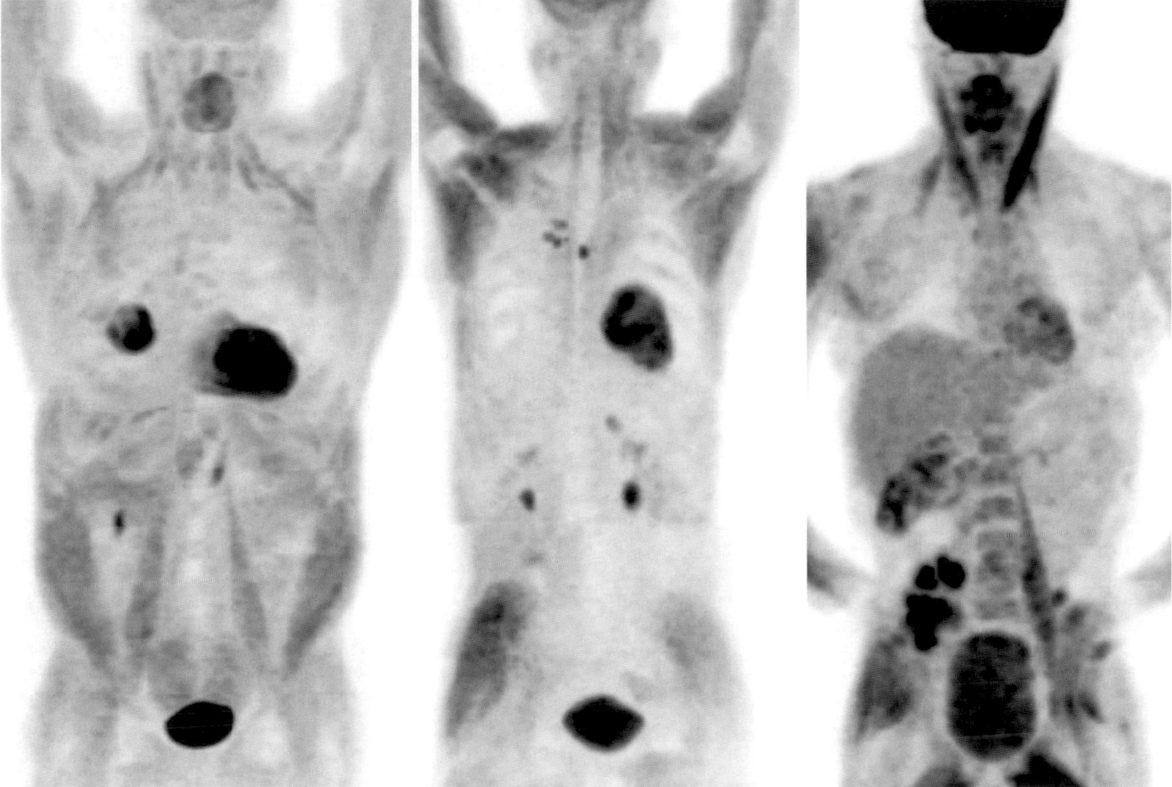

Fig. 12 Exogenous insulin administration in diabetic patients within 4 h of FDG PET imaging typically produces diffuse skeletal and cardiac muscle uptake (*left*). Exercise prior to PET/CT imaging produces regional muscle uptake. This patient shows shoulder and pelvic girdle muscle uptake (*center*). Increased muscle tension produces single muscle uptake due to activation. The sternocleidomastoid muscles commonly have elevated FDG uptake in head and neck cancer patients (*right*)

FDG is readily excreted in the urine, which is the principal route of FDG clearance from the body. High levels of FDG activity are routinely seen in the renal collecting system, ureters, and urinary bladder. Adequate hydration and frequent voiding should be encouraged to enhance FDG excretion and lower the patient's absorbed radiation dose. Urine stasis within redundant ureter, bladder diverticula, and in the prostatic urethra should not be misinterpreted as pathological findings (El-Haddad et al. 2004; Kamel et al. 2006) (Fig. 11a).

Physiological endometrial and ovarian activity varies cyclically in premenopausal women, peaking during the ovulatory and menstrual phases. Menstrual history should be documented in all premenopausal women to provide corroborative clinical information (Lerman et al. 2004). Symmetric uptake within the testes of variable intensity is common, especially in younger men (Kitajima et al. 2007) (Fig. 11b).

5.5 Extremities/Musculoskeletal

Exercise should be avoided for 24 h prior to scanning to avoid increased skeletal muscle uptake. The muscles of the neck and forearms often have increased activity due to increased muscle tension hanging on to the chair. In patients with COPD, intercostal and sternocleidomastoid muscle uptake can be seen due to excessive use to facilitate respiration (El-Haddad et al. 2004). Increased muscle tension often causes increased FDG uptake in the longus coli and sternocleidomastoid muscles of head and neck cancer patients following therapy (Zhuang et al. 2004) (Fig. 12).

References

ACR practice guideline for performing FDG-PET/CT in oncology. http://www.acr.org/SecondaryMainMenuCategories/quality_safety/guidelines/nuc_med/fdg_pet_ct.aspx. Accessed 10 Jan 2012

Agress H Jr, Wong TZ, Shreve P (2008) Interpretation and reporting of positron emission tomography-computed tomographic scans. Semin Ultrasound CT MR 29(4):283–90

Ak I, Stokkel MP, Pauwels EK (2000) Positron emission tomography with 2-[18F]fluoro-2-deoxy-D-glucose in oncology. Part II. The clinical value in detecting and staging primary tumours. J Cancer Res Clin Oncol 126(10):560–74

Brink I, Reinhardt MJ, Hoegerle S, Altehoefer C, Moser E, Nitzsche EU (2001) Increased metabolic activity in the thymus gland studied with 18F-FDG PET: age dependency and frequency after chemotherapy. J Nucl Med 42(4):591–5

CMS released Transmittals R108 NCD; R1833 CP rescinding transmittals R106 NCD and R1817 CP. http://www.cms.gov/transmittals/downloads/R108NCD.pdf. Accessed 10 Jan 2012

Coleman RE, Hillner BE, Shields AF et al (2010) PET and PET/CT reports: observations from the National Oncologic PET Registry. J Nucl Med 51:158–163

Culverwell AD, Scarsbrook AF, Chowdhury FU (2011) False--positive uptake on 2-[^{18}F]-fluoro-2-deoxy-D-glucose (FDG) positron-emission tomography/computed tomography (PET/CT) in oncological imaging. Clin Radiol 66(4):366–82

Dilsizian V, Bacharach SL, Khin MM, Smith MF (2001) Fluorine-18-deoxyglucose SPECT and coincidence imaging for myocardial viability: clinical and technologic issues. J Nucl Cardiol 8(1):75–88

El-Haddad G, Alavi A, Mavi A, Bural G, Zhuang H (2004) Normal variants in [18F]-fluorodeoxyglucose PET imaging. Radiol Clin North Am 42(6):1063–81

Ferdinand B, Gupta P, Kramer EL (2004) Spectrum of thymic uptake at 18F-FDG PET. Radiographics 24(6):1611–6

Goerres GW, Von Schulthess GK, Hany TF (2002) Positron emission tomography and PET/CT of the head and neck: FDG uptake in normal anatomy, in benign lesions, and in changes resulting from treatment. AJR Am J Roentgenol 179(5):1337–43

Gontier E, Fourme E, Wartski M, Blondet C, Bonardel G, Le Stanc E, Mantzarides M, Foehrenbach H, Pecking AP, Alberini JL (2008) High and typical 18F-FDG bowel uptake in patients treated with metformin. Eur J Nucl Med Mol Imaging 35(1):95–9

Hicks RJ, Binns D, Stabin MG (2001) Pattern of uptake and excretion of (18)F-FDG in the lactating breast. J Nucl Med 42(8):1238–42

Israel O, Yefremov N, Bar-Shalom R, Kagana O, Frenkel A, Keidar Z, Fischer D (2005) PET/CT detection of unexpected gastrointestinal foci of 18F-FDG uptake: incidence, localization patterns, and clinical significance. J Nucl Med 46(5):758–62

Kamel EM, Jichlinski P, Prior JO, Meuwly JY, Delaloye JF, Vaucher L, Malterre J, Castaldo S, Leisinger HJ, Delaloye AB (2006) Forced diuresis improves the diagnostic accuracy of 18F-FDG PET in abdominopelvic malignancies. J Nucl Med 47(11):1803–7

Karantanis D, Bogsrud TV, Wiseman GA, Mullan BP, Subramaniam RM, Nathan MA, Peller PJ, Bahn RS, Lowe VJ (2007) Clinical significance of diffusely increased 18F-FDG uptake in the thyroid gland. J Nucl Med 48(6):896–901

Kitajima K, Nakamoto Y, Senda M, Onishi Y, Okizuka H, Sugimura K (2007) Normal uptake of 18F-FDG in the testis: an assessment by PET/CT. Ann Nucl Med 21(7):405–10

Kostakoglu L, Agress H Jr, Goldsmith SJ (2003) Clinical role of FDG PET in evaluation of cancer patients. Radiographics 23(2):315–40

Lerman H, Metser U, Grisaru D, Fishman A, Lievshitz G, Even-Sapir E (2004) Normal and abnormal 18F-FDG endometrial and ovarian uptake in pre- and postmenopausal patients: assessment by PET/CT. J Nucl Med 45(2):266–71

Nakamoto Y, Tatsumi M, Hammoud D, Cohade C, Osman MM, Wahl RL (2005) Normal FDG distribution patterns in the head and neck: PET/CT evaluation. Radiology 234(3):879–85

Ozülker T, Ozülker F, Mert M, Ozpaçaci T (2010) Clearance of the high intestinal (18)F-FDG uptake associated with metformin after stopping the drug. Eur J Nucl Med Mol Imaging 37(5):1011–7

Reiner BI, Knight N, Siegel EL (2007) Radiology reporting, past, present, and future: the radiologist's perspective. J Am Coll Radiol 4:313–319

Skehan SJ, Brown AL, Thompson M, Young JE, Coates G, Nahmias C (2000) Imaging features of primary and recurrent esophageal cancer at FDG PET. Radiographics 20(3):713–23

SNM PET pros, elements of PET/CT reporting. http://www.snm.org/docs/PET_PROS/ElementsofPETCTReporting.pdf. Accessed 10 Jan 2012

Tatlidil R, Jadvar H, Bading JR, Conti PS (2002) Incidental colonic fluorodeoxyglucose uptake: correlation with colonoscopic and histopathologic findings. Radiology 224(3):783–7

Townsend DW (2008) Combined positron emission tomography-computed tomography: the historical perspective. Semin Ultrasound CT MR 29(4):232–5

Vranjesevic D, Schiepers C, Silverman DH, Quon A, Villalpando J, Dahlbom M, Phelps ME, Czernin J (2003) Relationship between 18F-FDG uptake and breast density in women with normal breast tissue. J Nucl Med 44(8):1238–42

Zhuang H, Kumar R, Mandel S, Alavi A (2004) Investigation of thyroid, head, and neck cancers with PET. Radiol Clin North Am 42(6):1101–11

Part II

Oncologic Applications

Central Nervous System

Jeffrey A. Miller and Terence Z. Wong

Contents

J. A. Miller · T. Z. Wong (✉)
Division of Nuclear Medicine,
Department of Radiology,
Duke University Medical Center,
Box 3949 Durham, NC 27710, USA
e-mail: wong0015@mc.duke.edu

Abstract

FDG-PET imaging has a defined role in the management of primary brain tumors. In contrast to other tumors, the primary role of FDG-PET imaging is to identify high-grade tumor. This task is complicated by the high background glucose metabolism present in normal cerebral cortex and gray matter structures. In general, high-grade brain neoplasms have FDG accumulation similar to cortical gray matter, while low-grade tumors have uptake more similar to white matter. As a consequence, accurate anatomic localization (preferably MRI) is necessary to identify areas of suspected tumor, so that corresponding FDG uptake within the abnormality can be evaluated. Tumor grade assessment by FDG-PET has prognostic implications for initial evaluation of brain tumor patients, and can be useful for evaluating patients for high-grade tumor recurrence following therapy. Other PET tracers under investigation will potentially have an increasingly important role as new treatment strategies are developed to manage primary brain tumors.

1 Keypoints

Like many other soft tissue tumors, malignant brain tumors demonstrate increased glucose metabolism that is reflected on FDG-PET imaging. The high background glucose metabolism of normal gray matter presents unique challenges in identifying and interpreting potential abnormalities. Accurate evaluation of brain tumors requires the registration of anatomic and FDG-PET images. FDG-PET imaging is useful for

P. Peller et al. (eds.), *PET-CT and PET-MRI in Oncology*, Medical Radiology. Diagnostic Imaging,
DOI: 10.1007/174_2011_431,

characterizing primary brain tumors with respect to both tumor grade and prognosis. Metabolic activity within a heterogeneous glioma can be used to identify the most active targets for stereotactic biopsy and thereby improve diagnostic accuracy of such procedures. FDG-PET may also be used to evaluate residual or recurrent tumor following therapy and, if necessary, define appropriate targets for biopsy. Hypermetabolic activity in a previously low-grade malignancy can provide sentinel information about degeneration into high-grade malignancy. Current limitations of FDG-PET include lack of sensitivity (compared to contrast-enhanced MRI) for detecting intracranial metastases, limited detection of low-grade primary brain tumors and occasional difficulty in distinguishing radiation necrosis from recurrent high-grade tumor. Although this chapter has emphasized the applications of FDG-PET for the evaluation of primary brain tumors, other tracers, in particular those, which take advantage of the relatively long half-life of ^{18}F, are potentially useful in certain clinical situations and may become more widely available for clinical use.

2 Introduction

Primary brain tumors are relatively uncommon malignancies with an annual worldwide incidence of between 3.7 per 100,000 men and 2.6 per 100,000 women (Bondy et al. 2008). An estimated 22,070 new cases of malignant primary central nervous system (CNS) tumors were diagnosed in the United States in 2009 (Jemal et al. 2009). In adults, metastatic tumors are much more common than primary CNS lesions. More than 100,000 people die every year with symptoms of intracranial metastases, the majority due to lung, breast and melanoma primary malignancies. In the pediatric population, primary brain tumors are the second most common childhood malignancy. CNS tumors are the second leading cause of cancer death (following leukemia) for men between the ages of 20 and 39 years and the fifth leading cause of cancer deaths in women in this age group (Jemal et al. 2009). Most primary brain tumors occur in the elderly and these tend to be more aggressive at initial presentation (Bondy et al. 2008). As with other cancers, there has been an overall decrease in death rates in the United States due to CNS tumors from 1990 to 2005 (Jemal et al. 2009).

2.1 Primary Brain Tumors

Brain tumor classification is derived from cell of origin, although many malignancies express heterogeneous histological features. The majority of central nervous system tumors are gliomas. The World Health Organization (WHO) recognizes three main types of gliomas: astrocytomas, oligodendrogliomas and mixed oligoastrocytomas. Tumor grade is based on the most malignant region of a tumor and is broadly divided into low-grade (WHO grades I and II) and high-grade (WHO grades III and IV) malignancies.

Low-grade tumors include pilocytic astrocytomas (grade I), astrocytomas (grade II) and oligodendrogliomas (grade II). Low-grade tumors are well-differentiated and lack the high cellularity, pleomorphism, mitosis, vascular endothelial proliferation and necrosis that characterize high-grade tumors (Daumas-Duport et al. 1988). These tumors are found more frequently in younger patients and are associated with longer median survival times compared to high-grade malignancies. For example, astrocytomas and oligodendrogliomas have 37 and 70% five year survival rates, respectively. However, with the exception of pilocytic astrocytomas, these tumors will progress to higher grade variants and are frequently fatal. Pilocytic astrocytomas, which are found most commonly in children and young adults, grow slowly, stabilize spontaneously and rarely undergo malignant transformation. In most cases, resectable pilocytic astrocytomas are cured following surgery and have an 80% twenty-year survival rate.

High-grade tumors include anaplastic astrocytomas (grade III), anaplastic oligodendrogliomas (grade III) and glioblastoma multiforme (grade IV). Of these, glioblastoma multiforme is the most frequent and aggressive subtype, accounting for 45–50% of all gliomas. These tumors have a male predominance with a mean age at onset of 61 years. They are associated with the poorest prognosis and a median survival of less than 1 year. Fewer than 3% of glioblastoma patients are alive after 5 years, with older age and tumor necrosis being the most significant and consistent prognostic factors of poorer outcome (Nelson et al. 1983; Ohgaki 2009). Anaplastic tumors occur in younger patients (mean age at onset of 40 years) and carry a median survival of 2–3 years.

High-grade gliomas may be further categorized as primary or secondary malignant astrocytomas

(Behin et al. 2003). Primary malignant astrocytomas are found in older patients without a preceding low-grade tumor. Secondary malignant astrocytomas result from the degeneration of low-grade gliomas and are usually found in younger patients.

Numerous biological and environmental factors have been implicated in the development of primary brain tumors and in the progression from low- to high-grade gliomas. Genetic causes of brain tumors, apart from well-known syndromes such as neurofibrosis and tuberous sclerosis, are not yet clarified. However, polymorphisms in DNA repair, carcinogen metabolism and immune function genes may increase inherited glioma risk (Bondy et al. 2008). Established risk factors for the development of intracranial gliomas include high-dose radiation exposure, hereditary syndromes, male sex, increasing age and, possibly, seizure history. Allergies, viruses, mutagen sensitivity and family history are all probable risk factors without precise associations (Bondy et al. 2008).

2.2 The Role of Positron Emission Tomography Imaging (PET)

Since its introduction in the 1990s, PET imaging has played a significant and increasing clinical role in the diagnosis and management of primary brain tumors. Current routine clinical applications include grading and evaluating prognoses based on metabolic tumor characteristics, targeting biopsy sites, defining target volumes for radiotherapy, assessing response to treatment and identifying recurrent disease.

PET imaging of brain tumors has become the standard of care at many institutions in the United States and is now recognized as indication for routine reimbursement by the Centers for Medicare and Medicaid Services.

2.2.1 Complementary Imaging Modalities

Anatomic imaging modalities such as magnetic resonance imaging (MRI) and computed tomography (CT) provide important information in the diagnosis and effects of therapy in patients with brain tumors. MR imaging, in particular, provides high spatial resolution, exceptional soft tissue contrast and excellent delineation of gray and white matter structures. MRI is also important in evaluating mass effect, edema, hemorrhage, increased intracranial pressure and necrosis that may accompany both primary and metastatic brain tumors. For these reasons, MRI has become the primary imaging modality for assessing suspected brain lesions.

Enhancement of tumors following intravenous contrast administration on both MRI and CT reflect disruption of the blood–brain barrier. High-grade tumors typically demonstrate ring-like contrast enhancement surrounding an area of central necrosis following gadolinium administration, whereas low-grade tumors have minimal enhancement. Low-grade tumors may be further distinguished by increased signal on T2-weighted images. Enlarging tumor size and increasing or new contrast enhancement usually establishes the diagnosis of disease progression. However, these patterns have limited utility in clinical practice, especially following surgical or radiation therapy, and are often more suggestive than definitive. Treatment-induced changes, especially radiation necrosis, may be difficult to distinguish from recurrent tumor (Alexiou et al. 2009).

2.2.2 Treatment Options

Treatment of high-grade gliomas typically consists of early, aggressive multimodality therapy that includes surgery, radiation therapy and chemotherapy (Croteau and Mikkelsen 2001; Burton and Prados 2000). Maximal resection to reduce the tumor burden is the first step before initiation of other adjuvant therapies. This is typically followed by external beam radiation therapy using conventional dosage and fractionation; stereotactic radiosurgery is used in selected cases. No curative chemotherapy exists for high-grade gliomas; however, standard cytotoxic agents, such as temozolomide alone or combined with 13-cis-retinoic acid, may be used in patients with relatively good prognostic factors (Croteau and Mikkelsen 2001). Anaplastic oligodendrogliomas are managed similarly in terms of surgery and radiation therapy but appear to respond to single agent or combination chemotherapy.

When possible, low-grade gliomas, including pilocytic astrocytomas, oligodendrogliomas and mixed oligo-astrocytomas are also initially treated with gross total resection, which has shown to improve survival (Stieber 2001). Corticosteroids are used to manage edema and vasogenic effects with anticonvulsants given prophylactically for seizures. Adjuvant radiotherapy is recommended for patients with incompletely resected grade II tumors or for patients older than age 40 regardless of extent of resection.

Treatment of intracranial metastatic disease has traditionally been whole-brain radiation due to the frequent presence of multiple lesions. For patients with solitary metastases, surgery with whole-brain radiation has demonstrated a survival advantage (Vecht et al. 1993). Stereotactic radiosurgery has emerged as an alternative therapy to treat patients with surgically inaccessible or multiple lesions. High-dose radiation is delivered to a defined target in a single treatment session. The greatest benefit of stereotactic radiosurgery is found in younger patients with two to four brain metastases (Kaal et al. 2005).

2.3 PET Imaging of Brain Tumors

Relatively uniform radiographic attenuation characteristics of the tissues surrounding the brain as well as immobilization of the brain in the skull provide a unique environment for PET imaging. PET images of the brain may be accurately registered with other imaging modalities such as computed tomography (CT) or magnetic resonance imaging (MRI).

Currently, the most widely used and readily available radiopharmaceutical for PET imaging is 2-[18F]-fluoro-2-deoxy-D-glucose (FDG). The long half-life (110 min), wide availability and use in evaluating other cancers currently makes FDG the most important agent for imaging primary brain tumors.

2.3.1 FDG Localization and Glucose Metabolism

As a glucose analog, FDG is transported across the blood–brain barrier into metabolically active cells where, like glucose, it is phosphorylated. However, once phosphorylated, no further metabolization occurs and FDG accumulates intracellularly at a rate proportional to glucose utilization. Since the brain utilizes glucose almost exclusively to meet its metabolic energy requirements, this results in very high background accumulation of FDG in normal brain tissues, particularly in gray matter structures such as the cerebral cortex and basal ganglia. There is an approximately 2.5–1 ratio of accumulation of FDG in the gray matter compared to white matter.

Since high-grade malignancies avidly accumulate FDG due to their high glucose metabolism and often have abnormal hypermetabolic activity similar to that of normal gray matter, detecting such lesions, especially if they are small, can be challenging. Even high-grade brain tumors may be less conspicuous in the brain than malignancies elsewhere in the body due high background activity in the normal brain. This difficulty may be partially overcome by adjusting acquisition parameters to obtain delayed images (Spence et al. 2004). In addition, other pathologies which are often present at the gray-white matter junction, such as infections and metastatic lesions, are often FDG-avid. Characterization and differentiation of these entities requires precise anatomical localization; correlation with CT or MRI anatomical imaging is necessary for accurate interpretation. This can now be done with commercially available software programs which electronically coregister anatomic images with three-dimensional FDG-PET data.

Low-grade tumors within deep white matter may be especially difficult to identify on FDG-PET images alone. Anatomic correlation is essential for evaluating and correctly localizing small tumors and for distinguishing the often heterogeneous elements of large tumors.

2.3.2 Scanning Protocols

Patients are instructed to have no caloric intake for at least 4 h before their FDG-PET examination; however, they are encouraged to drink water. A standard dose of FDG (10 mCi for adults; scaled weight-based doses for children) is injected and the patient is allowed to rest quietly in a dimly lit room for at least 30 min during the uptake phase. Auditory and visual stimulation is minimized to avoid extraneous cortical activation. At our institution, the scan is obtained using a single table position on a dedicated PET/CT scanner. An emission scan is obtained for 6 minutes using 3D acquisition, and a low-dose CT scan (140 kVp, 5 mAs) obtained for attenuation-correction. Iterative reconstruction (OSEM) is used to produce the final images: 25.6 cm FOV, 3.27 mm slice thickness, 128x128 pixel matrix. The PET images are electronically co-registered with axial MR images using commercially available software (MIM Software, Cleveland, OH). Coregistered axial PET/MR images, most commonly the postgadolidium T1-weighted data set, are used for interpretation. The original MRI series is independently reviewed to distinguish genuine areas of enhancement from regions of high intrinsic T1 signal (for example, in areas of hemorrhage following recent surgery). Coregistration with T2-weighted sequences is less commonly performed. Patients who are unable to complete an MRI examination undergo a combined contrast-enhanced CT and PET examination in which the two image sets are intrinsically coregistered.

2.4 Role of PET-MRI

2.4.1 Initial Diagnosis of Primary Brain Tumors

The majority of primary brain tumors are diagnosed using anatomic imaging, especially MRI. FDG-PET imaging may be used to differentiate common enhancing brain tumors such as high-grade gliomas, lymphomas and metastases. Based on semi-quantitative standardized uptake values (SUV), lymphomas demonstrate significantly higher metabolic activity than both high-grade gliomas and metastases (Kosaka et al. 2008). However, other studies have found substantial variation in FDG uptake across tumors and recommend visual assessment of activity when attempting to distinguish tumor type (Hustinx et al. 1999). FDG-PET has also been successfully used to distinguish lymphoma from non-malignant (presumably infectious) lesions in patients with AIDS (Hoffman et al. 1993).

An example of a patient with a new high-grade tumor, in this case a glioblastoma multiforme, is shown in Fig. 1. The patient underwent a prior resection of a left parietal GBM, followed by radiation and chemotherapy. No abnormal metabolic activity was present in or surrounding the resection cavity. However, a new left frontal mass with enhancement on MRI demonstrated intense metabolic activity on the coregistered PET study.

Evaluation of tumor grade, based on the correlation of FDG metabolism with histopathological characteristics of malignant lesions, is the major focus of PET imaging of primary brain tumors. FDG metabolism within gray and white matter structures serves as a convenient subjective reference with intrinsic comparison of the tumor to the (presumably) normal contralateral unaffected side. Low-grade tumors have FDG uptake similar to or below that of normal white matter; FDG accumulation in high-grade tumors approaches or exceeds that of normal gray matter. Qualitatively, tumor to white matter ratios of greater than 1.5 and tumor to gray matter ratios greater than 0.6 have been found to indicate high-grade tumors with a sensitivity of 94% and a specificity of 77% (Delbeke et al. 1995). An exception to this usual pattern is found with pilocytic astrocytomas which, despite their low grade, demonstrate avid FDG accumulation and significant enhancement on MRI.

A low-grade tumor, in this case a right optic chiasm glioma, is shown in Fig. 2. Regions of linear enhancement on MRI do not demonstrate significant metabolic activity on the coregistered FDG-PET study. Diffuse low-level metabolic activity throughout the mass does not exceed the intensity of white matter.

Grading may be further improved with dual time point imaging of tumors which renders high-grade tumors more conspicuous on delayed scanning following reduction in normal brain parenchymal uptake (Kim et al. 2010).

Borders of glial tumors are generally poorly defined, and the heterogeneous character of these lesions frequently results in geographic variation in tumor grade. The existence of rapidly growing focal high-grade regions result in an irregular contour of the tumor mass. Conventional anatomic imaging, such as MRI, is unable to distinguish high-grade features within the tumor. Even with MR or CT guidance, intrinsic tumor heterogeneity subjects stereotactic biopsy to significant sampling error and potential understaging. FDG-PET can map the metabolic pattern of heterogeneous tumors and aid in stereotactic biopsy targeting by identifying the subregions with the tumor with the greatest metabolic activity and, potentially, the highest grade (Hanson et al. 1991; Goldman et al. 1996; Pirotte et al. 2004). Such targeting may reduce the number of tissue samples required and improve the accuracy of the biopsy with respect to actual tumor grade.

2.4.2 Indicator of Prognosis

FDG metabolism carries prognostic significance for patients with primary brain tumors. Patients with hypermetabolic tumors have significantly shorter survival times than those with hypometabolic tumors and, within a subset of patients with high-grade gliomas, those with high tumor metabolism had significantly poorer prognosis than those with low tumor metabolism (Alavi et al. 1988; Patronas et al. 1985).

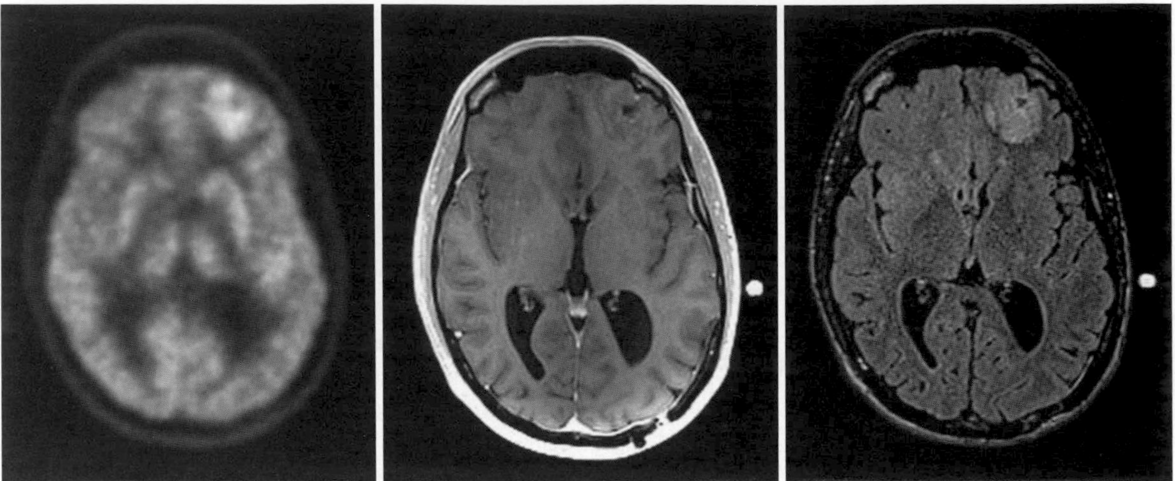

Fig. 1 A 44-year-old woman with a new enhancing mass in the left frontal lobe on MRI. Coregistered FDG-PET images demonstrates intense metabolic activity greater than cortical gray matter, compatible with high-grade tumor. The patient previously had a resected left parietal GBM followed by radiation and chemotherapy. There was no evidence of high-grade tumor recurrence at the resection site

Fig. 2 An 11-year-old boy with neurofibromatosis type I and a glioma of the right optic chiasm. The predominantly low T1-signal mass on MRI demonstrates areas of linear enhancement. Low-level metabolic activity within the mass on the coresgistered FDG-PET image does not exceed the intensity of adjacent white matter

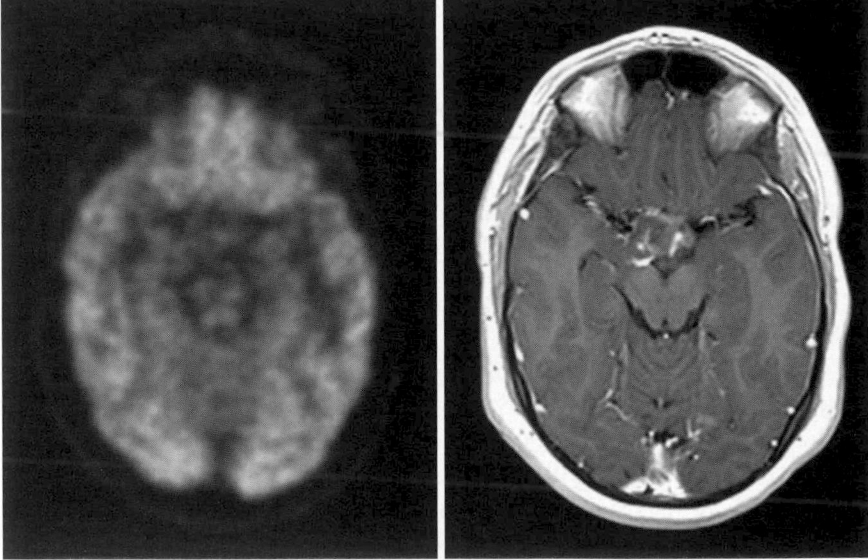

Inverse correlation of high tumor metabolism and survival is independent of the timing of PET scanning within the treatment cycle (Padma et al. 2003; Pardo et al. 2004).

FDG-PET findings carry prognostic significance for patients with low-grade brain tumors. The development of hypermetabolic features, defined as uptake greater than in white matter, in patients with low-grade gliomas, is correlated with malignant degeneration and poorer prognosis (De Witte et al. 1996; Minn 2005). The relationship between metabolic activity on the FDG-PET scan and biologic aggressiveness of the primary brain tumor, whether low or high-grade, is independent of prior therapy.

Figure 3 illustrates malignant degeneration of a previously diagnosed low-grade glioma in the left frontotemporal lobes treated with temozolomide. The FDG-PET scan revealed multiple areas of focal

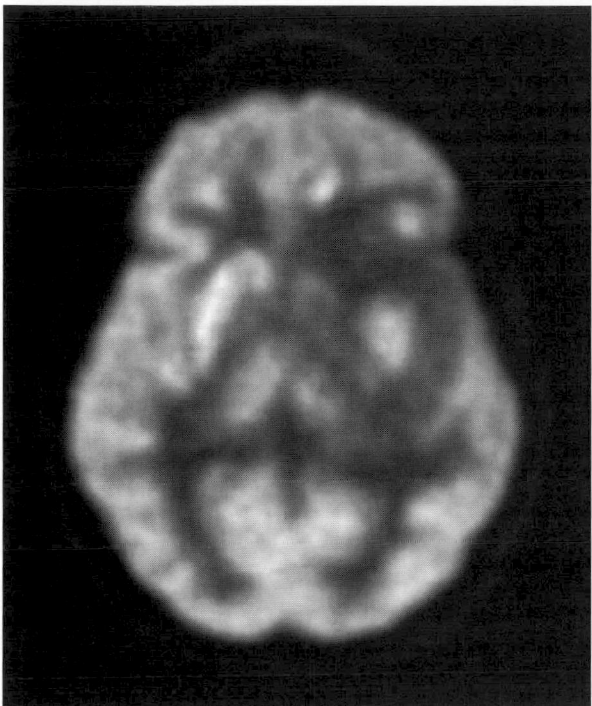
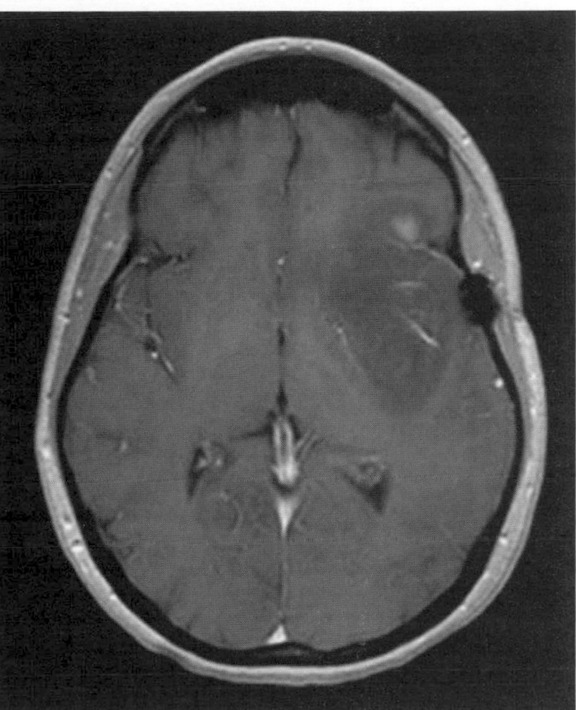

Fig. 3 A 36-year-old woman with a history of a low-grade glioma of the left frontotemporal lobes for which she received chemotherapy. A predominantly low-signal mass on T1-weighted MR images shows an enhancing nodule in the anterior aspect of the lesion which correlates to an intense focus of metabolic activity on the coregister FDG-PET image. Additional focal areas of metabolic activity were without MRI correlates. These findings are compatible with transformation from low- to high-grade glioma

metabolic activity at the tumor site, one of which corresponded to a new enhancing nodule on a coregistered MRI study, compatible with transformation to a high-grade glioma.

2.4.3 Targeted Radiotherapy

Radiation therapy plays an important role in the management of both low- and high-grade primary brain tumors. Because FDG is not dependent on the disruption of the blood–brain barrier for transport, there is the potential to better define the extent of brain lesions based on accumulation within tumor compared to contrast enhancement on MRI.

2.4.4 Evaluation Following Therapy

Abnormal enhancement on MRI may be seen with both residual brain tumors and postsurgically in altered brain tissues following resection. FDG-PET is relatively unaffected in evaluating the postsurgical patient for residual tumor since surgical changes do not inherently result in increased metabolic activity. Following surgery, contrast enhancement on MRI is not associated with hypermetabolic activity on the coregistered FDG-PET image in patients without residual tumor. Both high-grade residual tumors and early recurrence appear as abnormal hypermetabolic activity.

An example of a patient with a recurrent tumor is shown in Fig. 4. This patient had a surgical resection of a left parietal GBM, followed by radiation and chemotherapy. Nodular enhancement at the anterior margins of the coregistered MRI corresponds with activity similar to cortical gray matter on the FDG-PET scan, consistent with high-grade recurrence. In additional example high-grade tumor recurrence, in this case in a patient with an anaplastic astrocytoma and more subtle findings on MR imaging, is presented in Fig. 5.

In comparison, Fig. 6 is from a patient who had a surgical resection of a left fontal lobe GBM, with subsequent radiation and chemotherapy. A large left frontal lobe resection cavity is observed without focal

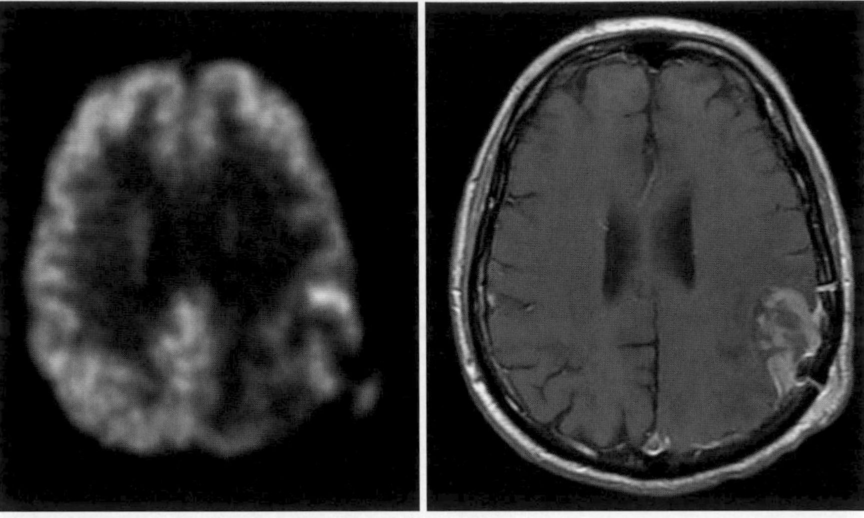

Fig. 4 A 75-year-old man with a history of a surgically resected left parietal GBM, and subsequent radiation and chemotherapy. Nodular enhancement at the anterior margins of the coregistered MRI corresponds with activity similar to cortical gray matter on the FDG-PET scan, consistent with high-grade recurrence

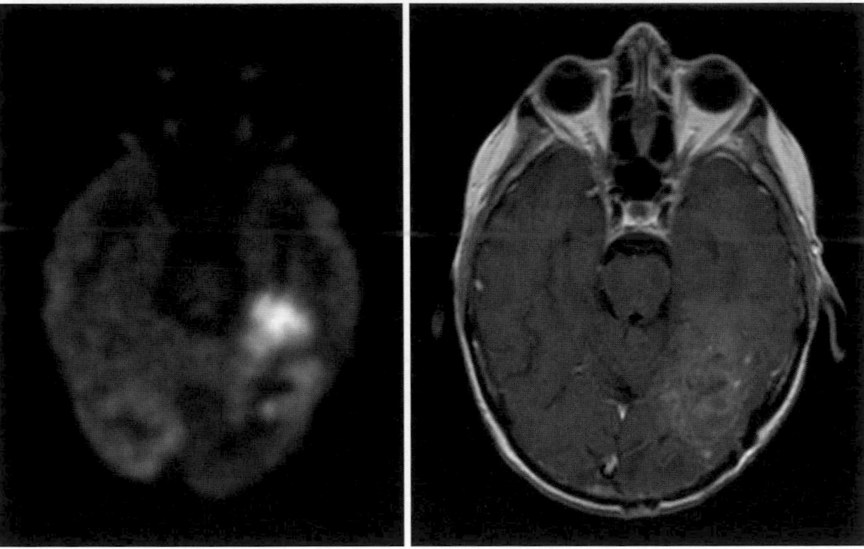

Fig. 5 A 67-year-old woman with a recurrent high-grade left occipital anaplastic astrocytoma following surgical resection, radiation and chemotherapy. There is minimal contrast enhancement on coregistered MRI but multiple areas of high FDG accumulation

nodular enhancement on the coregistered MRI and has no abnormal metabolic activity on the FDG-PET scan. Both imaging modalities demonstrate congruent lack of recurrent of high-grade tumor. An example of a patient with findings suspicious for high-grade tumor recurrence on MRI but without corresponding abnormalities on the FDG-PET scan is shown in Fig. 7. In this case, the patient had a treated anaplastic astrocytoma originating from a well-differentiated (grade II) astrocytoma. There is a nodular focus of enhancement present on MRI, whereas the FDG-PET scan shows a photopenic resection cavity without suspicious margins.

Radiation necrosis in the treated field following high-dose radiation therapy may present as abnormal enhancement on MRI (Di Chiro et al. 1988). This usually appears as moderate FDG activity intermediate between gray and white matter with a relatively uniform distribution that may be due to metabolically active macrophages that accumulate at the therapy site. However, occasionally nodular activity equal to or greater than gray matter may result in the inability to distinguish radiation necrosis from recurrent high-grade tumor. Radiation-induced changes in brain tissue at the therapy site require that potential recurrent lesions be evaluated with respect to local activity

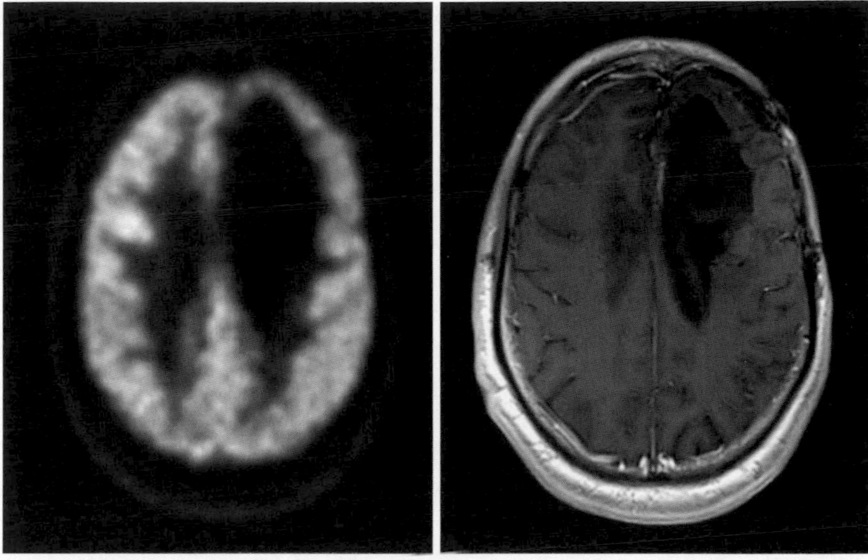

Fig. 6 A 24-year-old man with a history of surgically resected left frontal GBM, and subsequent radiation and chemotherapy. A large left frontal lobe resection cavity is without focal nodular enhancement on the coregisterd MRI and there are no areas of abnormally increased metabolic activity on the FDG-PET scan, compatible with absence of high-grade tumor recurrence

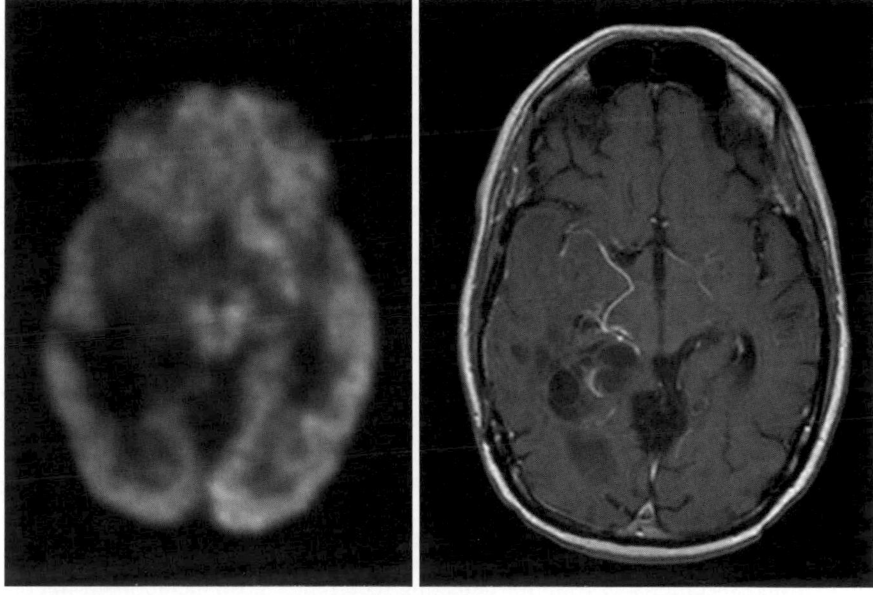

Fig. 7 A 49-year-old man with a history of a surgically resected anaplastic astrocytoma of the right temporal lobe originating from a well-differentiated (grade II) astrocytoma. A suspicious focus of enhancement is present on the coregistered MRI; no abnormality can be identified on the FDG-PET scan, which shows a photopenic resection cavity without elevated metabolic activity at the margins

and not against presumably more normal activity in the contralateral brain and correlated with anatomic information available from MRI. When such an approach is used the sensitivities and specificities of 96 and 77%, respectively, have been found in distinguishing radiation necrosis from tumor recurrence (Wang et al. 2006). The optimal time to perform FDG-PET studies following radiation therapy is not known but is probably not less than 6 weeks.

Examples of post-therapeutic radiation changes are shown in Figs. 8 and 9. Figure 8 shows the coregistered MRI and FDG-PET scans of a patient with a cerebellar-pontine angle anaplastic astrocytoma treated with radiation and chemotherapy. Both scans are without evidence for high-grade tumor. The FDG-PET scan further demonstrates decreased metabolic activity in the lesion compared to surrounding brain parenchyma, which also has less metabolic activity than tissue outside the radiation port. Radiation changes to the brain parenchyma surrounding a surgical resection cavity in a patient with a left frontal GBM is shown in Fig. 9. Diffuse FDG activity intermediate

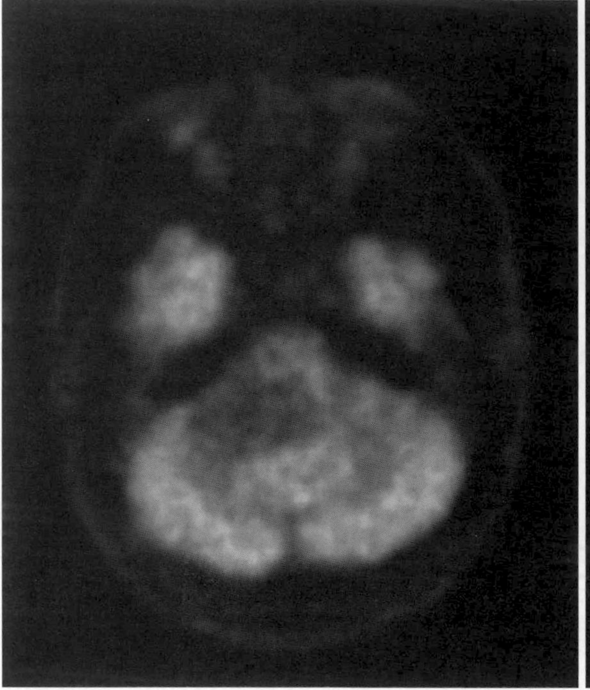
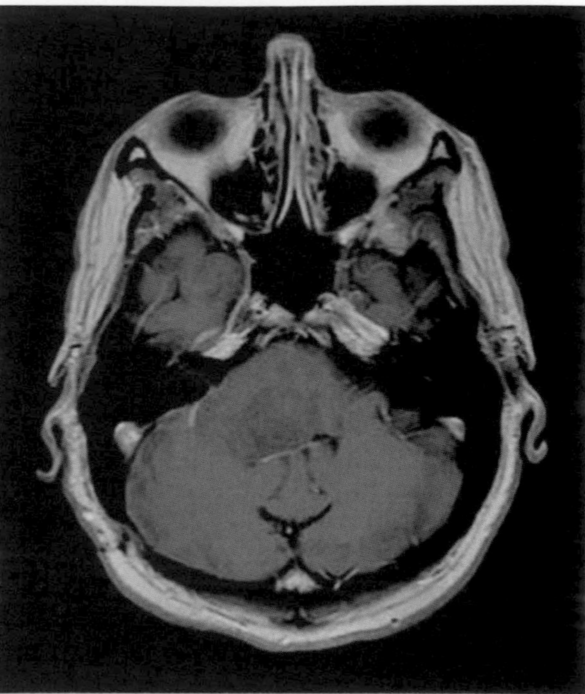

Fig. 8 A 38-year-old man with a cerebellar-pontine angle anaplastic astrocytoma treated with radiation and chemotherapy. Both the coregistered MRI scan and PET scan are without evidence for high-grade tumor. The FDG-PET scan further demonstrates decreased metabolic activity in the lesion compared to surrounding brain parenchyma, which also has less metabolic activity than tissue outside the radiation port. These changes are compatible with radiation-induced effects to the lesion and adjacent structures

between gray and white matter should not be mistaken for high-grade tumor recurrence.

High FDG accumulation in enlarging areas of enhancement on MRI following surgery and radiation therapy are correlated with significantly poorer prognosis compared to patients without hypermetabolic findings (Barker et al. 1997). Following stereotactic radiosurgery, FDG-PET was found to have a sensitivity of 75% and specificity of 81% for detecting recurrent tumor versus radiation necrosis (Chao et al. 2001).

FDG metabolism can be altered in brain tumor patients receiving corticosteroids with decreased cerebral glucose metabolism, possibly due to steroid-induced hyperglycemia (Fulham et al. 1995). Patients with brain tumors have decreased glucose metabolism in the contralateral cortex, an effect that is more closely related to tumor size than to corticosteroid dose (Roelcke et al. 1998). However, metabolism within brain tumors is not affected by corticosteroid therapy, even following high-dose administration (Glantz et al. 1991).

2.4.5 Metastatic Brain Tumors

Metastatic tumors in the brain generally demonstrate metabolic activity similar to that of normal cortical gray matter. Metastases can be readily indentified on FDG-PET imaging when metabolism exceeded that of normal gray matter. However, mildly or moderately hypermetabolic intracranial metastases are difficult to identify due to the high baseline glucose metabolism in cortical brain tissues. In addition, hematogenous seeding has a propensity to develop at the cortical gray-white junction which makes these metastases difficult to distinguish from adjacent cerebral cortex. Cytotoxic edema, which frequently surrounds metastatic deposits, has relatively low FDG accumulation and resulting volume-averaging effects may further decrease the conspicuity of these lesions.

The addition of FDG brain scanning to routine whole-body imaging detects few clinically relevant lesions and is not recommended as a routine part of the metastatic evaluation of primary extracranial malignancies (Larcos and Maisey 1996).

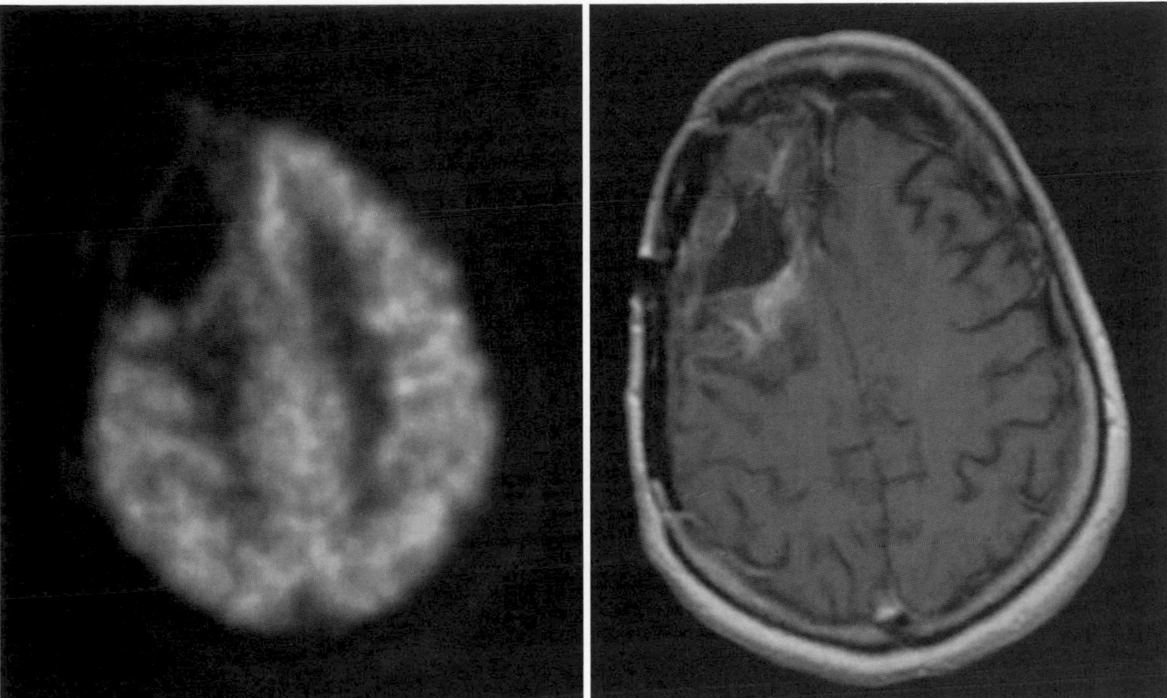

Fig. 9 A 29-year-old woman with a history of a surgically resected left frontal GBM who subsequently received radiation and chemotherapy. Diffuse enhancement is seen surrounding the resection cavity on coregistered MRI. Intermediate uptake between gray and white matter on the PET in areas of enhancement is compatible with post-therapeutic radiation changes. There is no evidence of high-grade tumor recurrence

2.5 Additional PET Radiopharmaceuticals

Although FDG is the most common PET imaging agent, other radiotracers have been used to study primary brain tumor pathology and to obtain important information about tumor physiology.

2.5.1 Amino Acid Analogues

Tumor growth and development is characterized by increased protein synthesis and, in turn, increased utilization of amino acids. Although amino acids may simply diffuse into cells, there are more than 20 membrane transport systems which are often overexpressed on tumor cell membranes (Vallabhajosula 2007). Radiolabeled amino acids, including ^{11}C-tyrosine and ^{11}C-methionine (MET), have been investigated as markers for brain tumor metabolism (Goldman et al. 1997; Jager et al. 2008; Singhal et al. 2008). Since background accumulation in normal brain tissue tends to be low, use of these agents results in excellent contrast between malignant lesions and surrounding structures with increased amino acid transport in malignant transformation mediated by type L amino acid carriers (Miyagawa et al. 1998). MET-PET is particularly promising for the evaluation of low-grade gliomas and oligodendrogliomas (Derlon et al. 2000; Ribom et al. 2001; Chung et al. 2002) as well as in defining areas of tumor with more malignant features and detecting early progression to a higher grade (Nariai et al. 2005). Reported sensitivity and specificity for the detection of tumor tissue using MET-PET has been as high as 87 and 89%, respectively (Kracht et al. 2004). Quantitative information derived from MET-PET studies performed to differentiate tumor recurrence from radiation necrosis have been used to guide further management of irradiated brain tumors (Terakawa et al. 2008). Although these ^{11}C-based radiotracers are more sensitive and specific for evaluation of primary brain tumors than FDG, their short half-lives (20 min) limit their use in routine clinical practice and require an onsite cyclotron for synthesis.

Longer lived ^{18}F-radiolabeled amino acids have been developed for tumor imaging (Laverman et al. 2002). Tumor uptake of radiolabeled amino acids based on ^{18}F-fluoroethyl-L-tyrosine (FET) and ^{18}F-fluoro-L-phenylalanine (FDOPA) is primarily based on carrier-mediated transport, and not protein synthesis (Vallabhajosula 2007). These agents have reported tumor uptake similar to ^{11}C-methionine (Weber et al. 2000; Becherer et al. 2003). The sensitivity of FET-PET imaging of high-grade gliomas has been as high as 93% with a negative predictive value of 89%; the authors of this study suggest that, due to the high negative predictive value of FET-PET, a conservative strategy of watchful waiting may be taken in patients with an MRI-demonstrated brain lesion of indeterminate significance and a negative FET study (Pichler et al. 2010). In a small study, combination imaging with MRI and FET-PET demonstrated a high predictive value for both low- and high-grade gliomas. A circumscribed growth pattern on MRI with low or normal FET uptake on PET was associated with low-grade tumors while a diffuse growth pattern and elevated FET uptake indicated high risk for high-grade glioma (Floeth et al. 2008). FET-PET is a robust imaging technique for patient receiving radiation therapy with a sensitivity of 100% and a specificity of 92.3% compared to 93.5 and 50% sensitivity and specificity, respectively, for MRI (Rachinger et al. 2005). When focal and high ^{18}F-FET uptake is considered suggestive of tumor recurrence, FET-PET was found to have 100% accuracy in distinguishing recurrent tumor from benign, radiation-induced changes (Pöpperl et al. 2004). Low background uptake also makes FET-PET useful both in delineating tumor extent to guide biopsy and in treatment planning (Pauleit et al. 2009).

^{18}F-FDOPA has demonstrated greater sensitivity and specificity, and is more accurate than FDG-PET, in detecting recurrent tumors, particularly recurrent low-grade gliomas that are usually not visualized on FDG imaging (Chen et al. 2006). The high contrast between tumor and normal brain tissue in PET scans using ^{18}F-FDOPA results in excellent visualization of both high- and low-grade lesions. In a small, prospective comparison for FDOPA, FLT and FDG, FDOPA was found to be superior for the visualization of primary and recurrent low-grade gliomas (Tripathi et al. 2009).

2.5.2 Nucleotide Metabolism

Radiolabeled thymidine analogues provide a measure of DNA synthesis and cell proliferation, ^{18}F-thymidine (FLT), an analogue substrate of thymidine carried by specific nucleoside transporters from the blood pool into brain tissue, is used to monitor cell proliferation at the molecular level. Once phosphorylated, FLT phosphates are impermeable to the cell membrane and are metabolically trapped inside cells (Vallabhajosula 2007). Since there is limited activity in normal brain tissue, brain tumors are visualized with high contrast, resulting in a high tumor-to-normal tissue ratio. In addition, uptake of ^{18}F-FLT in tumors correlates with Ki-67, a common proliferative index used in vivo, and provides a means of differentiating low- and high-grade tumors as well as planning and monitoring response to treatment (Choi et al. 2005; Saga et al. 2006; Salskov et al. 2007). Kinetic analysis of FLT uptake has shown promise in the assessment of high-grade gliomas and in the early evaluation of response to treatment (Ullrich et al. 2008). However, benign brain lesions that disrupt the blood–brain barrier cannot be reliably distinguished from malignancies using ^{18}F-FLT (Saga et al. 2006).

2.5.3 Cell Membrane Components

Choline is a precursor in the synthesis of phospholipids, which are essential components of cell membranes. Within the cell, choline can be phosphorylated, acetylated or oxidized. Phosphorylated choline is further incorporated into phosphatidylcholine (lecithin), a major phospholipid of all membranes, which demonstrates increased levels following malignant cell transformation. ^{18}F-labeled choline analogues (FCH) have been developed with a biodistribution similar to choline (Vallabhajosula 2007). Differences in ^{18}F-FCH uptake have been found to differentiate high-grade gliomas, solitary metastases and benign lesions with increased peritumoral uptake distinguishing high-grade gliomas (Kwee et al. 2007).

2.5.4 Hypoxia

Increasing tumor size results in reduced ability of local vasculature to supply adequate blood flow to meet the demands of rapidly growing cells. The resulting hypoxia may inhibit new cell division and lead to cell death, but it may also provoke an adaptive response that may help tumor cells progress. Hypoxia in tumors has been established as an important factor in tumor progression and in resistance to both radiation and chemotherapy (Foo et al. 2004).

^{15}O-labeled compounds have been used to study tumor hypoxia by quantifying blood flow and tissue oxygen utilization. Patients with higher regional cerebral blood flow, blood volume or metabolic oxygen utilization have significantly longer survival times than those with lower values (Mineura et al. 1994). In gliomas, and most head and neck cancers, low oxygen tension levels are associated with resistance to chemotherapy and radiation therapy, and subsequent development of local recurrence.

^{18}F-fluoromisonidazole (FMISO) provides an estimate of hypoxia within tumors by selectively binding to hypoxic cells (Vallabhajosula 2007). Substantial uptake is found in high-grade, but not low-grade gliomas and is related to expression of the angiogenesis marker VEGF-R1 (Cher et al. 2006). The intensity of increased uptake of ^{18}F-FMISO appears to be correlated with poorer survival and may have a role in monitoring response to targeted hypoxic therapies (Spence et al. 2008).

3 Conclusion

The primary role of FDG-PET imaging in primary brain tumors is to define regions of high tumor grade, either as part of the initial workup or in the evaluation for tumor recurrence. Accurate correlation with MRI is an important part of this evaluation. Treatment strategies for high-grade gliomas have significantly improved over the past several years. Concurrently, imaging follow-up with conventional MRI has become more complicated, with issues of false positive contrast-enhancement (pseudo progression), as well as potential suppression of enhancement by anti-angiogenic agents. PET imaging, using FDG or other tracers, may therefore have an increasingly important role in following brain tumor patients as these treatment strategies evolve.

References

Alavi JB, Alavi A, Chawluk J, Kushner M, Powe J, Hickey W, Reivich M (1988) Positron emission tomography in patients with glioma. A predictor of prognosis. Cancer 62(6): 1074–1078

Alexiou GA, Tsiouris S, Kyritsis AP, Voulgaris S, Argyropoulou MI, Fotopoulos AD (2009) Glioma recurrence versus radiation necrosis: accuracy of current imaging modalities. J Neurooncol 95(1):1–11

Barker FG 2nd, Chang SM, Valk PE, Pounds TR, Prados MD (1997) 18-Fluorodeoxyglucose uptake and survival of patients with suspected recurrent malignant glioma. Cancer 79(1):115–126

Becherer A, Karanikas G, Szabó M, Zettinig G, Asenbaum S, Marosi C, Henk C, Wunderbaldinger P, Czech T, Wadsak W, Kletter K (2003) Brain tumour imaging with PET: a comparison between [18F]fluorodopa and [11C]methionine. Eur J Nucl Med Mol Imaging 30(11):1561–1567

Behin A, Hoang-Xuan K, Carpentier AF, Delattre JY (2003) Primary brain tumours in adults. Lancet 361(9354):323–331

Bondy ML et al (2008) Brain tumor epidemiology: consensus from the brain tumor epidemiology consortium. Cancer 113(7 Suppl):1953–1968

Burton EC, Prados MD (2000) Malignant gliomas. Curr Treat Options Oncol 1(5):459–468

Chao ST, Suh JH, Raja S, Lee SY, Barnett G (2001) The sensitivity and specificity of FDG PET in distinguishing recurrent brain tumor from radionecrosis in patients treated with stereotactic radiosurgery. Int J Cancer 96(3):191–197

Chen W, Silverman DH, Delaloye S, Czernin J, Kamdar N, Pope W, Satyamurthy N, Schiepers C, Cloughesy T (2006) 18F-FDOPA PET imaging of brain tumors: comparison study with 18F-FDG PET and evaluation of diagnostic accuracy. J Nucl Med 47(6):904–911

Cher LM, Murone C, Lawrentschuk N, Ramdave S, Papenfuss A, Hannah A, O'Keefe GJ, Sachinidis JI, Berlangieri SU, Fabinyi G, Scott AM (2006) Correlation of hypoxic cell fraction and angiogenesis with glucose metabolic rate in gliomas using 18F-fluoromisonidazole, 18F-FDG PET, and immunohistochemical studies. J Nucl Med 47(3):410–418

Choi SJ, Kim JS, Kim JH, Oh SJ, Lee JG, Kim CJ, Ra YS, Yeo JS, Ryu JS, Moon DH (2005) [18F]3'-deoxy-3'-fluorothymidine PET for the diagnosis and grading of brain tumors. Eur J Nucl Med Mol Imaging 32(6):653–659

Chung JK, Kim YK, Kim SK, Lee YJ, Paek S, Yeo JS, Jeong JM, Lee DS, Jung HW, Lee MC (2002) Usefulness of 11C-methionine PET in the evaluation of brain lesions that are hypo- or isometabolic on 18F-FDG PET. Eur J Nucl Med Mol Imaging 29(2):176–182

Croteau D, Mikkelsen T (2001) Adults with newly diagnosed high-grade gliomas. Curr Treat Options Oncol 2(6):507–515

Daumas-Duport C, Scheithauer B, O'Fallon J, Kelly P (1988) Grading of astrocytomas. A simple and reproducible method. Cancer 62(10):2152–2165

De Witte O, Levivier M, Violon P, Salmon I, Damhaut P, Wikler D Jr, Hildebrand J, Brotchi J, Goldman S (1996) Prognostic value positron emission tomography with [18F]fluoro-2-deoxy-D-glucose in the low-grade glioma. Neurosurgery 39(3):470–476; discussion 476–477

Delbeke D, Meyerowitz C, Lapidus RL, Maciunas RJ, Jennings MT, Moots PL, Kessler RM (1995) Optimal cutoff levels of F-18 fluorodeoxyglucose uptake in the differentiation of low-grade from high-grade brain tumors with PET. Radiology 195(1):47–52

Derlon JM, Chapon F, Noël MH, Khouri S, Benali K, Petit-Taboué MC, Houtteville JP, Chajari MH, Bouvard G (2000)

Non-invasive grading of oligodendrogliomas: correlation between in vivo metabolic pattern and histopathology. Eur J Nucl Med 27(7):778–787

Di Chiro G, Oldfield E, Wright DC, De Michele D, Katz DA, Patronas NJ, Doppman JL, Larson SM, Ito M, Kufta CV (1988) Cerebral necrosis after radiotherapy and/or intraarterial chemotherapy for brain tumors: PET and neuropathologic studies. Am J Roentgenol 150(1):189–197

Floeth FW, Sabel M, Stoffels G, Pauleit D, Hamacher K, Steiger HJ, Langen KJ (2008) Prognostic value of 18F-fluoroethyl-L-tyrosine PET and MRI in small nonspecific incidental brain lesions. J Nucl Med 49(5):730–737

Foo SS, Abbott DF, Lawrentschuk N et al (2004) Functional imaging of intra-tumoral hypoxia. Mol Imaging Biol 6:291–305

Fulham MJ, Brunetti A, Aloj L, Raman R, Dwyer AJ, Di Chiro G (1995) Decreased cerebral glucose metabolism in patients with brain tumors: an effect of corticosteroids. J Neurosurg 83(4):657–664

Glantz MJ, Hoffman JM, Coleman RE, Friedman AH, Hanson MW, Burger PC, Herndon JE 2nd, Meisler WJ, Schold SC Jr (1991) Identification of early recurrence of primary central nervous system tumors by [18F]fluorodeoxyglucose positron emission tomography. Neurology 29(4):347–355

Goldman S, Levivier M, Pirotte B, Brucher JM, Wikler D, Damhaut P, Stanus E, Brotchi J, Hildebrand J (1996) Regional glucose metabolism and histopathology of gliomas. A study based on positron emission tomography-guided stereotactic biopsy. Cancer 78(5):1098–1106

Goldman S, Levivier M, Pirotte B, Brucher JM, Wikler D, Damhaut P, Dethy S, Brotchi J, Hildebrand J (1997) Regional methionine and glucose uptake in high-grade gliomas: a comparative study on PET-guided stereotactic biopsy. J Nucl Med 38(9):1459–1462

Hanson MW, Glantz MJ, Hoffman JM, Friedman AH, Burger PC, Schold SC, Coleman RE (1991) FDG-PET in the selection of brain lesions for biopsy. J Comput Assist Tomogr 15(5):796–801

Hoffman JM, Waskin HA, Schifter T, Hanson MW, Gray L, Rosenfeld S, Coleman RE (1993) FDG-PET in differentiating lymphoma from nonmalignant central nervous system lesions in patients with AIDS. J Nucl Med 34(4): 567–575

Hustinx R, Smith RJ, Benard F, Bhatnagar A, Alavi A (1999) Can the standardized uptake value characterize primary brain tumors on FDG-PET? J Nucl Med 26(11):1501–1509

Jager PL, Vaalburg W, Pruim J, de Vries EG, Langen KJ, Piers DA (2008) Radiolabeled amino acids: basic aspects and clinical applications in oncology. J Nucl Med 42(3):432–445

Jemal A, Siegel R, Ward E, Hao Y, Xu J, Thun MJ (2009) Cancer statistics, 2009. CA Cancer J Clin 59(4):225–249

Kaal EC, Niël CG, Vecht CJ (2005) Therapeutic management of brain metastasis. Lancet Neurol 4(5):289–298

Kim DW, Jung SA, Kim CG, Park SA (2010) The efficacy of dual time point F-18 FDG PET imaging for grading of brain tumors. Clin Nucl Med 35(6):400–403

Kosaka N, Tsuchida T, Uematsu H, Kimura H, Okazawa H, Itoh H (2008) 18F-FDG PET of common enhancing malignant brain tumors. Am J Roentgenol 190(6):W365–W369

Kracht LW, Miletic H, Busch S, Jacobs AH, Voges J, Hoevels M, Klein JC, Herholz K, Heiss WD (2004) Delineation of brain tumor extent with [11C]L-methionine positron emission tomography: local comparison with stereotactic histopathology. Clin Cancer Res 10(21):7163–7170

Kwee SA, Ko JP, Jiang CS, Watters MR, Coel MN (2007) Solitary brain lesions enhancing at MR imaging: evaluation with fluorine 18 fluorocholine PET. Radiology 244(2): 557–565

Larcos G, Maisey MN (1996) FDG-PET screening for cerebral metastases in patients with suspected malignancy. Nucl Med Commun 17(3):197–198

Laverman P, Boerman OC, Corstens FH, Oyen WJ (2002) Fluorinated amino acids for tumour imaging with positron emission tomography. Eur J Nucl Med Mol Imaging 29(5): 681–690

Mineura K, Sasajima T, Kowada M, Ogawa T, Hatazawa J, Shishido F, Uemura K (1994) Perfusion and metabolism in predicting the survival of patients with cerebral gliomas. Cancer 73(9):2386–2394

Minn H (2005) PET and SPECT in low-grade glioma. Eur J Radiol 56(2):171–178

Miyagawa T, Oku T, Uehara H, Desai R, Beattie B, Tjuvajev J, Blasberg R (1998) "Facilitated" amino acid transport is upregulated in brain tumors. J Cereb Blood Flow Metab 18(5):500–509

Nariai T, Tanaka Y, Wakimoto H, Aoyagi M, Tamaki M, Ishiwata K, Senda M, Ishii K, Hirakawa K, Ohno K (2005) Usefulness of L-[methyl-11C] methionine-positron emission tomography as a biological monitoring tool in the treatment of glioma. J Neurosurg 103(3):498–507

Nelson JS, Tsukada Y, Schoenfeld D, Fulling K, Lamarche J, Peress N (1983) Necrosis as a prognostic criterion in malignant supratentorial, astrocytic gliomas. Cancer 52(3): 550–554

Ohgaki H (2009) Epidemiology of brain tumors. Methods Mol Biol 472:323–342

Padma MV, Said S, Jacobs M, Hwang DR, Dunigan K, Satter M, Christian B, Ruppert J, Bernstein T, Kraus G, Mantil JC (2003) Prediction of pathology and survival by FDG PET in gliomas. J Neurooncol 64(3):227–237

Pardo FS, Aronen HJ, Fitzek M, Kennedy DN, Efird J, Rosen BR, Fischman AJ (2004) Correlation of FDG-PET interpretation with survival in a cohort of glioma patients. Anticancer Res 24(4):2359–2365

Patronas NJ, Di Chiro G, Kufta C, Bairamian D, Kornblith PL, Simon R, Larson SM (1985) Prediction of survival in glioma patients by means of positron emission tomography. J Neurosurg 62(6):816–822

Pauleit D, Stoffels G, Bachofner A, Floeth FW, Sabel M, Herzog H, Tellmann L, Jansen P, Reifenberger G, Hamacher K, Coenen HH, Langen KJ (2009) Comparison of (18)F-FET and (18)F-FDG PET in brain tumors. Nucl Med Biol 36(7):779–787

Pichler R, Dunzinger A, Wurm G, Pichler J, Weis S, Nußbaumer K, Topakian R, Aigner RM (2010) Is there a place for FET PET in the initial evaluation of brain lesions with unknown significance? Eur J Nucl Med Mol Imaging. 16 Apr 2010. [Epub ahead of print]

Pirotte B, Goldman S, Massager N, David P, Wikler D, Vandesteene A, Salmon I, Brotchi J, Levivier M (2004) Comparison of 18F-FDG and 11C-methionine for PET-guided stereotactic brain biopsy of gliomas. J Nucl Med 45(8):1293–1298

Pöpperl G, Götz C, Rachinger W, Gildehaus FJ, Tonn JC, Tatsch K (2004) Value of O-(2-[18F]fluoroethyl)- L-tyrosine PET for the diagnosis of recurrent glioma. Eur J Nucl Med Mol Imaging 31(11):1464–1470

Rachinger W, Goetz C, Pöpperl G, Gildehaus FJ, Kreth FW, Holtmannspötter M, Herms J, Koch W, Tatsch K, Tonn JC (2005) Positron emission tomography with O-(2-[18F]fluoroethyl)-L-tyrosine versus magnetic resonance imaging in the diagnosis of recurrent gliomas. Neurosurgery 57(3):505–511; discussion 505–511

Ribom D, Eriksson A, Hartman M, Engler H, Nilsson A, Långström B, Bolander H, Bergström M, Smits A (2001) Positron emission tomography (11)C-methionine and survival in patients with low-grade gliomas. Cancer 92(6):1541–1549

Roelcke U, Blasberg RG, von Ammon K, Hofer S, Vontobel P, Maguire RP, Radü EW, Herrmann R, Leenders KL (1998) Dexamethasone treatment and plasma glucose levels: relevance for fluorine-18-fluorodeoxyglucose uptake measurements in gliomas. J Nucl Med 39(5):879–884

Saga T, Kawashima H, Araki N, Takahashi JA, Nakashima Y, Higashi T, Oya N, Mukai T, Hojo M, Hashimoto N, Manabe T, Hiraoka M, Togashi K (2006) Evaluation of primary brain tumors with FLT-PET: usefulness and limitations. Clin Nucl Med 31(12):774–780

Salskov A, Tammisetti VS, Grierson J, Vesselle H (2007) FLT: measuring tumor cell proliferation in vivo with positron emission tomography and 3′-deoxy-3′-[18F]fluorothymidine. Semin Nucl Med 37(6):429–439

Singhal T, Narayanan TK, Jain V, Mukherjee J, Mantil J (2008) 11C-L-methionine positron emission tomography in the clinical management of cerebral gliomas. Mol Imaging Biol 10(1):1–18

Spence AM, Muzi M, Mankoff DA, O'Sullivan SF, Link JM, Lewellen TK, Lewellen B, Pham P, Minoshima S, Swanson K, Krohn KA (2004) 18F-FDG PET of gliomas at delayed intervals: improved distinction between tumor and normal gray matter. J Nucl Med 45(10):1653–1659

Spence AM, Muzi M, Swanson KR, O'Sullivan F, Rockhill JK, Rajendran JG, Adamsen TC, Link JM, Swanson PE, Yagle KJ, Rostomily RC, Silbergeld DL, Krohn KA (2008) Regional hypoxia in glioblastoma multiforme quantified with [18F]fluoromisonidazole positron emission tomography before radiotherapy: correlation with time to progression and survival. Clin Cancer Res 14(9):2623–2630

Stieber VW (2001) Low-grade gliomas. Curr Treat Options Oncol 2(6):495–506

Terakawa Y, Tsuyuguchi N, Iwai Y, Yamanaka K, Higashiyama S, Takami T, Ohata K (2008) Diagnostic accuracy of 11C-methionine PET for differentiation of recurrent brain tumors from radiation necrosis after radiotherapy. J Nucl Med 49(5):694–699

Tripathi M, Sharma R, D'Souza M, Jaimini A, Panwar P, Varshney R, Datta A, Kumar N, Garg G, Singh D, Grover RK, Mishra AK, Mondal A (2009) Comparative evaluation of F-18 FDOPA, F-18 FDG, and F-18 FLT-PET/CT for metabolic imaging of low grade gliomas. Clin Nucl Med 34(12):878–883

Ullrich R, Backes H, Li H, Kracht L, Miletic H, Kesper K, Neumaier B, Heiss WD, Wienhard K, Jacobs AH (2008) Glioma proliferation as assessed by 3′-fluoro-3′-deoxy-L-thymidine positron emission tomography in patients with newly diagnosed high-grade glioma. Clin Cancer Res 14(7):2049–2055

Vallabhajosula S (2007) (18)F-labeled positron emission tomographic radiopharmaceuticals in oncology: an overview of radiochemistry and mechanisms of tumor localization. Semin Nucl Med 37(6):400–419

Vecht CJ, Haaxma-Reiche H, Noordijk EM, Padberg GW, Voormolen JH, Hoekstra FH, Tans JT, Lambooij N, Metsaars JA, Wattendorff AR et al (1993) Treatment of single brain metastasis: radiotherapy alone or combined with neurosurgery? Ann Neurol 33(6):583–590

Wang SX, Boethius J, Ericson K (2006) FDG-PET on irradiated brain tumor: ten years' summary. Acta Radiol 47(1):85–90

Weber WA, Wester HJ, Grosu AL, Herz M, Dzewas B, Feldmann HJ, Molls M, Stöcklin G, Schwaiger M (2000) O-(2-[18F]fluoroethyl)-L-tyrosine and L-[methyl-11C]methionine uptake in brain tumours: initial results of a comparative study. Eur J Nucl Med 27(5):542–549

Head and Neck

Rathan M. Subramaniam, J. M. Davison, Ujas Parikh, and M. Abou-Zied

Contents

R. M. Subramaniam · J. M. Davison · U. Parikh
Boston University School of Medicine,
Boston, USA

M. Abou-Zied
Department of Nuclear Medicine,
State University of New York at Buffalo,
105 Parker Hall South Campus, 3435 Main Street,
Buffalo, NY 14214, USA

R. M. Subramaniam (✉)
Russell H Morgan Departments of Radiology and Radiological Sciences Institutions,
The Johns Hopkins Medical,
601 N. Caroline Street/ JHOC 3235,
Baltimore, MD 21287, USA
e-mail: rsubram4@jhmi.edu

Abstract

The hybrid technique of PET/CT has significantly impacted the imaging and management of head and neck squamous cell cancer (HNSCC) since its introduction and has become the technique of choice for imaging of this cancer. Diagnostic FDG PET/CT is useful for identification of an unknown primary tumor, delineation of extent of primary tumor, detection of regional lymph node involvement even in a normal-sized node, detection of distant metastases and occasional synchronous primary tumor, assessment of therapy response, and long-term surveillance for recurrence and metastases. The role of PET/CT is evolving in radiation therapy planning. Combined diagnostic PET/CT provides the best anatomic and metabolic in vivo information for the comprehensive management of HNSCC. FDG PET/CT is the modality of choice in detecting metastasis of differentiated thyroid cancer, when the disease is iodine negative. It is valuable in staging and prognosis of anaplastic and medullary thyroid cancer.

1 Introduction

Worldwide, head and neck cancers (HNC) are the sixth most common types of cancers, 90% of which are squamous cell carcinomas (HNSCC). In the United States in 2008, approximately 47,000 new cases of HNSCC were diagnosed. Prognosis and treatment planning is primarily based on TNM staging as well as tumor subsite in the head and neck. Patients presenting with early stage primary tumor at the time of diagnosis

P. Peller et al. (eds.), *PET-CT and PET-MRI in Oncology*, Medical Radiology. Diagnostic Imaging,
DOI: 10.1007/174_2012_603,

(T1 or T2, N0, and M0) have an excellent prognosis. However, the majority of patients at the time of presentation have regional nodal metastasis and upto 10% have distant metastases. Patients with recurrent or metastatic disease have a median survival of approximately 6–9 months. Effective disease control is difficult to achieve in patients with advanced stage HNC. Studies have shown that, after demonstrating complete response on clinical exam, residual cancer can be found in the neck nodes of 16–39% of patients with N2 or N3 disease. Another factor to consider in these patients is that second primary tumors are common and can be detected even in patients with early stage HNC. Accurate staging and early detection of recurrence in patients with head and neck malignancies is essential to assure locoregional control and increase survival benefit. Furthermore, detection of metastatic spread can spare patients' overly aggressive treatments and guarantee the best chance at a better quality of life.

Imaging modalities have proved essential in the initial staging, assessment of response to therapy, and post-treatment surveillance of patients with HNC. There has been increasing interest in the use of functional imaging with FDG PET rather than conventional cross-sectional modalities, such as computed tomography (CT) or magnetic resonance imaging (MRI), in the initial assessment and subsequent follow-up of malignancies in the head and neck. Combined FDG PET/CT has revolutionized HNC imaging by offering an integration of metabolic as well as anatomic information that allows for better localization of abnormalities in the complex anatomy of the head and neck as well as superior accuracy in distinguishing residual disease from post-therapy changes.

2 Head and Neck PET/CT Protocol

PET/CT imaging was developed to improve PET imaging by expediting attenuation correction and improving lesion localization. Hence, initial protocols for PET/CT imaging were designed to optimize the acquisition of the PET scan at the expense of the CT scan. For head and neck imaging, this meant that no intravenous contrast was used; a low-dose CT technique was common; and CT scans were reconstructed with a section thickness to match the PET scan (approximately 3–5 mm). Commonly, the imaging report emphasized the FDG PET findings with CT findings described only if they were related to PET findings, were significant, or were obvious. The advantage of this approach is its simplicity and shorter time. The limitation is that most patients will need high-quality anatomic imaging for surgical planning, and this often requires a separate visit.

With experience and improvement in technology, it is now possible to acquire a high-quality diagnostic CT (DCT) scan for surgical planning and PET for metabolic imaging at the time of PET/CT imaging. This examination is referred to as PET/DCT-neck. The advantage of this study is to perform a comprehensive evaluation of patients with HNSCC in a single visit to the imaging department. The addition of a diagnostic-level CT scan to FDG PET scanning affords hardware fusion of the images and the opportunity for a single report to incorporate results from both imaging studies. In general, nodal status and distant metastases are best evaluated by the PET component of the examination, but the morphology and relation of the primary lesion to critical anatomic structures are best evaluated by the CT component of the examination. The tradeoff is an examination that takes longer to perform and interpret and requires technical and interpretive expertise in both PET and CT modalities. At our institution, the head and neck surgeons have gravitated from the routine PET/CT to the more comprehensive PET/DCT. It not only images the neck with a diagnostic-quality CT scan but also includes the chest, abdomen, and pelvis to complete a CT scanning that matches a PET scanning from the skull base to the mid-thigh, providing both metabolic and high-quality anatomic imaging, the workhorse of oncology imaging. This examination provides a one-stop shopping experience that simplifies scheduling, allows staging, and surgical planning at the same time (Fig. 1), and is convenient for the patient. A single report is provided by an attending radiologist who has expertise in both PET and CT modalities.

The PET/DCT is performed in two parts. A dedicated PET/DCT for the neck is performed with the arms down and with thinner CT sections (1.25 cm), by using a 256 PET matrix and 60 ml of non-iodinated intravenous contrast agent. It covers from the skull base to the arch of the aorta, including the nodal chains draining the head and neck. The body part of the PET/

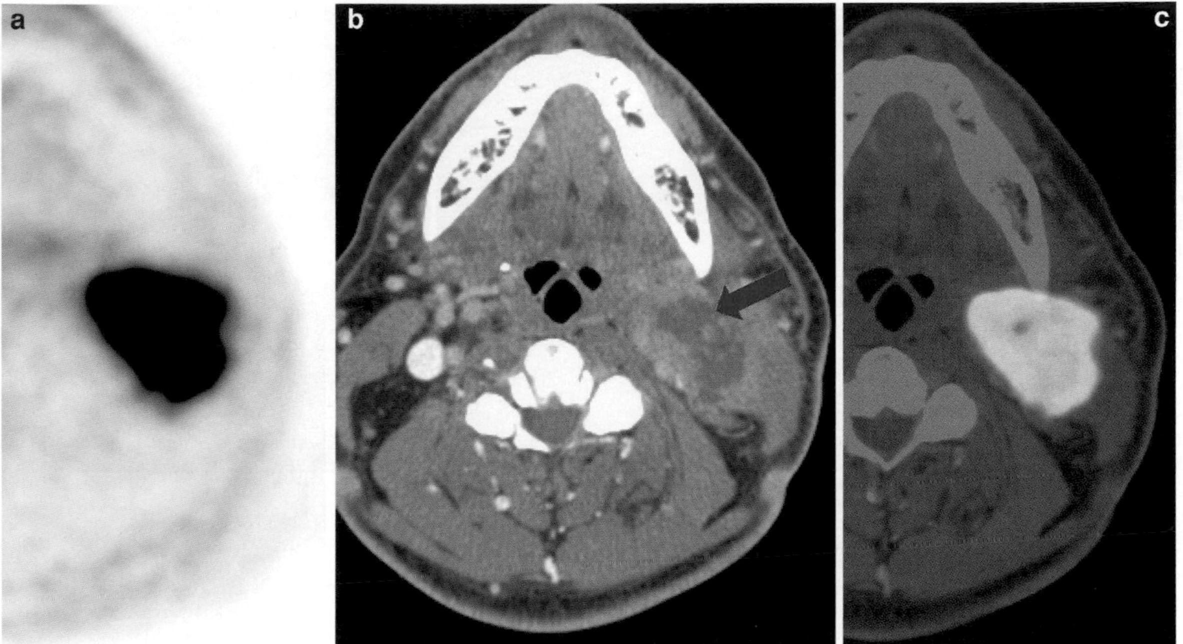

Fig. 1 Contrast enhanced PET/DCT. **a** PET, **b** Contrast-enhanced CT, **c** PET/DCT. The dedicated contrast-enhanced PET/DCT provides the anatomic details needed for surgical planning and metabolic information of the tumor. The left level IIA necrotic lymphadenopathy demonstrates left carotid sheath involvement, pericapsular spread, and invasion of the left sternocleidomastoid muscle, and is intensely FDG avid. All this information was integrated into patient's management from this single dedicated contrast-enhanced PET/CT

DCT study covers from just above the clavicles to the midthigh with 100 ml of non-iodinated intravenous contrast agent. The body part is performed with the arms up first followed by head and neck part of the study.

3 Detection of Unknown Primary

Not uncommonly, a patient will present with an enlarging neck mass, which, on FNA or excisional biopsy reveals metastatic SCC. Clinical exam with laryngoscopy or panendoscopy will frequently reveal the primary tumor site, however, upto 10% will go undetected on clinical exam or conventional imaging techniques. This is especially true if the tumor is too small to be seen on endoscopy or CT or located in areas difficult to assess by these methods such as the tonsils or tongue. FDG PET/CT has been shown to be accurate in determining location of the primary tumor in patients that present with locoregional metastasis. In a meta-analysis by Dong et al. (2008), the pooled sensitivity of FDG PET/CT across eight studies was 18% and the specificity was 83% in detecting unknown primary tumors of the head and neck. FDG PET detected 29% of tumors that were not apparent after workup with clinical exam and conventional imaging modalities (Fig. 2). It should be noted that care must be taken when assessing for malignancy in the base of the tongue and tonsils. FDG PET also exhibited a lower sensitivity with respect to the tumors at the base of the tongue and tonsils than at other sites, which was 68.2 and 76.7%, respectively. Dong et al. also found that tumors of the tongue base accounted for 20.7% of all false-positive FDG PET scans. In a meta-analysis, Rusthoven et al. (2004) noted a similarly high false-positive rate in the tonsils. FDG PET/CT can be a valuable tool in the assessment of an unknown primary as it can guide the clinicians toward suspicious sites, but does not have sufficient sensitivity and PPV to eliminate the need for a careful panendoscopy with directed biopsies and tonsillectomy.

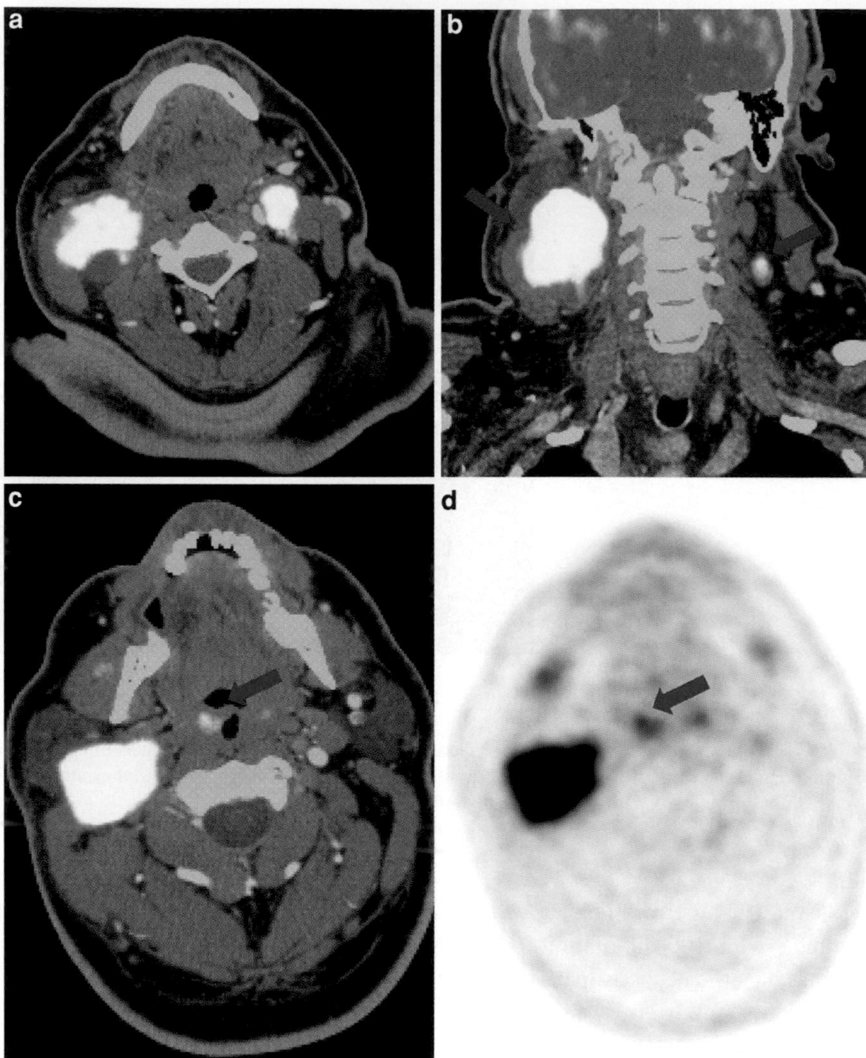

Fig. 2 Unknown primary Patient presented with a large right side neck mass with an unknown primary. The laryngoscopic examination failed to identify a primary site. The FDG PET/DCT demonstrated bilateral intense FDG-avid cervical lymphadenopathy (**a**, **b**) and a small FDG-avid primary tumor in the right tongue base/tonsil (**c**, **d**). This allowed appropriate tumor delineation for concurrent chemoradiation and to reduce morbidity related to radiation therapy

4 Initial Staging

4.1 Primary Tumor Staging

According to international staging guidelines, staging with CT and/or MRI is the current standard for HNC. Criteria for defining the T stage in patients with HNSCC vary slightly according to the site of primary tumor. Accurate and complete assessment of the T stage requires knowledge of the size of the primary lesion as well as depth of invasion and involvement of surrounding structures. While FDG PET is highly accurate in detection of malignant lesions, metabolic information alone is not sufficient to provide the information required to completely stage the primary tumor. The advent of combined FDG PET/CT allowed for synchronous image acquisition and comparison of functional anatomic data, increased interobserver agreement and superior localization of FDG-avid lesions in the head and neck when compared to PET alone.

With a dedicated HNC protocol with contrast enhanced PET/DCT-neck, T staging with PET/CT is as accurate as CT alone (Fig. 3). MRI may add value at certain primary sites, such as nasopharynx/skull base, parotid gland where tissue planes are better depicted than with a contrast-enhanced dedicated head and neck PET/DCT. Perineural spread can be better characterized by MRI.

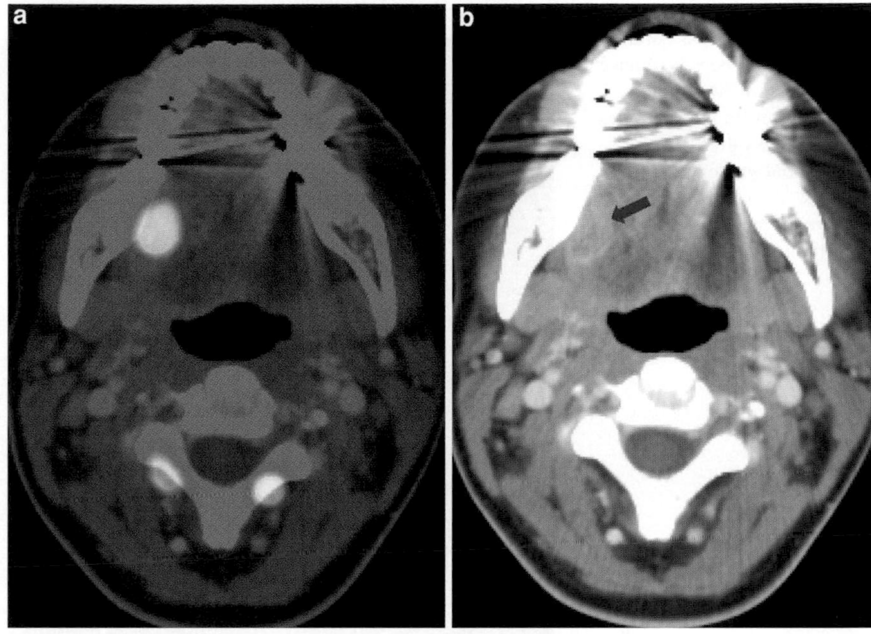

Fig. 3 Primary tumor staging—PET/DCT. **a** PET/DCT and **b** CT of neck demonstrating the primary tumor located in the right lateral tongue with homogeneous enhancement. The maximum diameter of the tumor was less than 2 cm (T1) with no evidence to involve muscle or the lingual cortex of the right hemimandible. The fused PET/CT demonstrates intense FDG hypermetabolism. The contrast enhanced PET/DCT was useful to exclude extrinsic muscle involvement of tongue

4.2 Nodal Staging

The most important prognostic factor in HNSCC is spread to regional lymph nodes. Staging for nodal metastases in HNSCC is uniform across sub-sites according to the AJCC system with the only exception being nasopharyngeal carcinoma. Important features in evaluation in involved lymph nodes include: the number of nodes with disease, the nodal levels, whether unilateral or bilateral, and morphology. Accurate determination of cervical nodal involvement is essential for future management. Imaging has clear superiority over clinical assessment for detecting nodal metastases. Both CT and MRI have similar rates of detection with sensitivities ranging from 14 to 80% for CT and 29 to 85% for MRI, and specificities for both modalities between 80 and 100%. Using CT, size criteria are most commonly employed to identify lymph nodes as suspicious for harboring cancerous cells with size thresholds of 15 mm in short axis for jugulodigastric nodes and of 10 mm for all other cervical nodes. However, in HNSCC, there is a high frequency of smaller lymph nodes that are positive for tumor and in fact approximately 25% of nodes greater than 10 mm will harbor metastases. Conventional imaging thus may lead to understaging.

PET has been shown to be superior to conventional imaging modalities for the detection of regional nodal metastases as it relies on functional rather than anatomic parameters such as size. Increased tumor cell glycolytic activity can be identified by FDG PET in affected nodes even when not pathologically enlarged by conventional size criteria (Fig. 4). While PET alone is limited by lack of spatial resolution, PET/CT combines metabolic and anatomic information allowing for the accurate assessment of the presence of malignant cells while simultaneously localizing the site of locoregional spread within the complex anatomy of the head and neck. Schwartz et al. (2005) found that the nodal level staging sensitivity and specificity for FDG PET/CT was 96 and 98.5%, respectively. In addition, the authors demonstrated that agreement between radiologic findings and pathology was stronger for FDG PET/CT than for CT alone.

With more sensitive and specific delineation of locoregional metastasis, FDG PET/CT has the ability to significantly alter further management through more accurate staging of disease (Fig. 5). It has been demonstrated that FDG PET/CT was able to provide additional information that confirmed the treatment plan in 69% of patients and altered the treatment plan in 31%. In those with an altered treatment plan, 55% were actually upstaged based on PET/CT data. Similarly Gourdin et al. showed that in 57% of patient studies, FDG PET/CT eliminated the need for

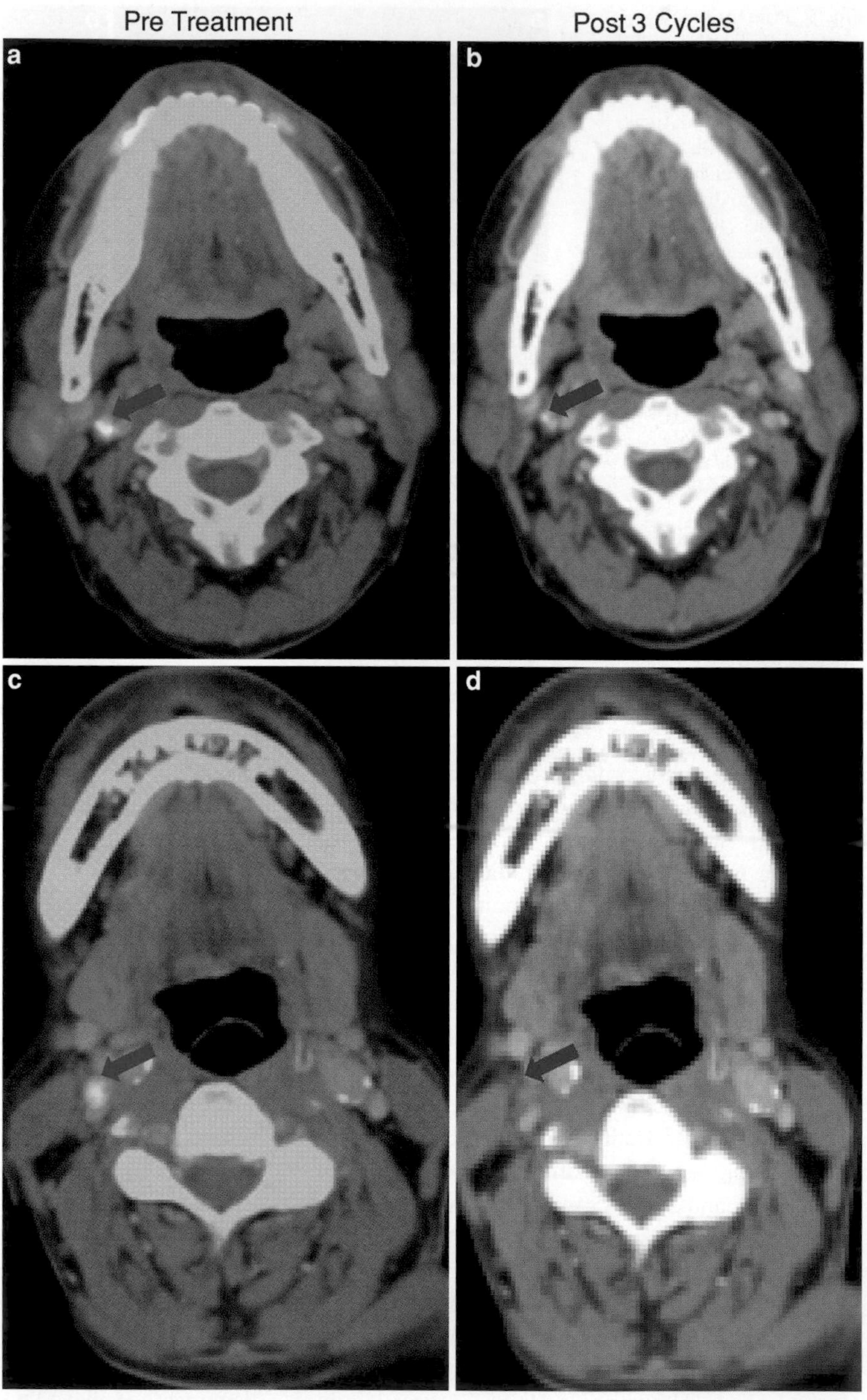

Fig. 4 Nodal staging. **a**, **c** PET/DCT and **b**, **d** contrast enhanced CT. There is intense FDG uptake in two right cervical level IIa lymph nodes which are less than 10 mm in size without evidence of necrosis. These nodes proved positive for nodal metastasis on pathology

previously planned diagnostic procedures in 33%, induced a change in the planned therapeutic approach in 15% of patients, and guided biopsy to a specific metabolically active area inside an edematous region in 3% of patients.

However, care must be taken due to technical limitations of FDG PET in detecting small deposits of tumor metastasis. In a study assessing the utilization of FDG PET/CT in detecting nodal metastases in the neck designated N0 on exam and conventional

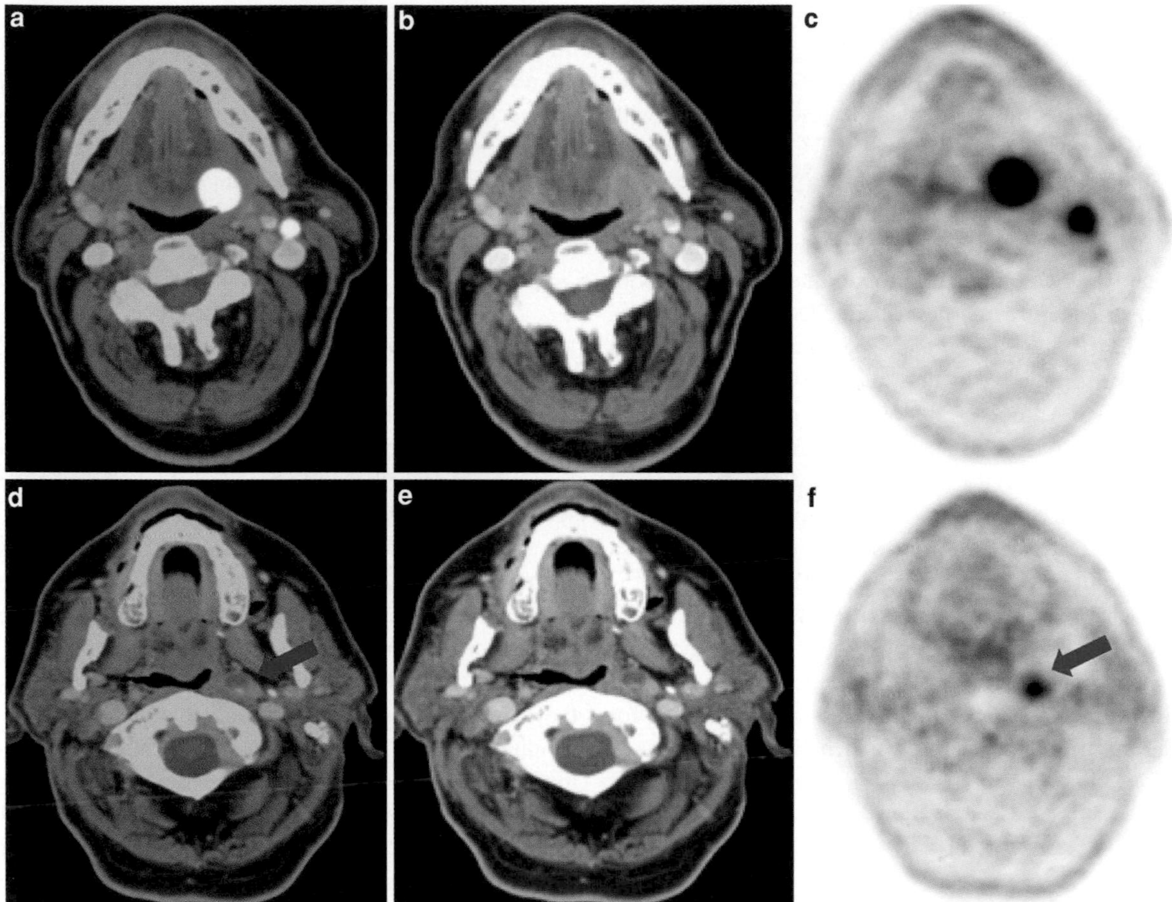

Fig. 5 Nodal staging—retropharyngeal node. **a**, **d** PET/DCT, **b**, **e** contrast enhanced CT and **c**, **f** PET. There is intense FDG uptake in the left tongue base primary tumor and left cervical level IIa metastatic lymph node. There is also central hypodensity and moderate FDG uptake in a left lateral retropharyngeal lymph node consistent with a necrotic metastatic lymph node. Identification of the retropharyngeal node changed the primary therapy to concurrent chemoradiation in this patient

imaging. PET/CT had high overall accuracy, but limited sensitivity for metastatic deposits less than 3 mm and a relatively high number of false-negative findings.

4.3 Detecting Distant Metastases (M-staging)

In patients with HNC, there is a high prevalence of synchronous and metachronous distant metastasis. On initial staging, 10–15% of patients with primary HNSCC will have distant metastases. The presence of distant spread portends a poor prognosis regardless of the time of diagnosis and significantly impacts future clinical management. Most commonly, metastases are found in the lungs, followed by the liver and skeletal system. Patients at risk for distant metastasis at the time of diagnosis and during follow-up include those with advanced T/N stage, poorly differentiated tumors on pathological examination, metastasis to level IV/V lymph nodes, laryngeal/hypopharyngeal primary sites, and increased SUV_{max}. Screening for distant metastasis is indicated in patients that have: more than four metastatic lymph nodes, metastases demonstrated in bilateral lymph nodes, nodal metastases measuring greater than 6 cm, level IV lymph node metastases, recurrent HNSCC, and those with a second primary tumor. Chest CT is better than plain radiography in detecting pulmonary involvement but will still miss a significant number of thoracic metastases.

A notable advantage of FDG PET is the ability to improve detection of distant disease in patients with HNSCC. Whole body FDG PET/CT, with superior spatial resolution, has been shown to be more accurate than conventional modalities in the identification of distant metastases and more accurate than PET alone. Haerle et al. (2011) found that, in patients with high-risk features as described, FDG PET/CT had a sensitivity of 96.8% and specificity of 95.4%, a positive predictive value of 69.8%, and negative predictive value of 99.6%, in detecting distant metastases on initial staging. FDG PET/CT, with its increased sensitivity and specificity for detection of locoregional as well as distant spread, provides a more accurate depiction of overall TNM staging in a significant percentage of patients. This information is critical for future management as it guides clinicians toward possibly curative surgery while avoiding overtreatment of those with advanced stage disease. FDG PET/CT has become the modality of choice for staging of patients with advanced HNSCC.

5 Treatment Planning

Depending on AJCC staging, patients with HNSCC will undergo surgical resection, often combined with radiation and/or chemotherapy. Radiation therapy, though effective in obtaining locoregional control, can have serious side effects in the head and neck such as osteonecrosis of the jaw and severe dysphagia secondary to tissue fibrosis. Newer treatment modalities, such as intensity-modulated radiation therapy (IMRT) and image-guided stereotactic radiosurgery, can offer effective and more targeted delivery of radiation. Accurate delineation of the radiation field is key in planning these forms of radiotherapy. Utilization of conventional imaging modalities, such as CT and MRI is standard due to excellent spatial resolution.

There has been increasing use of FDG PET/CT for planning radiation treatment. Several studies have shown combined PET/CT to be superior to CT in delineation of gross tumor volume (GTV). It should be noted that the choice of segmentation tool for target-volume definition of HNC based on FDG PET images is important as it influences the volume and shape of the resulting GTV. However, with adequate delineation, incorporation of PET data has been shown to add significantly to CT- and physical examination-based GTV definition. The role and value of FDG PET/CT in head and neck radiation therapy is discussed in detail in the chapter on radiation therapy planning later in this book (Chapter entitled in "Assessment of Response to Therapy").

6 Response to Treatment and Follow-up

Evaluation of patient response during therapy and restaging after completion of treatment is critical in determining whether alternate methods should be sought and in planning additional therapeutic measures. With postsurgical and postradiation alterations of anatomy, clinical examination alone is ineffective in monitoring response to treatment. In addition, conventional imaging modalities, while more accurate than clinical findings, are often sub-optimal as they are not sensitive for detecting recurrent or residual disease, especially in the setting of inflammation and altered anatomic planes postresection or postradiation. FDG PET is advantageous as malignant tumor cells in the surgical bed or radiation field, will be more hypermetabolic than benign tissues. In one study (Andrade et al. 2006), 8 weeks after definitive radiation therapy for HNC, the overall sensitivity and specificity of FDG PET/CT was 76.9 and 93.3%, respectively, while that of contrast enhanced CT was 92.3 and 46.7%. Hence, FDG PET/CT is the modality of choice for therapy response assessment in HNSCC (Fig. 6).

Radiologic surveillance after therapy allows for early and accurate detection of recurrent disease, offering a survival benefit if the patient is a potential candidate for surgery or re-irradiation. Surveillance after definitive therapy for HNC is of particular importance as these patients develop second primary tumors with a higher frequency than patients with other types of malignancy. FDG PET/CT is the modality of choice for surveillance of patients with HNSCC. Early detection of residual disease after incomplete resection or failed radiotherapy, recurrent tumor, distant metastases or secondary tumors can be critical in planning further management. FDG PET/CT may provide the most accurate assessment of treatment response. However, uncertainty exists in

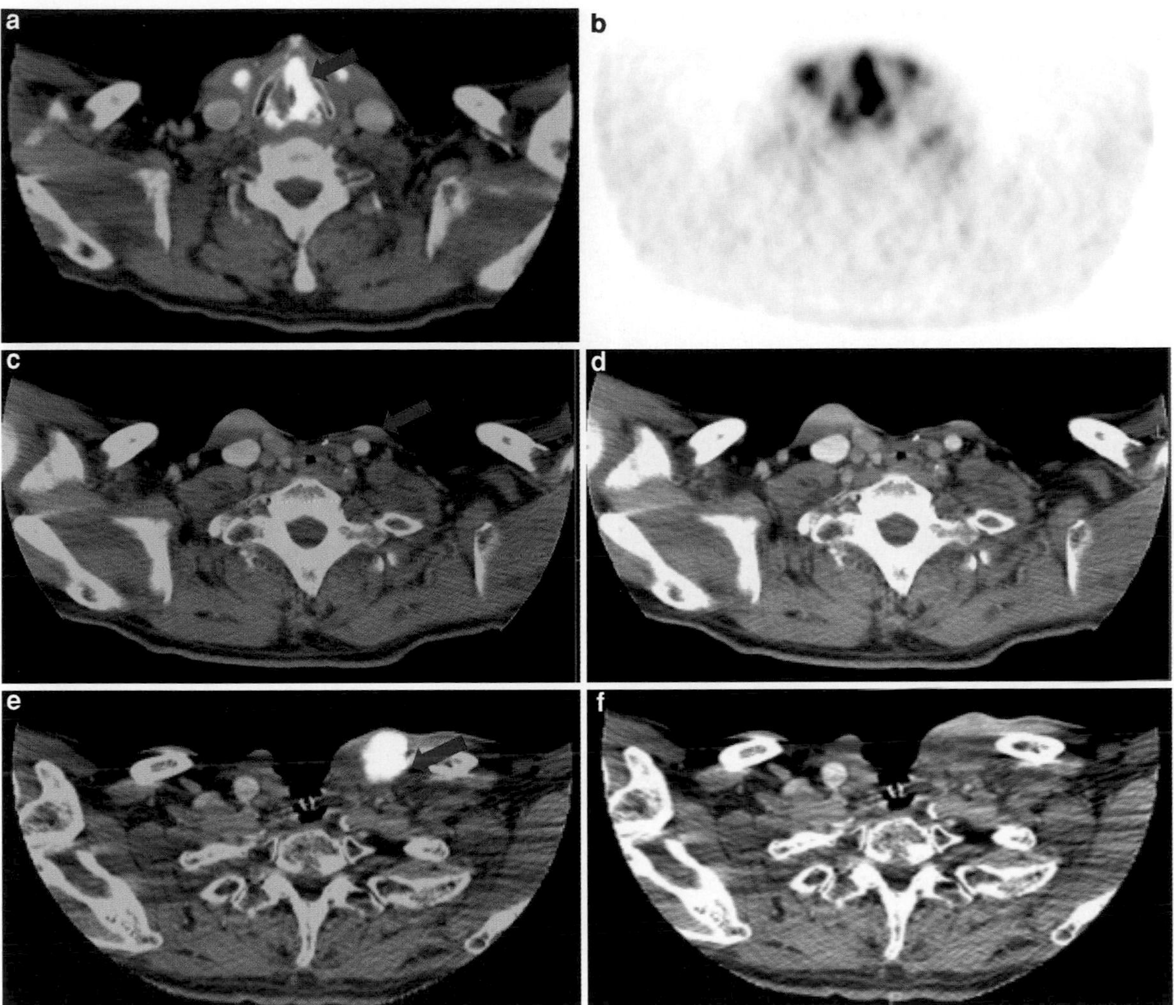

Fig. 6 Follow-up local nodal metastatic disease. **a**, **c**, **e** PET/DCT, **b** PET and **d**, **f** contrast enhanced CT. Patient presented with an intensely FDG-avid left vocal cord mass (**a**, **b**) and underwent total laryngectomy and left neck dissection. A follow-up PET/CT demonstrated a left level IV nodal metastasis that is only seen in the PET/CT (**c**) but not in the contrast-enhanced CT (**d**). This was resected and proven pathologically to be metastatic. A further follow-up PET/DCT demonstrated a local metastatic FDG-avid left supraclavicular mass. Patient underwent stereotactic radiation therapy

the literature in regards to optimal timing of the first surveillance scan after completion of treatment for head and neck tumors. The sensitivity of FDG PET/CT may be compromised early after therapy as residual tumor deposits may be too small to resolve on PET. In addition, FDG hypermetabolism is not specific for malignant cells and can also occur in tissues inflamed secondary to irradiation or surgical manipulation. All false-negative and false-positive FDG PET/CT results occurred between 4 and 8 weeks after treatment. FDG PET/CT provided the most accurate assessment for treatment response when performed later than 8 weeks after the conclusion of radiation therapy. However, Clavien et al. (2005) studied patients with more advanced Stage II and IV HNC and found that follow-up PET scans performed 6 weeks after combined radiation and chemotherapy had 90.9% sensitivity and 93.3%

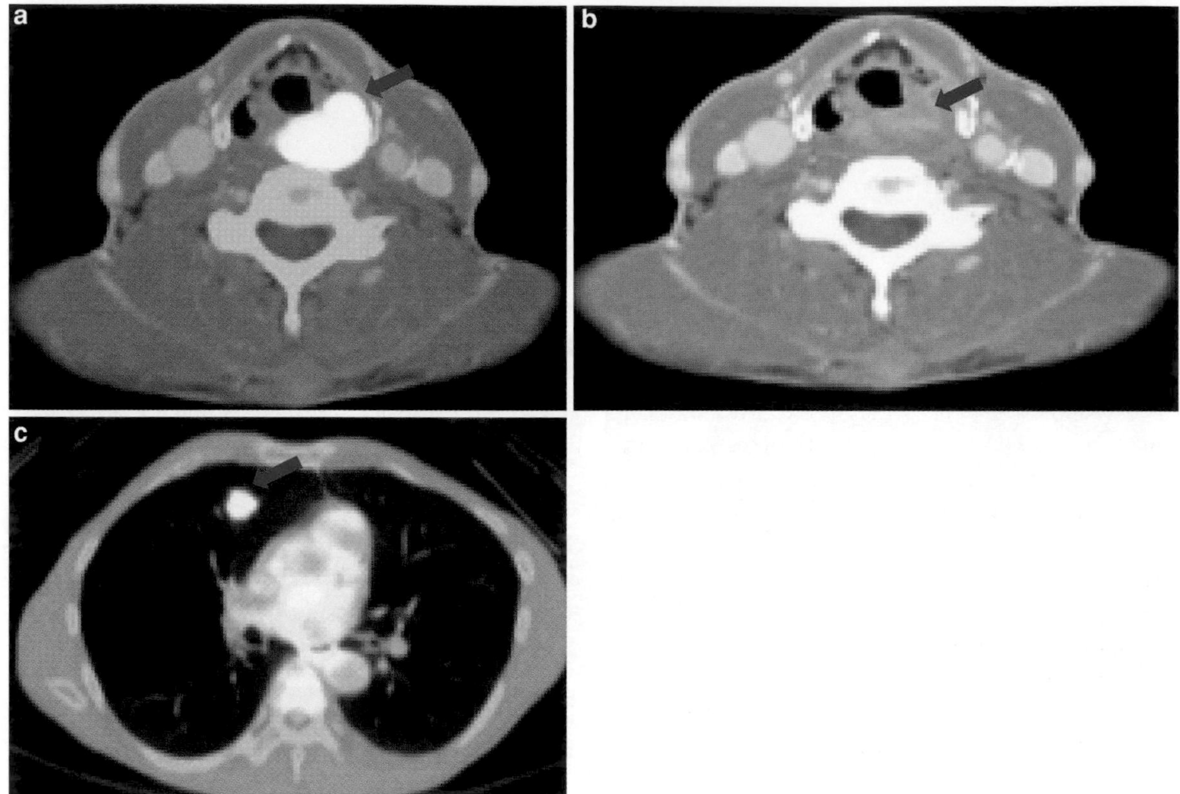

Fig. 7 Follow-up distant lung metastasis. **a**, **c** PET/DCT and **b** contrast-enhanced CT. There is an intensely FDG-avid left hypopharyngeal mass. Patient was treated with concurrent chemoradiation. The follow-up PET/CT demonstrated no recurrence at the primary site but an FDG-avid lung metastasis in the right upper lobe

specificity in detecting locoregional residual cancer, distant metastases, or secondary tumors. In practice, many clinicians perform the first surveillance FDG PET scan 8–12 weeks posttherapy to reduce the rate of false-positive findings.

The appropriate length of follow-up after the patient has undergone curative therapy is as yet unclear and there currently exist no data in the literature specifically addressing optimal length of radiologic surveillance using FDG PET imaging. In our institution, patients are followed up every 6 months with a PET/CT for the first 2 years after primary treatment as more than 90% of the progression in head and neck SCC occur during this period. Since HNSCC patients have a high incidence of developing non head and neck malignancies and distant metastasis (especially for patients with stage III or IV), FDG PET/CT is essential in follow-up to identify these second primary tumors and distant metastases (Fig. 7).

7 Prognosis

Features, such as TNM stage and histology, are predictive of outcome in patients with HNSCC. With increasing use of functional imaging in the initial staging of patient with HNC, there has been increasing interest in the utilization of FDG PET parameters, such as the standardized uptake value (SUV), a semiquantitiave measure of tumor FDG uptake, in determining prognosis. The SUV in the primary lesion at the time of diagnosis has, in fact, been shown to predict locoregional control and disease-free survival in patients with HNSCC. Machtay et al. (2009) examined HNSCC patients treated with either chemotherapy or radiation therapy and found that SUV prognosis remained a predictor of disease-free survival, independent of patient age and tumor stage.

There is increasing interest in the utilization of volumetric parameters in both treatment planning and predicting patient outcome. Furthermore, functional rather than anatomic parameters in tumor volume delineation may be superior in predicting prognosis. Incorporation of metabolic parameters has the potential to significantly improve determination of true lesion volume while also taking into account variability within the tumor itself. In several types of malignancies, including HNC, metabolic tumor volume (MTV), a volumetric parameter of FDG PET, has emerged as a highly prognostic factor for overall survival and local control of disease. Murphy et al. (2011) in a study including patients status postradiation therapy for head and neck cancer, comparison of multivariate analysis of MTV, maximum SUV and integrated tumor volume showed that the most robust predictor of disease progression and death was MTV. La et al. (2009) found that, even after controlling for Karnofsky performance status, an increase in MTV was significantly associated with an increased risk of recurrence or death. FDG PET/CT primary metabolic tumor has also been demonstrated to add value to AJCC staging in predicting the prognosis of oral and oropharyngeal patients (Dibble et al. 2011).

8 Thyroid Cancers

The prevalence of palpable thyroid nodules is approximately 5% in women and 1% in men living in iodine-sufficient parts of the world. Differentiated thyroid cancer (DTC), which includes papillary and follicular cancer, comprises the vast majority (90%) of all thyroid cancers. Medullary thyroid cancer (MTC) accounts for 5% of all thyroid cancers, but represents 13.4% of deaths attributed to thyroid cancer. Anaplastic thyroid cancer (ATC) is one of the most aggressive and lethal solid tumors known to affect humans. ATC along with other undifferentiated thyroid cancers account for only 1–1.5% of thyroid malignancies (Nanni et al. 2006).

In clinical practice it is well known that the whole body scan (WBS) with I-131 is more sensitive for localizing recurrent or metastatic disease when TSH levels are elevated, either as the result of withdrawal of thyroid hormone-replacement therapy or the administration of exogenous recombinant human TSH (rhTSH) (Abraham and Schoder 2011). It has also been suggested that when used in combination, ^{18}F-FDG PET and I-131 WBS may result in tumor foci being missed in as few as 7% of cases, suggesting a complementary role for the two imaging modalities (Conti et al. 1999; Grunwald et al. 1997).

PET with FDG has been able to improve the diagnostic work-up of patients when iodine scan is negative and serum Tg increased (Grunwald et al. 1997). Several studies on ^{18}F-FDG PET evaluated patients with negative radioiodine scintigraphy and an increase of serum Tg levels after radical treatment. FDG PET turned out to be accurate in this situation, and sensitivities and specificities range between 85% and 94% (Grunwald et al. 1997). This has been attributed to the fact that less-differentiated thyroid cancers lose the ability to concentrate iodine, due to disruption of the sodium iodide symporter, and tend to utilize more glucose. It has been demonstrated that the sensitivity of ^{18}F-FDG PET is higher when performed with TSH stimulation (Chin et al. 2004).

Attempts to identify patients at highest risk of death and to localize their disease with FDG PET have been made. Consistent with FDG uptake being a marker of more aggressive tumor dedifferentiation, Pryma et al. (2006) reported that each increase in intensity by SUV_{max} unit was associated with a 6% increase in mortality among patients with Hürthle cell carcinoma (HTC). The 5-year overall survival in patients with an SUV_{max} of less than 10 was 92%, whereas it declined to 64% in those with SUV_{max} greater than 10.

PET examination of patients with MTC is performed at least 2 months after initial treatment, when tumor markers are usually elevated and conventional imaging modalities are either negative or inconclusive to detect recurrent or metastatic disease. A study conducted by Seng Ong et al. (2007) focused on MTC demonstrated a sensitivity of 62% for ^{18}F-FDG PET in patients with elevated calcitonin levels and suspected residual, recurrent or metastatic MTC. However, the sensitivity for lesion detection was 78% when the calcitonin level was greater than 1,000 pg (Ong et al. 2007). In contrast to prior studies, Ong et al. specifically investigated and attempted to quantify the relationship between ^{18}F-FDG PET positivity and serum calcitonin. The results suggested that ^{18}F-FDG PET rarely detects disease in patients with calcitonin levels below 500 pg/ml.

Staging and re-staging of anaplastic carcinoma shows intense FDG uptake, and in selected cases FDG PET may be helpful in directing treatment and evaluating the efficacy of therapy. Data from the Mayo Clinic confirm this clinical impression. In a study of 16 patients with anaplastic thyroid cancer, all primary tumors showed intense FDG uptake, as well as all nine patients with lymph node metastases and the majority (7/10) of patients with distant metastases. PET findings had a direct impact on patient management in 50% of cases. Similar findings were reported by Poisson et al. from the Institute Gustave Roussy (Poisson et al. 2010). Metastatic disease was shown by FDG PET/CT or DCT in 63 organs in 18 of 20 evaluable patients. In 35% of involved organs, disease was shown only by FDG scan (Poisson et al. 2010). PET/CT findings changed patient management in 25% of cases. Of note, although the prognosis is generally poor in ATC, even in this group of patients, a high volume of FDG positive disease (300 ml) and an SUV_{max} of 18 or more identified patients with shorter survival (Abraham and Schoder 2011).

9 Novel Radiotracers and Head and Neck Oncology

9.1 3′-Deoxy-3′-^{18}F-Fluorothymidine

^{18}F-Fluorothymidine (^{18}F-FLT) has emerged as a noninvasive approach to image tumor cell proliferation, as uptake of this tracer occurs in cells undergoing active proliferation and DNA synthesis. Early studies by Been et al. (2009) compared this tracer to FDG PET scans in patient with primary laryngeal cancer. While uptake of ^{18}F-FDG was significantly higher than ^{18}F-FLT in these patients, the tumor to background ratios were similar. Furthermore, while ^{18}F-FDG was more sensitive in detecting disease recurrence in this small cohort, ^{18}F-FLT yielded fewer false positives. In monitoring response to radiation therapy, Troost et al. (2010) demonstrated that signal changes in ^{18}F-FLT actually precede volumetric tumor response. The authors compared scans of 10 oropharyngeal cancers before treatment and then twice more during radiotherapy and found FLT to be suitable for evaluation of early treatment response. However, other studies have expressed concerns over the accuracy of FLT in the detection of nodal metastasis. In a series of 10 patients with squamous cell carcinoma of the head and neck, Troost et al. found that FLT tends to accumulate in nonmetastatic lymph nodes, due to reactive B-lymphocyte proliferation.

9.2 ^{18}F-Fluoromisonidazole

While FDG PET is based on tumor glucose metabolism, ^{18}F-Fluoromisonidazole (FMISO) correlates with tumor hypoxia, a variable that has been associated with tumor resistance to treatment. The prospect of noninvasive imaging predicting treatment outcomes has been greatly anticipated. One early testament to the great potential of FMISO was a study performed by Dammann et al. (2005) in which a cohort of 26 advanced head and neck cancer patients were evaluated with FMISO before radiation treatment. Differences in FMISO SUVs, tumor-to-muscle ratios, tumor-to-mediastinum ratios, and accumulation-type curves were demonstrated between patients with and without postradiotherapy disease recurrence. Rischin et al. (2006) found that in patients treated with a standard chemotherapy regimen for HNSCC of cisplatin and infusional fluorouracil, tumor hypoxia on FMISO PET imaging was associated with a high risk of locoregional failure. These results suggest that FMISO may be predictive of incomplete treatment response, which may have implications for future management decisions. However, there are conflicting data as to the correlation of tumor hypoxia as detected by FMISO PET/CT. In a prospective study, Lee et al. (2009) found that, in patients with advanced head and neck cancer treated with concurrent platinum-based chemotherapy and IMRT, excellent locoregional control was achieved despite evidence of detectable hypoxia on the pretreatment FMISO PET/CT scans in 18 of the 20 patients studied. Neither presence nor absence of hypoxia correlated with patient outcome.

Some studies suggest that FMISO has the potential to add valuable information to therapy planning. Hendrickson et al. (2011) found that combined FMISO PET imaging and IMRT planning can allow delivery of higher radiation doses to hypoxic regions, increasing the predicted tumor control without increasing complications.

10 Limitations and Pitfalls

While the SUV has been shown to be accurate in predicting outcome in patients with head and neck cancer, the SUV is limited by a certain amount of variability as it is influenced by factors such as weight, plasma glucose level, incubation time, partial volume effect, and reconstruction algorithm. In addition, pitfalls arise when using SUV cutoff values to diagnose malignancy in the head and neck. Proposed threshold values for discriminating benign from malignant uptake in the literature range from 2.5 to 3.9. Using SUV cutoff values to diagnose head and neck malignancies is difficult as the amount of benign hypermetabolism, especially in the area of Waldeyer's ring, can vary greatly, often with SUVs that exceed cutoff values for diagnosing malignancy.

11 Conclusions

PET/CT has utility in the initial staging, therapy planning, and surveillance of patient with HNSCC. Accurate staging and early detection of recurrence in patients with head and neck malignancies is essential to assure locoregional control and to plan the therapeutic approach. Detection of metastatic spread can spare patients' overly aggressive treatments and improve quality of life. Functional imaging with FDG PET/CT is effective in primary tumor delineation, improves accuracy of nodal staging when compared to conventional cross sectional modalities such as CT or MRI, and has become the modality of choice for staging of patients with advanced HNSCC.

In the assessment of unknown primary tumors of the head and neck, FDG PET/CT cannot replace conventional workup, but may be a valuable adjunct in evaluating these patients. In radiation treatment planning, incorporation of FDG PET adds significantly to CT- and physical examination-based GTV definition. Radiologic surveillance after therapy allows for early and accurate detection of recurrent disease as well as early recognition of second primary. FDG PET/CT is the modality of choice for surveillance of patients with HNSCC. In predicting prognosis, SUV in the primary lesion at the time of diagnosis has been shown to predict locoregional control and disease-free survival in patients with HNSCC, independent of patient age. MTV, a volumetric parameter of FDG PET, has recently emerged as a highly prognostic factor for overall survival and local control of disease. FDG PET/CT plays a crucial role in detecting iodine-negative thyroid cancer metastasis and in the prognosis of these patients. FLT uptake occurs in cells undergoing active proliferation and DNA synthesis and use of this tracer may have promise in detection of tumor cell proliferation. Tumor hypoxia, a variable associated with tumor resistance to treatment, as imaged on FMISO PET may predict locoregional failure and may be useful in radiotherapy planning.

References

Abraham T, Schoder H (2011) Thyroid cancer—indications and opportunities for positron emission tomography/computed tomography imaging. Semin Nucl Med 41(2):121–138

Andrade RS, Heron DE, Degirmenci B et al (2006) Posttreatment assessment of response using FDG-PET/CT for patients treated with definitive radiation therapy for head and neck cancers. Int J Radiat Oncol Biol Phys 65(5):1315–1322

Been LB, Hoekstra HJ, Suurmeijer AJ, Jager PL, van der Laan BF, Elsinga PH (2009) [18F]FLT-PET and [18F]FDG-PET in the evaluation of radiotherapy for laryngeal cancer. Oral Oncol 45(12):e211–e215

Chin BB, Patel P, Cohade C, Ewertz M, Wahl R, Ladenson P (2004) Recombinant human thyrotropin stimulation of fluoro-D-glucose positron emission tomography uptake in well-differentiated thyroid carcinoma. J Clin Endocrinol Metab 89(1):91–95

Clavien PA, Heinrich S, Goerres GW et al (2005) Positron emission tomography/computed tomography influences on the management of resectable pancreatic cancer and its cost-effectiveness. Ann Surg 242(2):235–243

Conti PS, Durski JM, Bacqai F, Grafton ST, Singer PA (1999) Imaging of locally recurrent and metastatic thyroid cancer with positron emission tomography. Thyroid 9(8):797–804

Dammann F, Horger M, Mueller-Berg M et al (2005) Rational diagnosis of squamous cell carcinoma of the head and neck region: comparative evaluation of CT, MRI, and 18FDG PET. AJR Am J Roentgenol 184(4):1326–1331

Dibble E, Lara Alvarez A, Truong M, Mercier G, Cook E, Subramaniam R (2011) FDG Metabolic tumor volume and total glycolytic activity: prognostic imaging biomarkers of oral and oropharyngeal squamous cell cancers. J Nucl Med (in press)

Dong MJ, Zhao K, Lin XT, Zhao J, Ruan LX, Liu ZF (2008) Role of fluorodeoxyglucose-PET versus fluorodeoxyglucose-PET/computed tomography in detection of unknown primary tumor: a meta-analysis of the literature. Nucl Med Commun 29(9):791–802

Grunwald F, Menzel C, Bender H et al (1997) Comparison of 18FDG-PET with 131iodine and 99mTc-sestamibi scintigraphy in differentiated thyroid cancer. Thyroid 7(3): 327–335

Haerle SK, Schmid DT, Ahmad N, Hany TF, Stoeckli SJ (2011) The value of (18)F-FDG PET/CT for the detection of distant metastases in high-risk patients with head and neck squamous cell carcinoma. Oral Oncol 47 (7):653–659

Hendrickson K, Phillips M, Smith W, Peterson L, Krohn K, Rajendran J (2011) Hypoxia imaging with [F-18] FMISO-PET in head and neck cancer: Potential for guiding intensity modulated radiation therapy in overcoming hypoxia-induced treatment resistance. Radiother Oncol 101(3):369–375

La TH, Filion EJ, Turnbull BB et al (2009) Metabolic tumor volume predicts for recurrence and death in head-and-neck cancer. Int J Radiat Oncol Biol Phys 74(5):1335–1341

Lee N, Nehmeh S, Schoder H et al (2009) Prospective trial incorporating pre-/mid-treatment [18F]-misonidazole positron emission tomography for head-and-neck cancer patients undergoing concurrent chemoradiotherapy. Int J Radiat Oncol Biol Phys 75(1):101–108

Machtay M, Natwa M, Andrel J et al (2009) Pretreatment FDG-PET standardized uptake value as a prognostic factor for outcome in head and neck cancer. Head Neck 31(2): 195–201

Murphy JD, Chisholm KM, Daly ME et al (2011) Correlation between metabolic tumor volume and pathologic tumor volume in squamous cell carcinoma of the oral cavity. Radiother Oncol

Nanni C, Zamagni E, Farsad M et al (2006) Role of 18F-FDG PET/CT in the assessment of bone involvement in newly diagnosed multiple myeloma: preliminary results. Eur J Nucl Med Mol Imaging 33(5):525–531

Ong SC, Schoder H, Patel SG et al (2007) Diagnostic accuracy of 18F-FDG PET in restaging patients with medullary thyroid carcinoma and elevated calcitonin levels. J Nucl Med 48(4):501–507

Poisson T, Deandreis D, Leboulleux S et al (2010) 18F-fluorodeoxyglucose positron emission tomography and computed tomography in anaplastic thyroid cancer. Eur J Nucl Med Mol Imaging 37(12):2277–2285

Pryma DA, Schoder H, Gonen M, Robbins RJ, Larson SM, Yeung HW (2006) Diagnostic accuracy and prognostic value of 18F-FDG PET in Hurthle cell thyroid cancer patients. J Nucl Med 47(8):1260–1266

Rischin D, Hicks RJ, Fisher R et al (2006) Prognostic significance of [18F]-misonidazole positron emission tomography-detected tumor hypoxia in patients with advanced head and neck cancer randomly assigned to chemoradiation with or without tirapazamine: a substudy of Trans-Tasman Radiation Oncology Group Study 98.02. J Clin Oncol 24(13):2098–2104

Rusthoven K, Koshy M, Paulino A (2004) The role of fluorodeoxyglucose positron emission tomography in cervical lymph node metastases from an unknown primary tumor. Cancer 101(11):2641–2649

Schwartz DL, Ford E, Rajendran J et al (2005) FDG-PET/CT imaging for preradiotherapy staging of head-and-neck squamous cell carcinoma. Int J Radiat Oncol Biol Phys 61(1):129–136

Troost EG, Bussink J, Hoffmann AL, Boerman OC, Oyen WJ, Kaanders JH (2010). 18F-FLT PET/CT for early response monitoring and dose escalation in oropharyngeal tumors. J Nucl Med 51(6):866–874

Chest

Rathan M. Subramaniam, J. M. Davison, D. S. Surasi, G. Russo, and P. J. Peller

Contents

R. M. Subramaniam · J. M. Davison · D. S. Surasi
Boston University School of Medicine,
Boston, MA 02118, USA

P. J. Peller
Department of Radiology, Mayo Clinic College of Medicine,
200 First Street SW, Rochester, MN 55901, USA

G. Russo
Department of Radiation Oncology, Boston University
School of Medicine, 3rd Floor, Boston, MA 02118, USA

R. M. Subramaniam (✉)
Russell H Morgan Department of Radiology and
Radiological Sciences Institutions,
The Johns Hopkins Medical,
601 N. Caroline Street/ JHOC 3235,
Baltimore, MD 21287, USA
e-mail: rsubram4@jhmi.edu

Abstract

FDG PET/CT has become the standard-of care for staging, therapy assessment and follow-up of patients with lung cancers. It improves the staging, provides a road map for selective invasive mediastinal nodal biopsy and surgical planning (especially contrast-enhanced PET/CT) and accurately identifies distant metastasis. It improves the tumor delineation for radiation therapy planning by identifying tumor from atelectasis and involved mediastinal nodes. The maximum SUV of lung tumor correlates strongly with patient outcome. It is the modality of choice for identifying distant metastasis and valuable in loco-regional nodal staging for malignant pleural tumors.

1 Introduction

Worldwide, thoracic malignancies are the most common cause of cancer mortality for both men and women with approximately 1.2 million deaths per year attributable to lung cancer alone (Jemal et al. 2009). Cigarette smoking is the primary risk factor in the development of cancers within the chest and is

P. Peller et al. (eds.), *PET-CT and PET-MRI in Oncology*, Medical Radiology. Diagnostic Imaging,
DOI: 10.1007/174_2011_421, © Springer-Verlag Berlin Heidelberg 2012

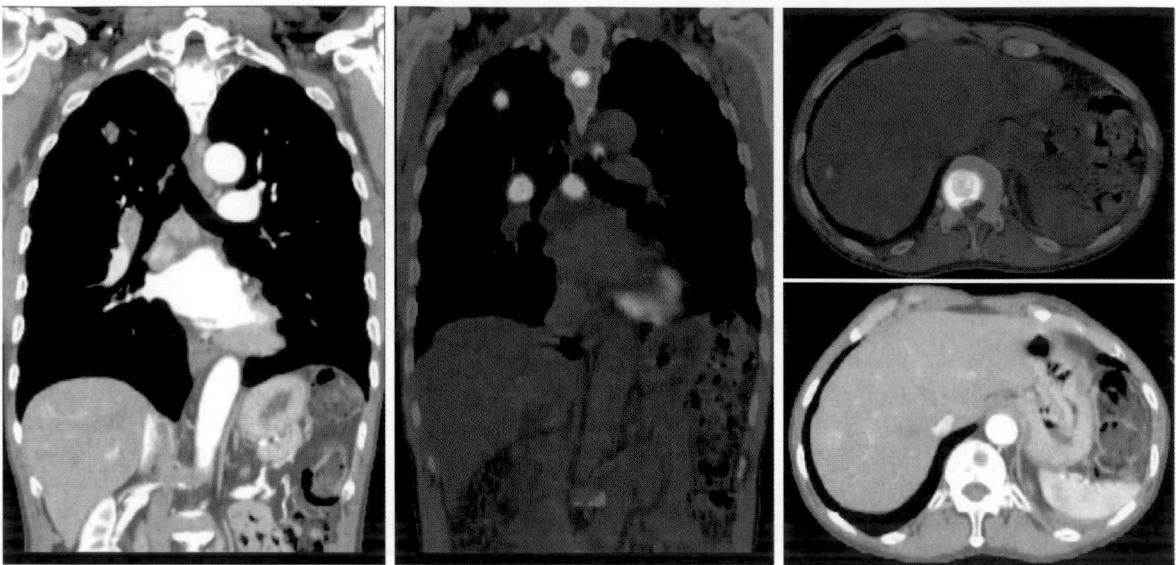

Fig. 1 *Dedicated contrast-enhanced PET/CT*. Anatomic and metabolic information is provided by a single dedicated contrast-enhanced PET/CT of a 54-year-old man with a hypermetabolic right upper lobe tumor, mediastinal nodal disease, and distant skeletal and hepatic metastases. The patient underwent chemotherapy for stage IV NSCLC

estimated to account for 90% of all lung cancers (Jemal et al. 2009). Other risk factors include exposure to asbestos, polycyclic aromatic hydrocarbons, nickel, radon gas, and arsenic. The frequency of lung cancer rose dramatically in the last century, emerging as the most common cause of cancer deaths in men in the 1950s (Jemal et al. 2008). As more women began to smoke, lung cancer death rates in women also began to rise, and by 1985 lung cancer had become the leading cause of cancer deaths in women (Jemal et al. 2008). With decreases in the smoking rate, lung cancer incidence rates and death rates have decreased among men in all age groups since 1990 (Jemal et al. 2008). The rise in the death rate in women continued after 1990, and only recently appears to have reached a plateau (Jemal et al. 2008). Almost 50% of all lung cancer deaths now occur in women (Jemal et al. 2008).

2 Thoracic PET/CT Protocols

2.1 Non-Contrast Enhanced PET/CT

Routine PET/CT scan for evaluation of lung cancer is performed from skull base to midthigh with arms up and without intravenous contrast. A full inspiration chest CT for detailed evaluation of lung parenchyma often follows this. PET scans are usually done using 3D imaging with emission scans that range from 2 to 4 min with a field of view (FOV) of 50 cm. The CT scans are obtained to match the PET scans' FOV and slice thickness. The low dose CT scan is only for attenuation correction and lesion localization of the PET data. Attenuation correction CT scans use a 512 × 512 matrix. The pitch is approximately 1.75 and collimation is 10 mm. Slices are reconstructed at 3.75 mm thickness and with 3.27 mm spacing. The X-ray beam is set at 120 kV and the mAs is modulated.

2.2 Contrast-Enhanced Dedicated PET/CT

The purpose of a contrast-enhanced dedicated CT is to provide the anatomical details needed for surgical resection and metabolic information about the lung tumor and staging in the same setting. It has the advantage of an integrated information flow to the physicians but requires dual expertise in interpreting contrast-enhanced CT and fluorodeoxyglucose (FDG) PET (Fig. 1). High dose CT scans are similar to low dose scans except for the use of oral and intravenous contrast material and higher X-ray dose. A total of 100 cc of Optiray 320 (Covidien, Dublin, Ireland) is given by intravenous injection at a rate of 3 cc/s, followed by a saline chase of 30 cc at the same rate. The SmartPrep (GE Healthcare, Milwaukee) is used to trigger imaging once the celiac trunk reaches a density of 180–200 Hounsfield units (HU).

3 Solitary Pulmonary Nodule

A solitary pulmonary nodule (SPN) is defined as a single, well-defined pulmonary opacity with a diameter of <3 cm surrounded by normal lung tissue that is not associated with atelectasis or adenopathy. Approximately 30–50% of solitary pulmonary nodules are malignant. Accurate and efficient diagnostic evaluation of SPNs facilitates prompt resection of malignant tumors when curative removal is possible. Invasive procedures, which allow histologic evaluation of SPNs, include fiber-optic bronchoscopy, transthoracic needle-aspiration biopsy, video-assisted thoracoscopy, video-assisted thorascopic surgery, or thoracotomy. These procedures are associated with high costs and morbidity. SPNs are also evaluated noninvasively with chest radiography, CT, MRI, and PET. Observation with serial chest radiographs avoids unnecessary surgery in cases of benign disease but can delay diagnosis and treatment when malignancy is present. In most cases, benign lesions meet the following criteria: central, concentric calcifications, round, or no nodule growth on CT after 2 years of observation (Gurney and Swensen 1995). Malignant features of a nodule typically include poorly demarcated borders, eccentric appearance, spiculated pattern, and a doubling time of less than 10 months (Gurney and Swensen 1995). CT provides excellent anatomic and morphologic information and can confirm whether a lesion is truly solitary, but it is frequently indeterminate, failing to differentiate benign from malignant nodules (Swensen et al. 2003).

FDG PET/CT appears to be an accurate, noninvasive imaging test for the characterization of SPNs (Fig. 2). Due to increased metabolism, malignant tissues typically demonstrate higher FDG uptake than both benign lesions and normal tissue. One meta-analysis reported a pooled sensitivity and specificity of 96.8 and 77.8% respectively for the characterization of SPNs (Gould et al. 2001). However, this systematic review was weakened by including studies with small sample sizes, incomplete masking, and biased patient selection. To address the limitations of previous studies, the Solitary Nodule Accuracy Project (SNAP), a prospective study conducted at 10 Veterans Administration hospitals nationwide in the United States, compared the accuracy of PET and CT in the characterization of pulmonary nodules ranging in size from 7 to 30 mm (Fletcher et al. 2008). In this study, sensitivity, and specificity were estimated for each level of diagnostic confidence (definitely benign, probably benign, indeterminate, probably malignant, and definitely malignant) (Fletcher et al. 2008). The authors found that PET had a sensitivity of 91.7% in the characterization of SPNs, which was similar to CT with 95.6% sensitivity (Fletcher et al. 2008). However, PET had superior specificity when compared to CT, with a specificity of 82.3% but only 40.2% for CT (Fletcher et al. 2008). Nodules that were described as probably or definitely benign were strongly associated with a benign final diagnosis regardless of imaging modality. However, definitely malignant results on PET were much more predictive of malignancy than were these results on CT. Receiver-operating characteristic (ROC) analysis yielded an area under the curve of 0.93 (95% CI, 0.90–0.95) for PET and 0.82 (95% CI, 0.77–0.86) for CT, confirming that PET is more accurate than CT (Fletcher et al. 2008). PET demonstrated better inter- and intra-observer variability than CT (Fletcher et al. 2008).

4 Non-Small Cell Lung Cancer (NSCLC)

Non-small cell lung cancers (NSCLC) comprise 80% of malignant lung tumors. NSCLCs are a heterogeneous group of neoplasms including adenocarcinoma, squamous cell carcinoma (SCC), and large cell lung carcinoma. Twenty percent of lung cancers are small cell lung cancers (SCLC). Centrally located tumors are generally squamous cell carcinomas or small cell carcinomas and most commonly present with cough, dyspnea, atelectasis, postobstructive pneumonia, wheezing, and hemoptysis. Peripheral tumors are usually adenocarcinomas or large cell carcinomas and in addition to cough and dyspnea, can cause pleural effusion and severe pleuritic chest pain due to infiltration of the parietal pleura and chest wall. Adenocarcinomas tend to develop peripherally and may not be symptomatic until extrathoracic metastases have developed. In this setting, they may present with signs

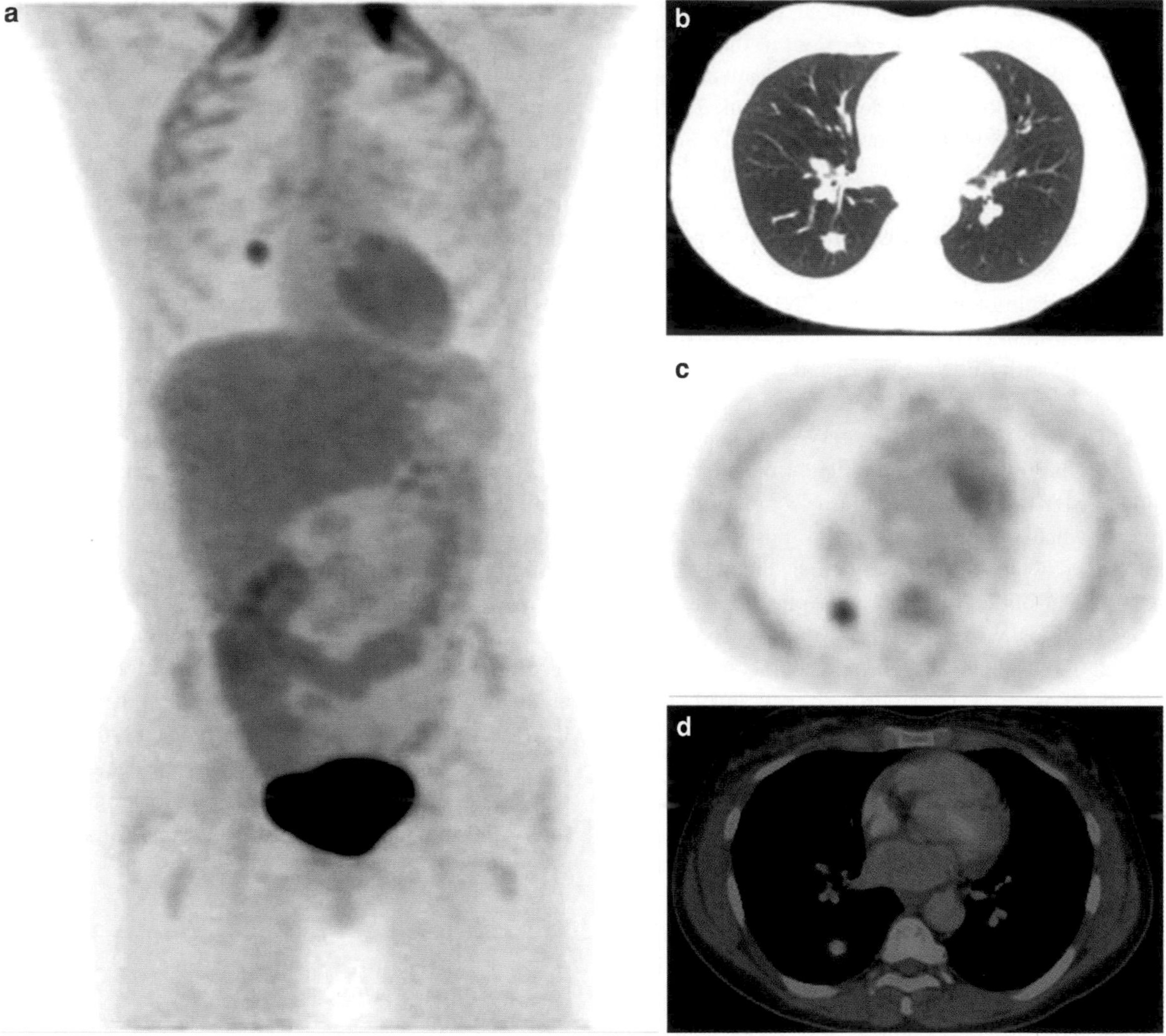

Fig. 2 *Evaluation of a pulmonary nodule*. Maximum intensity projection **a** and transaxial CT **b**, PET **c**, and fused images **d**. This patient is a 53-year-old woman with a history of smoking for 15 years, with a CT showing the interval increase in the size of a right lower lobe pulmonary nodule to 1.3 cm. PET/CT images demonstrate increased FDG uptake in the nodule with an SUVmax of 5.7. Pathology at biopsy was consistent with non-small cell lung carcinoma. Since she was a poor surgical candidate, she received Cyberknife stereotactic radiosurgery-56 Gy in 4 fractions. There was a dramatic reduction in the metabolic activity and size of the tumor within a month following completion of treatment

of osteolytic bone lesions or intracranial metastatic disease.

4.1 Diagnosis

CT plays a limited but important role in the initial evaluation of patients with pulmonary lesions. It provides morphologic information regarding the extent of disease, but it is not very good at differentiating benign from malignant lesions at the primary site or in the lymph nodes. Compared to conventional imaging, whole-body FDG PET has a higher rate of detection of mediastinal lymph node metastases and of extrathoracic metastases (Dwamena et al. 1999; Pieterman et al. 2000; Steinert et al. 1997; Al-Sugair and Coleman 1998). Furthermore, integrated PET/CT has better diagnostic accuracy than CT alone, PET alone, or visual correlation of PET and CT (Lardinois et al. 2003). Integrated PET-CT also has a high level of reliability in identifying hilar lymph nodes, mediastinal lymph nodes, and supraclavicular lymph nodes, and providing precise information on chest wall or mediastinal invasion (Lardinois et al. 2003). Pulmonary malignancies generally are differentiated from benign lesions by greater metabolic activity than the mediastinum (Patz et al. 1993). For solid pulmonary lesions with low uptake, semiquantitative approaches (using a maximum standardized uptake value (SUV) cutoff of 2.5) do not improve the accuracy of FDG PET over visual analysis (Hashimoto et al. 2006). Hashimoto et al. (2006) found that using faint visual uptake as the cutoff for positive FDG PET results, receiver-operating-characteristic (ROC) analysis yielded a sensitivity of 100% and specificity of 63%. When an SUVmax of 1.59 was used as the threshold for positive results, FDG PET had 81% sensitivity and 85% specificity according to ROC analysis. Thus, lack of visible uptake in pulmonary lesions indicates that the probability of malignancy is very low.

4.2 Staging

Tumor, node, and metastasis (TNM) staging plays an important role in determining prognosis and choosing a treatment strategy. Multimodality treatment of NSCLC is common, with surgery, chemotherapy, and radiotherapy alone, concurrently, or in an adjuvant or neoadjuvant setting (Chansky et al. 2009; Nestle et al. 2006). Complete surgical resection offers the best opportunity for long-term survival and cure in patients with early stage NSCLC, assuming that the patients are fit to undergo such a procedure. The standard-of-care for patients with stage I and II cancers is a lobectomy or pneumonectomy, with some patients receiving additional neoadjuvant or adjuvant chemotherapy and/or radiation therapy depending on risk factors and characteristics of the cancer. Patients who are not fit for surgery—usually due to poor pulmonary reserve—are often treated with alternative therapies such as radiofrequency ablation, stereotactic body radiation therapy, or subanatomic surgical resection (e.g. wedge resection or anatomic segmentectomy). Patients with stage III disease often are not considered appropriate candidates for surgery and are treated primarily with chemoradiotherapy. Some patients with stage IIIA disease may be treated with neoadjuvant chemoradiotherapy followed by surgical resection.

Chansky et al. (2009) assessed the prognostic impact of pathologic stage, age, gender, and specific histologic cell type on surgically managed stage I-IIIA NSCLC cases from the international staging database of the International Association for the Study of Lung Cancer. This study confirmed that age and gender are important prognostic factors in surgically resected NSCLC (Chansky et al. 2009). Pathologic TNM category is the most important prognostic factor (Chansky et al. 2009).

4.3 T Stage

Tumor designation (T) is based on tumor size, involvement of contiguous structures, and the presence or absence of satellite nodules (Goldstraw et al. 2007). While T1–T3 tumors are potentially resectable, many T4 tumors are considered inoperable (Goldstraw et al. 2007). Primary tumor extension with NSCLC is usually evaluated with thoracic CT. MRI is commonly used to evaluate tumors extending to the superior sulcus; involvement of the brachial plexus helps determines resectability. MRI is also used with centrally located tumors (e.g. paramediastinal tumor) where the relationship with the heart or large vessels is of importance (Schrevens et al. 2004). Their superior anatomic detail makes CT and MRI very useful for evaluating the proximity of the tumor to local structures. Precise anatomic localization is limited with PET, due to the lower resolution, and it offers little extra benefit (Schrevens et al. 2004). However, CT and MRI are limited by their reliance solely on morphology for detection of malignancy.

Hybrid FDG PET/CT is becoming the preferred method for noninvasive staging of NSCLC. FDG PET/CT (Fig. 3) can more accurately determine T designation than either PET or CT alone (Lardinois et al. 2003). One meta-analysis found that PET/CT accurately predicted the T stage in patients with NSCLC in 82% of cases compared with 55% for PET alone and 68% for CT alone (De Wever et al. 2007). PET/CT can readily differentiate central tumors from post-obstructive atelectasis because a tumor is more hypermetabolic than an atelectatic lung (De Wever et al. 2007). PET/CT also improves detection of subtle

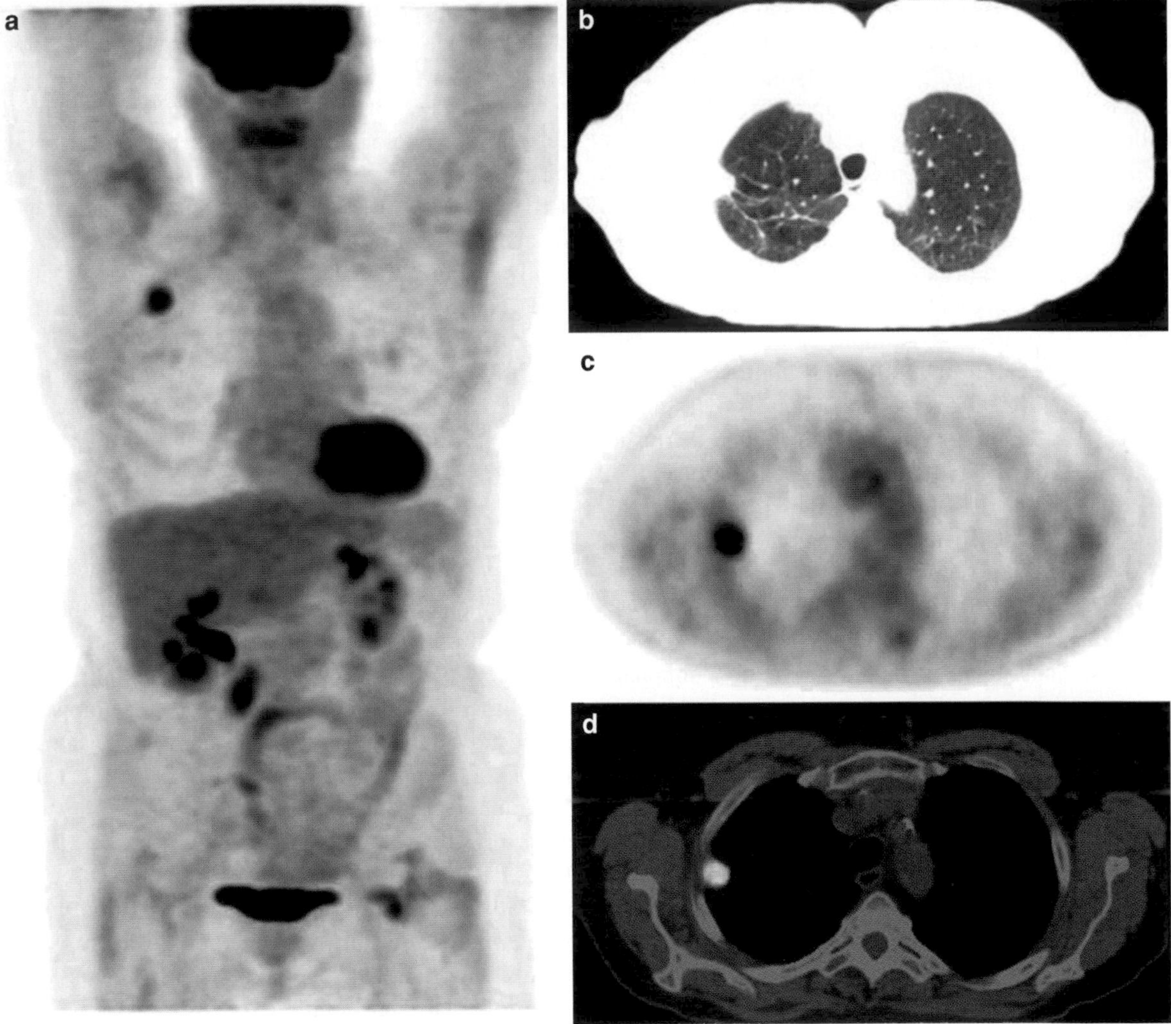

Fig. 3 *Non-small cell lung carcinoma tumor staging*. Maximum intensity projection **a** and transaxial CT **b**, PET **c**, and fused images **d**. This patient is a 64-year-old woman with severe emphysema being followed for nodular scarring in the right upper lobe apex. A recent CT showed a spiculated nodule measuring 1.5 × 1.4 in the right upper lobe. PET and PET/CT images show hypermetabolism in the right upper lobe lesion abutting the pleura with an SUVmax of 8.7, but no evidence of metastasis. A CT-guided biopsy was positive for adenocarcinoma and the patient underwent right upper lobectomy, mediastinal lymph node dissection and chest wall resection which proved to be a Stage IIB (T3N0) moderately differentiated adenocarcinoma. Due to the chest wall involvement, she was given four cycles of adjuvant chemotherapy

areas of invasion into adjacent structures that may not be apparent on CT alone (Halpern et al. 2005).

4.4 N Stage

A principal advantage of FDG PET lies in improved mediastinal staging of NSCLC. In the absence of distant metastases, locoregional lymph node spread will determine therapy and prognosis. While evaluation with CT has been the method of choice in pre-therapeutic lymph node staging of NSCLC (Quint and Francis 1999), use of this modality assumes a correlation between node size and metastatic infiltration. A lymph node with a short-axis diameter >1 cm on conventional imaging methods is considered enlarged and predictive of metastasis. However, diagnosing nodal metastases based on morphological characteristics has limitations

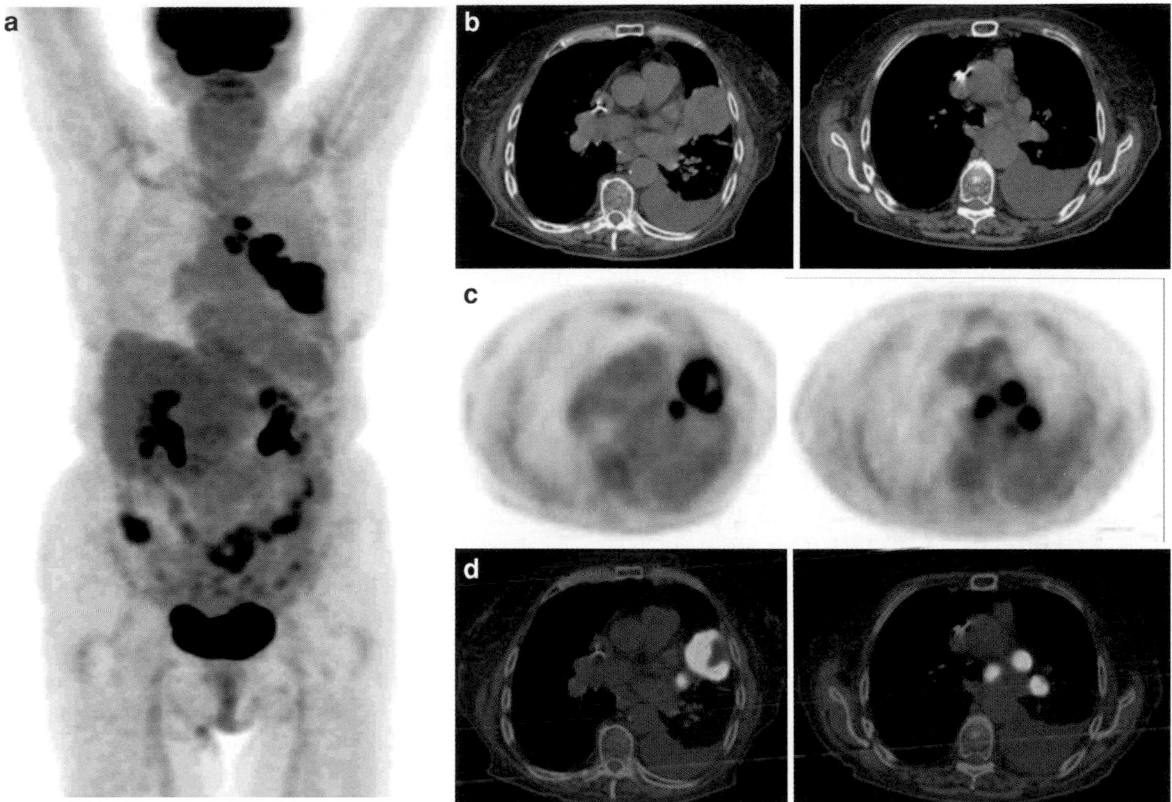

Fig. 4 *Non-small cell lung carcinoma with mediastinal nodal staging*. Maximum intensity projection **a** and transaxial CT **b**, PET **c** and fused images **d**. This 82-year-old woman with 60-year smoking history presented with chest congestion and hemoptysis. On CT, she had a 5.5 cm mass in the lingula of the left upper lobe abutting the mediastinum with gross nodal disease in the left hilar region and the anterior mediastinum. PET/CT images demonstrate an intensely hypermetabolic mass (SUVmax of 17.7) within the lingula and more than 3 cm contact of the tumor to the chest wall suggestive of chest wall invasion. There is FDG uptake in station 4L (*left paratracheal*), 5 (aortopulmonary window), and 10L (*left hilar*) nodes typical for metastatic disease. The left pleural effusion demonstrated no significant FDG uptake

as infectious or inflammatory causes can result in lymph node enlargement. Furthermore, small- or normal-sized nodes, even with a fatty hilum, can contain metastatic deposits leading to misdiagnosis and inaccurate staging with CT (Arita et al. 1996). No statistically significant relationship has been found between the size of the lymph nodes and the likelihood of malignancy (Kerr et al. 1992). Because of the moderate accuracy of CT in detecting metastatic lymph node involvement (Prenzel et al. 2003), invasive staging bronchoscopy or esophageal endoscopy with ultrasound-guided biopsies or mediastinoscopy are often used to assess locoregional lymph node spread (Schrevens et al. 2004).

FDG PET is an effective, noninvasive method for staging thoracic lymph nodes in patients with NSCLC and is superior to CT in the evaluation of hilar and mediastinal nodal metastases (Birim et al. 2005; Graeter et al. 2003; Gould et al. 2003; Halter et al. 2004). FDG PET can also differentiate between patients with N1/N2 disease and those with unresectable N3 disease (Halter et al. 2004). By combining functional and anatomic data, integrated PET/CT significantly increases the number of patients with correctly staged NSCLC and is the best noninvasive method for the detection of nodal metastases (Antoch et al. 2003; Cerfolio et al. 2004) (Fig. 4). Integrated PET/CT has been shown to improve diagnostic accuracy in the assessment of locoregional lymph nodes when compared to contrast-enhanced CT (Yang et al. 2008). Furthermore, integrated PET/CT is more accurate for the detection of total N2 nodes and for total N1 nodes than dedicated PET, more sensitive at the mediastinal stations 4R, 5, 7, 10L, and 11, and more accurate at the 7 and 11 lymph node stations (Cerfolio et al. 2004).

One retrospective study found that, compared to surgical resection, the overall sensitivity, specificity, positive and negative predictive values, and accuracy of PET/CT for detecting metastatic lymph nodes were 54.2, 91.9, 74.3, 82.3, and 80.5% when evaluated on a per-patient basis, and 57.7, 98.5, 74.5, 96.8, and 95.6% on per-nodal-station basis (Bille et al. 2009). The high negative predictive value of PET in mediastinal lymph node staging may allow PET-negative patients to be staged without invasive procedures and to proceed directly to thoracotomy (Graeter et al. 2003; Vansteenkiste et al. 1997), especially patients with T1 disease. Many centers will perform mediastinoscopy immediately prior to thoracotomy, in patients with T2 disease or above.

False-positive findings in regional lymph nodes can be a problem with FDG PET (Cerfolio et al. 2003; Nakamura et al. 2008), particularly in cases of anthracosilicosis, infection, or granulomatous disease (Schrevens et al. 2004; Bille et al. 2009) found that the sensitivity of PET/CT in detecting malignant involvement was 32.4% in nodes less than 10 mm, and 85.3% in nodes greater than or equal to 10 mm. Thus, mediastinoscopy may be necessary to confirm N2 or N3 disease to ensure that no patient with resectable N0 or N1 disease is denied the chance of curative surgery (Schrevens et al. 2004; Nakamura et al. 2008).

Meyers et al. (2006), analyzed the cost-effectiveness of routine mediastinoscopy in patients with stage I lung cancer staged with CT and PET and concluded that such patients benefit little from mediastinoscopy. However, for patients with stage II and III disease, mediastinoscopy is necessary as false positives do occur with PET/CT. Thus, PET/CT does not necessarily obviate the need for mediastinoscopy but can provide anatomical guidance prior to biopsy.

4.5 M Stage

Detection of distant metastases in patients with NSCLC has major implications on management and prognosis. Forty percent of patients with NSCLC have distant metastases at presentation, most commonly in the adrenal glands, bones, liver, or brain (Quint et al. 1996). On initial staging, CT alone can show definitive evidence of metastatic disease in 11–36% of patients (Quint et al. 1996).

4.5.1 Adrenal Metastases

Nearly 10% of NSCLC patients initially present with enlarged adrenal glands as visualized on CT, approximately two-thirds of which are non-malignant (Ettinghausen and Burt 1991). Thus, in a patient with otherwise operable NSCLC, treatment decisions should not be made in the presence of an isolated adrenal mass without pathologic proof of metastatic disease. PET has a high sensitivity (100%) and specificity (80–100%) for the detection of malignant adrenal metastases (Fig. 5) (Erasmus et al. 1997; Marom et al. 1999), which can reduce the number of unnecessary adrenal biopsies. Careful interpretation of PET is required for lesions less than 1 cm, as experience with smaller adrenal lesions is limited (Schrevens et al. 2004). Recently, Brady et al. (2009) developed an algorithm to maximize the diagnostic yield of PET/CT in the identification of adrenal metastases in patients who underwent PET/CT for known or suspected lung cancer. The authors found that a value for the SUV ratio (nodule SUVmax/liver SUVmean) of >2.5 allowed correct identification of 22 of 37 metastatic lesions and exclusion of all FDG-avid benign nodules (Brady et al. 2009). Alternatively, a mean attenuation >10 HU and SUVmax >3.1 had 97.3% sensitivity and 86.2% specificity in correctly identifying adrenal metastases (Brady et al. 2009).

4.5.2 Bone Metastases

For patients with NSCLC, bone involvement previously was assessed by bone scintigraphy, with a sensitivity of 90% (Bury et al. 1998). The specificity of bone scanning is only 60% as false-positive findings occur with non-selective uptake of the radionuclide tracer in any area of increased bone turnover (Bury et al. 1998). Confirmatory imaging by bone X-ray, CT, or MRI is often required. PET has been found to have similar sensitivity to bone scintigraphy but a higher specificity of approximately 98% (Marom et al. 1999; Bury et al. 1998).

FDG PET detection of unexpected metastatic spread is particularly valuable (Fig. 6). Unknown metastases are found with FDG PET in 8–24% of patients with negative conventional imaging (MacManus et al. 2001). The incidence of occult metastatic lesions increases with advancing stage from 8% in stage I, to 18% in stage II, to 24% in stage III (MacManus et al. 2001). If only a single metastatic lesion is detected with FDG PET additional imaging

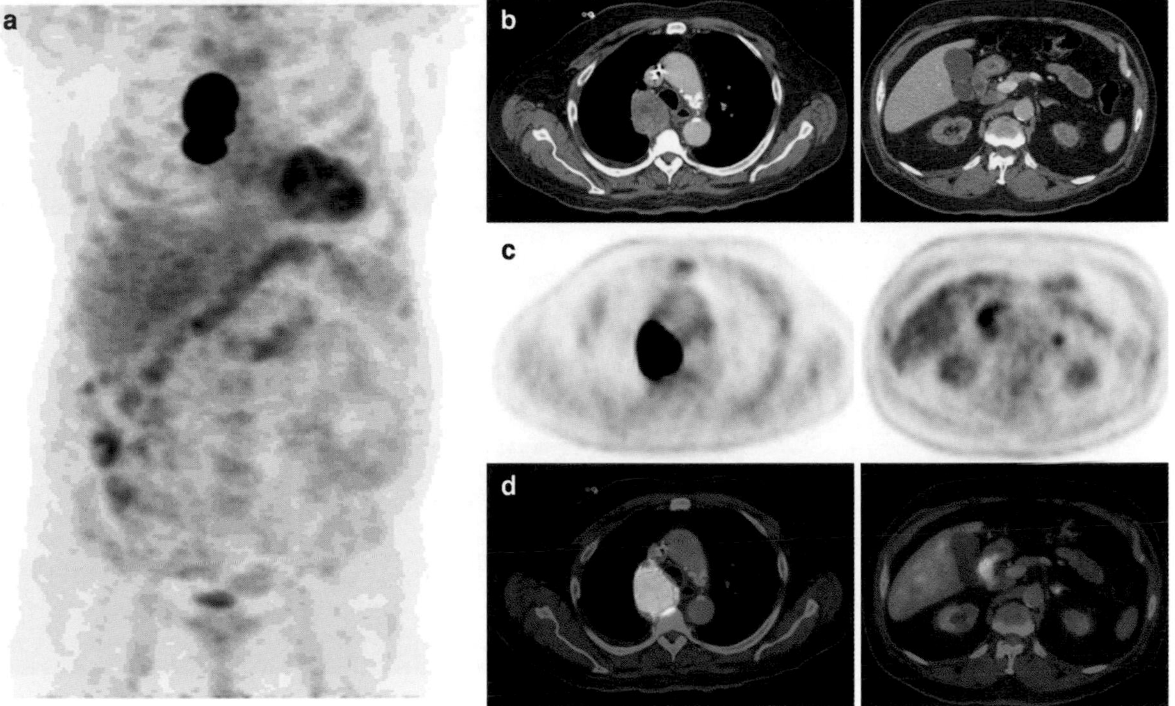

Fig. 5 *Non-small cell lung carcinoma with adrenal metastasis*. Maximum intensity projection **a** and transaxial CT **b**, PET **c**, and fused images **d**. This is an 80-year-old man who initially presented with chest discomfort. On CT, a heterogeneously enhancing 5.4 × 4.7 × 8.2 cm right perihilar mass was noted. PET and PET/CT images demonstrate a large hypermetabolic lung lesion with an SUVmax of 50. A focal region of abnormal radiotracer uptake was noted within the left adrenal gland with an SUVmax of 3.4 which was highly concerning for metastatic disease. Fine needle aspiration of the lung mass confirmed squamous cell carcinoma. Surgery and chemotherapy were not options due to his medical comorbidities, and therefore the patient was treated with radiation therapy

or pathological confirmation is warranted, to avoid a false-positive FDG PET result from preventing surgery with curative intent (MacManus et al. 2001).

4.6 Staging FDG PET/CT and Patient Management

As a single, noninvasive examination, FDG PET/CT from orbits to thighs is an attractive staging tool, due to its overall greater diagnostic accuracy when compared to conventional imaging procedures (Pieterman et al. 2000; Antoch et al. 2003; Hicks et al. 2001a; Brink et al. 2004). Clinical staging is often altered by PET/CT results in patients with NSCLC (Hicks et al. 2001a; Hoekstra et al. 2003; Schmucking et al. 2003). Upstaging is more frequent than down staging and is generally due to the detection of unexpected distant metastases by FDG PET (Brink et al. 2004). PET/CT findings that will alter management occur in 25–52% of NSCLC patients, (Bury et al. 1998; Hicks et al. 2001a; Schmucking et al. 2003; Hoekstra et al. 2002; Saunders et al. 1999).

Van Tinteren et al. (2002) reported a randomized control trial to assess the role of FDG PET in the management of patients in routine clinical practice. In the PET in Lung Cancer Staging study, better known as the PLUS study, patients were evaluated preoperatively with either conventional workup or conventional workup plus PET. The primary outcome measure was futile thoracotomy, defined as thoracotomy in a patient with benign disease, explorative thoracotomy, pathological stage IIIA-N2/IIIB, or postoperative relapse or death within 12 months of randomization. In one out of five patients with suspected NSCLC, adding PET to conventional workup prevented futile thoracotomies (van Tinteren et al. 2002). In a recent randomized study by Fischer et al.

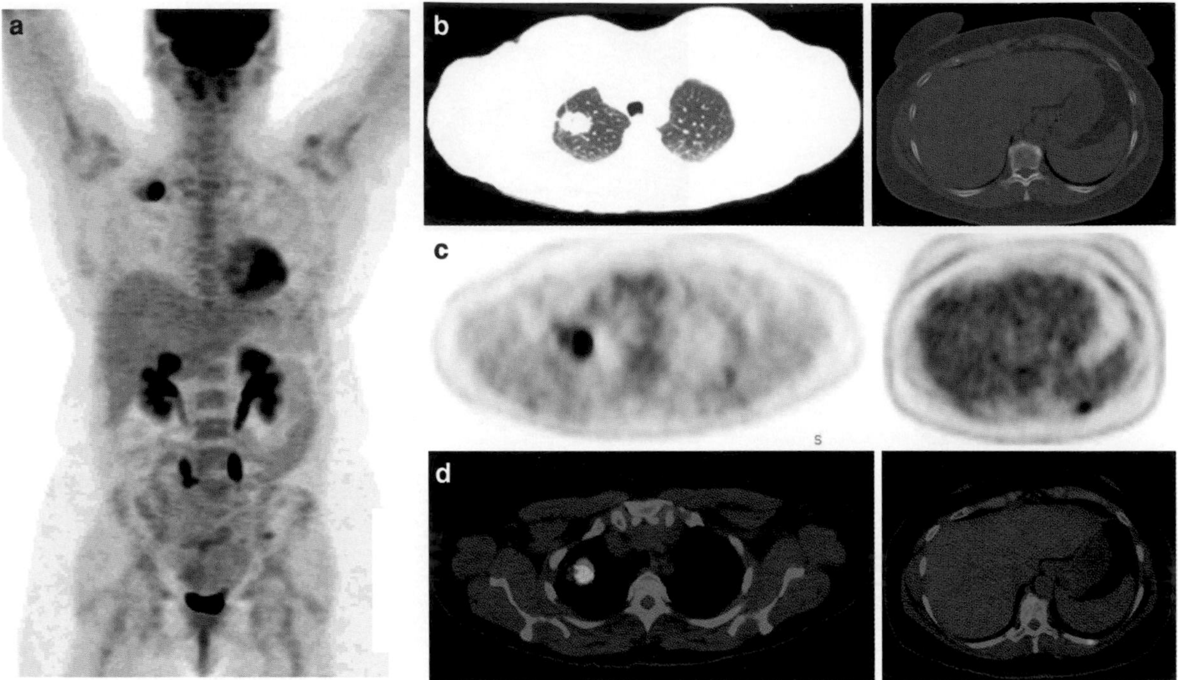

Fig. 6 *Non-small cell lung carcinoma with skeletal metastasis*. Maximum intensity projection **a** and transaxial CT **b**, PET **c**, and fused images **d**. This is a 50-year-old woman with an incidentally discovered right upper lobe nodule during a chest pain workup. The CT, PET, and PET/CT images demonstrate a 3.2 cm mass in the right upper lobe, which is intensely hypermetabolic with an SUVmax of 18.5. A focus of moderate activity was also noted in the posterior left 10th rib with an SUVmax of 4.1 compatible with metastatic disease. A CT-guided core biopsy of the right upper lobe (RUL) lung lesion confirmed adenocarcinoma. Brain MRI revealed four enhancing lesions consistent with metastasis. Stereotactic radiosurgery was planned

(2009), the clinical effect of combined PET/CT on preoperative staging of NSCLC was compared to conventional staging alone (medical history, physical examination, blood test, contrast-enhanced CT scan of the chest and upper abdomen, and bronchoscopy). The authors found that while the number of justified thoracotomies after staging was similar in both groups, the use of PET/CT for preoperative staging of NSCLC reduced both the total number of thoracotomies and the number of futile thoracotomies (Fischer et al. 2009).

4.7 Response to Therapy and Surveillance

NSCLC commonly presents with advanced stage disease and chemotherapy is often integral to treatment. Despite chemotherapy, tumor progression occurs in up to one-third of patients. Early determination of therapeutic failure allows prompt discontinuation of ineffective treatment and initiation of alternative therapies. Image-based serial measurements of tumor size before and after treatment based on recommendations of the World Health Organization (WHO) or Response Evaluation Criteria in Solid Tumors (RECIST) are commonly used to determine response (Wahl et al. 2009). Morphologic alterations on CT do not correlate with pathologic response and tumor viability. Treatment protocols that target tumor biology including tumor cell proliferation and invasion, angiogenesis, and metastasis further complicate objective assessment of response using morphological parameters. The antitumor effect in these regimens can be cytostatic and therefore may not result in a reduction in tumor size. Early and sensitive assessment of anticancer regimen effectiveness may be achieved with PET as FDG uptake is not only a function of proliferative activity but is also related to viable tumor cell number (Duhaylongsod et al. 1995; Higashi et al. 1993).

Recommendations by the European Organization for Research and Treatment of Cancer (EORTC) PET Study Group include patient preparation, timing of scans, and methods to measure FDG uptake, as well as definitions of tumor response (Young et al. 1999). More recently, Positron Emission Response Evaluation Criteria in Solid Tumors (PERCIST) has been proposed for use in clinical trials (Wahl et al. 2009).

Post-therapy assessment with CT or MRI may be complicated by the inability to distinguish persistent or recurrent tumor from necrosis, post-treatment scarring or fibrosis (Frank et al. 1995). FDG PET can detect local tumor recurrence after definitive treatment with surgery, chemotherapy, or radiotherapy with a sensitivity of 98–100% and specificity of 62–92% (Ryu et al. 2002; Inoue et al. 1995; Hicks et al. 2001b; Bury et al. 1999; Hellwig et al. 2006) and months earlier than conventional imaging. In particular, 3D conformal radiotherapy frequently produces opacities on CT, which are difficult to distinguish from tumor recurrence. The inflammatory changes associated with radiation can also result in increased FDG uptake and potential false positives on PET. However, in a study by Hicks et al. (2004), when patients with NSCLC were treated with radical radiotherapy and reevaluated with FDG PET at a median of 70 days after therapy completion, the ability of FDG PET to assess therapeutic response was not confounded by radiation-induced inflammatory changes. In addition, in a pilot study by Kong et al. (2007) a significant reduction in tumor FDG uptake in patients with NSCLC was observed during the course of treatment with fractionated radiotherapy without a significant confounding effect in the surrounding irradiated lung. In this study, radiation-induced hypermetabolism secondary to pneumonitis did not occur during treatment but rather was observed after completion of radiotherapy. This suggests that obtaining an FDG PET scan during treatment with radiotherapy may allow identification of targets for individualized adaptive therapy (Kong et al. 2007).

Determining a favorable response to chemotherapy early in the course of treatment also allows continuation with greater confidence in patients with NCSLC. Prospective studies have shown that, in patients with stage IIIB or IV unresectable NSCLC, restaging FDG PET scans could predict progressive disease after just one cycle of chemotherapy (Lee et al. 2009a, b; Weber et al. 2003). In one study, a fall in the primary tumor SUVmax of >20% was an independent predictor of long-term survival (Weber et al. 2003). Response on FDG PET had a tight correlation with the best response to therapy as determined on serial CT scans according to RECIST and was associated with a higher overall survival (Weber et al. 2003). In a prospective study, a restaging FDG PET showing a decrease in FDG uptake >35% after 1 cycle of induction chemotherapy correlated with increased overall and disease-free survival in patients with locally advanced but potentially resectable stage IIIA N2 NSCLC receiving neoadjuvant chemotherapy (Hoekstra et al. 2005). In this study, FDG PET was better than CT in monitoring response to therapy and enabled a prediction of survival early in therapy (Hoekstra et al. 2005). A currently ongoing multicenter study, ACRIN 6678 (American College of Radiology Imaging Network), is evaluating the value of FDG PET/CT in therapy assessment of stages IIIB and IV NSCLC.

4.8 Prognosis

Several studies suggest PET has a role as a prognostic marker in NSCLC patients. The degree of FDG uptake in the primary lesion at the time of diagnosis is inversely related to survival rate (Ahuja et al. 1998; Higashi et al. 2002; Jeong et al. 2002; Vansteenkiste et al. 1999). Threshold pretreatment FDG PET maximum SUV prognosis used for univariate analysis in the literature range from 3.3 to 20. These cut-off values used to predict prognosis are significantly associated with histological subtype (Casali et al. 2009). Casali et al. determined that patient outcome could be most accurately predicted with a threshold SUVmax of 5 for adenocarcinoma and 10.7 for other non-adenocarcinoma NSCLC subtypes. In one study by Higashi et al. (2002), patients with an SUVmax <5 had a better disease-free survival than did patients with an SUVmax >5. In patients with pathologic stage I the expected 5-year disease-free survival rate was 88% if the SUVmax was <5 and 17% if the SUVmax was >5 (Higashi et al. 2002). Multivariate analysis identified the SUVmax as a more significant independent factor for disease-free survival than pathologic stage (Higashi et al. 2002). Nair et al. (2010), found that, in patients with surgically treated clinical stage IA NSCLC, high pretreatment FDG uptake (defined as SUVmax >5) identified individuals at increased risk of death due to disease following surgery.

Post-therapy FDG uptake is also of prognostic significance for NSCLC. One prospective study evaluated the utility of FDG PET in determining prognosis after completion of definitive radiotherapy or chemoradiotherapy in patients with unresectable NSCLC (Mac Manus et al. 2003). There was a significant association between qualitative decrease in FDG uptake within the primary tumor and mediastinal lymph nodes and patient survival (Mac Manus et al. 2003). Furthermore, a single early post-treatment PET scan was found to be a better predictor of survival than CT response, stage, or pretreatment performance status (Mac Manus et al. 2003). For patients with locally advanced but potentially resectable NSCLC who have completed neoadjuvant therapy, FDG PET is also of value. FDG PET can identify patients who have had a pathologic response to treatment and may benefit from further locoregional therapy (Vansteenkiste et al. 1998; De Leyn et al. 2006; Eschmann et al. 2007; Cerfolio et al. 2006). In a prospective study by Cerfolio et al. (2006), integrated FDG PET/CT was superior to CT in evaluating patients with NSCLC and biopsy-proven stage IIIA N2 disease after induction chemoradiation therapy. The authors found that a decrease of 75% or more in primary tumor SUVmax after therapy indicates a high likelihood of a complete response, and a decrease of more than 50% in the N2 lymph node SUVmax is indicative of a high likelihood of no residual metastatic disease (Cerfolio et al. 2006). The authors did recommend nodal biopsies in the setting of a persistently high SUVmax, as this did not reliably equate with residual nodal metastatic disease (Cerfolio et al. 2006). In patients with advanced NSCLC, the difference between initial FDG uptake and uptake after induction chemotherapy was found to be highly predictive for long-term survival. Patients with a 60% or more decrease in SUVmax had a significantly longer survival than those below this threshold (Eschmann et al. 2007).

4.9 Considerations for Specific Histological Subtypes of NSCLC

4.9.1 Bronchioloalveolar Carcinoma

Bronchioloalveolar carcinoma (BAC) is a peripheral, well-differentiated adenocarcinoma, usually arising beyond a recognizable bronchus and demonstrating a growth pattern along intact alveolar septa (Higashi et al. 1998; Kim et al. 1998). BACs, particularly the focal form, typically show only mild FDG uptake which can lead to false-negative interpretations for malignancy (Higashi et al. 1998; Kim et al. 1998). This may be due to the low metabolic activity of this generally slow-growing tumor or to the presence of a relatively small number of metabolically active malignant cells with abundant mucin (Higashi et al. 1998; Kim et al. 1998). Awareness of the radiologic appearance of BAC (ground glass opacities with or without a solid component on CT, solitary, or multiple pulmonary nodules) in the setting of low FDG uptake is important to prevent misinterpretation (Truong et al. 2006) (Fig. 7). Compared to CT alone, PET/CT may be more accurate for the diagnosis of BAC as the characteristic appearance of BAC on CT can be integrated with metabolic parameters (Goudarzi et al. 2008). Many BACs have low values for SUVmax, generally less than 2.0, but proper identification is facilitated by their low HU on CT (Goudarzi et al. 2008). Goudarzi et al. (2008) found that integrated PET/CT can help differentiate between pure BAC and adenocarcinoma with a BAC component by using tumor size, CT density, and metabolic activity. They found that pure BAC exhibits smaller size, lower FDG uptake, and lower tumor density than adenocarcinoma with BAC. In the presence of multifocal BAC, however, FDG PET appears to be highly sensitive (Heyneman and Patz 2002).

4.9.2 Carcinoid Tumors

Carcinoid tumors of the respiratory tract are rare neoplasms of neuroendocrine origin that account for only 2–3% of primary pulmonary malignancies (Davila et al. 1993). Typical carcinoid tumors are comprised of small, regularly arranged polygonal cells with abundant eosinophilic cytoplasm (de Rosado Christenson et al. 1999). Typical carcinoid tumors generally have few mitoses and lack marked nuclear pleomorphism. Atypical carcinoid tumors demonstrate more irregular architecture, increased mitoses, nuclear pleomorphism, and areas of necrosis. Typical carcinoid tumors account for 85–90% of carcinoid tumors, and are diagnosed at an earlier age than atypical carcinoid tumors (mean 35–50 years vs. 55–60 years) (de Rosado Christenson et al. 1999). They are generally small, centrally located, and rarely spread beyond the thorax (de Rosado Christenson et al. 1999). Atypical carcinoid tumors are

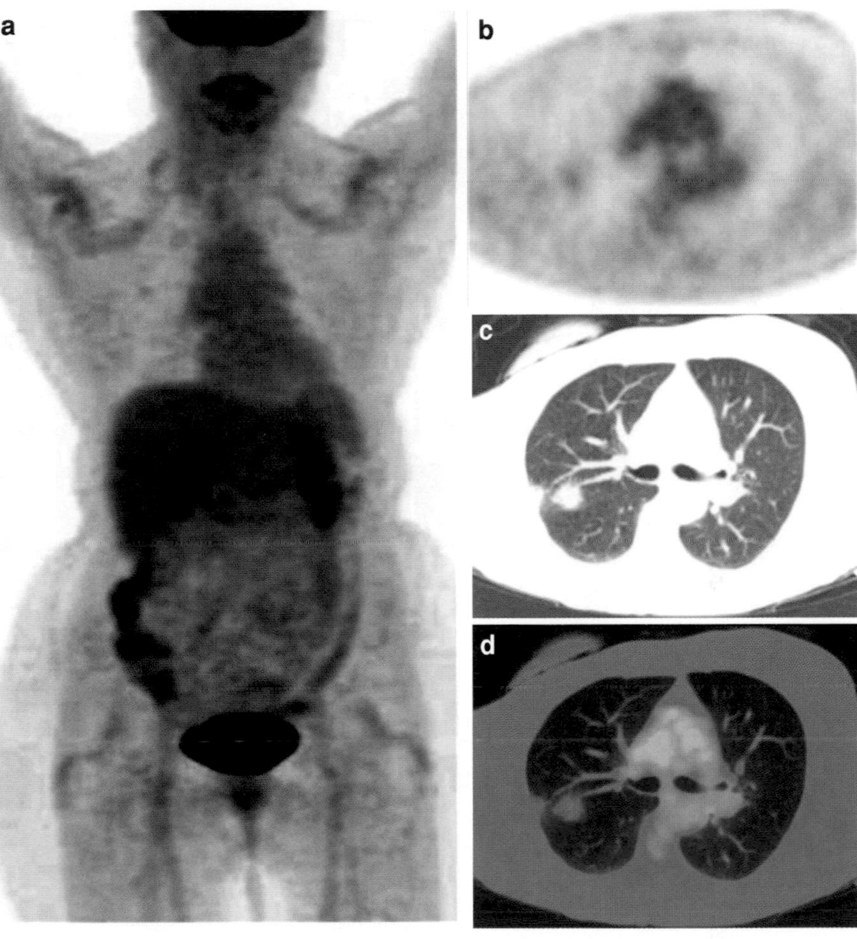

Fig. 7 *Brochioloalveolar Carcinoma*. Maximum intensity projection **a** and transaxial PET **b**, CT **c**, and fused images **d**. This is a 68-year-old woman with a history of breast cancer who developed a ground glass density in the right mid lung. The lung lesion slowly became denser over 18 months. PET/CT demonstrated a 2.5 cm nodule with mild FDG uptake (SUVmax = 2.3). No nodal or distant metastases were identified. CT-guided biopsy showed bronchioloalveolar carcinoma and the patient underwent a segmental resection with negative nodes

larger, located centrally and peripherally with equal frequency, more aggressive and commonly metastasize to regional nodes, liver, and bone (de Rosado Christenson et al. 1999).

The sensitivity of FDG PET in the diagnosis of pulmonary carcinoid is generally considered to be limited due to slow growth and therefore low metabolic activity of these tumors (de Rosado Christenson et al. 1999; Erasmus et al. 1998). In one retrospective study, only one of the seven carcinoid tumors that were evaluated demonstrated FDG uptake greater than background mediastinal activity and was correctly classified as positive for malignancy on PET scan (Erasmus et al. 1998). However, a more recent retrospective study evaluated pretreatment FDG PET scans from 16 patients with pulmonary carcinoid and found that, while overall metabolic activity of carcinoid tumors was lower and is generally observed in other histological subtypes of lung neoplasms, PET had a sensitivity of 75% for detecting malignancy in this cohort (Daniels et al. 2007). PET sensitivity was somewhat higher for atypical carcinoid tumors (80%) than for typical carcinoid tumors (72.7%) (Daniels et al. 2007). Thus, carcinoid tumors may not be universally PET-negative malignancies (Fig. 8).

5 Small Cell Lung Cancer

Small cell lung carcinomas (SCLC) account for nearly 20% of all lung cancers and are almost universally associated with smoking (Govindan et al. 2006). According to the National Institute of Health SEER database, the incidence of SCLC decreased in the United States between 1986 and 2002, possibly due to the decrease in smoking and the change to low-tar filter cigarettes (Govindan et al. 2006). Modest improvements in survival have been seen over the last

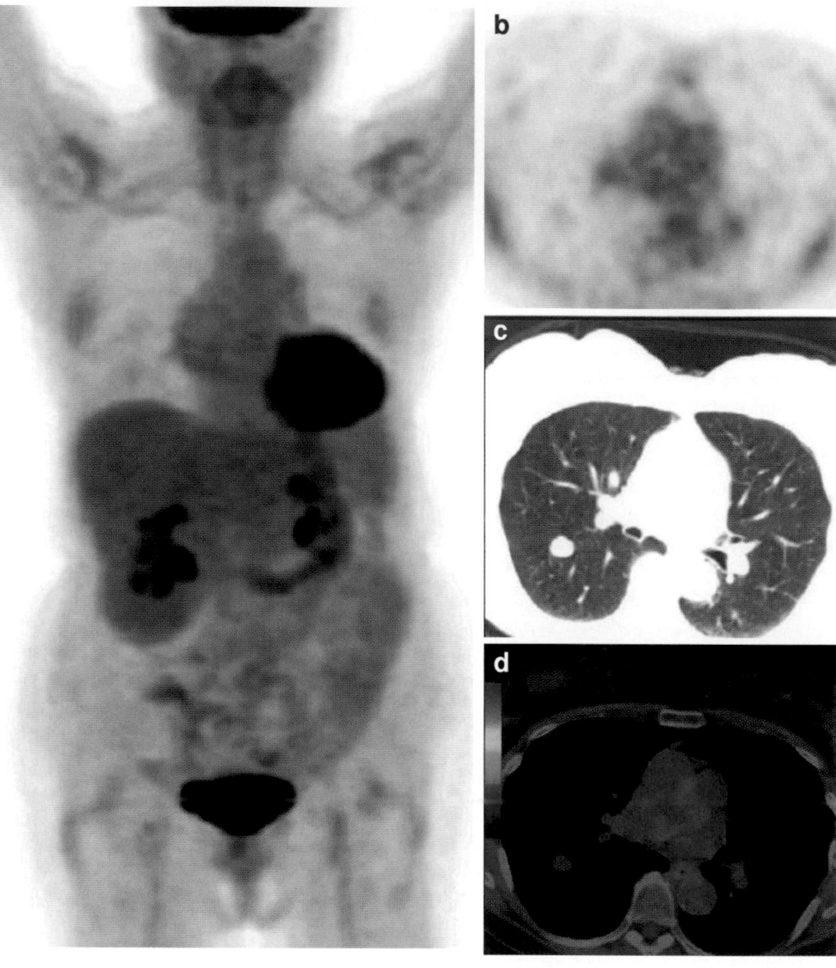

Fig. 8 *Carcinoid Tumor.* Maximum intensity projection **a** and transaxial PET **b**, CT **c**, and fused images **d**. This is a 62-year-old woman with an incidentally discovered right lower lobe nodule. PET/CT demonstrates a 2.0 cm nodule with minor FDG uptake (SUVmax = 1.3). CT-guided biopsy showed carcinoid histology. A wedge resection was performed without recurrence

30 years, although despite this trend, the outcome remains very poor. SCLCs are generally centrally located neoplasms arising from neuroendocrine cell precursors. SCLC is more clinically aggressive than NSCLC, with a rapid doubling time and propensity for widespread metastatic disease at presentation (Govindan et al. 2006). SCLC is sensitive to radiation therapy and chemotherapy, and generally surgery has no role in management. Though a large percentage of patients demonstrate an initial response to chemotherapy, there is a high rate of local and systemic recurrence.

In the staging of SCLC, TNM stages conventionally have been collapsed into a simple binary classification: limited disease (LD) and extensive disease (ED) (Schumacher et al. 2001). LD is defined as disease confined to the ipsilateral hemithorax that can be encompassed by a single radiotherapy port; ED is defined as disease beyond the ipsilateral hemithorax (Lally et al. 2007). Recent data suggests that clinical staging of SCLC should be based on TNM staging (Shepherd et al. 2007). Shepherd et al. (2007), using the International Association for the Study of Lung Cancer database, performed survival analyses for 8,088 patients with SCLC for which TNM staging was available. Survival was directly correlated to both tumor and node stage, with differences more pronounced in patients without mediastinal or supraclavicular nodal involvement. Stage grouping according to the sixth edition of the American Joint Committee on Cancer's staging manual also differentiated survival except between IA and IB (Shepherd et al. 2007). Thus, while LD and ED are still commonly referred to in the literature, TNM staging has replaced classification according to LD and ED in the current evaluation of SCLC.

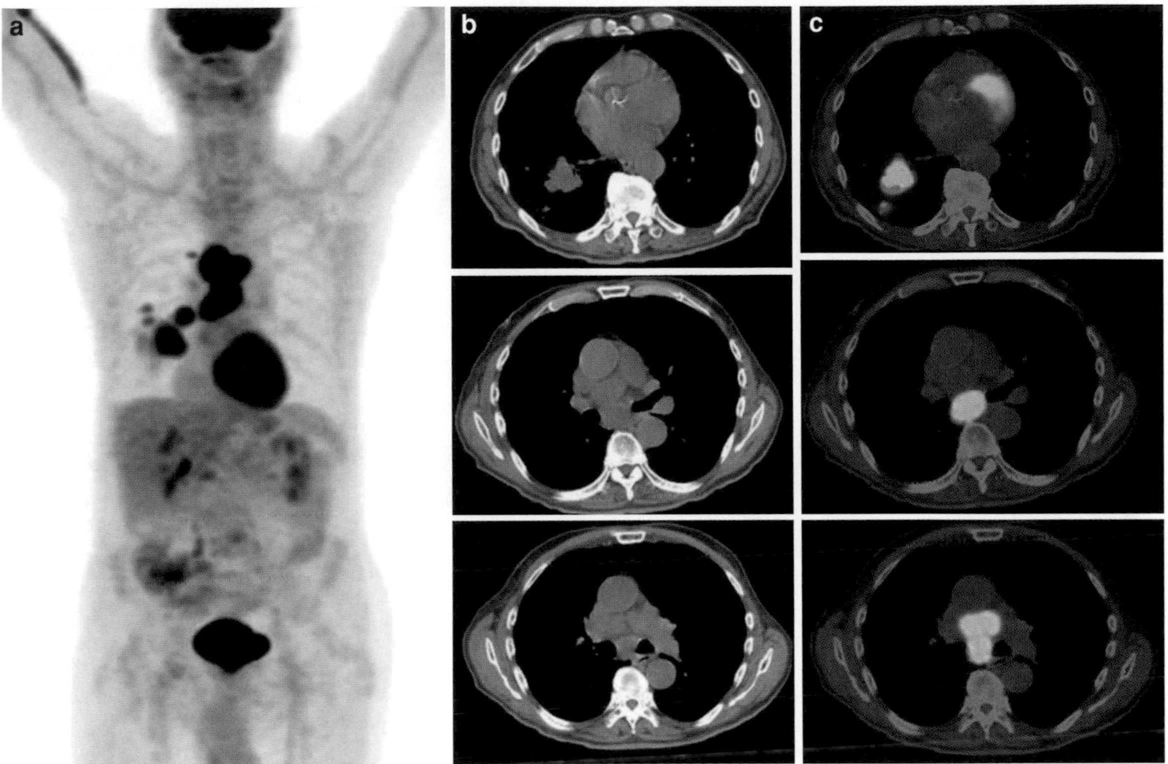

Fig. 9 *PET/CT Small cell lung carcinoma staging*. Maximum intensity projection **a**, transaxial CT **b**, and fused images **c**. This is an 87-year-old man with a positive tuberculin skin test. A chest X-ray revealed a right lower lobe mass. On CT, a right lower lobe spiculated mass with significant mediastinal and hilar lymphadenopathy was noted. A CT-guided lung biopsy was consistent with undifferentiated small cell carcinoma. PET/CT images demonstrate a hypermetabolic mass in the right lower lobe with an SUVmax of 14. Multiple hypermetabolic lymph nodes were identified particularly in the pretracheal region (SUVmax: 17.8), AP window (SUVmax = 17.1), subcarinal region (SUVmax = 17), and in the right hilum (SUVmax = 10). The patient refused chemotherapy and was being followed in hospice

Studies have shown that FDG PET when compared to conventional imaging procedures allows faster, more accurate differentiation between LD and ED, sparing the need for additional invasive diagnostic studies (Schumacher et al. 2001; Shen et al. 2002; Hauber et al. 2001) (Fig. 9). In a retrospective study, Vinjamuri et al. (2008) found that FDG PET was more accurate in the initial staging of SCLC than CT. In this study, the PET results from 8 of 51 patients (16%) resulted in a change in disease management. PET results accurately down staged 6 of 51 patients (12%) allowing these patients to be treated with radiation (Vinjamuri et al. 2008). Thus PET can ensure that over staging by CT scan does not deny potentially curative treatment for limited-stage SCLC. In patients with SCLC, FDG PET appears to be more sensitive for the detection of metastatic mediastinal and hilar lymph nodes as well as distant metastases (Schumacher et al. 2001; Shen et al. 2002). FDG PET is particularly effective in the identification of unsuspected regional nodal metastases, which can have a significant impact on therapy planning (Bradley et al. 2004). PET has been shown to identify occult adrenal metastases and metastases to supraclavicular lymph nodes missed by CT (Vinjamuri et al. 2008). Whole-body FDG PET may be useful as a simplified staging tool for small cell lung cancer (Schumacher et al. 2001). Evidence suggests that whole-body FDG PET may be able to replace the combination of conventional imaging modalities for staging SCLC in a cost-effective manner even when CT or MRI is included to rule out brain metastases (Chin et al. 2002).

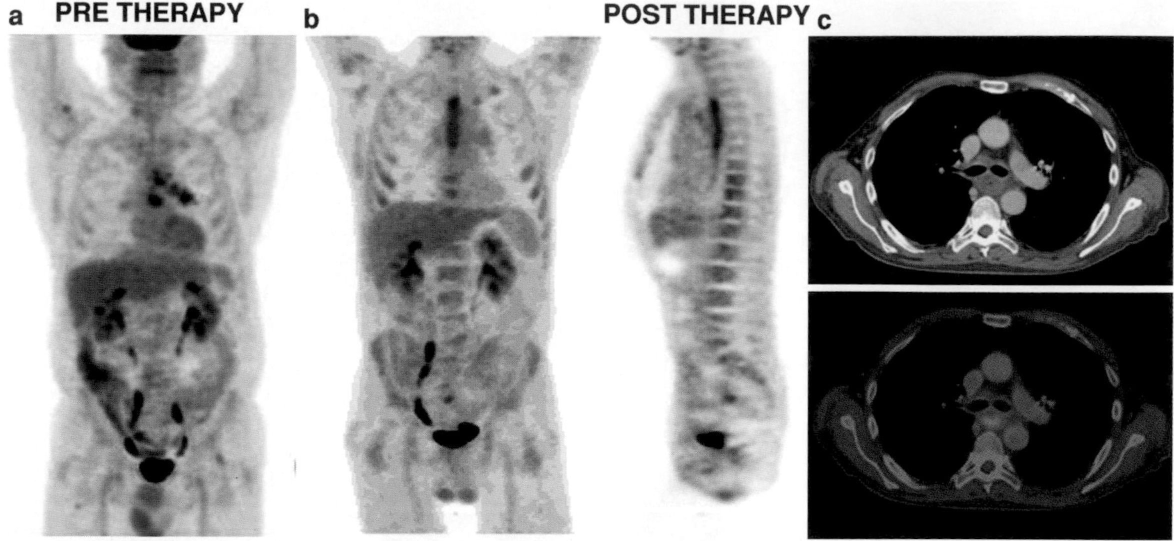

Fig. 10 *Therapy assessment of small cell lung carcinoma by PET/CT*. Pretherapy maximum intensity projection **a** and post-therapy MIP and transaxial CT, fused images **b** and **c**. This 62-year-old man with a 40-year smoking history presented with syndrome of inappropriate secretion of antidiuretic hormone. He was found to have a left upper lobe nodule with hilar and mediastinal lymphadenopathy. The staging PET/CT demonstrated a hypermetabolic lingular mass with an SUVmax of 3.9 and multiple hypermetabolic lymph nodes. Bronchoscopic biopsy of the station 4L and level 7 mediastinal lymph nodes was positive for poorly differentiated small cell carcinoma. He was treated with concurrent chemoradiation (six cycles of chemotherapy and 66 Gy in 33 fractions radiotherapy). A restaging PET/CT 3 months after treatment showed complete metabolic response and diffuse esophageal thickening with increased uptake consistent with the esophagitis

5.1 Response to Therapy

FDG PET is an accurate method for restaging after therapy for SCLC as it can correctly identify patients in total remission, those with residual disease, and patients with progressive disease (Kamel et al. 2003) (Fig. 10). In predicting residual disease, FDG PET has been shown to be more effective than CT (Onitilo et al. 2008). With SCLC, dissolution and shrinkage of residual tumor mass after therapy may occur, even after all viable tumor cells have been eradicated.

5.2 Prognosis

In a prospective study, Lee et al. (2009a, b) found that pretreatment of tumor metabolic activity as assessed by FDG PET is a significant prognostic factor for SCLC and could identify subgroups of patients at higher risk of death in both LD and ED SCLC. For patients with both LD and ED, a high SUVmax defined as a value >8.7 was associated with significantly poorer survival outcomes as compared to the low SUVmax group. Additionally, post-therapy PET findings may be of prognostic value in patients with SCLC (Pandit et al. 2003). Patients with positive PET scans after completion of treatment have significantly worse survival profiles than patients with negative studies (Onitilo et al. 2008; Pandit et al. 2003) and PET-negative patients have significantly longer progression-free survival times compared to PET-positive patients with SCLC (Onitilo et al. 2008). A good correlation between lesion SUVmax and patient survival has also been observed, with high maximum SUVs associated with poor survival (Pandit et al. 2003). In patients receiving treatment, a persistently high SUVmax may indicate a poor response, indicating a need for a change in treatment, while a low SUVmax suggests a good response to therapy (Pandit et al. 2003).

6 Pleural Disease

6.1 Pleural Effusion

Pleural involvement is relatively common in patients with lung cancer and differentiation between benign and malignant effusion is important in determining resectability and use of radiotherapy. Pleural thickening or nodularity on CT may indicate the presence of metastases in the pleural cavity, but CT is often unable to distinguish between benign or malignant pleural disease. Similarly, MRI has failed to show high accuracy in differentiating benign from malignant pleural effusions. FDG PET may be better at evaluating pleural effusions than conventional imaging. In one study, 35 patients with lung cancer and abnormal pleural findings on CT underwent PET (Gupta et al. 2002). Sensitivity, specificity, and accuracy of FDG PET were 89, 94, and 91%, respectively. The high negative predictive value of PET in pleural effusions may be of help in reducing the number of repeat thoracocenteses or thoracoscopic biopsies in patients with negative PET findings and benign effusion.

6.2 Malignant Pleural Mesothelioma

Malignant pleural mesothelioma (MPM) is a neoplasm arising from the mesothelial cells of the pleural cavities. In the United States, approximately 2500–3000 cases of MPM are diagnosed per year. The incidence of mesothelioma in the United States peaked around the year 2000, after which a decline has been observed secondary to control of exposure to asbestos (Teta et al. 2008). Mesothelioma is almost always fatal with a median survival of 11 months. Asbestos is the principal carcinogen implicated in the pathogenesis, with 80% of patients in the United States reporting history of asbestos exposure. There is a long latency period (30–40 years) from the time of asbestos exposure to the development of clinically apparent mesothelioma. Malignant mesothelioma usually begins as discrete plaques and nodules, which subsequently coalesce to produce a sheet-like neoplasm. Tumor growth most often begins at the lower part of the chest and may invade the diaphragm and encase the surface of the lung and interlobar fissures.

Early identification of the extent of the disease is essential for treatment planning and prognosis. CT was considered the standard diagnostic study for staging MPM and is the primary modality in assessing local extent and identifying nodal and distant metastases (Heelan et al. 1999). MRI can be used to complement CT in the evaluation of patients with mesothelioma when resection is being considered as a treatment option. MRI is superior to CT in the differentiation of malignant from benign pleural disease and in revealing solitary foci of chest wall invasion, endothoracic fascia involvement, and diaphragmatic muscle invasion (Heelan et al. 1999). CT and MRI are, however, limited in that diffuse pleural thickening can represent either malignancy or a benign process caused by asbestos exposure, hemorrhagic effusion, or infectious processes such as tuberculosis or empyema (Ho et al. 2001). Benign pleural plaques caused by asbestos exposure can also complicate evaluation based on anatomic parameters alone (Haberkorn 2004). Thus, the accuracy of CT in predicting the malignant nature of diffuse pleural lesions is not optimal (Haberkorn 2004). Thoracoscopy has a high sensitivity (>90%) with a mortality rate of less than 0.1%, but non-fatal complications occur in up to 10% of patients. Despite this high morbidity, thoracoscopy remains the primary diagnostic modality for mesothelioma, but it is invasive and cannot always accurately stage the mediastinal nodes or transdiaphragmatic extension (Haberkorn 2004).

Imaging with FDG PET/CT is noninvasive and can accurately and reliably differentiate MPM from benign pleural disease (Yildirim et al. 2009; Duysinx et al. 2004). FDG PET/CT can make this distinction with high sensitivity and specificity as the FDG uptake of pleural malignancies is significantly greater than that of benign processes (Yildirim et al. 2009).

6.3 T Staging

MPM is typically detected by PET as moderate to high FDG uptake in areas of pleural thickening observed on anatomic imaging modalities (Subramaniam et al. 2009). Early stage tumors usually have focal or linear patterns of uptake, while diffuse and heterogeneous patterns are indicative of advanced disease, regardless of histological type or grade (Gerbaudo 2003) (Fig. 9). However, due to the poor spatial resolution of PET alone, FDG uptake in the parietal pleura cannot be differentiated from hypermetabolism in the visceral pleura in the absence of a pleural effusion

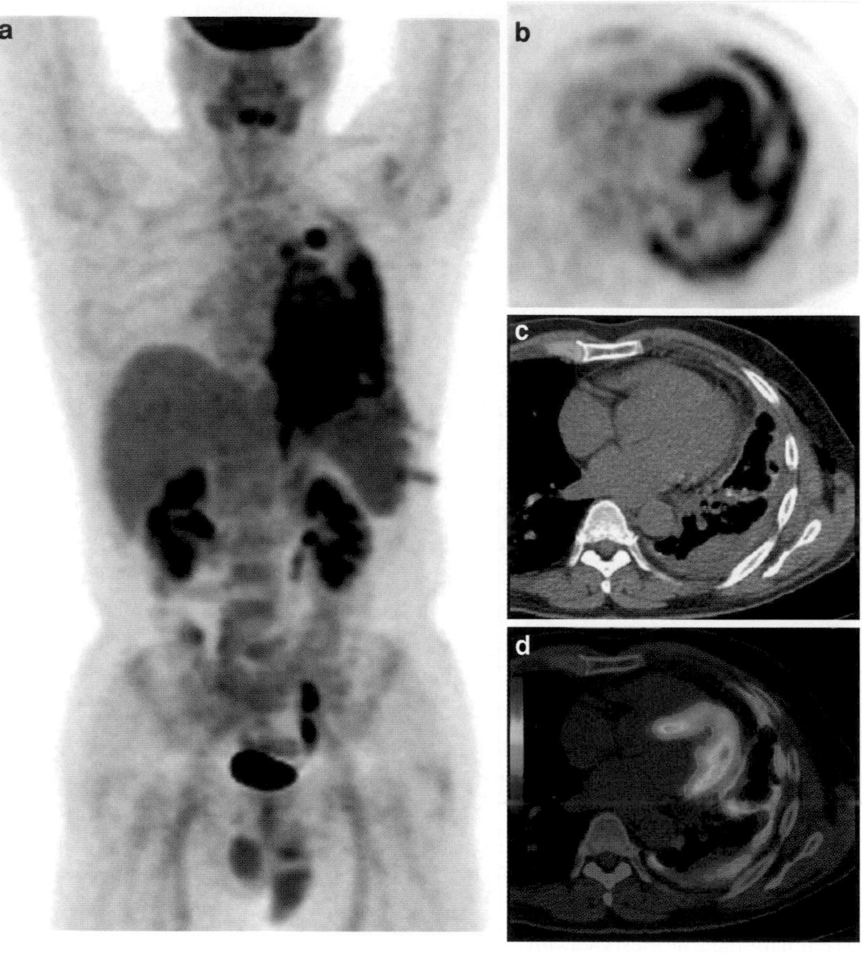

Fig. 11 *Pleural Mesothelioma*. Maximum intensity projection **a** and transaxial PET **b**, CT **c**, and fused images **d**. This is an 86-year-old man with a remote history of asbestos exposure who presented with shortness of breath. Pleural thickening in the left hemithorax prompted a PET/CT. The PET/CT demonstrates diffuse, intense hypermetabolism throughout the thickened pleura (SUVmax = 17.8). The hypermetabolic pleural thickening involves the major fissure, which is a hallmark of mesothelioma. An extrapleural pneumonectomy was successfully performed. Left chest wall recurrence was detected 3 years after surgery

(Erasmus et al. 2005). It is also difficult to determine the extent of local invasion into the chest wall, diaphragm, or pericardium (Erasmus et al. 2005). The use of integrated PET/CT substantially improves primary tumor staging (Fig. 11).

6.4 N Staging

MPM metastasizes to intrathoracic lymph nodes in 22–50% of patients (Sugarbaker et al. 1999; Rusch and Venkatraman 1996). Metastasis to N2 nodes is associated with a far worse prognosis than N1 disease (Sugarbaker et al. 1999). Supraclavicular nodal involvement has the worst prognosis (Subramaniam et al. 2009). While the accuracy of MRI and CT in differentiating between N1 and N2 disease is approximately 50% (Marom et al. 2002), the sensitivity of FDG PET for staging the mediastinum in patients with malignant mesothelioma ranges from 83 to 88% with a specificity between 75 and 82% (Duysinx et al. 2004; Marom et al. 2002).

6.5 M Staging

Systemic metastases are common with MPM and can occur in the contralateral lung, liver, adrenal glands, kidneys, bone, anterior and posterior abdominal wall, peritoneum, brain, and leptomeninges (Benard et al. 1998; Duysinx et al. 2004; Kramer et al. 2004). The detection of distant metastases is important in directing the course of management, as these patients are not considered candidates for surgery (Erasmus et al. 2005). FDG PET may be superior to routine clinical and conventional radiological evaluation in correctly identifying distant metastases (Erasmus et al. 2005; Schneider et al. 2000).

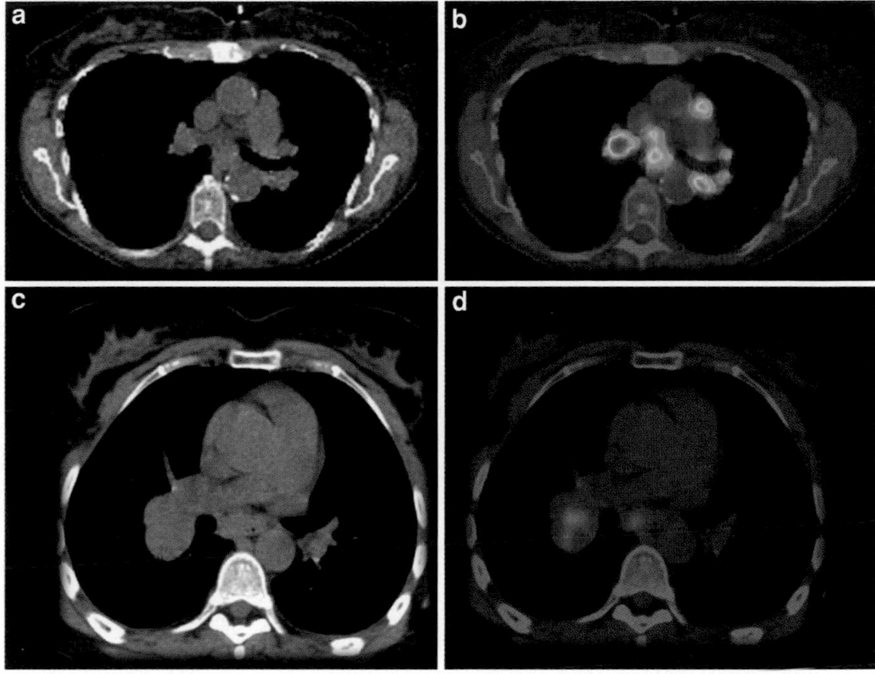

Fig. 12 *Granulomatous disease*. **a** CT and **b** PET/CT demonstrate multiple mediastinal and hilar FDG hypermetabolic lymph nodes. Mediastinoscopy-directed biopsy proved sarcoidosis rather than metastatic lymph nodes. **c** and **d** demonstrate FDG hypermetabolic right hilar and subcarinal lymph nodes which biopsy proven to be tuberculosis

6.6 Prognosis

FDG PET may be useful for determining the prognosis in patients with MPM. In one study, median survivals were significantly lower in patients with lesion maximum SUV >10 compared to patients with an SUVmax of <10 (Flores et al. 2006). In this study, low SUVmax (<10) and epithelial histology had the best prognosis, whereas high SUVmax (>10) and non-epithelial histology resulted in the worst survival prognosis (Flores et al. 2006). In another study, the intensity of tumor uptake correlated poorly with histological grade but correlated well with surgical stage (Gerbaudo et al. 2003). Lesion FDG uptake increased over time at a higher rate in patients with more advanced disease and the increment of FDG lesion uptake over time was a better predictor of disease aggressiveness than the histological grade (Gerbaudo et al. 2003).

6.7 Response to Therapy

Measuring response with CT is challenging in patients with MPM due to the circumferential pattern of tumor growth. There is growing evidence that therapy-induced changes in tumor FDG uptake may predict response and patient outcome early in the course of treatment (Ceresoli et al. 2006). In one prospective study, patients were evaluated by both FDG PET and CT at baseline and after two cycles of a pemetrexed-based regimen of palliative chemotherapy (Ceresoli et al. 2006). A decrease of 25% or more in tumor FDG uptake as measured by the maximum SUV was defined as a metabolic response (Ceresoli et al. 2006). Early metabolic response was significantly correlated to median time-to-tumor progression while no correlation was found between time-to-tumor progression and radiologic response evaluated by CT (Ceresoli et al. 2006). Patients with a metabolic response also had a trend toward longer overall survival (Ceresoli et al. 2006). In another recent study, a statistically significant relationship was observed between a fall in total glycolytic volume of the tumor after one cycle of chemotherapy and improved patient survival (Francis et al. 2007) while neither a reduction in the maximum SUV nor CT demonstrated a statistically significant association with patient survival (Francis et al. 2007). Thus, metabolic imaging can improve the care of patients receiving chemotherapy for mesothelioma through the early identification of favorable response to therapy.

7 Limitations of FDG PET/CT Imaging of the Chest

When evaluating the chest, the interpreter must be mindful of potential artifacts and pitfalls (see PET/CT Pitfalls and Artifacts). Inflammatory false positives on FDG PET are not uncommon and can occur with anthracosilicosis, infection, granulomatous disease (Fig. 10) (Schrevens et al. 2004), or reactive hyperplasia in the mediastinal lymph nodes (Pieterman et al. 2000). In patients with malignancies of the lung, false-positive interpretations can occur due to hypermetabolism from inflammation secondary to obstructing endobronchial tumors (Pieterman et al. 2000). False-negative interpretations can occur due to microscopic tumor residue or due to the inability to distinguish between a paramediastinal primary tumor and mediastinal lymph nodes (Pieterman et al. 2000). Imaging cannot detect microscopic lymph node metastases (Lardinois et al. 2003) (Fig. 12).

8 Conclusion

Over the last decade, FDG PET/CT has become the standard-of care for staging, therapy assessment and follow-up of patients with thoracic malignancies. It improves the staging, provides a road map for selective invasive mediastinal biopsy and surgical planning (especially contrast-enhanced PET/CT) and accurately identifies distant metastasis. The maximum SUV correlates strongly with patient survival. PET/CT allows accurate assessment of therapy response for patients with cancer within the chest. PET/CT detects early recurrence and identifies the extent of the recurrent disease. Further research is ongoing to determine the effects on outcomes, but PET/CT is currently the best imaging modality for thoracic malignancies.

References

Ahuja V, Coleman RE, Herndon J, Patz Jr EF (1998) The prognostic significance of fluorodeoxyglucose positron emission tomography imaging for patients with nonsmall cell lung carcinoma. Cancer 83:918–924

Al-Sugair A, Coleman RE (1998) Applications of PET in lung cancer. Semin Nucl Med 28:303–319

Antoch G, Stattaus J, Nemat AT et al (2003) Non-small cell lung cancer: dual-modality PET/CT in preoperative staging. Radiology 229:526–533

Arita T, Matsumoto T, Kuramitsu T et al (1996) Is it possible to differentiate malignant mediastinal nodes from benign nodes by size? Reevaluation by CT, transesophageal echocardiography, and nodal specimen. Chest 110:1004–1008

Benard F, Sterman D, Smith RJ, Kaiser LR, Albelda SM, Alavi A (1998) Metabolic imaging of malignant pleural mesothelioma with fluorodeoxyglucose positron emission tomography. Chest 114:713–722

Bille A, Pelosi E, Skanjeti A et al (2009) Preoperative intrathoracic lymph node staging in patients with non-small-cell lung cancer: accuracy of integrated positron emission tomography and computed tomography. Eur J Cardiothorac Surg 36:440–445

Birim O, Kappetein AP, Stijnen T, Bogers AJ (2005) Meta-analysis of positron emission tomographic and computed tomographic imaging in detecting mediastinal lymph node metastases in nonsmall cell lung cancer. Ann Thorac Surg 79:375–382

Bradley JD, Dehdashti F, Mintun MA, Govindan R, Trinkaus K, Siegel BA (2004) Positron emission tomography in limited-stage small-cell lung cancer: a prospective study. J Clin Oncol 22:3248–3254

Brady MJ, Thomas J, Wong TZ, Franklin KM, Ho LM, Paulson EK (2009) Adrenal nodules at FDG PET/CT in patients known to have or suspected of having lung cancer: a proposal for an efficient diagnostic algorithm. Radiology 250:523–530

Brink I, Schumacher T, Mix M et al (2004) Impact of [18F]FDG-PET on the primary staging of small-cell lung cancer. Eur J Nucl Med Mol Imaging 31:1614–1620

Bury T, Barreto A, Daenen F, Barthelemy N, Ghaye B, Rigo P (1998) Fluorine-18 deoxyglucose positron emission tomography for the detection of bone metastases in patients with non-small cell lung cancer. Eur J Nucl Med 25: 1244–1247

Bury T, Corhay JL, Duysinx B et al (1999) Value of FDG-PET in detecting residual or recurrent nonsmall cell lung cancer. Eur Respir J 14:1376–1380

Casali C, Cucca M, Rossi G et al (2009) The variation of prognostic significance of Maximum Standardized Uptake Value of [18F]-fluoro-2-deoxy-glucose positron emission tomography in different histological subtypes and pathological stages of surgically resected Non-Small Cell Lung Carcinoma. *Lung Cancer* 69(2):187–193

Ceresoli GL, Chiti A, Zucali PA et al (2006) Early response evaluation in malignant pleural mesothelioma by positron emission tomography with [18F]fluorodeoxyglucose. J Clin Oncol 24:4587–4593

Cerfolio RJ, Ojha B, Bryant AS, Bass CS, Bartalucci AA, Mountz JM (2003) The role of FDG-PET scan in staging patients with nonsmall cell carcinoma. Ann Thorac Surg 76:861–866

Cerfolio RJ, Ojha B, Bryant AS, Raghuveer V, Mountz JM, Bartolucci AA (2004) The accuracy of integrated PET-CT compared with dedicated PET alone for the staging of patients with nonsmall cell lung cancer. Ann Thorac Surg 78:1017–1023 discussion 1017–1023

Cerfolio RJ, Bryant AS, Ojha B (2006) Restaging patients with N2 (stage IIIa) non-small cell lung cancer after neoadjuvant chemoradiotherapy: a prospective study. J Thorac Cardiovasc Surg 131:1229–1235

Chansky K, Sculier JP, Crowley JJ, Giroux D, Van Meerbeeck J, Goldstraw P (2009) The international association for the study of lung cancer staging project: prognostic factors and pathologic TNM stage in surgically managed non-small cell lung cancer. J Thorac Oncol 4:792–801

Chin R Jr, McCain TW, Miller AA et al (2002) Whole body FDG-PET for the evaluation and staging of small cell lung cancer: a preliminary study. Lung Cancer 37:1–6

Daniels CE, Lowe VJ, Aubry MC, Allen MS, Jett JR (2007) The utility of fluorodeoxyglucose positron emission tomography in the evaluation of carcinoid tumors presenting as pulmonary nodules. Chest 131:255–260

Davila DG, Dunn WF, Tazelaar HD, Pairolero PC (1993) Bronchial carcinoid tumors. Mayo Clin Proc 68:795–803

De Leyn P, Stroobants S, De Wever W et al (2006) Prospective comparative study of integrated positron emission tomography-computed tomography scan compared with remediastinoscopy in the assessment of residual mediastinal lymph node disease after induction chemotherapy for mediastinoscopy-proven stage IIIA-N2 Non-small-cell lung cancer: a Leuven Lung Cancer Group Study. J Clin Oncol 24:3333–3339

de Rosado Christenson ML, Abbott GF, Kirejczyk WM, Galvin JR, Travis WD (1999) Thoracic carcinoids: radiologic-pathologic correlation. Radiographics 19:707–736

De Wever W, Ceyssens S, Mortelmans L et al (2007) Additional value of PET-CT in the staging of lung cancer: comparison with CT alone, PET alone and visual correlation of PET and CT. Eur Radiol 17:23–32

Duhaylongsod FG, Lowe VJ, Patz EF Jr, Vaughn AL, Coleman RE, Wolfe WG (1995) Lung tumor growth correlates with glucose metabolism measured by fluoride-18 fluorodeoxyglucose positron emission tomography. Ann Thorac Surg 60:1348–1352

Duysinx B, Nguyen D, Louis R et al (2004) Evaluation of pleural disease with 18-fluorodeoxyglucose positron emission tomography imaging. Chest 125:489–493

Dwamena BA, Sonnad SS, Angobaldo JO, Wahl RL (1999) Metastases from non-small cell lung cancer: mediastinal staging in the 1990 s–meta-analytic comparison of PET and CT. Radiology 213:530–536

Erasmus JJ, Patz EF Jr, McAdams HP et al (1997) Evaluation of adrenal masses in patients with bronchogenic carcinoma using 18F-fluorodeoxyglucose positron emission tomography. Am J Roentgenol 168:1357–1360

Erasmus JJ, McAdams HP, Patz EF Jr, Coleman RE, Ahuja V, Goodman PC (1998) Evaluation of primary pulmonary carcinoid tumors using FDG PET. Am J Roentgenol 170:1369–1373

Erasmus JJ, Truong MT, Smythe WR et al (2005) Integrated computed tomography-positron emission tomography in patients with potentially resectable malignant pleural mesothelioma: staging implications. J Thorac Cardiovasc Surg 129:1364–1370

Eschmann SM, Friedel G, Paulsen F et al (2007) Repeat 18F-FDG PET for monitoring neoadjuvant chemotherapy in patients with stage III non-small cell lung cancer. Lung Cancer 55:165–171

Ettinghausen SE, Burt ME (1991) Prospective evaluation of unilateral adrenal masses in patients with operable non-small-cell lung cancer. J Clin Oncol 9:1462–1466

Fischer B, Lassen U, Mortensen J et al (2009) Preoperative staging of lung cancer with combined PET-CT. N Engl J Med 361:32–39

Fletcher JW, Kymes SM, Gould M et al (2008) A comparison of the diagnostic accuracy of 18F-FDG PET and CT in the characterization of solitary pulmonary nodules. J Nucl Med 49:179–185

Flores RM, Akhurst T, Gonen M et al (2006) Positron emission tomography predicts survival in malignant pleural mesothelioma. J Thorac Cardiovasc Surg 132:763–768

Francis RJ, Byrne MJ, van der Schaaf AA et al (2007) Early prediction of response to chemotherapy and survival in malignant pleural mesothelioma using a novel semiautomated 3-dimensional volume-based analysis of serial 18F-FDG PET scans. J Nucl Med 48:1449–1458

Frank A, Lefkowitz D, Jaeger S et al (1995) Decision logic for retreatment of asymptomatic lung cancer recurrence based on positron emission tomography findings. Int J Radiat Oncol Biol Phys 32:1495–1512

Gerbaudo VH (2003) 18F-FDG imaging of malignant pleural mesothelioma: scientiam impendere vero. Nucl Med Commun 24:609–614

Gerbaudo VH, Britz-Cunningham S, Sugarbaker DJ, Treves ST (2003) Metabolic significance of the pattern, intensity and kinetics of 18F-FDG uptake in malignant pleural mesothelioma. Thorax 58:1077–1082

Goldstraw P, Crowley J, Chansky K et al (2007) The IASLC lung cancer staging project: proposals for the revision of the TNM stage groupings in the forthcoming (seventh) edition of the TNM classification of malignant tumours. J Thorac Oncol 2:706–714

Goudarzi B, Jacene HA, Wahl RL (2008) Diagnosis and differentiation of bronchioloalveolar carcinoma from adenocarcinoma with bronchioloalveolar components with metabolic and anatomic characteristics using PET/CT. J Nucl Med 49:1585–1592

Gould MK, Maclean CC, Kuschner WG, Rydzak CE, Owens DK (2001) Accuracy of positron emission tomography for diagnosis of pulmonary nodules and mass lesions: a meta-analysis. JAMA 285:914–924

Gould MK, Kuschner WG, Rydzak CE et al (2003) Test performance of positron emission tomography and computed tomography for mediastinal staging in patients with non-small-cell lung cancer: a meta-analysis. Ann Intern Med 139:879–892

Govindan R, Page N, Morgensztern D et al (2006) Changing epidemiology of small-cell lung cancer in the United States over the last 30 years: analysis of the surveillance, epidemiologic, and end results database. J Clin Oncol 24:4539–4544

Graeter TP, Hellwig D, Hoffmann K, Ukena D, Kirsch CM, Schafers HJ (2003) Mediastinal lymph node staging in suspected lung cancer: comparison of positron emission tomography with F-18-fluorodeoxyglucose and mediastinoscopy. Ann Thorac Surg 75:231–235 discussion 235–236

Gupta NC, Rogers JS, Graeber GM et al (2002) Clinical role of F-18 fluorodeoxyglucose positron emission tomography imaging in patients with lung cancer and suspected malignant pleural effusion. Chest 122:1918–1924

Gurney JW, Swensen SJ (1995) Solitary pulmonary nodules: determining the likelihood of malignancy with neural network analysis. Radiology 196:823–829

Haberkorn U (2004) Positron emission tomography in the diagnosis of mesothelioma. Lung Cancer 45(Suppl 1): S73–S76

Halpern BS, Schiepers C, Weber WA et al (2005) Presurgical staging of non-small cell lung cancer: positron emission tomography, integrated positron emission tomography/CT, and software image fusion. Chest 128:2289–2297

Halter G, Buck AK, Schirrmeister H et al (2004) Lymph node staging in lung cancer using [18F]FDG-PET. Thorac Cardiovasc Surg 52:96–101

Hashimoto Y, Tsujikawa T, Kondo C et al (2006) Accuracy of PET for diagnosis of solid pulmonary lesions with 18F-FDG uptake below the standardized uptake value of 2.5. J Nucl Med 47:426–431

Hauber HP, Bohuslavizki KH, Lund CH, Fritscher-Ravens A, Meyer A, Pforte A (2001) Positron emission tomography in the staging of small-cell lung cancer : a preliminary study. Chest 119:950–954

Heelan RT, Rusch VW, Begg CB, Panicek DM, Caravelli JF, Eisen C (1999) Staging of malignant pleural mesothelioma: comparison of CT and MR imaging. Am J Roentgenol 172:1039–1047

Hellwig D, Groschel A, Graeter TP et al (2006) Diagnostic performance and prognostic impact of FDG-PET in suspected recurrence of surgically treated non-small cell lung cancer. Eur J Nucl Med Mol Imaging 33:13–21

Heyneman LE, Patz EF (2002) PET imaging in patients with bronchioloalveolar cell carcinoma. Lung Cancer 38:261–266

Hicks RJ, Kalff V, MacManus MP et al (2001a) (18)F-FDG PET provides high-impact and powerful prognostic stratification in staging newly diagnosed non-small cell lung cancer. J Nucl Med 42:1596–1604

Hicks RJ, Kalff V, MacManus MP et al (2001b) The utility of (18)F-FDG PET for suspected recurrent non-small cell lung cancer after potentially curative therapy: impact on management and prognostic stratification. J Nucl Med 42: 1605–1613

Hicks RJ, Mac Manus MP, Matthews JP et al (2004) Early FDG-PET imaging after radical radiotherapy for non-small-cell lung cancer: inflammatory changes in normal tissues correlate with tumor response and do not confound therapeutic response evaluation. Int J Radiat Oncol Biol Phys 60:412–418

Higashi K, Clavo AC, Wahl RL (1993) Does FDG uptake measure proliferative activity of human cancer cells? In vitro comparison with DNA flow cytometry and tritiated thymidine uptake. J Nucl Med 34:414–419

Higashi K, Ueda Y, Seki H et al (1998) Fluorine-18-FDG PET imaging is negative in bronchioloalveolar lung carcinoma. J Nucl Med 39:1016–1020

Higashi K, Ueda Y, Arisaka Y et al (2002) 18F-FDG uptake as a biologic prognostic factor for recurrence in patients with surgically resected non-small cell lung cancer. J Nucl Med 43:39–45

Ho L, Sugarbaker DJ, Skarin AT (2001) Malignant pleural mesothelioma. Cancer Treat Res 105:327–373

Hoekstra CJ, Stroobants SG, Hoekstra OS, Smit EF, Vansteenkiste JF, Lammertsma AA (2002) Measurement of perfusion in stage IIIA-N2 non-small cell lung cancer using H(2)(15)O and positron emission tomography. Clin Cancer Res 8:2109–2115

Hoekstra CJ, Stroobants SG, Hoekstra OS et al (2003) The value of [18F]fluoro-2-deoxy-D-glucose positron emission tomography in the selection of patients with stage IIIA-N2 non-small cell lung cancer for combined modality treatment. Lung Cancer 39:151–157

Hoekstra CJ, Stroobants SG, Smit EF et al (2005) Prognostic relevance of response evaluation using [18F]-2-fluoro-2-deoxy-D-glucose positron emission tomography in patients with locally advanced non-small-cell lung cancer. J Clin Oncol 23:8362–8370

Inoue T, Kim EE, Komaki R et al (1995) Detecting recurrent or residual lung cancer with FDG-PET. J Nucl Med 36:788–793

Jemal A, Thun MJ, Ries LA et al (2008) Annual report to the nation on the status of cancer, 1975–2005, featuring trends in lung cancer, tobacco use, and tobacco control. J Natl Cancer Inst 100:1672–1694

Jemal A, Siegel R, Ward E, Hao Y, Xu J, Thun MJ (2009) Cancer statistics, 2009. CA Cancer J Clin 59:225–249

Jeong HJ, Min JJ, Park JM et al (2002) Determination of the prognostic value of [(18)F]fluorodeoxyglucose uptake by using positron emission tomography in patients with non-small cell lung cancer. Nucl Med Commun 23:865–870

Kamel EM, Zwahlen D, Wyss MT, Stumpe KD, von Schulthess GK, Steinert HC (2003) Whole-body (18)F-FDG PET improves the management of patients with small cell lung cancer. J Nucl Med 44:1911–1917

Kerr KM, Lamb D, Wathen CG, Walker WS, Douglas NJ (1992) Pathological assessment of mediastinal lymph nodes in lung cancer: implications for non-invasive mediastinal staging. Thorax 47:337–341

Kim BT, Kim Y, Lee KS et al (1998) Localized form of bronchioloalveolar carcinoma: FDG PET findings. AJR Am J Roentgenol 170:935–939

Kong FM, Frey KA, Quint LE et al (2007) A pilot study of [18F]fluorodeoxyglucose positron emission tomography scans during and after radiation-based therapy in patients with non small-cell lung cancer. J Clin Oncol 25:3116–3123

Kramer H, Pieterman RM, Slebos DJ et al (2004) PET for the evaluation of pleural thickening observed on CT. J Nucl Med 45:995–998

Lally BE, Urbanic JJ, Blackstock AW, Miller AA, Perry MC (2007) Small cell lung cancer: have we made any progress over the last 25 years? Oncologist 12:1096–1104

Lardinois D, Weder W, Hany TF et al (2003) Staging of non-small-cell lung cancer with integrated positron-emission tomography and computed tomography. N Engl J Med 348:2500–2507

Lee DH, Kim SK, Lee HY et al (2009a) Early prediction of response to first-line therapy using integrated 18F-FDG PET/CT for patients with advanced/metastatic non-small cell lung cancer. J Thorac Oncol 4:816–821

Lee YJ, Cho A, Cho BC et al (2009b) High tumor metabolic activity as measured by fluorodeoxyglucose positron emission tomography is associated with poor prognosis in limited and extensive stage small-cell lung cancer. Clin Cancer Res 15:2426–2432

Mac Manus MP, Hicks RJ, Matthews JP et al (2003) Positron emission tomography is superior to computed tomography scanning for response-assessment after radical radiotherapy or chemoradiotherapy in patients with non-small-cell lung cancer. J Clin Oncol 21:1285–1292

MacManus MP, Hicks RJ, Matthews JP et al (2001) High rate of detection of unsuspected distant metastases by pet in apparent stage III non-small-cell lung cancer: implications for radical radiation therapy. Int J Radiat Oncol Biol Phys 50:287–293

Marom EM, McAdams HP, Erasmus JJ et al (1999) Staging non-small cell lung cancer with whole-body PET. Radiology 212:803–809

Marom EM, Erasmus JJ, Pass HI, Patz EF Jr (2002) The role of imaging in malignant pleural mesothelioma. Semin Oncol 29:26–35

Meyers BF, Haddad F, Siegel BA et al (2006) Cost-effectiveness of routine mediastinoscopy in computed tomography- and positron emission tomography-screened patients with stage I lung cancer. J Thorac Cardiovasc Surg 131:822–829 discussion 822–829

Nair VS, Barnett PG, Ananth L, Gould MK (2010) PET scan 18F-fluorodeoxyglucose uptake and prognosis in patients with resected clinical stage IA non-small cell lung cancer. Chest 137:1150–1156

Nakamura H, Taguchi M, Kitamura H, Nishikawa J (2008) Fluorodeoxyglucose positron emission tomography integrated with computed tomography to determine resectability of primary lung cancer. Gen Thorac Cardiovasc Surg 56:404–409

Nestle U, Kremp S, Grosu AL (2006) Practical integration of [18F]-FDG-PET and PET-CT in the planning of radiotherapy for non-small cell lung cancer (NSCLC): the technical basis, ICRU-target volumes, problems, perspectives. Radiother Oncol 81:209–225

Onitilo AA, Engel JM, Demos JM, Mukesh B (2008) Prognostic significance of 18 F-fluorodeoxyglucose—positron emission tomography after treatment in patients with limited stage small cell lung cancer. Clin Med Res 6:72–77

Pandit N, Gonen M, Krug L, Larson SM (2003) Prognostic value of [18F]FDG-PET imaging in small cell lung cancer. Eur J Nucl Med Mol Imaging 30:78–84

Patz EF Jr, Lowe VJ, Hoffman JM et al (1993) Focal pulmonary abnormalities: evaluation with F-18 fluorodeoxyglucose PET scanning. Radiology 188:487–490

Pieterman RM, van Putten JW, Meuzelaar JJ et al (2000) Preoperative staging of non-small-cell lung cancer with positron-emission tomography. N Engl J Med 343:254–261

Prenzel KL, Monig SP, Sinning JM et al (2003) Lymph node size and metastatic infiltration in non-small cell lung cancer. Chest 123:463–467

Quint LE, Francis IR (1999) Radiologic staging of lung cancer. J Thorac Imaging 14:235–246

Quint LE, Tummala S, Brisson LJ et al (1996) Distribution of distant metastases from newly diagnosed non-small cell lung cancer. Ann Thorac Surg 62:246–250

Rusch VW, Venkatraman E (1996) The importance of surgical staging in the treatment of malignant pleural mesothelioma. J Thorac Cardiovasc Surg 111:815–825 discussion 825–826

Ryu JS, Choi NC, Fischman AJ, Lynch TJ, Mathisen DJ (2002) FDG-PET in staging and restaging non-small cell lung cancer after neoadjuvant chemoradiotherapy: correlation with histopathology. Lung Cancer 35:179–187

Saunders CA, Dussek JE, O'Doherty MJ, Maisey MN (1999) Evaluation of fluorine-18-fluorodeoxyglucose whole body positron emission tomography imaging in the staging of lung cancer. Ann Thorac Surg 67:790–797

Schmucking M, Baum RP, Griesinger F et al (2003) Molecular whole-body cancer staging using positron emission tomography: consequences for therapeutic management and metabolic radiation treatment planning. Recent Results Cancer Res 162:195–202

Schneider DB, Clary-Macy C, Challa S et al (2000) Positron emission tomography with f18-fluorodeoxyglucose in the staging and preoperative evaluation of malignant pleural mesothelioma. J Thorac Cardiovasc Surg 120:128–133

Schrevens L, Lorent N, Dooms C, Vansteenkiste J (2004) The role of PET scan in diagnosis, staging, and management of non-small cell lung cancer. Oncologist 9:633–643

Schumacher T, Brink I, Mix M et al (2001) FDG-PET imaging for the staging and follow-up of small cell lung cancer. Eur J Nucl Med 28:483–488

Shen YY, Shiau YC, Wang JJ, Ho ST, Kao CH (2002) Whole-body 18F-2-deoxyglucose positron emission tomography in primary staging small cell lung cancer. Anticancer Res 22:1257–1264

Shepherd FA, Crowley J, Van Houtte P et al (2007) The International Association for the Study of Lung Cancer lung cancer staging project: proposals regarding the clinical staging of small cell lung cancer in the forthcoming (seventh) edition of the tumor, node, metastasis classification for lung cancer. J Thorac Oncol 2:1067–1077

Steinert HC, Hauser M, Allemann F et al (1997) Non-small cell lung cancer: nodal staging with FDG PET versus CT with correlative lymph node mapping and sampling. Radiology 202:441–446

Subramaniam RM, Wilcox B, Aubry MC, Jett J, Peller PJ (2009) 18F-fluoro-2-deoxy-D-glucose positron emission tomography and positron emission tomography/computed tomography imaging of malignant pleural mesothelioma. J Med Imaging Radiat Oncol 53:160–169 quiz 170

Sugarbaker DJ, Flores RM, Jaklitsch MT et al (1999) Resection margins, extrapleural nodal status, and cell type determine postoperative long-term survival in trimodality therapy of malignant pleural mesothelioma: results in 183 patients. J Thorac Cardiovasc Surg 117:54–63 discussion 63–65

Swensen SJ, Jett JR, Hartman TE et al (2003) Lung cancer screening with CT: Mayo Clinic experience. Radiology 226:756–761

Teta MJ, Mink PJ, Lau E, Sceurman BK, Foster ED (2008) US mesothelioma patterns 1973–2002: indicators of change and insights into background rates. Eur J Cancer Prev 17: 525–534

Truong MT, Pan T, Erasmus JJ (2006) Pitfalls in integrated CT-PET of the thorax: implications in oncologic imaging. J Thorac Imaging 21:111–122

van Tinteren H, Hoekstra OS, Smit EF et al (2002) Effectiveness of positron emission tomography in the preoperative assessment of patients with suspected non-small-cell lung cancer: the PLUS multicentre randomised trial. Lancet 359:1388–1393

Vansteenkiste JF, Stroobants SG, De Leyn PR et al (1997) Mediastinal lymph node staging with FDG-PET scan in patients with potentially operable non-small cell lung cancer: a prospective analysis of 50 cases. Leuven Lung Cancer Group. Chest 112:1480–1486

Vansteenkiste JF, Stroobants SG, De Leyn PR, Dupont PJ, Verbeken EK (1998) Potential use of FDG-PET scan after induction chemotherapy in surgically staged IIIa-N2 non-small-cell lung cancer: a prospective pilot study. The Leuven Lung Cancer Group. Ann Oncol 9:1193–1198

Vansteenkiste JF, Stroobants SG, Dupont PJ et al (1999) Prognostic importance of the standardized uptake value on (18)F-fluoro-2-deoxy-glucose-positron emission tomography scan in non-small-cell lung cancer: An analysis of 125 cases. Leuven Lung Cancer Group. J Clin Oncol 17:3201–3206

Vinjamuri M, Craig M, Campbell-Fontaine A, Almubarak M, Gupta N, Rogers JS (2008) Can positron emission tomography be used as a staging tool for small-cell lung cancer? Clin Lung Cancer 9:30–34

Wahl RL, Jacene H, Kasamon Y, Lodge MA (2009) From RECIST to PERCIST: evolving considerations for PET response criteria in solid tumors. J Nucl Med 50(Suppl 1):122S–150S

Weber WA, Petersen V, Schmidt B et al (2003) Positron emission tomography in non-small-cell lung cancer: prediction of response to chemotherapy by quantitative assessment of glucose use. J Clin Oncol 21:2651–2657

Yang W, Fu Z, Yu J et al (2008) Value of PET/CT versus enhanced CT for locoregional lymph nodes in non-small cell lung cancer. Lung Cancer 61:35–43

Yildirim H, Metintas M, Entok E et al (2009) Clinical value of fluorodeoxyglucose-positron emission tomography/computed tomography in differentiation of malignant mesothelioma from asbestos-related benign pleural disease: an observational pilot study. J Thorac Oncol 4: 1480–1484

Young H, Baum R, Cremerius U et al (1999) Measurement of clinical and subclinical tumour response using [18F]-fluorodeoxyglucose and positron emission tomography: review and 1999 EORTC recommendations. European Organization for Research and Treatment of Cancer (EORTC) PET Study Group. Eur J Cancer 35:1773–1782

Breast Cancer

Gustavo A. Mercier, Felix-Nicolas Roy, and François Bénard

Contents

G. A. Mercier (✉)
Molecular Imaging and Nuclear Medicine, Boston Medical Center, Boston University School of Medicine, Boston, MA, USA
e-mail: Gustavo.Mercier@bmc.org

F.-N. Roy
Department of Radiology, Centre Hospitalier de l'Université de Montréal (CHUM), 3840 Saint Urbain Street, Montreal, QC H2W 1T8, Canada

F. Bénard
Department of Radiology, BC Cancer Agency, Functional Cancer Imaging, Centre of Excellence for Functional Cancer Imaging, University of British Columbia, Vancouver, Canada

Abstract

Breast cancer is a leading cause of death in women. Advance imaging, including radioisotope-based methods, plays a crucial role in the management of these patients. Current guidelines recommend 18-fluorodeoxyglucose PET (or PET/CT) imaging in patients with advanced disease or with suspected tumor recurrence. However, the development of breast-specific PET scanners is expanding the indications to surgical planning and to assist in the diagnosis of breast cancer. Today, these are applications where MRI is the main imaging modality. For this reason combined PET/MRI imaging, if developed as a small parts breast specific scanner, is likely to make dramatic changes in our imaging of breast cancer. This is particularly true when we consider the development of new tracers capable of in vivo receptor imaging, and advanced techniques to measure perfusion and hypoxia. We review the application of whole-body PET and PET/CT imaging in breast cancer, and the role of one of the dedicated PET breast scanners that is also approved for radioisotope guided biopsy. The chapter ends with a synopsis of new tracers and an introduction to breast MRI that speculates on the value of PET/MRI in breast cancer.

1 Key Points

The role of FDG PET/CT is well documented for staging of breast cancer patients with locally advanced disease (stage IIIc) or for those in whom recurrence is suspected because of equivocal CT

P. Peller et al. (eds.), *PET-CT and PET-MRI in Oncology*, Medical Radiology. Diagnostic Imaging,
DOI: 10.1007/174_2012_636, © Springer-Verlag Berlin Heidelberg 2012

scans, MRI, or bone scans. This fact is reflected in the guidelines of the National Comprehensive Cancer Network (NCCN). There is some data to suggest that patients with a high likelihood of metastatic disease, either because of axillary lymph node metastases, tumor histology such as triple negative tumors, or inflammatory cancer can benefit from FDG PET/CT imaging as part of staging. FDG PET/CT with whole-body scanners is inadequate for evaluating the axillae and does not replace sentinel lymph node biopsy. However, it may expand the role of sentinel lymph node biopsy in patients with large primary lesions if the axilla is PET negative. FDG PET/CT imaging is also of value in therapy assessment in those with advanced disease and documented uptake from a baseline scan. Reviewers must be careful with bone metastases because interpretation of FDG uptake in the bone/bone marrow may reflect a flare phenomenon in response to therapy, while sclerosis with poor uptake may reflect either healing in a bone metastasis or possibly a new metastasis with poor uptake.

Dedicated units for breast PET imaging, positron emission mammography (PEM) show great promise in evaluating the breast due to their high sensitivity and improved resolution. PEM can assist in the detection and characterization of breast cancer beyond what is possible with whole-body scanners. Recent comparisons with MRI also suggest that PEM can either compete or be complementary to MRI in the characterization of lesions in mammography and in surgical planning. Recent data shows that PEM imaging is more specific than MRI while MRI seems more sensitive in the detection of breast cancer. In this respect, a PET/MRI unit designed for breast imaging would represent a major advance. When this technology is coupled with the development of new tracers that can provide a molecular signature of the tumor without invasive sampling, it is clear that patients with breast cancer can expect a brighter future with more options than just mammography and biopsy.

2 Introduction

Breast cancer is a common malignancy that afflicts primarily women Cancer Facts and Figures 2010 and is a leading cause of cancer-related mortality for women (WHO I Cancer 2010). In the USA, the American Cancer Society estimates 207,090 women will be diagnosed with invasive breast cancer. Only 54,010 women will be diagnosed with the most curable form of the disease, carcinoma in situ; and approximately 39,840 women are expected to die of breast cancer each year (Cancer Facts and Figures 2010). Because it is a major health problem, significant resources are spent screening for the disease. Mammography is the primary means of screening, and in spite of much controversy (Evans et al. 2010; Kopans 2010a, b; Kopans et al. 2010; Lee et al. 2010; Marshall 2010) it is generally regarded as successful in helping to reduce deaths due to breast cancer (Berry et al. 2005). However, mammography has limitations as an imaging modality, and other technologies play a significant role, especially outside of the scope of screening. Most notable among these are sonography and MRI (Bartella et al. 2007). Imaging with positron emitters is the newest tool in breast imaging and in the management of breast cancer.

The molecular characterization of breast cancer is important in treating the disease. Chip analysis of tissue samples to probe a battery of molecular markers and provide a recurrence risk factor score is already in clinical use (Gene Expression Profiling 2010). A feature of PET imaging is the ability to query tumor biology at the molecular level in an individual patient in vivo, a feature critical to the concept of individualized medicine, and to monitor changes in the biologic profile of residual tissue that may be resistant to treatment (Dunphy and Lewis 2009). It is the increase in aerobic glycolysis (Warburg effect) with the associated increase in glucose transporters and hexokinase activity that is relevant for tumor detection using 18-fluorodeoxyglucose (FDG) (Goethals et al. 2010; Jadvar et al. 2009; Vander Heiden et al. 2009). The molecular biology of breast cancer suggests that this is a heterogeneous disease (Anderson and Matsuno 2006). The expression of estrogen, progesterone, and HER2/neu receptors affects prognosis. For example, "triple negative" tumors, tumors that fail to express any of these receptors, are associated with higher mortality rates (Basu et al. 2008). Currently, immunohistochemistry is used to detect the presence of these receptors in tissue samples. However, upon treatment and with time the tumors may change due to selection pressures; receptors that were present at the time of initial staging may be lost during the course of treatment. In vivo monitoring is an enticing alternative to help guide therapy because breast cancer chemotherapy includes agents that specifically bind to these receptors, and it is impractical to obtain multiple tissue samples for serial immunohistochemistry analysis.

The need to characterize tumor biology in vivo has led to a variety of experimental tracers and, due to their importance and the likelihood of their future use, these are included in this chapter. The characterization of tumor biology becomes even more relevant when we consider breast-specific PET imaging devices, which are able to see very small tumors not well identified with whole-body scanners. Tumor biomarker imaging will be integral to selecting the right therapy for patients and hopefully this imaging will provide the ability to predict response to specific agents.

The bulk of this chapter reviews the clinical applications of FDG PET imaging in the diagnosis, staging, restaging, and follow-up of therapy in breast cancer. The main focus is on the application of whole-body PET/CT scanners. A PEM unit that generates limited 3D images using tomosynthesis (limited angle tomography) technology has recently been approved by the Federal Drug Administration. We include an introduction to breast MRI, and a discussion of the role that PET/MR and PEM may have in a world where MRI dominates advanced breast imaging.

3 Clinical FDG PET and PET/CT Imaging

Most of the research and clinical experience with FDG and imaging of breast cancer stems from work using whole-body scanners, either PET or PET/CT scanners. This is the focus of this section. Although the technologies have significant differences, it is tacitly assumed that knowledge learned from PET scanners translates to PET/CT scanners. Moreover, the market for PET technology is dominated by sales of PET/CT equipment. For these reasons we will not attempt to distinguish between these two. When we refer to "PET imaging," we imply both PET and PET/CT imaging unless we state otherwise.

3.1 Diagnosis

Breast cancer is usually diagnosed through the biopsy of a palpable mass or an asymptomatic lesion identified at screening mammography. Although the specificity of screening mammography is poor and results in many false positive biopsies (Bartella et al. 2007), screening schemes are successful in detecting subcentimeter breast cancers (Kopans 2010a, b). The lack of adequate spatial resolution and the variable uptake seen with FDG, limits the value of whole-body scanners in assisting mammography in the diagnosis of breast cancer, unlike sonography and MRI.

Scheidhauer et al. has reviewed the use of FDG PET with whole-body scanners and other modalities in the diagnosis of breast cancer (Scheidhauer et al. 2004). For FDG PET, they report pooled sensitivity that ranges from 64 to 96 % and specificity that ranges from 73 to 100 %. They emphasize that most of the studies fail to include the small (T1a) cancers that have a better prognosis. Two factors are relevant to the poor performance of FDG PET imaging with whole-body scanners in the diagnosis of breast lesions that are suspicious for malignancy in mammography: the size of the lesion, and variations in the uptake of FDG.

Work by Avril et al. has shown that the sensitivity of FDG PET for diagnosis of malignant breast lesions decreases from 92 % for pT2 to 68 % for pT1 lesions (Avril et al. 2000). For pT1a lesions the sensitivity was zero. They also noted that the performance of FDG PET was worse for invasive lobular carcinoma (ILC) than for invasive ductal carcinoma (IDC), and that the sensitivity for noninvasive breast cancer was very low, 42 % with their high sensitivity analysis. The poor sensitivity for ILC could not be explained by the size of the tumor, and they suggested that the tumor biology of this histologic subtype is responsible for its poor affinity for FDG. Torizuka et al. have shown that breast cancer tumors show lower hexokinase activity than lung cancer cells (Torizuka et al. 1998) and this may explain the overall lower FDG affinity seen in breast cancer. Unfortunately, analysis of subtypes of breast cancer to investigate the clinical observations by Avril et al. has not been done. Avril's work is noteworthy for their use of a foam insert and the prone position with a dedicated breast emission scan time of 20 min using ECAT 951R/31 and ECAT EXACT scanners. This imaging protocol could be considered optimal for a single time-point whole-body scan. Heusner et al. used a similar protocol as a part of a comprehensive FDG PET/CT (contrast enhanced) scan that they call whole-body PET/CT mammography and which they compared against dedicated MRI breast imaging in the setting of initial staging, but not of diagnosis (Heusner et al. 2008a, b).

Two strategies have been used to improve the diagnostic ability of FDG PET imaging: dual time-point imaging with whole-body scanners and single time-point imaging with dedicated breast PET scanners. The first strategy exploits the fact that tumors show progressive FDG uptake while benign lesions and normal tissues show a plateau or decline in FDG uptake. Hence, contrast improves with delayed imaging for malignant lesions. The group led by Alavi supports this strategy with whole-body scanners (Kumar et al. 2005; Mavi et al. 2006). The second strategy aims at improving the diagnostic ability of FDP PET by improving the spatial resolution and sensitivity of the scanner. This strategy applies to a new technology, PEM, which we will discuss in a separate section.

The dual time-point imaging technique consists of two FDG PET scans that are acquired in the same imaging session but at different time points after the injection of tracer. Normally, the first scan covers the base of the skull to mid-thighs at 60 min after injection of tracer. At the conclusion of that scan, the breasts are again scanned using one or two additional bed-positions. Normally, this second scan starts about 100 min after the injection of tracer. Using this approach, Kumar et al. showed a sensitivity of 82 % and a specificity of 83 % in discriminating benign from malignant lesions using an increase of at least 3.75 % in SUV_{max} as a criterion for a malignant lesion (Kumar et al. 2005). The study included 57 lesions (39 malignant; average size of 18 mm $\pm$ 11 mm; range 2–40 mm), mostly invasive ductal carcinomas. There were six false negative lesions ranging in size from 2 to 35 mm. Three of the six T1a lesions were true positives. There were three false positive lesions with two of these showing significant signs of inflammation.

In summary, the use of FDG PET (or PET/CT) with whole-body scanners cannot be recommended for the diagnosis of breast cancer at this time. This is consistent with the current position of the Center for Medicare Services (CMS) in the United States and the NCCN guidelines. However, the dual time-point scheme of FDG PET imaging is promising. If the dual time-point scheme was coupled with small part scanners that provide better spatial resolution and sensitivity to tracer detection, the current applications of FDG imaging to the diagnosis of breast cancer might be expanded. It is also clear that there are limitations to the ability of breast cancer to accumulate FDG. Lobular cancers show lower tracer uptake than ductal cancers (Kumar et al. 2005; Mavi et al. 2006), and triple negative tumors show higher uptake than tumors that are ER+/PR +/HER2- (Basu et al. 2008). See Fig. 1 for these reasons, future studies should control not only the size of the lesions, but also their histology and receptor status. Researchers should also aim at developing and testing tracers that show higher uptake in primary breast cancers.

3.2 Staging

The initial staging of breast cancer is aimed at answering questions that are relevant to establishing the prognosis and selecting appropriate therapy. The locoregional extent of disease is important for the surgeon because it dictates the type of mastectomy, and possibly the likelihood of axillary lymph node dissection versus sentinel lymph node biopsy (Heusner et al. 2009). For the oncologist, the molecular biology of the tumors is important because it determines the success of hormonal therapy and anti-HER2/neu agents. Hence, staging depends on physical exam, imaging findings, and pathologic examination. Current NCCN guidelines emphasize conventional imaging, i.e. mammography, sonography, bone scan, CT, and MRI (NCCN Breast Cancer Clinical Practice Guidelines Updated 2010; NCCN Invasive Breast Cancer Clinical Practice Guidelines 2007). The use of FDG PET in staging is limited to locally advanced disease (i.e., clinical stage IIIc—primary tumor larger than 5 cm; skin or chest wall involvement; fixed axillary lymph nodes; positive infra/supraclavicular lymph nodes, or internal mammary lymph nodes), or for the case of equivocal conventional imaging (Fig. 3). Recently, Hodgson and Gulenchyn have reviewed the literature on the use of FDG PET imaging for staging of breast cancer (Hodgson and Gulenchyn 2008). They emphasize the lack of adequate trials and the limitations of FDG in staging breast cancer, particularly the limited sensitivity in staging the status of axillary lymph nodes. Next, we highlight some of these shortcomings. However, we also emphasize recent studies that provide preliminary support for the use of FDG PET in the staging of aggressive subtypes of breast cancer, such as inflammatory carcinomas (See Fig. 2) (Alberini et al. 2009; Lee et al. 2009a, b, Yang et al.

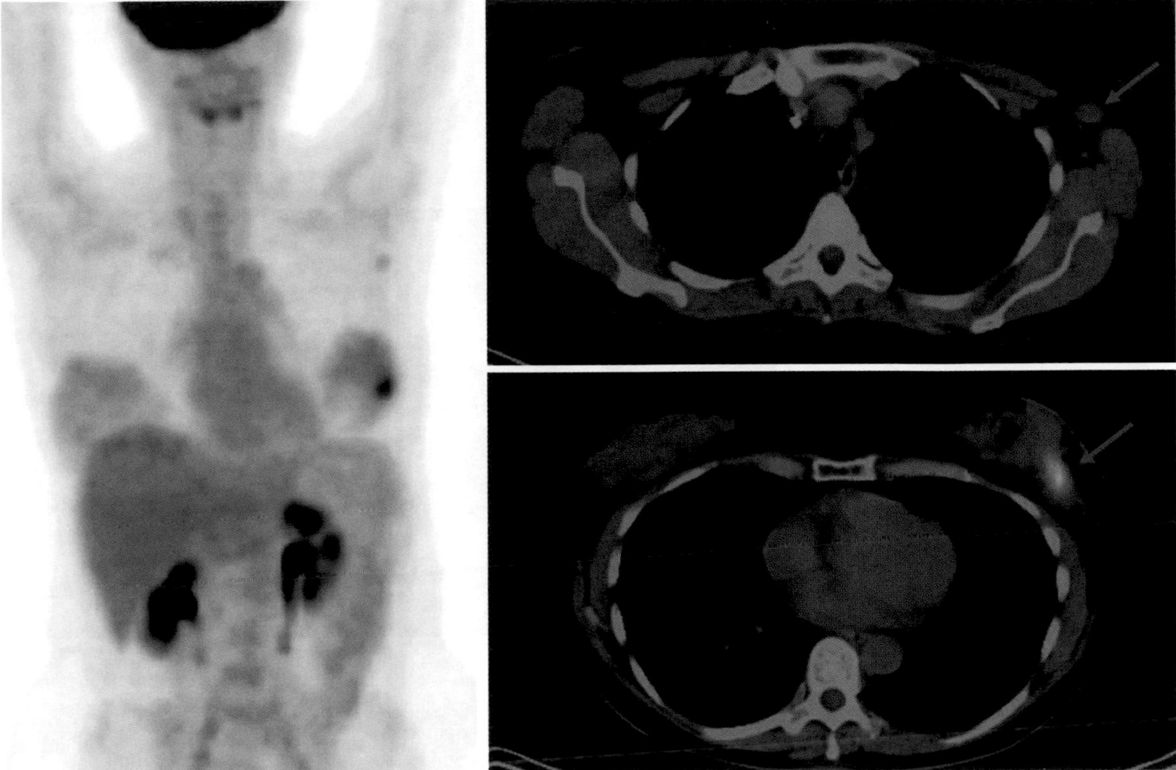

Fig. 1 Triple negative breast cancer. This 41-year-old woman presented for evaluation of a palpable mass in the left breast. Biopsy showed infiltrating ductal breast cancer, which was negative for estrogen, progesterone, and HER2/neu receptors. PET/CT shows single intensely FDG-avid lesion in the left breast. Nodal metastasis seen in the left axilla precluded sentinel node procedure. The patient received chemotherapy followed by a lumpectomy and axillary node dissection

2008) and triple negative tumors (Basu et al. 2008). We also note that the NCCN guidelines fail to recognize the value of a baseline exam to allow for follow-up of therapy, a promising area for FDG PET imaging (Dose-Schwarz et al. 2010; Avril et al. 2009; Lee et al. 2009a, b; Rousseau et al. 2006).

The same limitations that FDG PET has in the diagnosis of breast cancer also apply to the characterization of the extent of disease within the breast. For example, Uematsu et al. have shown that whole-body scanners consistently underestimate the extent of disease within the breast and that MRI is more accurate in this setting (Uematsu et al. 2009). This limitation still persists even when the technique is optimized (Heusner et al. 2008a, b). In performing T staging of the primary breast lesion, MRI was still more accurate than their dedicated FDG PET/CT scan (77 % for MRI vs. 54 % PET/CT). In general, FDG PET/CT imaging is not accurate enough to replace sentinel lymph node biopsy to determine the status of axillary lymph nodes. However, early reports to be discussed below suggest that FDG PET/CT scans may assist in surgical planning because the scans may stratify patients between those who should first undergo sentinel lymph node biopsy (SLNB), and those who should go directly to axillary lymph node dissection.

The review by Hodgson and Gulenchyn presents a nice summary of experience in using FDG PET to perform N staging in breast cancer (Hodgson and Gulenchyn 2008). The accuracy of FDG PET in staging the axilla is related to the size of the primary tumor and its histology (Avril et al. 1996). For this reason early reports, where larger tumors were common, frequently overestimated the accuracy of FDG PET in staging the axilla. Today, the consensus is that FDG PET imaging with whole-body scanners can not compete against the accuracy of axillary lymph node dissection (Hodgson and Gulenchyn 2008; Wahl et al. 2004) or even sentinel lymph node biopsy (Veronesi et al. 2007) in staging the axillary lymph nodes.

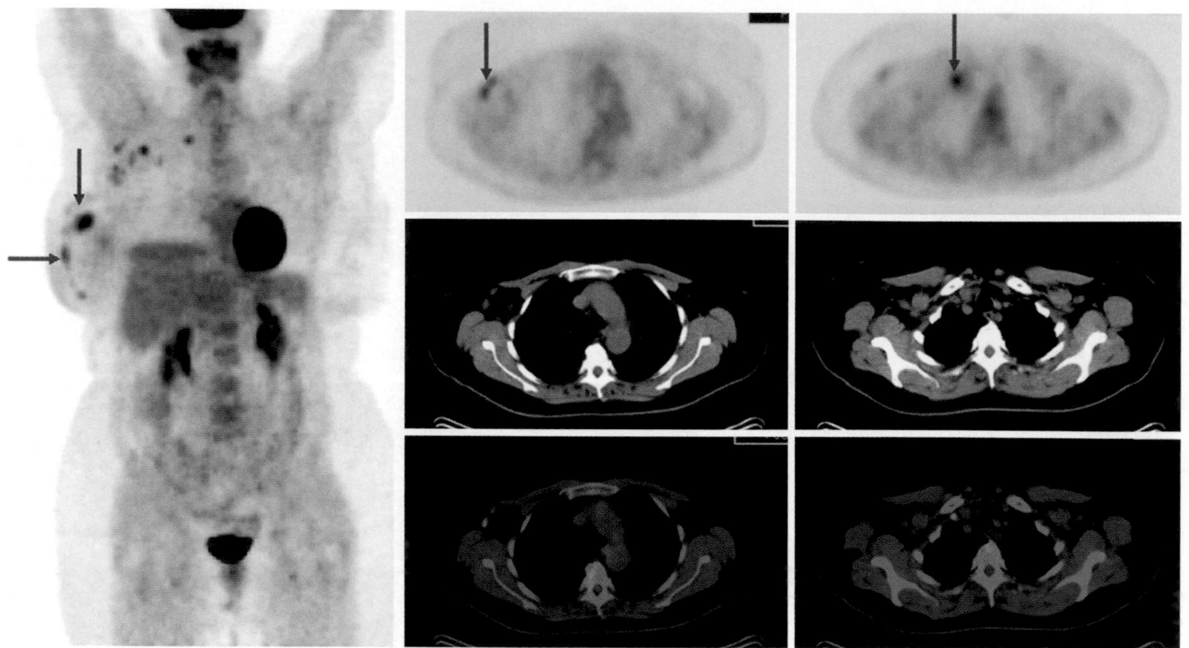

Fig. 2 Inflammatory breast cancer. This 46-year-old woman presented for redness and swelling of the right breast. Skin and breast biopsy were positive for tumor. PET/CT shows multiple intensely FDG-avid lesions scattered throughout the right breast. Nodal metastases are seen in the axilla extending into the supraclavicular region. Sonography-guided biopsy confirmed the right supraclavicular node metastasis. The patient received chemotherapy followed by a mastectomy

Critical to the development of this consensus was the prospective multicenter trial reported by Wahl because the cohort in that study was composed of women with early disease in whom axillary instrumentation could be avoided if the nodal status of the axilla could be determined accurately with noninvasive imaging.

In the multicenter trial reported by Wahl et al., 308 axillae were evaluated from an initial cohort of 360 women (Wahl et al. 2004). Fifty-six women were excluded because they received therapy before their scans or did not have surgery to sample their lymph nodes. The prevalence of axillary tumor involvement was 35 % and nearly 100 % of the patients were clinical stage T2 or less. In their analysis, the authors made no effort to do a lymph node by lymph node analysis. Instead, an axilla was judged true positive on PET imaging if in the scan at least one lymph node was hot enough above background to be judged probably malignant, and pathology confirmed metastases to that axilla. With this criterion, the sensitivity of FDG PET was 61 % (95 % CI: 54–67 %). The specificity, positive, and negative predictive values were 80, 62, and 79 %, respectively. Quantitative analysis did not improve the performance of PET. FDG PET underestimated the number of metastatic lymph nodes, a result also confirmed by others (Heusner et al. 2009), and as usual, lower uptake was seen with lobular carcinomas.

Although FDG PET is unable to stage the axilla and spare surgery, some have argued that FDG PET may be useful in selecting which women should go for direct axillary lymph node dissection and which should be spared from this extensive surgery and simply undergo sentinel lymph node biopsy (Heusner et al. 2009). Heusner et al. evaluated the performance of FDG PET in staging the axilla using both per-patient and per-lymph node analysis. They confirmed the poor performance of FDG PET in staging the axilla, but argued that the negative predictive value on a per patient basis is high enough that FDG PET can be used to increase the threshold for axillary lymph node dissection and expand the use of sentinel lymph node biopsy. Using their results, 58 % sensitivity and 92 % specificity in a population made largely of T1 and T2 tumors with a prevalence of axillary lymph node metastases of 39 %, they presented a statistical argument that supports a change in the threshold for determining whether to perform sentinel lymph node

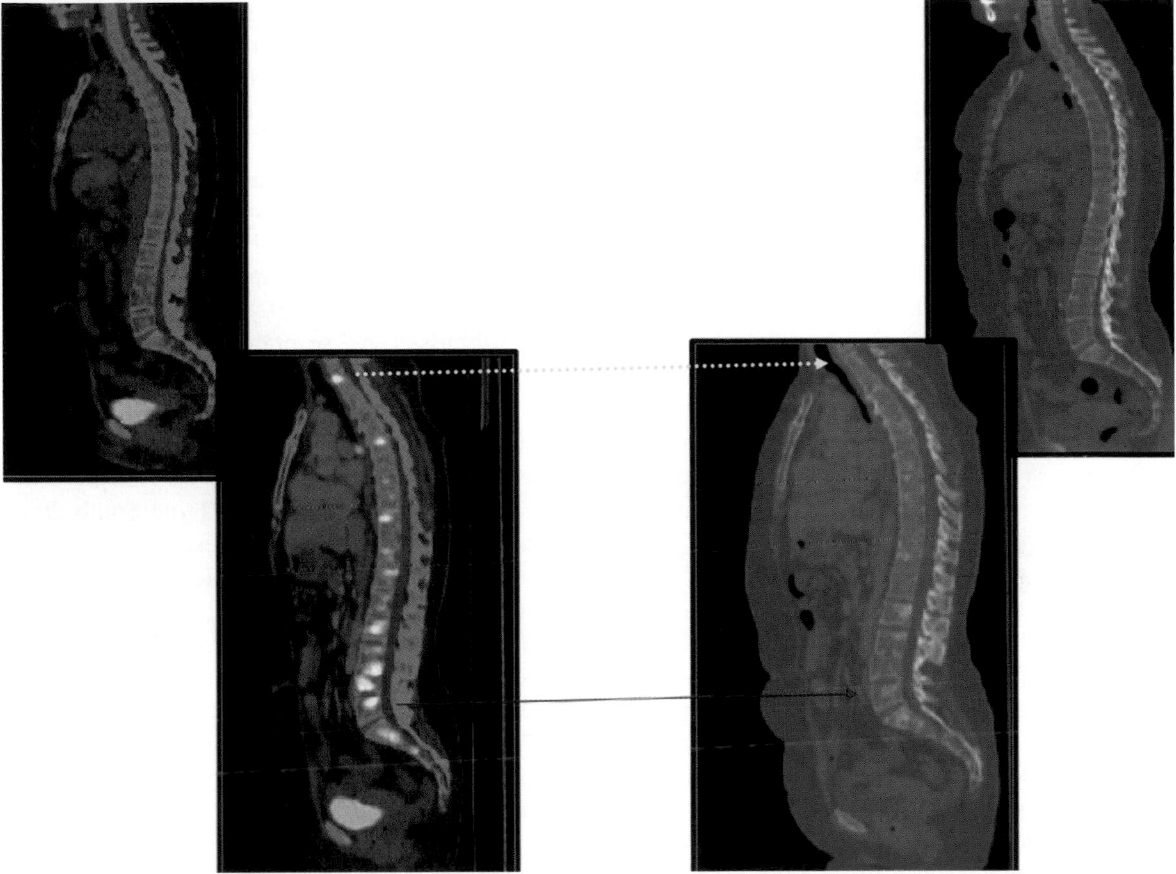

Fig. 3 Bone metastases and CT correlation FDG PET/CT fusion image in the sagittal plane along the spine and corresponding sagittal CT view. Images in the *upper outside* corners show no bone metastatic disease, while the images in the *middle* were taken 8 months later and show extensive bone metastases that are hypermetabolic in FDG PET/CT. Notice that on CT the spectrum of bone metastases include mixed sclerotic lytic lesions, and sclerotic lesions. A mixed lesion seen on both PET and CT is noted in the vertebral body of L5, while a lesion seen only on PET is visible in the lower cervical spine (see *arrows*). There is also a sclerotic lesion seen only on CT in the posterior aspect of the superior endplate vertebral body of L2; however, the central portion of L2 shows abnormal FDG uptake

biopsy or direct axillary lymph node dissection from a pretest probability of axillary metastasis of 40 % (tumors 2–3 cm in size) to 60 % (tumors 4–5 cm in size). This is possible because in patients with large tumors (>3 cm) but negative axilla, by FDG PET the sentinel lymph node biopsy technique will still retain a high negative predictive value (i.e., 95 % or better). A significant point in Heusner's study is that the clinical evaluation of the axilla included sonography. However, sonography was not used to guide biopsy of suspicious lymph nodes. Such a strategy would have spared women sentinel lymph node biopsy, and it is gaining momentum with recent promising results (Baruah et al. 2010).

Supraclavicular and internal mammary nodal stations are not usually biopsied in staging. However, they are relevant to staging because the presence of ipsilateral internal mammary lymph node metastases means at least N2 disease (at least stage IIIA), while supraclavicular malignant lymphadenopathy means N3 disease (stage IIIC). There are no good studies evaluating the performance of FDG PET in staging these nodal stations. The limitation stems from the lack of pathologic correlation. Bellon et al. 2004 have attempted to evaluate the performance of FDG PET in detecting metastasis to the ipsilateral internal mammary chain of lymph nodes in patients with locally advanced disease. Instead of using pathology as a standard, they did clinical follow-up and studied the pattern of subsequent metastatic disease to determine if internal mammary lymph nodes were involved with tumor. In this series with only 28 women, FDG PET identified 7 with ipsilateral internal mammary lymph node metastases and none of which was seen on chest CT. A total of 25 women had long-term follow-up (median 25 months) including six of the seven women with abnormal PET scans. Eight women had a pattern of failure consistent with involvement of the internal mammary nodal station, and four of these had uptake in the PET scan (50 % sensitivity). In 17 women, there was no failure to suggest internal mammary nodal station disease, and 15 of these had negative PET scans (88 % specificity). The positive predictive value was 67 % and the negative predictive value was 79 % Fig. 3.

The skeleton is the most common site of distant metastases in breast cancer with the spine and ribs most commonly affected (Even-Sapir 2005). Patients with bone-dominant metastatic disease have a very poor prognosis. The current NCCN guidelines recommend bone scans for patients with symptoms or high likelihood of bone metastases (Stage II or higher). The use of FDG PET or PET/CT imaging to detect bone metastases in breast cancer has been the subject of several reviews (Even-Sapir 2005; Fogelman et al. 2005; Rosen et al. 2007). Shie et al. have performed a meta-analysis of the literature from 1995 to 2006 to determine whether FDG PET (PET/CT was not included) or bone scintigraphy with Tc-99 m diphosphonate is better at detecting bone metastases in breast cancer (Shie et al. 2008). They found no conclusive evidence that either technology was superior in detecting bone metastases, although FDG PET had a higher specificity, or not. Their pooled patient based sensitivity and specificity for FDG PET was 81 % (95 % CI: 70–89 %) and 93 % (95 % CI: 84–97 %), respectively. For bone scintigraphy sensitivity was 78 % (95 % CI: 67–86 %) and specificity 79 % (95 % CI: 40–95 %). On a per-lesion analysis the pooled sensitivity and specificity for FDG PET was 69 % (95 % CI: 28–93 %) and 98 % (95 % CI: 87–100 %), respectively. For bone scintigraphy the pooled sensitivity and specificity on a per-lesion analysis was 88 % (95 % CI: 82–92 %) and 87 % (95 % CI: 29–99 %), respectively (Fig. 4).

The lack of clear superiority of FDG PET imaging over bone scan imaging may reflect the common observation in the literature that FDG PET imaging is more sensitive to osteolytic/mixed lesions than osteoblastic lesions (Cook et al. 1998; Du et al. 2007; Fogelman et al. 2005; Nakai et al. 2005; Rosen et al. 2007; Uematsu et al. 2005). The significance of this observation is controversial (Fogelman et al. 2005; Uematsu et al. 2005) and in some early studies such as the one by Yang et al. FDG PET imaging was superior to bone scintigraphy in detecting bone metastases (Yang et al. 2002).

As discussed by several authors, the apparent lower sensitivity of FDG PET for detection of sclerotic bone metastases in breast cancer may be an artifact of the study designs in which treated and untreated subjects were included as a single cohort (Fogelman et al. 2005; Williams and Smith 2005). Including patients who have received systemic therapy may result in an overestimate of the number of sclerotic bone lesions that show little or no uptake, as the natural history of metastatic bone lesions in breast cancer is to reduce their FDG uptake and become more sclerotic upon successful treatment (Du et al. 2007; Fogelman et al. 2005; Tateishi et al. 2008). This biology reflects a delayed bone response effect that is different from the better known flare phenomenon seen within 3 months of treatment, and that has the opposite effect of increasing FDG and Tc-99m diphosphonate uptake. Hence, the sensitivity of FDG PET would be unexpectedly low and for the bone scan it would be unexpectedly high (active sclerosis would have increased Tc-99 m diphosphonate uptake). The specificity of FDG PET imaging would improve because the fraction of false negatives would be low.

Recent work from our group in which the cohort was limited to untreated patients showed that although bone scans might be helpful, FDG PET/CT may be enough for the initial staging of the bones, particularly on a per-patient basis (Sacks et al. 2010). In a small series by our group that included six patients with 74 lesions of which 26 were malignant, the addition of Tc-99m MDP bone scan did not add value to the FDG PET/CT scan results. FDG PET/CT correctly identified all patients with bone metastases with only one false positive case; bone scans detected only three of the patients with bone metastases and had four false positive cases. Although the series is small, it is significant because it not only included patients with no prior treatment, but also because

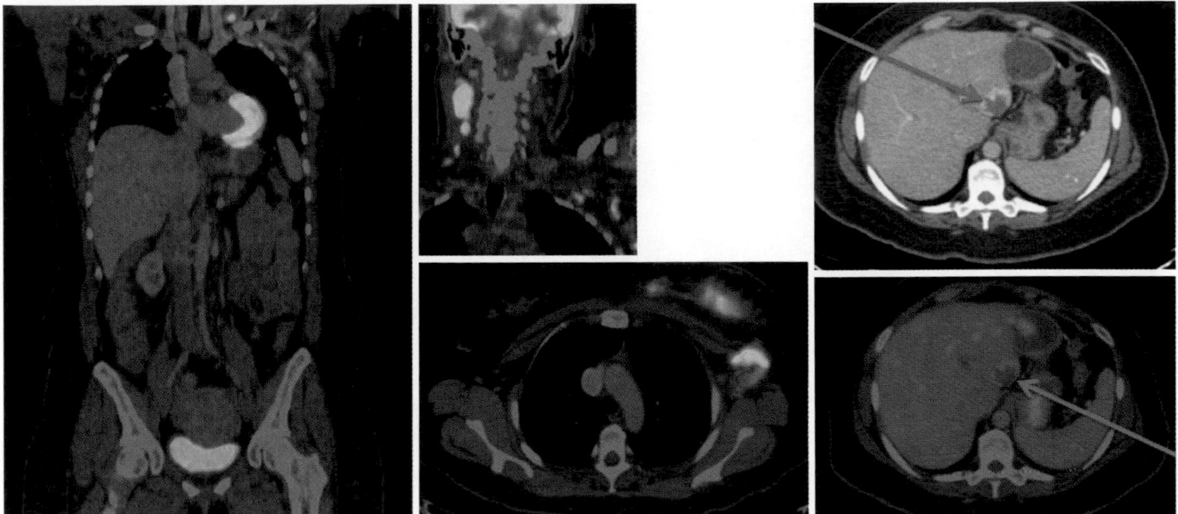

Fig. 4 Initial staging of advanced disease FDG PET/CT. A patient with extensive disease in the left breast and dramatic malignant lymphadenopathy in the left axilla, left supraclavicular nodal station, and lymphadenopathy on both sides of the neck. Note that the CT scan was obtained with diagnostic level parameters, including intravenous contrast. A liver lesion (*blue arrow*) is noted with no 18-FDG uptake and peripheral globular enhancement characteristic of a benign liver hemangioma

whole-body bone scanning included SPECT of the trunk for all patients and PET/CT was used instead of only PET (Sacks et al. 2010). SPECT imaging has been shown to improve the performance of bone scans (Savelli et al. 2001), and in the study by Uematsu et al. 2005 bone scan with SPECT imaging was shown to be superior to FDG PET while Ohta et al. 2001 found that planar bone scintigraphy had a similar or slightly inferior performance than FDG PET. The addition of CT as part of hybrid PET/CT has been shown to be synergistic. Many of the lesions that have abnormal uptake near a bone still represent soft tissue metastases when CT is used to localize the PET finding (for example pleural disease vs rib metastasis), and nearly 50 % of bone metastases are seen only in FDG PET (Nakamoto et al. 2005). More recently, a prospective study by Bristow et al. 2008 has shown that CT scan of the trunk may be a suitable replacement for bone scan with fewer false positive findings and only a few false negative results. The false negative findings where in areas not imaged by CT but included in the whole-body bone scans. Hence, FDG PET/CT should perform like a bone scan plus PET and it is not surprising that it is superior to even the best bone scan (i.e. SPECT) alone. This thought is also supported by the recent retrospective study by Morris et al. who showed that FDG PET/CT and bone scintigraphy were highly concordant in detecting bone metastases (81 %), but that upon follow-up or biopsy of discordant cases, FDG PET/CT was more accurate (Morris et al. 2010).

In an effort to improve bone imaging, investigators have explored the use of Fluoride PET and PET/CT. The expectation is that the lytic lesions that are not seen in bone scintigraphy with gamma emitters will be visible using positron emitters and PET technology. Early work by Petrén-Mallmin et al. 1998 confirmed this expectation in a small number of patients with breast cancer. More recently, Even-Sapir et al. using a cohort with a significant fraction of breast cancer, showed not only the ability of Fluoride PET to detect both lytic and sclerotic lesions, but that adding CT, as part of PET/CT, improved the specificity of the imaging (Even-Sapir 2005). In their study, the sensitivity of Fluoride PET/CT was significantly higher than Fluoride PET (88 % vs. 100 %) and the specificity showed a similar trend (56 % for PET vs. 88 % for PET/CT). Damle et al. 2007 studied 72 breast cancer patients as part of presurgical staging using Tc-99m MDP bone scintigraphy with SPECT, FDG PET/CT, and Fluoride PET/CT. The highest sensitivity and negative predictive value was seen with 18-Fluoride PET/CT (100 % for both), while FDG PET/CT had the lowest sensitivity and negative predictive

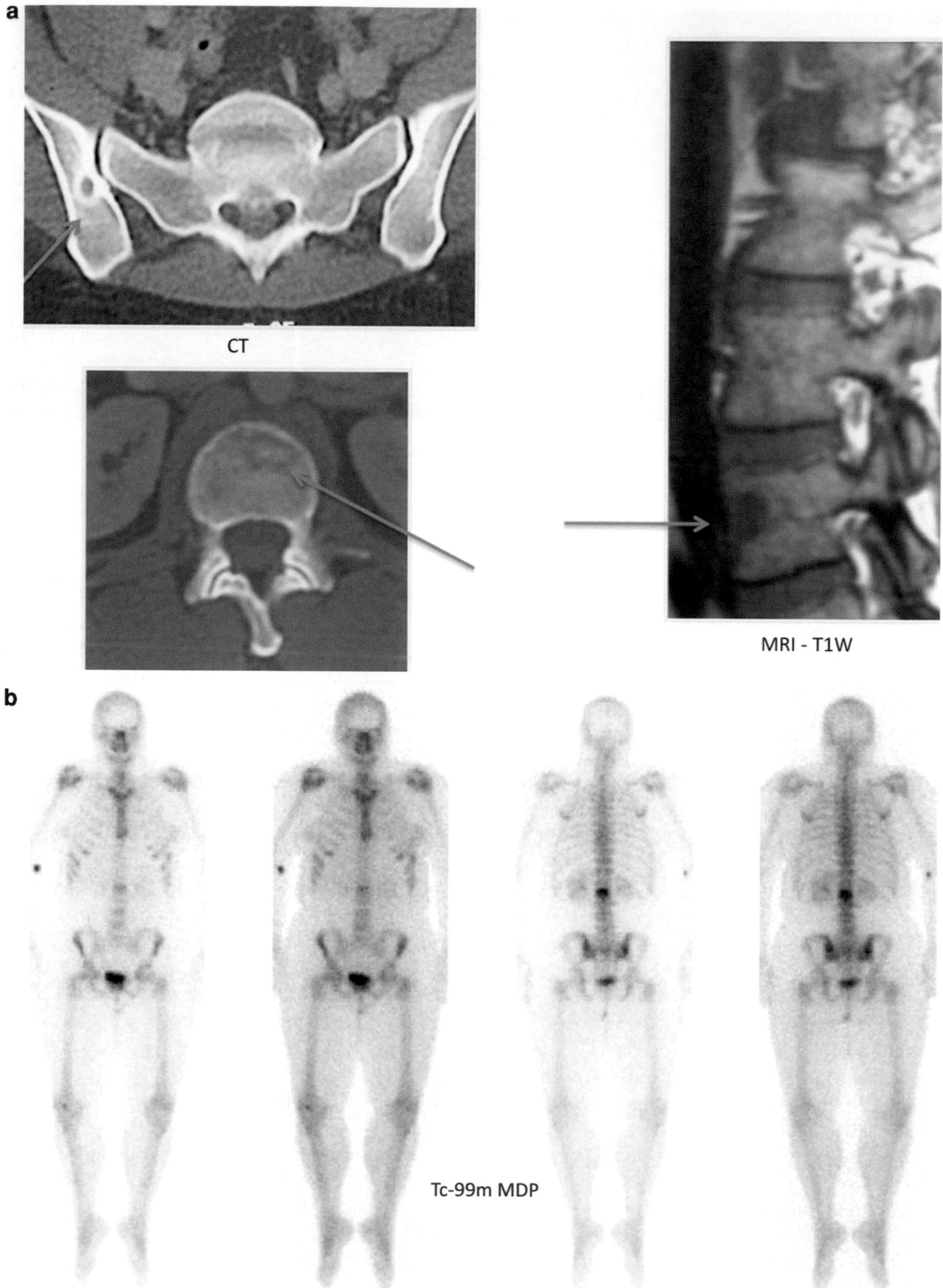

Fig. 5 (continued)

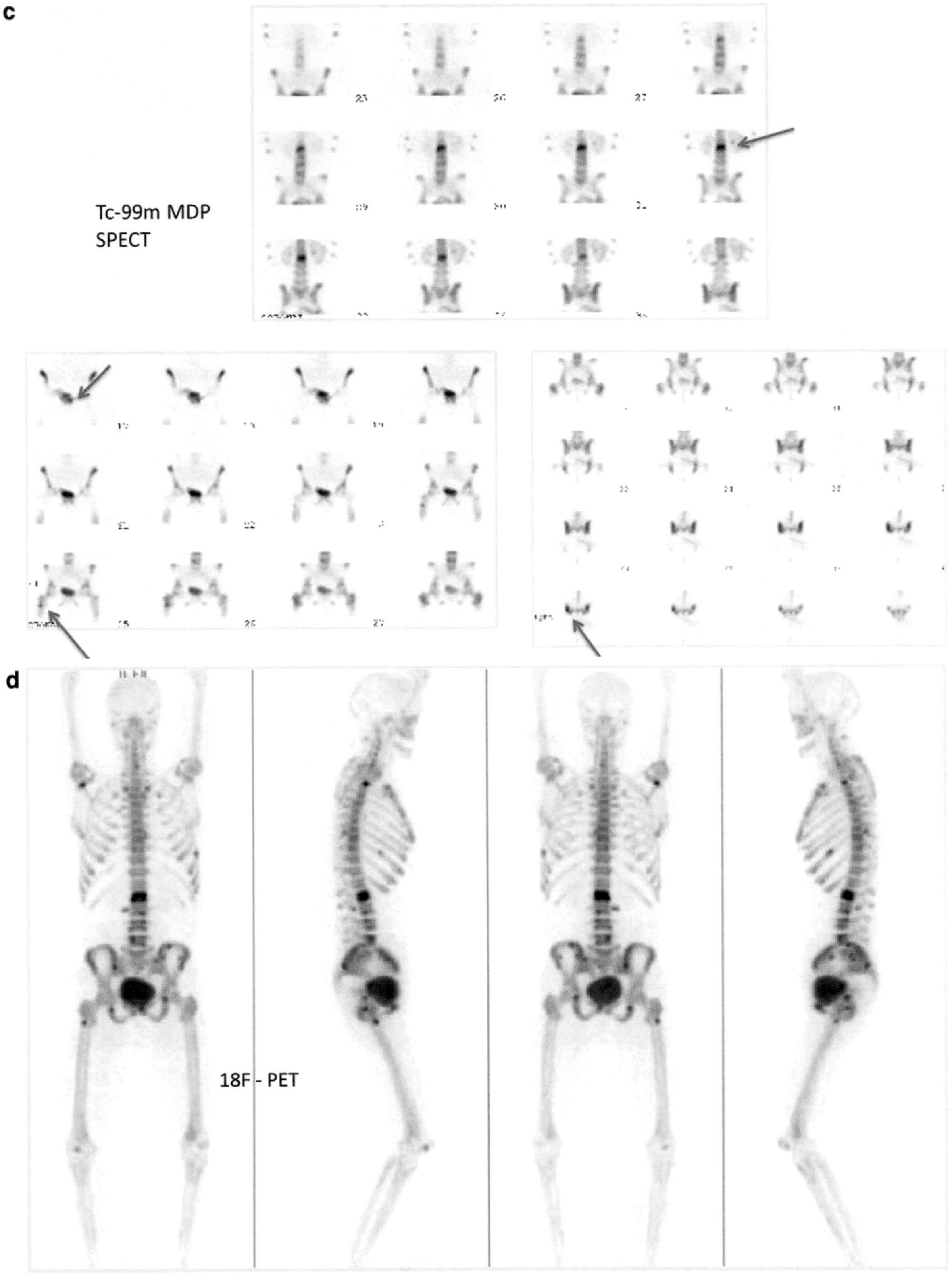

Fig. 5 (continued)

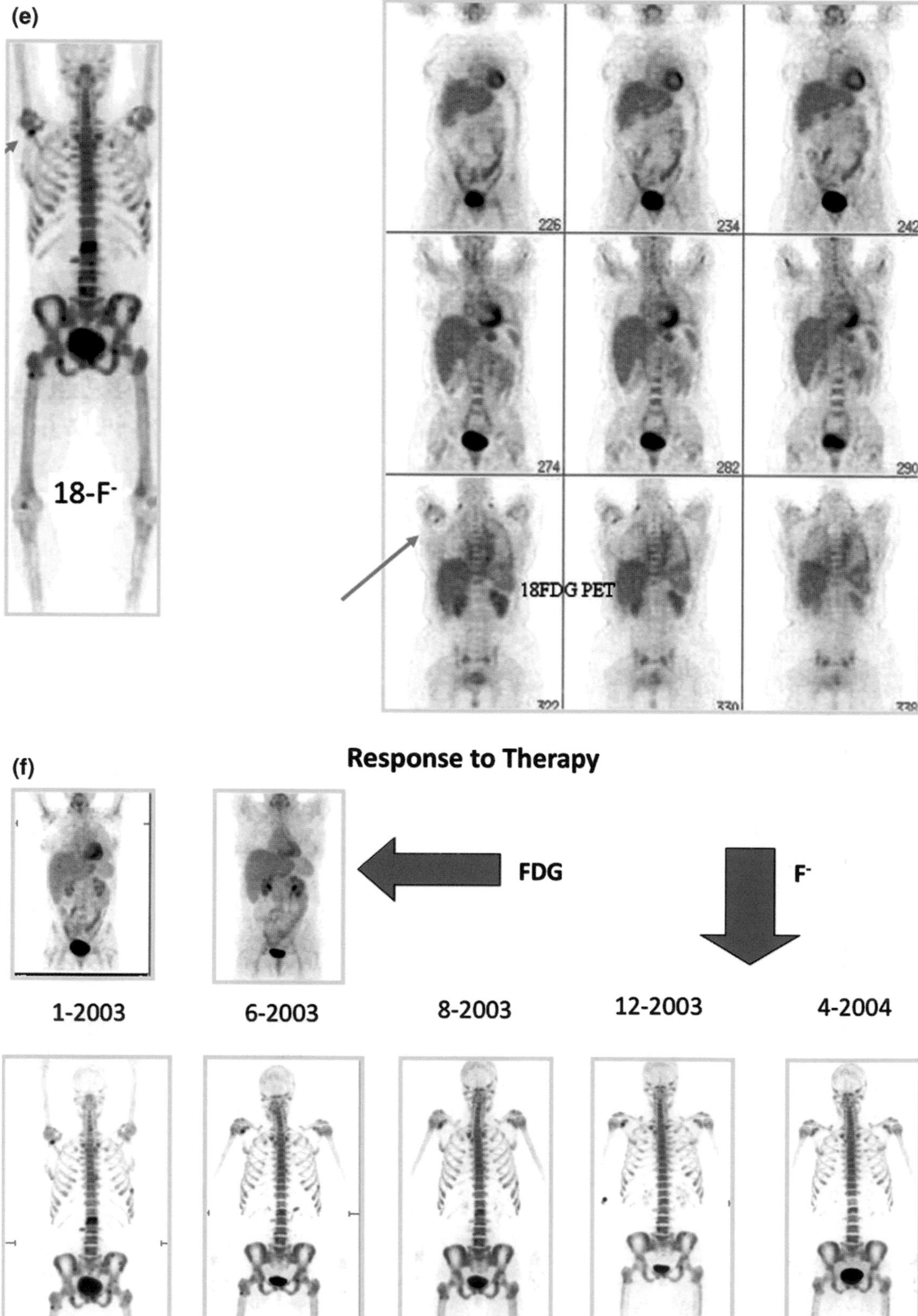

Fig. 5 (continued)

◀**Fig. 5** Bone metastases and PET imaging. This is a 36-year-old woman with intraductal carcinoma of the breast; positive for estrogen and progesterone receptors but HER2/neu negative. Treated with surgery and chemotherapy. The patient returned with back pain and there was concern for bone metastases. Radiographs and MRI were equivocal. Bone scan with Tc-99m MDP showed a single lesion in the thoracolumbar junction in routine planar views. SPECT imaging identified additional lesions. Subsequent Fluoride PET scan uncovered multiple discrete foci consistent with metastatic disease while FDG PET detected a single lesion in the right glenoid that was also seen in Fluoride PET. PET scans following treatment with chemotherapy showed prompt resolution of the FDG PET findings in the right glenoid and slower clearance of the abnormalities in Fluoride PET imaging. Biopsy of the thoracolumbar lesion confirmed metastatic breast cancer

value (44 and 47 %, respectively). However, FDG PET/CT had the highest specificity and positive predictive value (100 % for each). The best accuracy was seen with Fluoride 92 % and FDG PET/CT had the lowest accuracy at 63 %. Within these extremes Tc-99m bone scans with SPECT showed intermediate results (Fig. 5).

Even though FDG PET has a limited role in the initial staging of breast cancer, there is evidence that some subgroups of patients with breast cancer may benefit from early FDG PET imaging. Inflammatory breast cancer (IBC) represents a small group (1–3 %) of breast cancers that has very poor prognosis (median survival between 12–36 months) (Le-Petross et al. 2008; Levine and Veneroso 2008). A group at M.D. Anderson Cancer Center in Houston, Texas has recently reviewed their imaging experience in inflammatory breast cancer (Yang et al. 2008) with attention to FDG PET/CT (Carkaci et al. 2009). Because the cancer is so aggressive and a large proportion of patients have metastases at the time of presentation (20 %), a significant number of imaging studies are performed to determine the extent of disease. However, the 2009 report from the M.D. Anderson group suggests that FDG PET/CT imaging may provide a simple one-stop shopping imaging modality for initial staging of this cancer. For example, contrary to other histologies of breast cancer, FDG PET/CT had a high sensitivity in detecting ipsilateral axillary lymph node metastases (90 % sensitivity). The single false negative finding was in a subcentimeter lymph node with low SUV and micrometastasis. It is also noteworthy that the primary tumor in the breast was seen 98 % of the time, in addition to the expected uptake from skin inflammation. FDG PET/CT was also instrumental in the detection of distant metastatic disease because in 17 % of the patients PET/CT detected metastases not suspected after clinical examination and conventional imaging work-up. IBC is aggressive so it is not surprising that FDG PET imaging is able to detect many lesions (Fig. 2). The uptake is expected to be high and there is a high prevalence of widespread disease large enough to be seen without difficulty with a whole-body scanner. However, more common are the triple negative tumors and these also show significant uptake. They may represent another subtype of breast cancer where FDG PET/CT may make significant contributions to initial staging of the disease (Fig. 1). Unfortunately, we are not aware of a specific series evaluating the role of FDG PET/CT in the setting of staging triple negative breast cancers.

In summary, FDG does not match the accuracy of sentinel lymph node biopsy for detection of lymph node metastases and therefore is not recommended to evaluate the nodal status of the axilla in initial staging. However, FDG PET plays a role in evaluating infraclavicular, supraclavicular, or internal mammary lymphadenopathy that is not readily reached either by the sonographer or the surgeon. FDG PET is also important for detecting distant metastatic disease. For these reasons, FDG PET imaging is recommended by the NCCN for patients with advanced locoregional disease (stage III) (Fig. 4) and FDG PET/CT should be considered in patients with high-risk stage II disease, inflammatory breast cancer, and triple negative tumors due to the higher risk of FDG-avid metastasis. Because PET/CT has the ability to detect smaller lung nodules than PET, particularly when the CT of the chest is done in deep inspiration (Juergens et al. 2006), and is also able to detect sclerotic bone lesions, this modality is superior to PET in staging breast cancer. It is important to recognize that an initial staging exam not only assist with staging but also serves as a baseline to monitor the effects of therapy. This is particularly critical in following bone metastases because upon treatment they turn sclerotic and lose their 1FDG uptake. Without a baseline exam it is simply impossible to distinguish between a treated lesion and one responding to therapy, or simply a false negative sclerotic bone metastasis that is still viable. Bone scans with Tc-99 m diphosphonate are not useful in this setting because both untreated and treated metastases have high uptake. The jury is still out regarding the best way to detect skeletal metastases, although FDG PET/CT is again superior to FDG PET. However, it may still underestimate disease when compared to Fluoride PET/CT.

3.3 Response to Therapy

FDG PET imaging has also been proposed for monitoring tumor response to chemotherapy (Eubank et al. 2001; Kamel et al. 2003; Lee et al. 2009a, b; Rousseau et al. 2006; Wahl et al. 1993). observed a significant decrease in 18F-FDG uptake in responders after one cycle of chemotherapy and no significant decrease in nonresponders. In a series of 30 patients with large primary tumors or locally advanced disease treated with neoadjuvant chemotherapy, Smith et al. 2000 reported that after one cycle of chemotherapy, a reduction of FDG predicted a complete pathologic response. Schelling et al. 2000 reported similar results after three or four cycles of chemotherapy. Mankoff studied tumor blood flow and glucose metabolism by PET and found specific patterns that were predictive of the response to chemotherapy in locally advanced breast cancer (Mankoff et al. 2002). In a follow-up study in patients with locally advanced breast cancer, they found that a reduction in tumor perfusion midway through chemotherapy was associated with a longer disease-free survival and overall survival (Dunnwald et al. 2008).

Rousseau et al. 2006 conducted a prospective study in 64 patients with stage II and III breast cancer treated by neoadjuvant chemotherapy. Patients underwent PET imaging at baseline and after 1, 2, 3, and 6 cycles of chemotherapy. They found that a 40 % reduction in the SUV compared to baseline was highly predictive of response after two cycles of chemotherapy, with a sensitivity of 89 % and a specificity of 97 %. Of note, this study defined pathologic response as greater than 50 % therapeutic effect, and thus did not attempt to predict a complete or near-complete pathologic response.

Schwarz-Dose et al. 2009 recently published the results of a prospective multicenter study conducted in 104 patients with large and locally advanced breast cancers. They found that patients with a low baseline SUV (<3.0) did not achieve a pathologic response. Patients with high percentage decrease in SUV after one (>45 % decrease) or two cycles (>55 % decrease) of chemotherapy had a high likelihood of achieving a complete pathologic response. The negative predictive value for a smaller decrease was 90 %, suggesting a potential role in the decision to stop chemotherapy in patients who do not present an adequate metabolic response after one cycle of chemotherapy.

Initial reports suggested a potential role for FDG PET imaging in assessing response in patients with metastatic breast cancer (Dose-Schwarz et al. 2005; Schwarz-Dose et al. 2009). Couturier et al. 2006 in a prospective study of 20 patients with metastatic breast cancer treated by chemotherapy, showed that a FDG PET scan after three cycles of chemotherapy and compared to baseline was predictive of the clinical response at 6 months and overall survival. In patients with breast cancer and multiple bone metastases, FDG PET imaging has also been shown to be of value in measuring response because it correlated with outcome (Stafford et al. 2002) (Figs. 6, 7).

Overall, the data suggests that FDG PET is a valid tool to monitor response to therapy, both in locally advanced breast cancers and in the setting of metastatic breast cancer. In locally advanced breast cancer, other methods, such as even simple physical examination, as well as breast MRI, can provide valuable information so the precise clinical role of FDG PET imaging in this context remains to be defined. In metastatic breast cancer, FDG PET imaging can provide an earlier assessment of the response to chemotherapy than conventional imaging techniques, and is of value for assessing bone-dominant metastatic disease. The importance of a baseline study cannot be overstated. Small studies suggest that a successful response demonstrated by FDG PET imaging indicates a favorable outcome, providing valuable information, particularly when response is difficult to assess by conventional imaging methods.

3.4 Restaging

Guidelines from the NCCN recommend the use of PET imaging as an adjunct to other imaging modalities (i.e., CT, MRI, and bone scans) for the initial evaluation of recurrent or metastatic disease or as necessary when other modalities have equivocal results (Podoloff et al. 2007, 2009). Most of the current applications of whole-body PET imaging in breast cancer follow this recommendation, particularly when women have physical signs or biochemical markers suggestive of recurrent

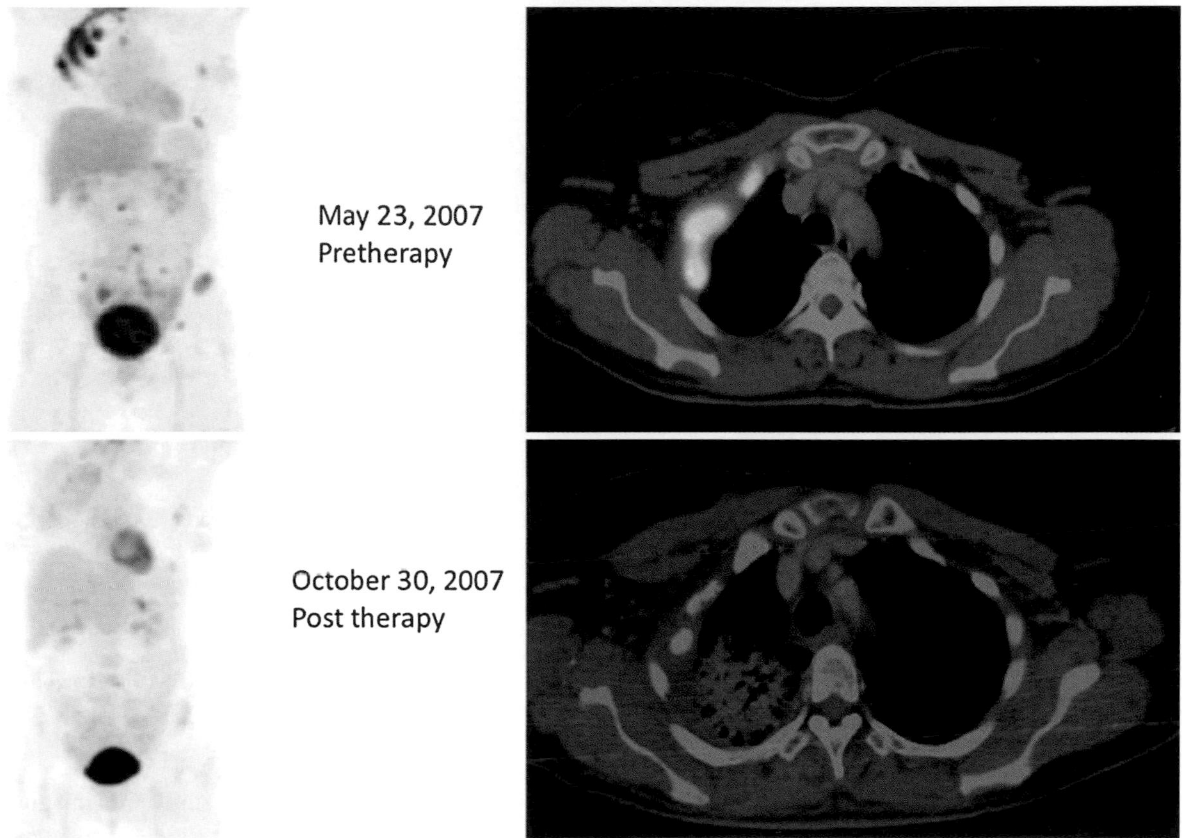

Fig. 6 Follow-up of therapy—bone metastases. The FDG PET/CT scan shows extensive metastatic disease, particularly to the upper right rib cage. Several months after local radiation and chemotherapy, there is marked improvement, particularly the rib activity has resolved with resultant sclerosis and underlying post radiation changes in the right lung

disease. However, PET imaging is not recommended for surveillance, and the NCCN guidelines recommend that surveillance be limited to physical examination, mammography, and blood work that includes liver function tests. Additional imaging such as chest imaging, bone scans, or CT/MRI is reserved for when there is concern about metastatic disease (Carlson et al. 2009; NCCN Clinical Practice Guidelines 2010). Although the NCCN guidelines do not readily embrace the use of FDG PET for the restaging of breast cancer in patients with suspected recurrence, it is in this clinical scenario where FDG PET imaging has the most impact.

Retrospective studies have long suggested that FDG PET can accurately detect recurrent breast cancer (Du et al. 2007; Fogelman et al. 2005; Tateishi et al. 2008). In a study by Kamel et al. 2003 the accuracy was 89 and 98 % for the detection of local and metastatic recurrences. Siggelkow et al. 2003 found a sensitivity of 81 % and a specificity of 98 % for FDG PET imaging. Eubank et al. 2004 also demonstrated the impact of FDG PET on management of breast cancer with locoregional disease in a retrospective study. In their work in 2004, FDG PET imaging led to a change in management in 44 % of the cases with suspected locoregional recurrence, but a similar change was seen in only 8 % of those with known distant metastatic disease. It is noteworthy that surgery was canceled in slightly over 20 % of the patients with locoregional disease due to the FDG PET findings alone. In a prospective study conducted on 118 patients with suspected recurrent breast cancer, reported in abstract form in 2008, Souvatzoglou et al. 2008 showed that PET/CT imaging detected recurrence in 67 % of patients and altered management in 33 %. Radan et al. 2006 reached a similar conclusion in an analysis of 47 consecutive patients with suspected recurrence. In their study, PET/CT changed management in 51 % of the cases.

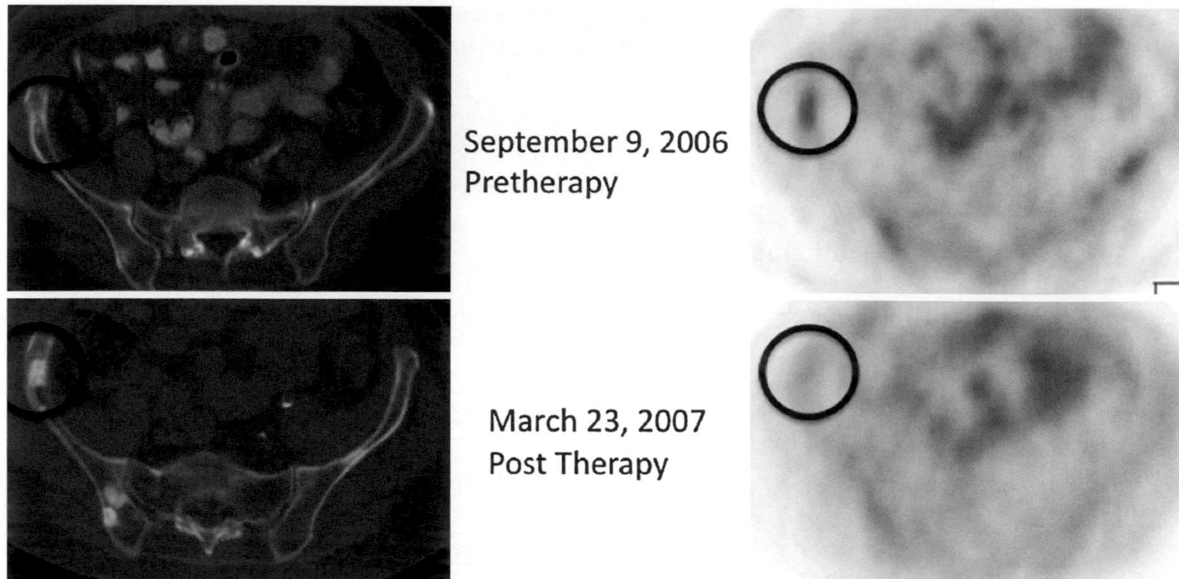

Fig. 7 Follow-up of therapy—bone metastases. FDG PET/CT scan shows metastatic disease in the pelvis. Several lesions are noted with varying degree of sclerosis in the pretherapy CT scan and mild activity in the FDG PET scan. One lesion is highlighted by the *black circle*. Several months after chemotherapy, the FDG uptake has returned to background bone marrow activity and the bone lesions have become sclerotic

The value of FDG PET imaging in detecting breast cancer recurrence has been demonstrated in studies involving patients with a variety of breast cancer histologies and with elevated tumor markers (carcinoembryonic antigen, CEA, and cancer antigen 15-3, CA 15-3), who were asymptomatic and showed no clear evidence of recurrence using NCCN recommended imaging modalities like Tc-99m MDP bone scans, mammography, sonography, and CT scans (Liu et al. 2002; Suarez et al. 2002). On a per-patient basis, the work by Suarez et al. and Liu et al. showed that FDG PET has sensitivity between 92 and 96 % for detection of recurrent disease, and a more variable specificity between 75 and 90 %. The work by Suarez et al. also reported a change in management in 63 % of the patients due to the FDG PET findings. False positive findings included inflammatory conditions, reactive mediastinal lymph nodes, benign tumors (e.g., thyroid colloid cyst), physiologic bowel uptake, and activity in a cystocele. False negatives were related to lymph node micrometastases, the low volume of incidental tumors such as adnexal neoplasm, or metastases outside the field of view such as brain lesions. In a group of 34 women with increased tumor markers, Haug et al. 2007 showed that FDG PET/CT imaging identified more lesions than CT imaging, with a similar patient sensitivity (96 %) and higher specificity compared to CT (89 % vs. 78 %). This specificity is in the high end of the range reported by Suarez et al. and Liu et al. for FDG PET imaging.

Several studies have looked into the additional value of integrated PET/CT imaging over PET imaging alone or read side-by-side with CT scans (Dirisamer et al. 2010; Fueger et al. 2005; veit-Haibach et al. 2007). Fueger et al. showed that the CT scans in PET/CT scans detected sclerotic bone lesions that were missed in FDG PET imaging. This resulted in a slight improvement in accuracy for restaging from 79 % for FDG PET to 90 % for FDG PET/CT. In work by veit-Haibach et al. and Dirisamer et al. the CT imaging included intravenous contrast. In a per-patient analysis, both studies showed improved accuracy in the restaging of breast cancer when the imaging was escalated from CT to integrated PET/CT, although the improvement was small between PET/CT and PET plus CT read side-by-side. The combined accuracy for restaging between these two studies was 94 % for PET/CT, 83 % for PET, and 77 % for CT. As expected, the advantage of PET imaging was the detection of metastases in normal sized lymph nodes, while CT detected lung metastases too small to see on PET. Although CT was able to detect sclerotic bone lesions not seen in PET, this feature of CT was not a dominant finding in the studies of veit-Haibach et al. and Dirisamer et al. Finally, it is interesting to note that Saad et al. 2008 compared FDG PET/CT imaging against measurements of tumor markers (i.e., CA 27.29 and circulating tumor cells) for the detection of metastatic disease, and found that FDG PET/CT was more sensitive and had a better negative predictive value.

Pan et al. published a meta-analysis evaluating the role of sonography, CT, MRI, scintimammography, and PET (with or without concurrent CT) in the detection of recurrent and/or metastatic breast cancer (Pan et al. 2010). This meta-analysis included the english and chinese literature from 1995 to 2008 as indexed in major databases such MEDLINE and EMBASE. A total of 1017 articles were extracted from the databases and evaluated using the Quality Assessment of Diagnostic Accuracy Studies (QUADAS) criteria as described by Whiting et al. (2003). Using strict inclusion criteria 43 original research articles were chosen for analysis. The analysis included computation of pooled sensitivities, specificities, diagnostic odd ratios (OR), and the area under the curve (AUC) for the summary receiver operator characteristic curves (ROC). A random effects model was used to estimate these parameters and to compensate for heterogeneity in the publications. This heterogeneity was most pronounced for the sonography and CT studies. Their results showed that MRI and PET imaging had similar and the highest pooled sensitivities—0.9530 and 0.9500, respectively. However, MRI retained a high-pooled specificity of 0.929 versus 0.8630 for PET. Only MRI and sonography showed better specificity than PET. Consistent with these findings was the observation that the AUC for MRI and PET was similar (0.9718 vs. 0.9604, respectively) and the calculation of a large diagnostic OR for both these modalities (131.7 % for MRI vs. 106.88 % for PET). The authors concluded that the overall diagnostic ability of MRI and PET for detection of recurrent disease was similar. However, they favored MRI because it lacks ionizing radiation, may be cheaper, and with the latest technology is also able to do full body (i.e., head-to-toe imaging) imaging in a short time. The latter feature is state-of-the-art MRI and may not be as readily available as FDG PET/CT (Kwee et al. 2010).

In summary, although NCCN guidelines favor the use of conventional imaging for detection of suspected recurrent breast cancer and leave FDG PET to evaluate equivocal cases, there is ample evidence to support the use of FDG PET/CT imaging as a sensitive tool in detecting recurrent disease. In light of the significant impact that FDG PET/CT has in the management of patients with suspected disease, we propose that FDG PET/CT be considered a firstline imaging modality in evaluating suspected recurrence. Issues of ionizing radiation may be a concern, and MRI may be an alternative. However, such MRI would require imaging from the base of the skull to mid-thighs using methods that may not be readily available (i.e., parallel body imaging and diffusion tensor imaging in the body). The FDG PET/CT scan would serve as a baseline to measure the response to new therapy earlier than methods that depend on changes in volume.

4 Positron Emission Mammography

Several devices for dedicated breast imaging using positron emitters are in different stages of development (Bowen et al. 2009; Judy et al. 2008; Lousa et al. 2006; MacDonald et al. 2009; Thompson et al. 1994). For example, Bowen et al. 2009 described a prototype PET/CT, called the dedicated breast PET/CT, which is not yet commercially available. On the other end of the spectrum a device developed by Naviscan (www.naviscanpet.com), the PEM Flex Solo II, is approved by the Federal Drug Administration in the USA and is the subject of multiple clinical trials (MacDonald et al. 2009; Thompson et al. 1994). This unit will be the focus of the remainder of this section (Fig. 8).

The PEM Flex Solo II is an annihilation energy scanner that looks like a mammography unit (Fig. 8). It is fitted with LYSO scintillators with a geometry that allows for coincidence imaging with high spatial resolution (Adler et al. 2005; MacDonald et al. 2009). The scanner uses the principle of tomosynthesis—tomography with limited angular sampling, to create from a series of projections a set of slices parallel to the detector that when stacked together recreate the 3D image of the object of interest (Grant 1972). The result is an image of the breast with voxels that have anisotropic resolution. In the case of the PEM unit, two detectors are placed in parallel with the breast

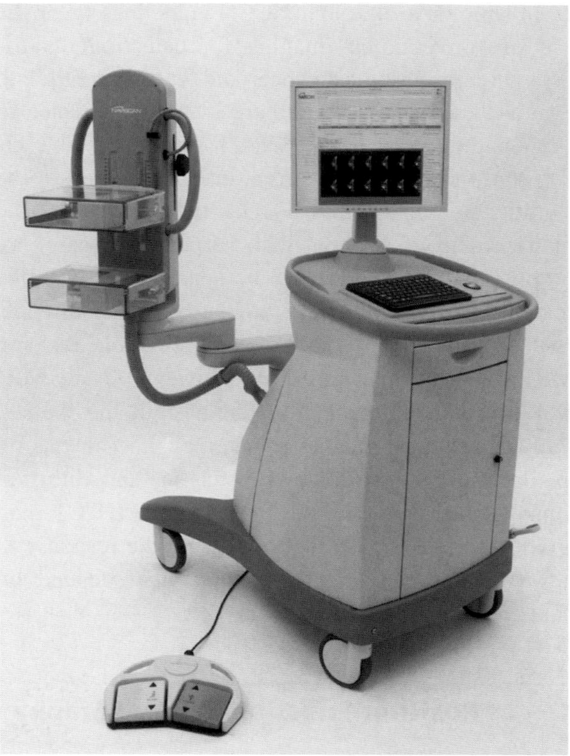

Fig. 8 PEM machine. Positron emission mammography unit, the PEM Flex Solo II. Notice similarity to mammography unit with two paddles to capture the breast and perform positron emission tomosynthesis, usually in the standard craniocaudal and mediolateral oblique planes that are common to mammography

between them on a platform that provides gentle fixation while imaging in the standard craniocaudal and mediolateral orientations used in mammography. The unit produces 12 slices along the plane of the orientations. The slice thickness depends on the breast thickness and the degree of fixation. The fixation consists of gentle pressure using about 15 lb of force as opposed to the compression used in mammography where it can reach up to 45 lb. The performance characteristics of the PEM unit have been published (MacDonald et al. 2009), and the main feature is its significant spatial resolution, approximately 2 mm in the plane of imaging, a significant improvement over whole-body scanners. The current commercially available unit does not perform attenuation or scatter corrections so it is unable to compute SUV like whole-body scanners. However, the manufacturer has developed a way to perform quantification using a measurement without these corrections called PEM uptake value (PUV). PUV_{mean} for fatty breast is about 0.3 gm/ml, while glandular breast tissue has a PUV_{mean} of approximately 0.85 gm/ml (Berg et al. 2006).

4.1 Image Acquisition

Patient preparation for FDG PEM imaging is similar to imaging with whole-body scanners. Patients should fast for at least 4 hours and preferably longer. It is also recommended that they avoid strenuous exercise. A common dose is 10 mCi of FDG and incubation time is at least 60 min, although contrast is improved with a longer incubation time of 90 min and there is evidence that a 5 mCi dose is adequate (Lu et al. 2010; MacDonald 2010). Emission scans are taken for at least 5 min per position, and preferably 10 min. Hence, the experience is much longer than mammography with total imaging time of about 20–40 min (craniocaudal and mediolateral orientations for each breast) in addition to the incubation time. Our initial results evaluating patient satisfaction with their PEM imaging experience when compared to mammography have shown that there is no significant preference between mammography and PEM imaging because although PEM takes longer, the breast fixation is much gentler than compression in mammography (Mercier et al. 2010a, b). Unfortunately, women with large cup sizes, normally D or above, need tiling of the breast to image the whole breast with the current units and this takes significantly longer time. The geometry of the imaging paddles makes it difficult to characterize the relationship between posterior lesions and the chest wall, and it has been suggested that a single bed whole-body PET scan be acquired, preferably using an insert that will allow prone imaging. In spite of these difficulties, an initial report using PEM as a tool to screen for breast cancer showed that PEM has a similar or possibly lower rate of nondiagnostic exams (i.e. BI-RADS 0) when compared to digital screening mammography (Mercier et al. 2010a, b).

4.2 Imaging Interpretation

There are multiple ongoing trials with PEM imaging, motivated by the high resolution and insensitivity to the density of the breasts and hormonal status of the woman. Breast density normally limits image interpretation in mammography while hormonal status affects MRI imaging of the breasts. Although several small series have been published on PEM imaging (Murthy et al. 2000; Ross et al. 2005; Tafra 2007; Zavarzin et al. 2003; Zujewski et al. 1996), the most comprehensive studies are the multicenter, multireader prospective trials published by Berg et al. 2006 on the use of PEM imaging to assist in the characterization of index mammographic lesion as malignancies, and a comparison of PEM against MRI in presurgical planning of breast cancer (Berg et al. 2011). Schilling et al. 2010 have also performed a comparison of PEM versus MRI for presurgical planning of breast cancer but it was limited to a single center.

A trial reported by Berg et al. evaluating PEM to characterize mammographic index lesions as benign or malignant, included 77 index lesions discovered during mammography plus 15 more lesions seen only at PEM imaging. All lesions had pathologic evaluation (52 % malignant; 42 % benign; and 3 % atypical ductal hyperplasia). Lesions that were clearly benign on conventional imaging (i.e., mammography and sonography) were not included. Patients with lymphoma of the breast and uncontrolled or type 1 diabetes were excluded. The median size of the lesions was 21 mm, but the sample included lesions less than 5 mm and multiple cases of ductal carcinoma in situ (DCIS). Although the readers had experience reading mammograms, their training for reading PEM scans was limited to viewing a sample of four cases of malignant lesions imaged with PEM. Because they used a computed attenuation correction, the PUV values in the study were labeled SUV. However, the analysis of tissue uptake focused on the computation of tumor to background ration. In PEM, this normally means the ratio of the PUV_{max} of the lesion to the PUV_{mean} of the normal glandular tissue in the background. Although overlap exists between benign and malignant lesions, a commonly accepted cut-off for this ratio is 1.5 to 2.0.

Using these criteria, the investigators found that PEM was 90 % sensitive and 86 % specific in detecting malignant lesions. The negative and positive predictive values were both 88 % while the overall accuracy was 88 %. More significant was the finding that PEM detected 9 out 11 cases of DCIS. Interestingly, the smallest lesion detected was 2 mm in size, but lesions as large as 10 mm were missed. This is consistent with the idea that FDG uptake in malignant breast lesions is variable, and that improvements in resolution are not enough to capture all the malignant lesions using this radiotracer. Nonetheless, PEM technology represents an improvement over optimized FDG PET imaging of the breasts with whole-body scanners, because PEM is able to detect smaller lesions. For example, the work from Avril et al. 2000 demonstrated a sensitivity of 68 % for pT1 lesions with whole-body FDG PET imaging in the prone position. However, Berg et al. reported a sensitivity of 67 and 100 % for T1b and T1c lesions using PEM (Figs. 9, 10, 11).

Both false positives and false negative were seen on PEM imaging. Noteworthy is the prominent uptake that can be seen with fat necrosis. Other false positive lesions included fibroadenoma and fibrocystic disease. False negative lesions included invasive ductal and lobular tumors, DCIS and some T2 tumors. Notably, the study confirmed that breast density or hormonal status did not affect the results and that the most important feature in predicting a malignant lesion was the degree of uptake and not the distribution of the activity.

The work by Schilling et al. confirmed the results of Berg et al., and provided the first comparison between PEM and MRI in the setting of surgical planning in patients with breast cancer (Schilling et al. 2010). This prospective and single institution trial by the group at Boca Raton Regional Hospital analyzed PEM, MRI, and whole-body PET scans in 182 women with newly diagnosed breast cancer who were scheduled for surgery. Most were diagnosed by core biopsy (92 %) and residual tumor was available for pathologic evaluation after surgery in 167 cases. In addition to the 182 index lesions, there were 67 ipsilateral breast lesions that were also analyzed as part of the evaluation before surgery. Thirty of the 167 lesions were DCIS. Of the 137 invasive cancers, 82 lesions were stage T1 with slightly over half of themT1c cancers. The remainders were overwhelmingly T2 lesions. The overall sensitivity of PEM and MRI for index lesions was 93 % while whole-body PET had a sensitivity of 68 %. The sensitivity of PEM for DCIS was 90 % and for MRI it was 83 %. For T1a and T1b lesions (greater than 1 mm and less than or equal to 10 mm), PEM and MRI had the same sensitivity (88 %). PEM and MRI both tended to overestimate the size of the lesions by similar margins

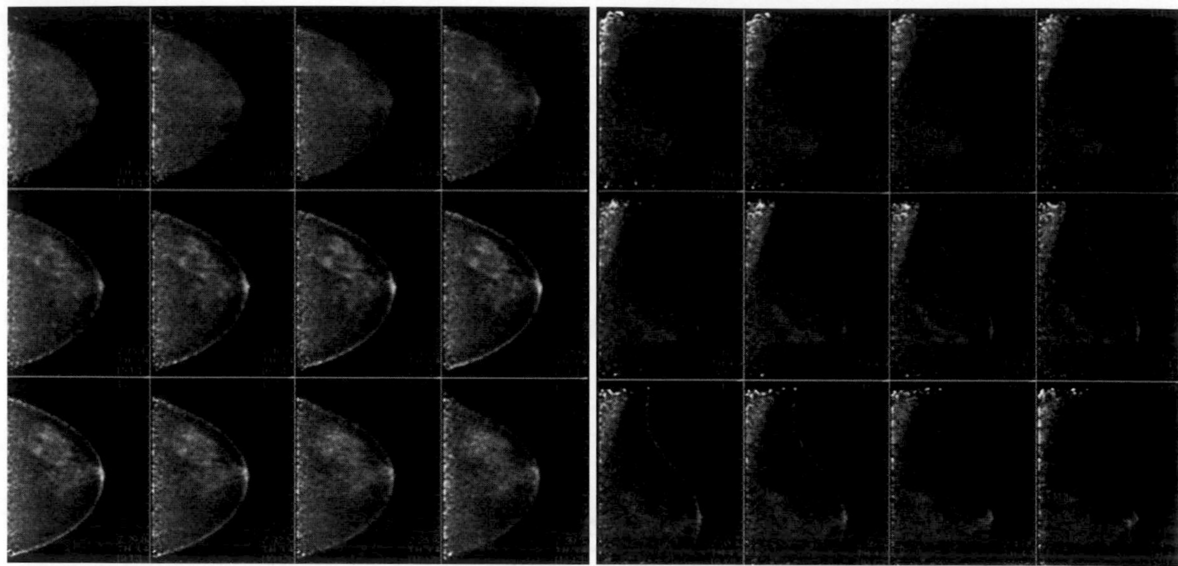

Fig. 9 Normal PEM breast images. There are craniocaudal (*left*) and mediolateral oblique (*right*) slices of the left breast in a normal subject. Notice faint activity of the glandular tissue. The skin, nipple, and pectoralis muscle are seen. The relative decreased activity in the mediolateral oblique slices is an artifact of the auto level choice by the software due to the relatively high activity in the pectoralis muscle

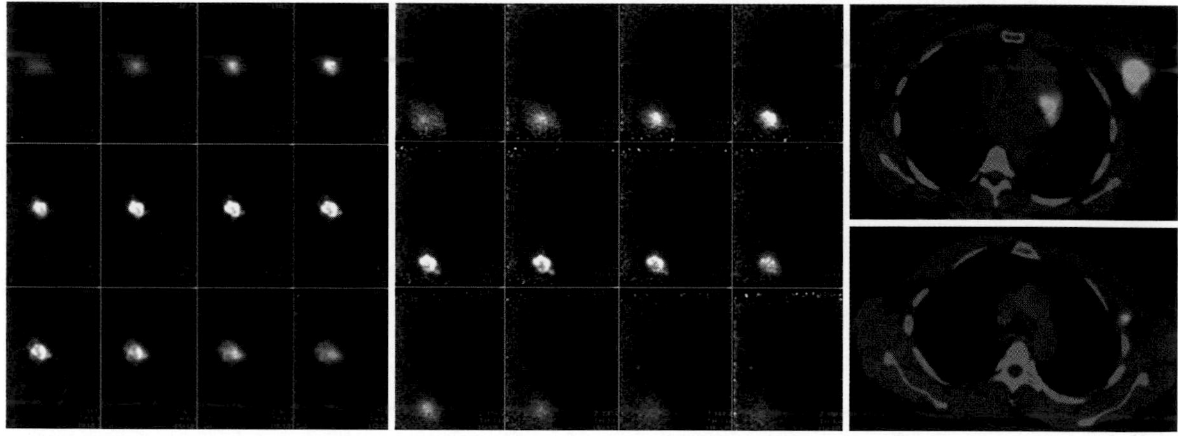

Fig. 10 Abnormal PEM scan with PET/CT correlate: Patient with recurrent breast cancer after lumpectomy, axillary lymph node dissection, and neoadjuvant chemotherapy evaluated while awaiting radiation therapy. Initial staging was T3, N2, MX. **a** Mediolateral oblique PEM views with single axial view of fused FDG PET/CT scan shows active tumor in the breast. Left axillary PEM view ("Cleopatra view") showing a possible tiny lymph node metastasis. However, a deep axillary lymph node metastasis is evident in the axial fused FDG PET/CT view

when compared to pathology. Menopausal status, breast density, and history of hormone replacement did not change the sensitivity of PEM or MRI. For the additional unexpected 67 lesions, PEM and MRI had similar performance although there was a trend for MRI to have higher sensitivity and PEM to have higher specificity (sensitivity: 85 % PEM vs. 98 % MRI; specificity: 74 % PEM vs. 48 % MRI). The authors concluded that PEM was a good alternative to MRI as an option for presurgical imaging.

In 2011, Berg et al. published the results of a multireader and multi-institutional trial to evaluate the performance of PEM and MRI in the presurgical planning of women who were candidates for breast

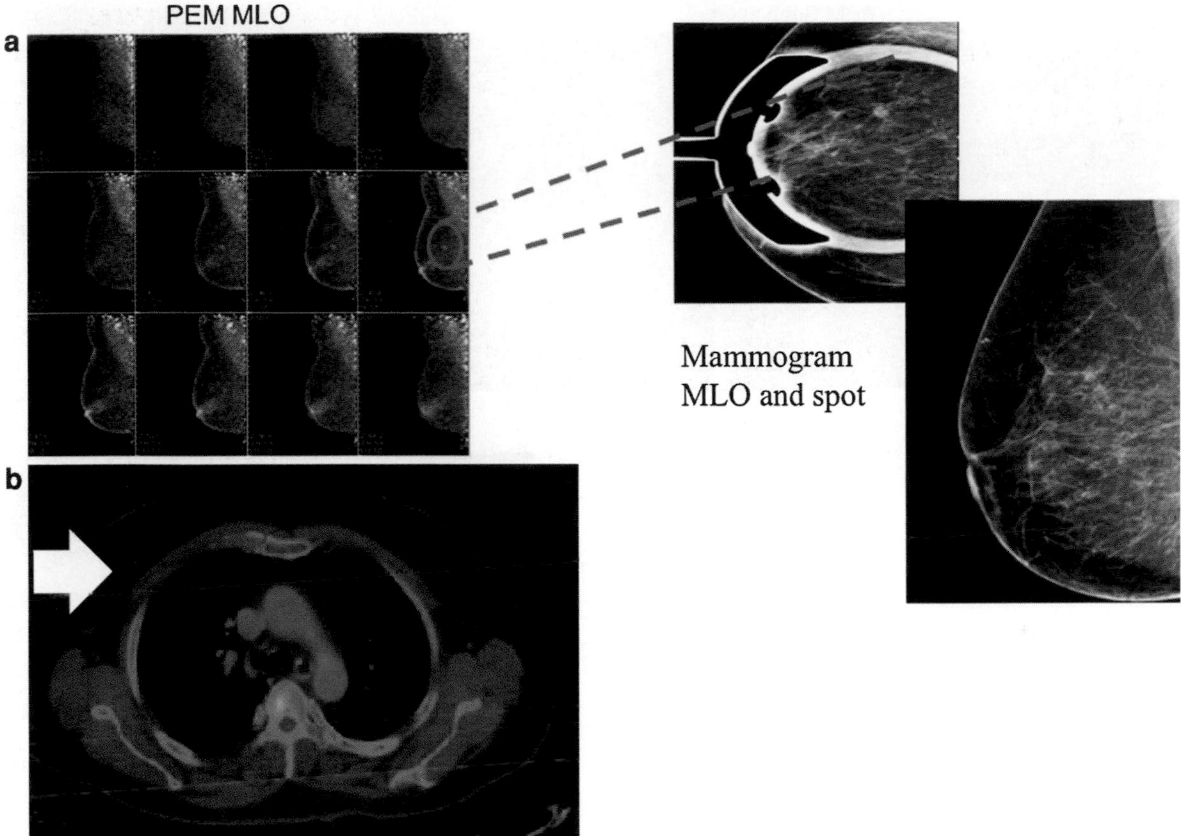

Fig. 11 Abnormal PEM scan small lesion without PET correlate. This lobular breast carcinoma was an incidental finding in a volunteer for a PEM study. Patient had a whole-body FDG PET/CT scan for initial staging of cervical cancer. PEM showed a small nodular lesion seen in retrospect in the whole-body PET/CT scan. Fused PET/CT image shows the subcentimeter lesion but detects no uptake (see *arrow*). PEM scan images with spot compression mammography correlation detects the lesion with uptake above background. Pathology showed a T1bN0M0 tumor that stained positive for estrogen and progesterone receptor, but not for HER2/neu receptor

conservation therapy on the basis of conventional imaging, i.e., mammography and sonography. Only the ipsilateral breast was evaluated in a cohort of 388 women who had index lesions that ranged from 0.4 to 6.9 cm with a median size of 1.5 cm (T1c lesion). Eighty-four women had DCIS, while 302 (78 %) had invasive cancer, largely invasive ductal cancer. In addition to the index lesions, there were 116 additional lesions that were evaluated using pathologic sampling as the standard. The analysis was done on a per-breast and per-lesion basis. When all lesions were included (index plus those not identified in conventional imaging), the sensitivity of PEM and MRI was similar, 81 % for both. However, for the nonindex lesions the sensitivity of MRI was superior (53 % for MRI vs. 41 % for PEM). PEM was more specific (80 %) than MRI (66 %). This pattern of higher sensitivity with MRI and higher specificity with PEM is consistent with findings reported by Schilling et al., although Schilling's group reported much higher sensitivities for PEM and MRI. The difference in sensitivity between the modalities was lost while PEM retained its superior specificity when a per-breast analysis was done. In general, performance was improved when either MRI or PEM was combined with conventional imaging; this improvement was most obvious in a per-breast analysis. When MRI plus conventional imaging versus PEM plus conventional imaging are compared for the evaluation of the non-index lesions, there was no statistical difference

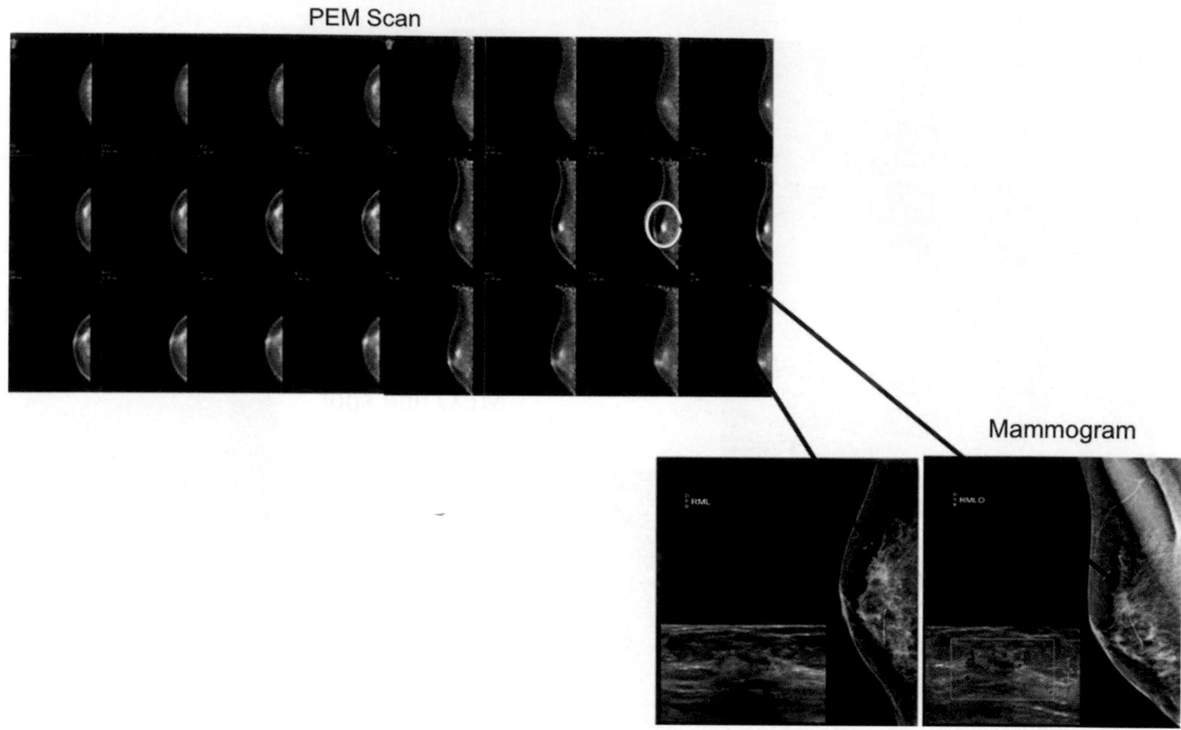

Fig. 12 Abnormal PEM scan in dense breast. New breast cancer at the site of a scar in dense breast tissue in a woman with remote (longer than 5 years) history of left breast cancer. Mammographic correlate with sonography as an insert with color doppler shows an area of density that had been called a stable scar. PEM showed a PUV_{max}/PUV_{mean} lesion-to-background ratio of 3.07, consistent with malignancy. Surgery discovered a DCIS grade III measuring 2.5 cm that stained negative for estrogen or progesterone receptors but positive for HER2/neu receptor

between the technologies in their accuracy or area under the receiver operator curve (ROC). However, PEM plus conventional imaging led to significantly higher specificity and positive predictive value. MRI plus conventional imaging was more sensitive, but this difference disappeared on a per-breast analysis. As expected the best performance was seen when all modalities were combined (Fig. 12).

The study also showed that MRI was superior to PEM for surgical planning because it was more accurate in outlining the extent of disease within the ipsilateral breast. However, MRI led to more unnecessary mastectomies, although the difference was not statistically significant. Both technologies were poor at determining the extent of disease within the ipsilateral breast when the disease was more extensive. Both techniques were equally likely to overestimate the extent of disease, but MRI resulted in fewer under estimates. The sensitivity of MRI and PEM increased with larger lesions. Hormone use or menopause did not affect the sensitivity of PEM or MRI.

The study by Berg et al. represents a major effort in comparative effectiveness research to define the role of PEM imaging in an environment where MRI is dominant. The authors conclude that PEM is an alternative for women who cannot undergo MRI. The added specificity with improved positive predictive value of PEM imaging is a significant advance. The combination of PEM plus conventional imaging is an adequate substitute for MRI plus conventional imaging, although when details of anatomy and extent of disease are necessary, MRI is preferred. The authors recognized the limitation of dealing only with the ipsilateral breast, and the effect of the lack of PEM-guided biopsy in the initial stages of the study.

Kalinyak et al. 2008 described a biopsy system designed for a PEM scanner developed by Naviscan. The system consists of software and grid systems that guide the placement of commercially available vacuum-assisted, large-bore core biopsy devices. Patients are injected with FDG and after incubation, imaging is performed in the craniocaudal plane with biopsy via a lateral or medial approach. A line source is also included to confirm the placement of the needle before deployment. With this system, 100 % of the 24 biopsies were successful. The median size of the lesions was 7.5 mm. There were no significant complications or complaints from the subjects. One significant advantage of PEM-guided biopsy over MRI was the ability to monitor the activity in real-time, including specimen imaging to help guide the pathologist's exam. Moreover, unlike X-ray stereotactic biopsy, repeat imaging did not expose the subjects to additional radiation.

In summary, PEM imaging is an exciting new technology that is already in clinical practice. We can expect this technology to become more popular if it is able to supplement or even replace MRI in selected situations. PEM is able to detect subcentimeter tumors using 18-FDG with good sensitivity and great specificity. Dual time-point imaging seems to improve sensitivity (Adler et al. 2007). Its relative low cost, small footprint, and similarity to mammography makes it an attractive alternative for breast centers that do not wish to invest in MRI. Future work will focus on using PEM for follow-up and molecular biology profiling of tumors by using the new tracers that are under development. Concerns regarding radiation exposure (Hendrick 2010; O'Connor et al. 2010) have been addressed and early data supports accurate imaging using half the dose used in the initial trials (i.e., 5 m Ci) with similar emission scan times (Lu et al. 2010; MacDonald 2010; MacDonald et al. 2010).

5 Breast MRI

Breast MRI is the dominant breast imaging modality after mammography and sonography. Recent reviews detail its application and future developments (Arlinghaus et al. 2010; Weinstein and Rosen 2010). Here, we provide a primer for nonspecialists and highlight comparisons between MRI and PET imaging beyond those already addressed under PEM.

The American College of Radiology recommends MRI imaging of the breast as a screening tool for women at high risk for breast cancer (i.e., >20–25 %); evaluation of indeterminate mammographic abnormalities; local staging of breast cancer (i.e., multifocal vs. multicenter disease and chest wall invasion); evaluating response to neoadjuvant chemotherapy; and detecting the primary lesion in women with adenocarcinoma metastatic to axillary lymph nodes and negative clinical breast exams, mammography, and breast sonography (MRI: Practice Guidelines and Technical Standards 2010). Even though there are new technologies in development such as diffusion tensor imaging and magnetic resonance spectroscopy, the workhorse in breast MRI is detection of the tumor by its characteristic dynamic contrast enhancement (Weinstein and Rosen 2010).

Dynamic contrast enhancement MRI of the breast depends on good temporal and spatial resolution. The temporal resolution is necessary to establish the kinetics of tumor enhancement. Spatial resolution is necessary to address subcentimeter lesions. In general, there is a trade off between achieving optimal temporal resolution and optimal spatial resolution. The practice guidelines developed by the ACR recommend imaging both breasts simultaneously with a dedicated breast coil and using a 1.5T scanner. T2 weighted images are part of the accreditation program (MRI: Practice Guidelines and Technical Standards 2010). However, emphasis is placed on pre- and postcontrast T1 weighted images. Gradient echo techniques are common because they are fast. Chemical shift fat suppression is preferred over subtraction of precontrast and postcontrast images to eliminate the signal from background fat. Imaging should be in the axial, sagittal, and coronal planes with no gap between slices. Slice thickness should be 3 mm or less while in plane pixel resolution should be 1 mm or less. Contrast injection should be a bolus of 0.1 mmol/kg of gadolinium based contrast agent followed by a 10 ml saline flush. For kinetic analysis, time points should be done within 5 min at less than 3 min apart (MRI: Practice Guidelines and Technical Standards 2010).

Image interpretation follows a Bi-RADS lexicon that parallels the one developed for mammography (Erguvan-Dogan et al. 2006). This lexicon has been adapted to include features unique to MRI such as contrast enhancement and internal structure. The lexicon includes statements about symmetry and findings in the chest wall, nipple, and skin. As with mammography the results are summarized into numbered categories, from 0 to 6. These categories reflect the likelihood of malignancy and the need for specific follow-up. A unique feature of MRI is the kinetic analysis of the enhancement of a mass. This analysis is confined to enhancing masses and focuses on the fastest enhancing part of the lesion with the most suspicious pattern. A 77 % positive predictive value for malignancy is seen for lesions with rapid or medium initial slope (slope within the first 2 min) and a plateau or washout in the delayed phase. Other features of malignancy include rim enhancement, central enhancement, or enhancement of internal septations. However, rim enhancement may also be seen with fat necrosis or a cyst with inflammation. Ductal and segmental distributions in nonmass enhancement are also consistent with malignancy, although benign lesions like sclerosing adenosis may also enhance this way. A reticular or dendritic pattern of enhancement with loss of the normal fat-glandular tissue interface is highly suspicious of inflammatory breast cancer or lymphangitic spread of tumor within the breast. Diffuse enhancement is usually benign and dark internal septations in an enhancing mass with smooth or lobulated borders is most consistent with a fibroadenoma. Again, as in mammography the morphology of a lesion is also important and spiculated borders are worrisome for malignancy.

An important aspect of breast MRI imaging is evaluation of the contralateral breast prior to surgery in women with newly diagnosed breast cancer. A study sponsored by the American College of Radiology Imaging Network (ACRIN 6667) looked at bilateral breast imaging in this context (Lehman et al. 2007). In this multicenter trial, women with newly diagnosed unilateral breast cancer and no abnormalities in the contralateral breast detected by mammography and physical exam were imaged with bilateral breast MRI and evaluated for the presence of cancer in the contralateral breast through biopsy or 1 year follow-up. A small number of occult breast cancers were detected in the contralateral breast (3.1 %). MRI had a high negative predictive value (99 %) but the positive predictive value was low (ca. 25 %). This reflects the common observation that MRI is sensitive for detection of breast cancer but not very specific. MRI was able to detect small tumors (mean diameter 10.9 mm, including a large proportion of invasive cancers). The sensitivity and negative predictive value was not affected by breast density, menopausal status, or the histology of the primary tumor. However, the positive predictive value (31 vs. 11 %) and specificity (91 vs. 84 %) were higher for postmenopausal women than premenopausal or perimenopausal women. Whole-body PET scanners can do no better than MRI in evaluating tumor within the breast during the surgical planning (Uematsu et al. 2009), but dedicated devices like PEM do much better and early evidence suggests that these devices can compete with breast MRI at a fraction of the cost (Berg et al. 2011; Schilling et al. 2010).

Because MRI is very sensitive but not very specific in detecting breast cancer but FDG PET is more specific and less sensitive, PET/MRI of the breast is an attractive tool in breast cancer imaging. However, to fully realize its potential the technology will require devices dedicated to breast imaging only. This is necessary to maximize signal detection in PET. In this regard, the recent work by Moy et al. 2010, 2007 is significant. In a small cohort of 23 women who had either newly diagnosed breast cancer or suspected recurrence, Moy used a breast insert to perform prone FDG PET imaging with a whole-body scanner, and then fused the images to MRI of the breast. The gold standard was either biopsy or 1-year clinical or radiologic follow-up. Forty-five lesions ranging from 6 to 100 mm were evaluated. On a per-lesion analysis, MRI alone had a sensitivity of 92 % and a specificity of 52 %. The fused images had a sensitivity of 63 % and specificity of 95 %. The positive predictive value for MRI was 69 versus 94 % for the fused images; the negative predictive value was 85 % for MRI versus 69 % for the fused images. As expected, fusion of FDG PET with MRI improved the specificity for detection of malignancy, but at a cost of sensitivity. Future work should focus on combining dedicated PET imaging devices like PEM or dbPET/CT with MRI, because these PET units have better sensitivity than the whole-body units used in the study by Moy.

6 Novel Tracers

Although FDG is the most common PET imaging agent, other radiotracers have been used to study breast cancer pathophysiology and to obtain important information about tumor biomarkers.

6.1 Steroid Hormone Receptor Imaging

Determining the estrogen receptor (ER) and progesterone receptor (PR) status of breast tumors is fundamental to the therapeutic approach. The presence of ER and PR is predictive of a successful response to hormone therapy (Berry et al. 2006). About 50–85 % of breast cancers contain measurable amounts of ER. The presence and concentration of ER increases with age, and is highest in postmenopausal patients. Because of its simplicity and the small amount of tissue required, immunohistochemistry is the most common method in use for hormone receptor measurement (Barnes et al. 1996; Elledge et al. 2000; Harvey et al. 1999). In advanced disease, a beneficial effect from first-line hormone therapy can be expected in 75–85 % of patients (Bezwoda et al. 1991; Dowsett et al. 2006). Because of phenotypic changes, the receptor status of metastatic sites differs from that of the primary in about 20 % of cases (Kuukasjarvi et al. 1996; Spataro et al. 1992). Conversion from ER-positive to ER-negative status and vice versa, have been reported in recurrent tumors with rates of 30 and 12–33 %, respectively (Lee 1982; Webster et al. 1978).

It is in this context of recurrent tumor ER status conversion and ER expression heterogeneity across metastatic sites that in vivo ER imaging could play a significant role. In vivo ER imaging adds little to the initial diagnosis of breast cancer where the ER status is almost always known from a histopathology specimen. Potential advantages of PET in vivo ER imaging include reducing tissue sampling errors, the ability to assess heterogeneity of ER expression across many sites with a single study (whole-body imaging), in particular sites that are difficult to biopsy (for example, bone). In vivo ER imaging offers the possibility of predicting and monitoring the response to hormone therapy noninvasively.

16-alpha-[fluorine-18]-fluoroestradiol-17 beta (FES), an analog of 17b-estradiol, is the most studied ER imaging radiopharmaceutical. Immediate precursors for radiolabeling are available commercially and automated synthesis methods have been refined (Kumar et al. 2007). In humans, FES is extensively protein bound, with typically about 45 % linked to sex hormone-binding globulin and 55 % linked to albumin (Tewson et al. 1999). This partially protects FES from being metabolized and may thus potentiate its ER-mediated uptake by ensuring that it is delivered to ER-positive tumor cells (Jonson et al. 1999). FES enters cells by passive diffusion and then binds to receptors α and β, with a preference for the receptor β subtype (Katzenellenbogen et al. 1993; Yoo et al. 2005). Images can be obtained in 30–90 min after injection. The effective dose in humans is 0.022 mSv/MBq, which translates into an absorbed dose of 6.2 mSv, comparable to other commonly performed nuclear medicine tests (Mankoff et al. 2001, Fig. 13).

Mintun et al. 1988 found excellent correlation between uptake within the primary tumor measured on the PET images and the tumor–estrogen concentration measured in vitro by radioligand binding after excision ($r = 0.96$). Excellent correlation was also found with immunohistochemistry measurement of ER expression, the method most often used in clinical practice (Peterson et al. 2008). Uptake in metastatic lesions was also demonstrated (McGuire et al. 1991). A comparison with FDG PET was unable to demonstrate any significant relationship between tumor FDG uptake and in vitro ER assays or between tumor FDG uptake and tumor FES uptake, indicating that FES PET provides unique direct information that cannot be obtained indirectly by FDG PET (Dehdashti et al. 1995).

6.2 HER2 Receptor Imaging

The human epidermal receptor type 2 (HER2), a member of the epidermal growth factor receptor (EGFR) family, is a transmembrane glycoprotein receptor with intracellular tyrosine kinase activity encoded for by the HER2 oncogene (King et al. 1985). HER2 is involved in tumor cell survival, proliferation, maturation, metastasis, and angiogenesis and has antiapoptotic effects (Moasser 2007). Overexpression is observed in approximately 20 % of human breast cancers (Owens et al. 2004). The activity of the HER2 oncogene is usually measured by immunohistochemistry, a semiquantitative method that measures the overexpression of the HER2 receptor, or fluorescence in situ hybridization (FISH), which directly measures the number of copies of the HER2 gene (Pauletti et al. 2000; Wolff et al. 2007). Patients whose cancers overexpress HER2 have a relatively poor prognosis independently of other clinical features like age, stage, or tumor grade (Slamon et al. 1987). The HER2 inhibitors trastuzumab (Herceptin), a humanized recombinant monoclonal antibody, and lapatinib (Tykerb), a tyrosine kinase inhibitor, have been shown to be beneficial in high risk HER2-positive breast cancers in randomized phase III clinical trials. The addition of trastuzumab to a combination chemotherapy regimen in the adjuvant and metastatic settings significantly improves outcomes and survival measures (Romond et al. 2005; Slamon et al. 2001). Lapatinib improves time to progression when

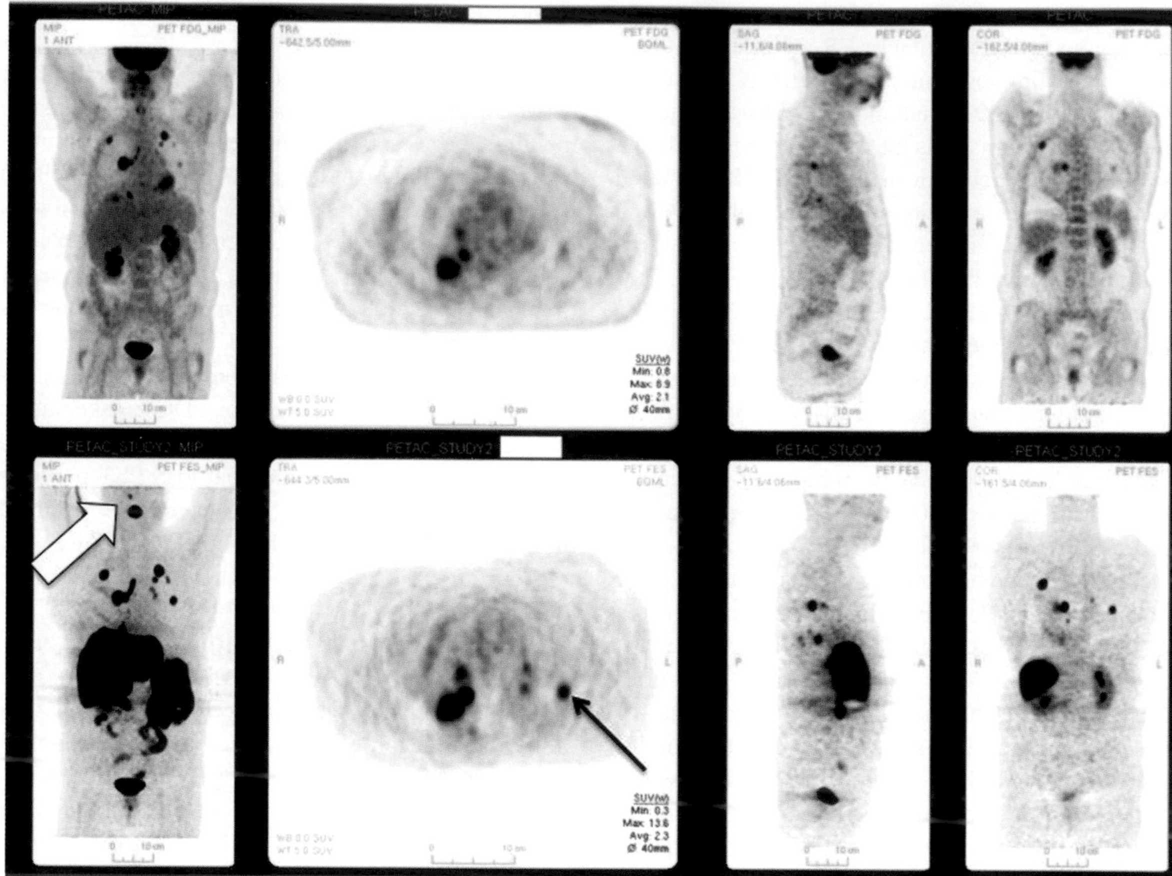

Fig. 13 Comparison 18-Fluorodeoxyglucose versus 18-Fluoroestradiol whole-body PET scans in patient with diffusely metastatic breast cancer. *Top* scan is with FDG and the *bottom* is with FES. Notice right maxillary bone metastasis (*block arrow*) in the FES scan is not readily seen in the FDG scan. Similarly, some lung lesions are more readily seen in FES (see *thin arrow*). Notice normal distribution of FES includes intense liver activity, which limits detection of liver metastases

combined with chemotherapy in the management of advanced breast cancer (Geyer et al. 2006).

However, HER2 tumor expression can vary during treatment and can differ across metastatic lesions within a patient, which of course can affect treatment response (Meng et al. 2004; Rasbridge et al. 1994; Sekido et al. 2003; Solomayer et al. 2006; Zidan et al. 2005). In vivo HER2 imaging could potentially improve patient management by its ability to noninvasively and repeatedly assess HER2 status in all lesions. For PET imaging, full-length HER2 monoclonal antibodies have been labeled with ^{124}I, ^{84}Y, ^{76}Br, and ^{89}Zr and smaller antibody fragments, proteins, and peptides have been labeled with ^{18}F, ^{68}Ga, ^{64}Cu, ^{124}I, and ^{76}Br (Dijkers et al. 2008).

HER2 PET may be useful for pharmacodynamic evaluation of HER2 down regulating therapies. A study comparing ^{68}Ga-DOTA-F(ab')(2)-herceptin and FDG in breast tumor xenografts treated with the HSP90 inhibitor 17-AAG demonstrated a significant decrease in HER2 as measured by ^{68}Ga-DOTA-F(ab')(2)-herceptin within 24 h after treatment, whereas FDG uptake was unchanged. This decrease in ^{68}Ga-DOTA-F(ab')(2)-herceptin uptake was an early predictor of marked growth inhibition that became evident only 11 days after treatment (Smith-Jones et al. 2006). Clinical-grade

^{89}Zr-trastuzumab showing high and HER2 specific tumor uptake at a good resolution was recently developed (Dijkers et al. 2009, 2010). PET tumor quantification showed a mean reduction of 41 % ($p = 0.0001$) in ^{89}Zr-trastuzumab uptake after treatment with the HSP90 inhibitor NVP-AUY922 and might thus be used as an early biomarker in HER2-positive metastatic breast cancer patients (Oude Munnink et al. 2009, 2010).

In summary, in vivo quantification of HER2 receptors and monitoring response to anti-HER2 therapy has been documented in preclinical models, but clinical studies demonstrating the value of HER2 PET imaging to predict and monitor response to therapy are needed.

6.3 DNA Synthesis Imaging

FDG is the most clinically useful radiotracer in breast cancer, but suffers from many pitfalls, not the least its nonspecific binding in inflammatory and infectious processes (Wang and Koch 2009). This can cause a particular problem in the assessment of tumor response. In this context, the ability of radiolabeled nucleosides to specifically evaluate deoxyribonucleic acid biosynthesis has triggered interest. Thymidine is a pyrimidine deoxynucleoside that is phosphorylated by thymidine kinase-1 and subsequently incorporated into DNA, but not RNA, and can therefore serve as a specific marker of cell growth (Livingston and Hart 1977).

Even though the tumor uptake as measured by SUV was lower with 18F-fluoro-L-thymidine (FLT) than FDG, a pilot study has demonstrated the ability of FLT to detect primary breast cancer and locoregional metastases with generally high tumor-to-background ratios, particularly in the mediastinum, due to its lower uptake in normal surrounding tissues (Smyczek-Gargya et al. 2004). Similar results were obtained in another pilot study, but the emphasis was on the low sensitivity of FLT for small axillary lymph node metastases (Been et al. 2006).

Early assessment of breast tumor response to therapy with FLT has been the focus of interest of a few studies. Mean change in FLT uptake in primary and metastatic tumors after the first course of chemotherapy was shown to correlate significantly with late changes in CA27.29 tumor marker levels ($p = 0.001$) and tumor size as measured by CT scans ($p = 0.01$) (Pio et al. 2006). In a study of 13 patients with stage II–IV breast cancer, a decrease in FLT uptake at 1 week after FEC chemotherapy could predict clinical response and stable disease assessed at 60 days (Kenny et al. 2007).

Overall, data regarding the utility of imaging DNA synthesis in breast cancer is still scarce, but early chemotherapy response assessment appears promising. Larger clinical trials with different tumor profiles and chemotherapeutic regimens are needed to identify the niche where imaging of DNA synthesis could have the most clinical impact.

6.4 Perfusion and Hypoxia Imaging

Oxygen is an essential metabolic substrate because of its critical role as the terminal electron acceptor in metabolic respiration. Hypoxia is characterized as a lack of oxygen required for cells to function normally and is defined as the oxygen tension at which the metabolic demand exceeds the supply (Ljungkvist et al. 2007). Tumor vessels are structurally and functionally abnormal. They are typically immature, tortuous, and leaky, contributing to heterogeneity in blood flow and thus varied levels of oxygenation in tumors (Jain 2005; Vaupel 2004). High interstitial pressure, caused by fluid accumulating in the tumor matrix and the rapidly proliferating cancer cells, may exacerbate the already inefficient vascularization within the tumor (Bhujwalla et al. 2001; Padera et al. 2004). Adverse diffusion geometry caused by abnormal vasculature, as well as tumor-related/therapy induced anemia also contribute to hypoxia (Vaupel 2004).

Data from oxygen electrodes suggests that up to 30 % of advanced breast cancers exhibit severe hypoxia in part of the tumor (Mankoff and Eubank 2006). Hypoxic cells have been shown to have an increased resistance to radiotherapy, some forms of chemotherapy and photodynamic therapy. In addition, hypoxia leads to an adaptive response, orchestrated by HIF-1 (hypoxia-inducible factor-1), that is crucial to tumor progression and therapy resistance, and a very poor patient outcome (Milani and Harris 2008).

The most physiologically robust, quantitative measures of tumor blood flow rely on freely diffusible imaging probes. ^{15}O-water PET has been shown to yield reliable estimates of tumor blood flow for breast carcinoma (Wilson et al. 1992). In 9 women with untreated primary breast carcinoma, a strong correlation between tumor blood flow measured with ^{15}O-water and FDG uptake

(SUV_{mean}) was demonstrated ($r = 0.82$, $p = 0.007$) (Zasadny et al. 2003). Another group in Seattle studied changes in blood flow (measured with ^{15}O-water PET) and metabolism in locally advanced breast cancer treated with neoadjuvant chemotherapy. In their group of patients, tumor blood flow and metabolism were correlated but highly variable. A low ratio of metabolic rate of FDG to blood flow was the best predictor of macroscopic complete response (Mankoff et al. 2002). After 2 months of chemotherapy, although both responders and nonresponders showed a decline in the metabolic rate of FDG, resistant tumors had an average increase in blood flow whereas responsive tumors had a decrease (+48 % vs. −32 %, $P < 0.005$) (Mankoff et al. 2003). A low ratio of glucose metabolism to glucose delivery after therapy was associated with a favorable response (Tseng et al. 2004). In a group of 53 women who underwent dynamic FDG PET and ^{15}O-water PET scans before and at midpoint of neoadjuvant therapy, tumor perfusion changes measured directly by ^{15}O-water or indirectly by dynamic FDG PET predicted disease-free survival and overall survival (Dunnwald et al. 2008).

^{18}F-Fluoromisonidazole (FMISO) is the most extensively studied PET radiotracer of hypoxia in both animals and humans (Hicks et al. 2006). It enters cells by passive diffusion. Then it is reduced by nitroreductase enzymes, and trapped in cells with reduced tissue oxygen partial pressure. FMISO, thus only accumulates in viable hypoxic cells with functional nitroreductase enzymes and not in necrotic cells (Lee and Scott 2007). A study comparing FDG and FMISO in different tumor types, including breast cancer, found that although acute hypoxia results in accelerated glycolysis, cellular metabolism is slowed in chronic hypoxia and can lead to discordance between FMISO and FDG uptake (Rajendran et al. 2004). In other words, hypoxia could not be predicted solely by FDG uptake.

References

Adler L, Narayanan D, Gammage L, Beylin D, Keen R (2007) Quantitative improvement in breast lesion detectability on delayed images using high resolution positron emission mammography. J Nucl Med 48(S2):369P

Adler L, Weinberg I, Beylin D, Zavarzin V, Yarnall S, Stepanov P, et al. (2005) Positron Emission Mammography: High-Resolution Biochemical Breast Imaging. Technol Cancer Res Trea 4(1):55-60

Anderson WF, Matsuno R (2006) Breast Cancer Heterogeneity: A Mixture of At Least Two Main Types. J Natl Cancer Inst 98(14):948−951

Alberini J, Lerebours F, Wartski M, Fourme E, Stanc EL, Gontier E et al (2009) 18F-fluorodeoxyglucose positron emission tomography/computed tomography (FDG-PET/CT) imaging in the staging and prognosis of inflammatory breast cancer. Cancer 115(21):5038–5047

Arlinghaus LR, Li X, Levy M, Smith D, Welch EB, Gore JC et al (2010) Current and future trends in magnetic resonance imaging assessments of the response of breast tumors to neoadjuvant chemotherapy. J Oncol [Internet] [cited 5 Jan 2011]. Available from: http://www.ncbi.nlm.nih.gov/pubmed/20953332

Avril N, Adler L (2007) F-18 Fluorodeoxyglucose-positron emission tomography imaging for primary breast cancer and loco-regional staging. Radiol Clin North Am 45(4):645–657

Avril N, Dose J, Jänicke F, Ziegler S, Römer W, Weber W et al (1996) Assessment of axillary lymph node involvement in breast cancer patients with positron emission tomography using radiolabeled 2-(fluorine-18)-fluoro-2-deoxy-D-glucose. J Natl Cancer Inst 88(17):1204–1209

Dose-Schwarz J, Tiling R, Avril-Sassen S, Mahner S, Lebeau A, Weber C, Schwaiger M, Jänicke F, Untch M, Avril N (2010) Assessment of residual tumour by FDG-PET: conventional imaging and clinical examination following primary chemotherapy of large and locally advanced breast cancer. Br J Cancer 102(1):35–41

Avril N, Rosé CA, Schelling M, Dose J, Kuhn W, Bense S et al (2000) Breast imaging with positron emission tomography and fluorine-18 fluorodeoxyglucose: use and limitations. J Clin Oncol 18(20):3495–3502

Avril N, Sassen S, Roylance R (2009) Response to therapy in breast cancer. J Nucl Med 50(Suppl 1):55S–63

Barnes DM, Harris WH, Smith P, Millis RR, Rubens RD (1996) Immunohistochemical determination of oestrogen receptor: comparison of different methods of assessment of staining and correlation with clinical outcome of breast cancer patients. Br J Cancer 74(9):1445–1451

Bartella L, Smith CS, Dershaw DD, Liberman L (2007) Imaging breast cancer. Radiol Clin North Am 45(1):45–67

Baruah BP, Goyal A, Young P, Douglas-Jones AG, Mansel RE (2010) Axillary node staging by ultrasonography and fine-needle aspiration cytology in patients with breast cancer. Br J Surg 97(5):680−683

Basu S, Chen W, Tchou J, Mavi A, Cermik T, Czerniecki B et al (2008) Comparison of triple-negative and estrogen receptor-positive/progesterone receptor-positive/HER2-negative breast carcinoma using quantitative fluorine-18 fluorodeoxyglucose/positron emission tomography imaging parameters. Cancer 112(5):995–1000

Been LB, Elsinga PH, de Vries J, Cobben DC, Jager PL, Hoekstra HJ et al (2006) Positron emission tomography in patients with breast cancer using (18)F-3'-deoxy-3'-fluoro-l-thymidine ((18)F-FLT)-a pilot study. Eur J Surg Oncol 32(1):39–43

Bellon JR, Livingston RB, Eubank WB, Gralow JR, Ellis GK, Dunnwald LK et al (2004) Evaluation of the internal mammary lymph nodes by FDG-PET in locally advanced breast cancer (LABC). Am J Clin Oncol 27(4):407–410

Berg WA, Madsen KS, Schilling K, Tartar M, Pisano ED, Larsen LH et al (2011) Breast cancer: comparative effectiveness of positron emission mammography and MR Imaging in presurgical planning for the ipsilateral breast. Radiology 258(1):59–72

Berg WA, Weinberg IN, Narayanan D, Lobrano ME, Ross E, Amodei L et al (2006) High-resolution fluorodeoxyglucose positron emission tomography with compression ("positron emission mammography") is highly accurate in depicting primary breast cancer. Breast J 12(4):309–323

Berry DA, Cirrincione C, Henderson IC, Citron ML, Budman DR, Goldstein LJ et al (2006) Estrogen-receptor status and outcomes of modern chemotherapy for patients with node-positive breast cancer. JAMA 295(14):1658–1667

Berry DA, Cronin KA, Plevritis SK, Fryback DG, Clarke L, Zelen M et al (2005) Effect of screening and adjuvant therapy on mortality from breast cancer. N Engl J Med 353(17):1784–1792

Bezwoda WR, Esser JD, Dansey R, Kessel I, Lange M (1991) The value of estrogen and progesterone receptor determinations in advanced breast cancer. Estrogen receptor level but not progesterone receptor level correlates with response to tamoxifen. Cancer 68(4):867–872

Bhujwalla ZM, Artemov D, Aboagye E, Ackerstaff E, Gillies RJ, Natarajan K et al (2001) The physiological environment in cancer vascularization, invasion and metastasis. Novartis Found Symp 240:23–38; discussion 38–45, 152–153

Bowen SL, Wu Y, Chaudhari AJ, Fu L, Packard NJ, Burkett GW et al (2009) Initial characterization of a dedicated breast PET/CT scanner during human imaging. J Nucl Med 50(9):1401–1408

Bristow A, Agrawal A, Evans A, Burrell H, Cornford E, James J et al (2008) Can computerised tomography replace bone scintigraphy in detecting bone metastases from breast cancer? A prospective study. Breast 17(1):98–103

Cancer Facts and Figures (2010) http://www.cancer.org/Research/CancerFactsFigures/CancerFactsFigures/cancer-facts-and-figures-2010. Accessed 20 Sept 2010

Carkaci S, Macapinlac HA, Cristofanilli M, Mawlawi O, Rohren E, Gonzalez Angulo AM et al (2009) Retrospective study of 18F-FDG PET/CT in the diagnosis of inflammatory breast cancer: preliminary data. J Nucl Med 50(2):231–238

Carlson RW, Allred DC, Anderson BO, Burstein HJ, Carter WB, Edge SB et al (2009) Breast cancer. Clinical practice guidelines in oncology. J Natl Compr Canc Netw 7(2):122–192

Cook GJ, Houston S, Rubens R, Maisey MN, Fogelman I (1998) Detection of bone metastases in breast cancer by 18FDG PET: differing metabolic activity in osteoblastic and osteolytic lesions. J Clin Oncol 16:3375–3379

Couturier O, Jerusalem G, N'Guyen J, Hustinx R (2006) Sequential positron emission tomography using [18F]fluorodeoxyglucose for monitoring response to chemotherapy in metastatic breast cancer. Clin Cancer Res 12(21):6437–6443

Damle N, Bal C, Bandopadhyaya G, Kumar L, Kumar P (2007) Role of 18F Fluoride PET/CT in the detection of bone metastases in breast cancer patients. J Nucl Med 48(Suppl 2):142P

Dehdashti F, Mortimer JE, Siegel BA, Griffeth LK, Bonasera TJ, Fusselman MJ et al (1995) Positron tomographic assessment of estrogen receptors in breast cancer: comparison with FDG-PET and in vitro receptor assays. J Nucl Med 36(10):1766–1774

Dijkers EC, de Vries EG, Kosterink JG, Brouwers AH, Lub-de Hooge MN (2008) Immunoscintigraphy as potential tool in the clinical evaluation of HER2/neu targeted therapy. Curr Pharm Des 14(31):3348–3362

Dijkers EC, Kosterink JG, Rademaker AP, Perk LR, van Dongen GA, Bart J et al (2009) Development and characterization of clinical-grade 89Zr-trastuzumab for HER2/neu immunoPET imaging. J Nucl Med 50(6):974–981

Dijkers EC, Oude Munnink TH, Kosterink JG, Brouwers AH, Jager PL, de Jong JR et al (2010) Biodistribution of 89Zr-trastuzumab and PET imaging of HER2-positive lesions in patients with metastatic breast cancer. Clin Pharmacol Ther 87(5):586–592

Dirisamer A, Halpern BS, Flöry D, Wolf F, Beheshti M, Mayerhoefer ME et al (2010) Integrated contrast-enhanced diagnostic whole-body PET/CT as a first-line restaging modality in patients with suspected metastatic recurrence of breast cancer. Eur J Radiol 73(2):294–299

Dose Schwarz J, Bader M, Jenicke L, Hemminger G, Jänicke F, Avril N (2005) Early prediction of response to chemotherapy in metastatic breast cancer using sequential 18F-FDG PET. J Nucl Med 46(7):1144–1150

Dowsett M, Houghton J, Iden C, Salter J, Farndon J, A'Hern R et al (2006) Benefit from adjuvant tamoxifen therapy in primary breast cancer patients according oestrogen receptor, progesterone receptor, EGF receptor and HER2 status. Ann Oncol 17(5):818–826

Du Y, Cullum I, Illidge TM, Ell PJ (2007) Fusion of metabolic function and morphology: sequential [18F]fluorodeoxyglucose positron-emission tomography/computed tomography studies yield new insights into the natural history of bone metastases in breast cancer. J Clin Oncol 25(23):3440–3447

Dunnwald LK, Gralow JR, Ellis GK, Livingston RB, Linden HM, Specht JM et al (2008) Tumor metabolism and blood flow changes by positron emission tomography: relation to survival in patients treated with neoadjuvant chemotherapy for locally advanced breast cancer. J Clin Oncol 26(27): 4449–4457

Dunphy MP, Lewis JS (2009) Radiopharmaceuticals in preclinical and clinical development for monitoring of therapy with PET. J Nucl Med 50(Suppl 1):106S–121

Elledge RM, Green S, Pugh R, Allred DC, Clark GM, Hill J et al (2000) Estrogen receptor (ER) and progesterone receptor (PgR), by ligand-binding assay compared with ER, PgR and pS2, by immuno-histochemistry in predicting response to tamoxifen in metastatic breast cancer: a southwest oncology group study. Int J Cancer 89(2):111–117

Erguvan-Dogan B, Whitman GJ, Kushwaha AC, Phelps MJ, Dempsey PJ (2006) BI-RADS-MRI: a primer. AJR Am J Roentgenol 187(2):W152–W160

Eubank WB, Mankoff D, Bhattacharya M, Gralow J, Linden H, Ellis G et al (2004) Impact of FDG PET on defining the extent of disease and on the treatment of patients with recurrent or metastatic breast cancer. AJR Am J Roentgenol 183(2):479–486

Eubank WB, Mankoff DA, Takasugi J, Vesselle H, Eary JF, Shanley TJ et al (2001) 18fluorodeoxyglucose positron emission tomography to detect mediastinal or internal mammary metastases in breast cancer. J Clin Oncol 19(15):3516–3523

Evans WP, Lee CH, Monsees BS, Monticciolo DL, Rebner M, Berlin L et al (2010) U.S. Preventive services task force: the unbalanced view. Radiology 257(1):297

Even-Sapir E (2005) Imaging of malignant bone involvement by morphologic, scintigraphic, and hybrid modalities. J Nucl Med 46(8):1356–1367

Fogelman I, Cook G, Israel O, Van der Wall H (2005) Positron emission tomography and bone metastases. Semin Nucl Med 35(2):135–142

Fogelman I (2005) Osteoblastic bone metastases in breast cancer: is not seeing believing? Eur J Nucl Med Mol Imaging 32(11):1250–1252

Fueger BJ, Weber WA, Quon A, Crawford TL, Allen-Auerbach MS, Halpern BS et al (2005) Performance of 2-deoxy-2-[F-18]fluoro-D-glucose positron emission tomography and integrated PET/CT in restaged breast cancer patients. Mol Imaging Biol 7(5): 369–376

Gene Expression Profiling of Breast Cancer to Select Women for Adjuvant Chemotherapy (2010) http://www.bcbs.com/blueresources/tec/vols/22/22_13.html. Accessed 21 Sept 2010

Geyer CE, Forster J, Lindquist D, Chan S, Romieu CG, Pienkowski T et al (2006) Lapatinib plus capecitabine for HER2-positive advanced breast cancer. N Engl J Med 355(26):2733–2743

Goethals I, Hanssens S, Kortbeek K, Smeets P, Van Belle S, Ham H (2010) Support for Warburg's hypothesis using dynamic 18F-FDG PET in oncology. Eur J Nucl Med Mol Imaging 37(4):833

Grant DG (1972) Tomosynthesis: a three-dimensional radiographic imaging technique. IEEE Trans Biomed Eng 19(1): 20–28

Harvey JM, Clark GM, Osborne CK, Allred DC (1999) Estrogen receptor status by immunohistochemistry is superior to the ligand-binding assay for predicting response to adjuvant endocrine therapy in breast cancer. J Clin Oncol 17(5):1474

Haug AR, Schmidt GP, Klingenstein A, Heinemann V, Stieber P, Priebe M et al (2007) F-18-fluoro-2-deoxyglucose positron emission tomography/computed tomography in the follow-up of breast cancer with elevated levels of tumor markers. J Comput Assist Tomogr 31(4):629–634

Hendrick RE (2010) Radiation doses and cancer risks from breast imaging studies1. Radiology 257(1):246–253

Heusner T, Freudenberg LS, Kuehl H, Hauth EAM, Veit-Haibach P, Forsting M et al (2008a) Whole-body PET/CT-mammography for staging breast cancer: initial results. Br J Radiol 81(969):743–748

Heusner TA, Kuemmel S, Umutlu L, Koeninger A, Freudenberg LS, Hauth EA et al (2008b) Breast cancer staging in a single session: whole-body PET/CT mammography. J Nucl Med 49(8): 1215–1222

Heusner TA, Kuemmel S, Hahn S, Koeninger A, Otterbach F, Hamami ME et al (2009) Diagnostic value of full-dose FDG PET/CT for axillary lymph node staging in breast cancer patients. Eur J Nucl Med Mol Imaging 36(10):1543–1550

Hicks RJ, Dorow D, Roselt P (2006) PET tracer development—a tale of mice and men. Cancer Imaging 6:S102–S106

Hodgson NC, Gulenchyn KY (2008) Is there a role for positron emission tomography in breast cancer staging? J Clin Oncol 26(5):712–720

Jadvar H, Alavi A, Gambhir SS (2009) 18F-FDG uptake in lung, breast, and colon cancers: molecular biology correlates and disease characterization. J Nucl Med 50(11):1820–1827

Jain RK (2005) Normalization of tumor vasculature: an emerging concept in antiangiogenic therapy. Science 307(5706):58–62

Jonson SD, Bonasera TA, Dehdashti F, Cristel ME, Katzenellenbogen JA, Welch MJ (1999) Comparative breast tumor imaging and comparative in vitro metabolism of 16alpha [18F]fluoroestradiol-17beta and 16beta-[18F]fluoromoxestrol in isolated hepatocytes. Nucl Med Biol 26(1):123–130

Judy CO, Kross B, Ramasubramanian S, Banta LE, Kinahan PE, Champley K et al (2008) The positron emission mammography/tomography breast imaging and biopsy system (PEM/PET): design, construction and phantom-based measurements. Phys Med Biol 53(3):637–653

Juergens KU, Weckesser M, Stegger L, Franzius C, Beetz M, Schober O et al (2006) Tumor staging using whole-body high-resolution 16-channel PET-CT: does additional low-dose chest CT in inspiration improve the detection of solitary pulmonary nodules? Eur Radiol 16(5):1131–1137

Kalinyak J, Kassab R, Payne S, Luo W, Narayanan D, Yarnall SA (2008) Clinical PET guided breast biopsy system: from bench to bedside. J Nucl Med 49(S1):411P

Kamel EM, Wyss MT, Fehr MK, von Schulthess GK, Goerres GW (2003) [18F]-Fluorodeoxyglucose positron emission tomography in patients with suspected recurrence of breast cancer. J Cancer Res Clin Oncol 129(3):147–153

Katzenellenbogen JA, Mathias CJ, vanBrocklin HF, Brodack JW, Welch MJ (1993) Titration of the in vivo uptake of 16 alpha-[18F]fluoroestradiol by target tissues in the rat:competition by tamoxifen, and implications for quantitating estrogen receptors in vivo and the use of animal models in receptor-binding radiopharmaceutical development. Nucl Med Biol 20(6): 735–745

Kenny L, Coombes RC, Vigushin DM, Al-Nahhas A, Shousha S, Aboagye EO (2007) Imaging early changes in proliferation at 1 week post chemotherapy: a pilot study in breast cancer patients with 3'-deoxy-3'-[18F]fluorothymidine positron emission tomography. Eur J Nucl Med Mol Imaging 34(9): 1339–1347

King CR, Kraus MH, Aaronson SA (1985) Amplification of a novel v-erbB-related gene in a human mammary carcinoma. Science 229(4717):974–976

Kopans DB, Berlin L, Hall FM (2010) The U.S. Preventive services task force guidelines are not supported by the scientific evidence. Radiology 257(1):294–295

Kopans DB (2010a) Re: "Saving lives: mammograms, breast cancer, and health insurance reform". J Am Coll Radiol 7(7):545; author reply 545–546

Kopans DB (2010b) The recent US preventive services task force guidelines are not supported by the scientific evidence and should be rescinded. J Am Coll Radiol 7(4):260–264

Kumar P, Mercer J, Doerkson C, Tonkin K, McEwan AJ (2007) Clinical production, stability studies and PET imaging with 16-alpha-[18F]fluoroestradiol ([18F]FES) in ER positive breast cancer patients. J Pharm Pharm Sci 10(2):256s–265s

Kumar R, Loving VA, Chauhan A, Zhuang H, Mitchell S, Alavi A (2005) Potential of dual-time-point imaging to improve breast cancer diagnosis with (18)F-FDG PET. J Nucl Med 46(11):1819–1824

Kuukasjarvi T, Kononen J, Helin H, Holli K, Isola J (1996) Loss of estrogen receptor in recurrent breast cancer is associated with poor response to endocrine therapy. J Clin Oncol 14(9):2584–2589

Kwee TC, Takahara T, Ochiai R, Koh D, Ohno Y, Nakanishi K et al (2010) Complementary roles of whole-body diffusion-weighted MRI and 18F-FDG PET: the state of the art and potential applications. J Nucl Med 51(10):1549–1558

Le-Petross CH, Bidaut L, Yang WT (2008) Evolving role of imaging modalities in inflammatory breast cancer. Semin Oncol 35(1):51–63

Lee CH, Dershaw DD, Kopans D, Evans P, Monsees B, Monticciolo D et al (2010) Breast cancer screening with imaging: recommendations from the Society of Breast Imaging and the ACR on the use of mammography, breast MRI, breast ultrasound, and other technologies for the detection of clinically occult breast cancer. J Am Coll Radiol 7(1):18–27

Lee JH, Rosen EL, Mankoff DA (2009a) The role of radiotracer imaging in the diagnosis and management of patients with breast cancer: part 1—overview, detection, and staging. J Nucl Med 50(4):569–581

Lee JH, Rosen EL, Mankoff DA (2009b) The role of radiotracer imaging in the diagnosis and management of patients with breast cancer: part 2—response to therapy, other indications, and future directions. J Nucl Med 50(5):738–748

Lee ST, Scott AM (2007) Hypoxia positron emission tomography imaging with 18f-fluoromisonidazole. Semin Nucl Med 37(6):451–461

Lee YT (1982) Variability of steroid receptors in multiple biopsies of breast cancer: effect of systemic therapy. Breast Cancer Res Treat 2(2):185–193

Lehman CD, Gatsonis C, Kuhl CK, Hendrick RE, Pisano ED, Hanna L et al (2007) MRI evaluation of the contralateral breast in women with recently diagnosed breast cancer. N Engl J Med 356(13):1295–1303

Levine PH, Veneroso C (2008) The epidemiology of inflammatory breast cancer. Semin Oncol 35(1):11–16

Liu C, Shen Y, Lin C, Yen R, Kao C (2002) Clinical impact of [(18)F]FDG-PET in patients with suspected recurrent breast cancer based on asymptomatically elevated tumor marker serum levels: a preliminary report. Jpn J Clin Oncol 32(7):244–247

Livingston RB, Hart JS (1977) The clinical applications of cell kinetics in cancer therapy. Annu Rev Pharmacol Toxicol 17:529–543

Ljungkvist AS, Bussink J, Kaanders JH, van der Kogel AJ (2007) Dynamics of tumor hypoxia measured with bioreductive hypoxic cell markers. Radiat Res 167(2):127–145

Lousa P, Martins M, Matela N, Mendes P, Moura R, Nobre J et al (2006) Design and evaluation of the clear-PEM scanner for positron emission mammography. IEEE Trans Nucl Sci 53(1):71–77

Lu X, Luo W, Kalinyak J (2010) Radiation dose reduction for personalized breast PET imaging. J Nucl Med 51(S2):358

MacDonald L, Edwards J, Lewellen T, Haseley D, Rogers J, Kinahan P (2009) clinical imaging characteristics of the positron emission mammography camera: PEM Flex Solo II. J Nucl Med 50(10):1666–1675

MacDonald L, Luo W, Lu X, Wang C, Rogers J (2010) TH-D-201B-09: low dose lesion contrast on PEM Flex Solo II. Med Phys 37(6):3473

MacDonald L (2010) WE-B-204C-01: postron emission mammography. Med Phys 37(6):3416

Magnetic Resonance Imaging (MRI) (2010) Practice guidelines and technical standards—american college of radiology http://www.acr.org/SecondaryMainMenuCategories/quality_safety/guidelines/mri.asx. Accessed 5 Jan 2011

Mankoff DA, Dunnwald LK, Gralow JR, Ellis GK, Charlop A, Lawton TJ et al (2002) Blood flow and metabolism in locally advanced breast cancer: relationship to response to therapy. J Nucl Med 43(4):500–509

Mankoff DA, Dunnwald LK, Gralow JR, Ellis GK, Schubert EK, Tseng J et al (2003) Changes in blood flow and metabolism in locally advanced breast cancer treated with neoadjuvant chemotherapy. J Nucl Med 44(11):1806–1814

Mankoff DA, Eubank WB (2006) Current and future use of positron emission tomography (PET) in breast cancer. J Mammary Gland Biol Neoplasia 11(2):125–136

Mankoff DA, Peterson LM, Tewson TJ, Link JM, Gralow JR, Graham MM et al (2001) [18F]fluoroestradiol radiation dosimetry in human PET studies. J Nucl Med 42(4):679–684

Marshall E (2010) Public health. Brawling over mammography. Science 327(5968):936–938

Mavi A, Urhan M, Yu JQ, Zhuang H, Houseni M, Cermik TF et al (2006) Dual time point 18F-FDG PET imaging detects breast cancer with high sensitivity and correlates well with histologic subtypes. J Nucl Med 47(9):1440–1446

McGuire AH, Dehdashti F, Siegel BA, Lyss AP, Brodack JW, Mathias CJ et al (1991) Positron tomographic assessment of 16 alpha-[18F] fluoro-17 beta-estradiol uptake in metastatic breast carcinoma. J Nucl Med 32(8):1526–1531

Meng S, Tripathy D, Shete S, Ashfaq R, Haley B, Perkins S et al (2004) HER-2 gene amplification can be acquired as breast cancer progresses. Proc Natl Acad Sci U S A 101(25): 9393–9398

Mercier G, Slanetz P, Kornguth P (2010a) Positron emission mammography vs. digital mammography—what do women prefer? J Nucl Med 51(S2):1198

Mercier GA, Slanetz PJ, Kornguth PJ (2010b) Does positron emission mammography result in a lower call back rate than digital screening mammography? Abstract Book: 24th Annual Northeast Regional Scientific Meeting of the Society of Nuclear Medicine. Oct 22:Poster #8

Milani M, Harris AL (2008) Targeting tumour hypoxia in breast cancer. Eur J Cancer 44(18):2766–2773

Mintun MA, Welch MJ, Siegel BA, Mathias CJ, Brodack JW, McGuire AH et al (1988) Breast cancer: PET imaging of estrogen receptors. Radiology 169(1):45–48

Moasser MM (2007) The oncogene HER2: its signaling and transforming functions and its role in human cancer pathogenesis. Oncogene 26(45):6469–6487

Morris PG, Lynch C, Feeney JN, Patil S, Howard J, Larson SM, et al (2010) Integrated positron emission tomography/ computed tomography may render bone scintigraphy unnecessary to investigate suspected metastatic breast cancer. J Clin Oncol 28(19):3154–3159

Moy L, Noz ME, Jr GQM, Melsaethe A, Deans AE, Murphy-Walcott AD et al (2010) Role of fusion of prone FDG-PET and magnetic resonance imaging of the breasts in the evaluation of breast cancer. Breast J [Internet]. [cited 2010 Apr 28] Available from: http://dx.doi.org/10.1111/j.1524-4741.2010.00927.x

Moy L, Ponzo F, Noz ME, Maguire GQ, Murphy-Walcott AD, Deans AE et al (2007) Improving specificity of breast MRI using prone PET and fused MRI and PET 3D volume datasets. J Nucl Med 48(4):528

Murthy K, Aznar M, Thompson CJ, Loutfi A, Lisbona R, Gagnon JH (2000) Results of preliminary clinical trials of the positron emission mammography system PEM-I: a dedicated breast imaging system producing glucose metabolic images using FDG. J Nucl Med 41(11):1851–1858

Nakai T, Okuyama C, Kubota T, Yamada K, Ushijima Y, Taniike K et al (2005) Pitfalls of FDG-PET for the diagnosis of osteoblastic bone metastases in patients with breast cancer. Eur J Nucl Med Mol Imaging 32(11):1253–1258

Nakamoto Y, Cohade C, Tatsumi M, Hammoud D, Wahl RL (2005) CT appearance of bone metastases detected with FDG PET as part of the same PET/CT examination. Radiology 237(2):627–634

NCCN Breast Cancer Guidelines Updated: SLNB and PET/CT Are Highlights (2010) http://www.medscape.com/viewarticle/718398?src=rss. Accessed 19 Mar 2010

NCCN Clinical Practice Guidelines in Oncology (2010) http://www.nccn.org/professionals/physician_gls/f_guidelines.asp. Accessed 13 Oct 2010

NCCN Invasive Breast Cancer Clinical Practice Guidelines (2007) J Natl Compr Cancer Netw (JNCCN) 5:246

O'Connor M, Li H, Rhodes D, Hruska C, Vetter R (2010) Comparison of radiation exposure and associated radiation-induced cancer risks from mammography and molecular imaging of the breast in a screening environment. J Nucl Med 51(S2):240

Ohta M, Tokuda Y, Suzuki Y, Kubota M, Makuuchi H, Tajima T et al (2001) Whole body PET for the evaluation of bony metastases in patients with breast cancer: comparison with 99Tcm-MDP bone scintigraphy. Nucl Med Commun 22(8):875–879

Oude Munnink TH, Korte MA, Nagengast WB, Timmer-Bosscha H, Schroder CP, Jong JR et al (2010) (89)Zr-trastuzumab PET visualises HER2 downregulation by the HSP90 inhibitor NVP-AUY922 in a human tumour xenograft. Eur J Cancer 46(3):678–84

Oude Munnink TH, Nagengast WB, Brouwers AH, Schröder CP, Hospers GA, Lub-de Hooge MN et al (2009) Molecular imaging of breast cancer. Breast 18(Suppl 3):S66–73

Owens MA, Horten BC, Da Silva MM (2004) HER2 amplification ratios by fluorescence in situ hybridization and correlation with immunohistochemistry in a cohort of 6556 breast cancer tissues. Clin Breast Cancer 5(1):63–69

Padera TP, Stoll BR, Tooredman JB, Capen D, di Tomaso E, Jain RK (2004) Pathology: cancer cells compress intratumour vessels. Nature 427(6976):695

Pan L, Han Y, Sun X, Liu J, Gang H (2010) FDG-PET and other imaging modalities for the evaluation of breast cancer recurrence and metastases: a meta-analysis. J Cancer Res Clin Oncol 136(7):1007–1022

Pauletti G, Dandekar S, Rong H, Ramos L, Peng H, Seshadri R, et al (2000) Assessment of methods for tissue-based detection of the HER-2/neu alteration in human breast cancer: a direct comparison of fluorescence in situ hybridization and immunohistochemistry. J Clin Oncol 18(21):3651–3664

Peterson LM, Mankoff DA, Lawton T, Yagle K, Schubert EK, Stekhova S et al (2008) Quantitative imaging of estrogen receptor expression in breast cancer with PET and 18F-fluoroestradiol. J Nucl Med 49(3):367–374

Petrén-Mallmin M, Andréasson I, Ljunggren O, Ahlström H, Bergh J, Antoni G et al (1998) Skeletal metastases from breast cancer: uptake of 18F-fluoride measured with positron emission tomography in correlation with CT. Skeletal Radiol 27(2):72–76

Pio BS, Park CK, Pietras R, et al (2006) Usefulness of 3'-[F-18]fluoro-3'-deoxythymidine with positron emission tomography in predicting breast cancer response to therapy. Mol Imaging Biol 8(1):36–42

Podoloff DA, Advani RH, Allred C, Benson AB, Brown E, Burstein HJ et al (2007) NCCN task force report: positron emission tomography (PET)/computed tomography (CT) scanning in cancer. J Natl Compr Canc Netw 5 (Suppl 1): S1–S22; quiz S23–22

Podoloff DA, Ball DW, Ben-Josef E, Benson AB, Cohen SJ, Coleman RE et al (2009) NCCN task force: clinical utility of PET in a variety of tumor types. J Natl Compr Canc Netw 7(Suppl 2):S1–S26

Radan L, Ben-Haim S, Bar-Shalom R, Guralnik L, Israel O (2006) The role of FDG-PET/CT in suspected recurrence of breast cancer. Cancer 107(11):2545–2551

Rajendran JG, Mankoff DA, O'Sullivan F, Peterson LM, Schwartz DL, Conrad EU et al (2004) Hypoxia and glucose metabolism in malignant tumors: evaluation by [18F]fluoromisonidazole and [18F]fluorodeoxyglucose positron emission tomography imaging. Clin Cancer Res 10(7):2245–2252

Rasbridge SA, Gillett CE, Seymour AM, Patel K, Richards MA, Rubens RD et al (1994) The effects of chemotherapy on morphology, cellular proliferation, apoptosis and oncoprotein expression in primary breast carcinoma. Br J Cancer 70(2):335–341

Romond EH, Perez EA, Bryant J, Suman VJ, Geyer CE, Davidson NE et al (2005) Trastuzumab plus adjuvant chemotherapy for operable HER2-positive breast cancer. N Engl J Med 353(16):1673–1684

Rosen EL, Eubank WB, Mankoff DA (2007) FDG PET, PET/CT, and Breast Cancer Imaging. Radiographics 27(Suppl 1):S215–S229

Ross E, Beylin D, Yarnall S, Keen R, Sawyer K, Van Geffen J et al (2005) Pilot clinical trial of 18F-fluorodeoxyglucose positron-emission mammography in the surgical management of breast cancer. Am J Surg 190(4):628–632

Rousseau C, Devillers A, Sagan C, Ferrer L, Bridji B, Campion L et al (2006) Monitoring of early response to neoadjuvant chemotherapy in stage II and III breast cancer by [18F]fluorodeoxyglucose positron emission tomography. J Clin Oncol 24(34):5366–5372

Saad A, Kanate A, Sehbai A, Marano G, Hobbs G, Abraham J (2008) Correlation among [18F]fluorodeoxyglucose positron emission tomography/computed tomography, cancer antigen 27.29, and circulating tumor cell testing in metastatic breast cancer. Clin Breast Cancer 8(4):357–361

Sacks A, Subramaniam R, Hayim M, Ozonoff A, Mercier G (2010) Value of FDG PET/CT and Tc-99 m MDP bone scan in initial staging of skeletal metastases in patients with breast cancer. In: Abstract Book RSNA, Chicago, IL, USA: 2010 http://rsna2010.rsna.org/search/search.cfm?action-add&filter=Author&value=101672. Accessed 29 Dec 2010

Scheidhauer K, Walter C, Seemann M (2004) FDG PET and other imaging modalities in the primary diagnosis of suspicious breast lesions. Eur J Nucl Med Mol Imaging 31:S70–S79

Savelli G, Maffioli L, Maccauro M, De Maccauro E, Bombardieri E (2001) Bone scintigraphy and the added value of SPECT (single photon emission tomography) in detecting skeletal lesions. Q J Nucl Med. 45(1):27–37

Schelling M, Avril N, Nährig J, Kuhn W, Römer W, Sattler D et al (2000) Positron emission tomography using [18F]Fluorodeoxyglucose for monitoring primary chemotherapy in breast cancer. J Clin Oncol 18(8):1689–1695

Schilling K, Narayanan D, Kalinyak JE, The J, Velasquez MV, Kahn S et al (2010) Positron emission mammography in breast cancer presurgical planning: comparisons with magnetic resonance imaging. Eur J Nucl Med Mol Imaging http://www.ncbi.nlm.nih.gov/pubmed/20871992. Accessed 25 Oct 2010

Schwarz-Dose J, Untch M, Tiling R, Sassen S, Mahner S, Kahlert S et al (2009) Monitoring primary systemic therapy of large and locally advanced breast cancer by using sequential positron emission tomography imaging with [18F]fluorodeoxyglucose. J Clin Oncol 27(4):535–541

Sekido Y, Umemura S, Takekoshi S, Suzuki Y, Tokuda Y, Tajima T et al (2003) Heterogeneous gene alterations in primary breast cancer contribute to discordance between primary and asynchronous metastatic/recurrent sites: HER2 gene amplification and p53 mutation. Int J Oncol 22(6):1225–1232

Shie P, Cardarelli R, Brandon D, Erdman W, Abdulrahim N (2008) Meta-analysis: comparison of F-18 Fluorodeoxyglucose-positron emission tomography and bone scintigraphy in the detection of bone metastases in patients with breast cancer. [Erratum appears in Clin Nucl Med. 2008 May 3(5):329]. Clin Nucl Med 33(2):97-101

Siggelkow W, Zimny M, Faridi A, Petzold K, Buell U, Rath W (2003) The value of positron emission tomography in the follow-up for breast cancer. Anticancer Res 23(2C):1859–67

Slamon DJ, Clark GM, Wong SG, Levin WJ, Ullrich A, McGuire WL (1987) Human breast cancer: correlation of relapse and survival with amplification of the HER-2/neu oncogene. Science 235(4785):177–182

Slamon DJ, Leyland-Jones B, Shak S, Fuchs H, Paton V, Bajamonde A et al (2001) Use of chemotherapy plus a monoclonal antibody against HER2 for metastatic breast cancer that overexpresses HER2. N Engl J Med 344(11):783–792

Smith IC, Welch AE, Hutcheon AW, Miller ID, Payne S, Chilcott F et al (2000) Positron emission tomography using [18F]-fluorodeoxy-D-glucose to predict the pathologic response of breast cancer to primary chemotherapy. J Clin Oncol 18(8):1676–1688

Smith-Jones PM, Solit D, Afroze F, Rosen N, Larson SM (2006) Early tumor response to Hsp90 therapy using HER2 PET: comparison with 18F-FDG PET. J Nucl Med 47(5):793–796

Smyczek-Gargya B, Fersis N, Dittmann H, Vogel U, Reischl G, Machulla HJ et al (2004) PET with [18F]fluorothymidine for imaging of primary breast cancer: a pilot study. Eur J Nucl Med Mol Imaging 31(5):720–724

Solomayer EF, Becker S, Pergola-Becker G, Bachmann R, Kramer B, Vogel U et al (2006) Comparison of HER2 status between primary tumor and disseminated tumor cells in primary breast cancer patients. Breast Cancer Res Treat 98(2):179–184

Souvatzoglou M, Buck A, Schmidt S, Quante S, Herrmann K, Scheidhauer K et al (2008) PET/CT for restaging breast cancer—impact on patient management and patient outcome. J Nucl Med Meet Abstr 49(MeetingAbstracts):18P

Spataro V, Price K, Goldhirsch A, Cavalli F, Simoncini E, Castiglione M et al (1992) Sequential estrogen receptor determinations from primary breast cancer and at relapse: prognostic and therapeutic relevance. The international breast cancer study group (formerly Ludwig Group). Ann Oncol 3(9):733–740

Stafford SE, Gralow JR, Schubert EK, Rinn KJ, Dunnwald LK, Livingston RB et al. (2002) Use of serial FDG PET to measure the response of bone-dominant breast cancer to therapy. Acad Radiol 9(8):913–921

Suarez M, Perez-Castejon MJ, Jimenez A, Domper M, Ruiz G, Montz R et al (2002) Early diagnosis of recurrent breast cancer with FDG-PET in patients with progressive elevation of serum tumor markers. Q J Nucl Med 46(2):113–121

Tafra L (2007) Positron emission tomography (PET) and mammography (PEM) for breast cancer: importance to surgeons. Ann Surg Oncol 14(1):3–13

Tateishi U, Gamez C, Dawood S, Yeung HWD, Cristofanilli M, Macapinlac HA (2008) Bone metastases in patients with metastatic breast cancer: morphologic and metabolic monitoring of response to systemic therapy with integrated PET/CT. Radiology 247(1):189–196

Tewson TJ, Mankoff DA, Peterson LM, Woo I, Petra P (1999) Interactions of 16alpha-[18F]fluoroestradiol (FES) with sex steroid binding protein (SBP). Nucl Med Biol 26(8):905–913

Thompson CJ, Murthy K, Weinberg IN, Mako F (1994) Feasibility study for positron emission mammography. Med Phys 21(4):529–538

Torizuka T, Zasadny KR, Recker B, Wahl RL (1998) Untreated primary lung and breast cancers: correlation between F-18 FDG kinetic rate constants and findings of in vitro studies. Radiology 207(3):767–774

Tseng J, Dunnwald LK, Schubert EK, Link JM, Minoshima S, Muzi M et al (2004) 18F-FDG kinetics in locally advanced breast cancer: correlation with tumor blood flow and changes in response to neoadjuvant chemotherapy. J Nucl Med 45(11):1829–1837

Uematsu T, Kasami M, Yuen S (2009) Comparison of FDG PET and MRI for evaluating the tumor extent of breast cancer and the impact of FDG PET on the systemic staging and prognosis of patients who are candidates for breast-conserving therapy. Breast Cancer 16(2):97–104

Uematsu T, Yuen S, Yukisawa S, Aramaki T, Morimoto N, Endo M et al (2005) Comparison of FDG PET and SPECT for detection of bone metastases in breast cancer. Am J Roentgenol 184(4):1266–1273

Vander Heiden MG, Cantley LC, Thompson CB (2009) Understanding the Warburg effect: The metabolic requirements of cell proliferation. Science 324(5930):1029–1033

Vaupel P (2004) Tumor microenvironmental physiology and its implications for radiation oncology. Semin Radiat Oncol 14(3):198–206

Veit-Haibach P, Antoch G, Beyer T, Stergar H, Schleucher R, Hauth EA, et al (2007) FDG-PET CT in restaging of patients with recurrent breast cancer: possible impact on staging and therapy. Brit J Radiol 80(955):508-515

Veronesi P, Berrettini A, Paganelli G, Veronesi U, De Cicco C, Galimberti VE et al (2007) A comparative study on the value of FDG-PET and sentinel node biopsy to identify occult axillary metastases. Ann Oncol 18(3):473–478

Wahl RL, Siegel BA, Coleman RE, Gatsonis CG (2004) Prospective multicenter study of axillary nodal staging by positron emission tomography in breast cancer: a report of the staging breast cancer with PET study group. J Clin Oncol 22(2):277–285

Wahl RL, Zasadny K, Helvie M, Hutchins GD, Weber B, Cody R (1993) Metabolic monitoring of breast cancer chemohormonotherapy using positron emission tomography: initial evaluation. J Clin Oncol 11(11):2101–2111

Wang X, Koch S (2009) Positron emission tomography/computed tomography potential pitfalls and artifacts. Curr Probl Diagn Radiol 38(4):156–169

Webster DJ, Bronn DG, Minton JP (1978) Estrogen receptor levels in multiple biopsies from patients with breast cancer. Am J Surg 136(3):337–338

Weinstein S, Rosen M (2010) Breast MR imaging: current indications and advanced imaging techniques. Radiol Clin North Am 48(5):1013–1042

Whiting P, Rutjes AWS, Reitsma JB, Bossuyt PMM, Kleijnen J (2003) The development of QUADAS: a tool for the quality assessment of studies of diagnostic accuracy included in systematic reviews. BMC Med Res Methodol 10(3):25

WHO | Cancer (2010) http://www.who.int/mediacentre/factsheets/fs297/en/index.html. Accessed 19 April 2010

Wolff AC, Hammond ME, Schwartz JN, Hagerty KL, Allred DC, Cote RJ et al (2007) American Society of Clinical Oncology/College of American Pathologists guideline recommendations for human epidermal growth factor receptor 2 testing in breast cancer. J Clin Oncol 25(1):118–145

Williams HT, Smith S (2005) FDG PET and SPECT of bone metastases in breast cancer. Am J Roentgenol 185(6):1651-a-1653

Wilson CB, Lammertsma AA, McKenzie CG, Sikora K, Jones T (1992) Measurements of blood flow and exchanging water space in breast tumors using positron emission tomography: a rapid and noninvasive dynamic method. Cancer Res 52(6):1592–1597

Yang SN, Liang JA, Lin FJ, Kao CH, Lin CC, Lee CC (2002) Comparing whole body (18)F-2-deoxyglucose positron emission tomography and technetium-99 m methylene diphosphonate bone scan to detect bone metastases in patients with breast cancer. J Cancer Res Clin Oncol 128(6):325–328

Yang W, Le-Petross H, Macapinlac H, Carkaci S, Gonzalez-Angulo A, Dawood S et al (2008) Inflammatory breast cancer: PET/CT, MRI, mammography, and sonography findings. Breast Cancer Res Treat 109(3):417–426

Yoo J, Dence CS, Sharp TL, Katzenellenbogen JA, Welch MJ (2005) Synthesis of an estrogen receptor beta-selective radioligand: 5-[18F]fluoro-(2R,3S)-2,3-bis(4 hydroxyphenyl) pentanenitrile and comparison of in vivo distribution with 16alpha [18F]fluoro-17beta-estradiol. J Med Chem 8(20):6366–6378

Zasadny KR, Tatsumi M, Wahl RL (2003) FDG metabolism and uptake versus blood flow in women with untreated primary breast cancers. Eur J Nucl Med Mol Imaging 30(2):274–280

Zavarzin V, Weinberg IN, Stepanov PY, Beylin D, Lauckner K, Doss M et al (2003) Positron emission mammography: initial clinical results. Ann Surg Oncol 10(1):86–91

Zidan J, Dashkovsky I, Stayerman C, Basher W, Cozacov C, Hadary A (2005) Comparison of HER-2 overexpression in primary breast cancer and metastatic sites and its effect on biological targeting therapy of metastatic disease. Br J Cancer 93(5):552–556

Zujewski J, Chow C, Jones E, Chang V, Berg W, Frank J et al (1996) Preliminary results for positron emission mammography: real-time functional breast imaging in a conventional mammography gantry. Eur J Nucl Med Mol Imaging 23(7):804–806

Gastrointestinal

Roland Hustinx

Contents

R. Hustinx (✉)
Division of Nuclear Medicine,
University Hospital of Liège,
Domaine Universitaire du Sart Tilman B35,
4000, Liège 1, Belgium
e-mail: rhustinx@chu.ulg.ac.be

Abstract

PET-CT combines in a single imaging session both anatomical and metabolic information. Depending on the strategy, the CT part of the study may yield only crude anatomical information and attenuation correction for the PET part, or it may offer full radiological diagnostic features. Regarding the radiotracers for gastrointestinal oncology, FDG remains the mainstay but alternative compounds aimed at more specific biological targets are actively tested. In particular Ga-68-labelled DOTA derivatives image somastostatin receptors with exquisite sensitivity and specificity. In clinical practice, several indications are well recognized for FDG PET-CT. These include the initial staging of esophageal, pancreatic and rectal cancers with a clinical impact in a significant proportion of patients. The metabolic activity, as recorded prior to any treatment, holds prognostic information in esophageal cancer and hepatocarcinomas. Furthermore, the metabolic response assessed early on during chemotherapy and/or radiotherapy may be very valuable in esophageal and rectal cancers, as well as in GISTs. Methodological issues remain to be solved, but the potential is clearly present so that an increased clinical role is highly likely in the near future. FDG PET-CT is a major clinical tool in the detection and staging of recurrent colorectal cancer, and for determining the resectability of liver metastases. Ongoing developments include technological advances, in particular the combined PET-MR devices, and alternative tracers, such as those imaging angiogenesis.

P. Peller et al. (eds.), *PET-CT and PET-MRI in Oncology*, Medical Radiology. Diagnostic Imaging,
DOI: 10.1007/174_2011_432,

1 Key Points

Among all cancers, approximately one out of five arises in the digestive tract, and almost one-fourth of all cancer deaths are due to digestive cancers. The clinical role of PET-CT depends on the tumor type, location and clinical indication. FDG-PET-CT is considered as a standard of care for assessing suspected recurrences of colorectal cancer and in the preoperative staging of liver metastases. It is clearly useful for ruling out malignancy in equivocal pancreatic masses, staging esophageal and rectal cancers, assessing the resectability of pancreatic cancer and assessing the response to tyrosine kinase inhibitors in GISTs. FDG-PET-CT has an independent prognostic value in hepatocellular carcinoma and neuroendocrine tumors, but the direct clinical implications are not fully clarified. Similarly, it is very effective at evaluating the response to neo-adjuvant treatment in esophageal and rectal cancers but unanswered methodological issues prevent its widespread application in this setting. Determination of the tumor metabolic volume for radiation therapy planning is increasingly used and ligands to the somatostatin receptors labeled with ^{68}Ga may become standard diagnostic and staging procedures in neuroendocrine tumors in the future. Although attractive as a concept for GI oncology imaging, combined PET-MRI needs to be investigated both from a clinical and methodological perspective.

2 Introduction

In the USA, the estimated number of new cancer cases in 2009 was 275,720 for the entire digestive system, which represents 18.6% of the total number of new cancers (American_Cancer_Society 2009). Regarding the mortality of these cancers, 135,830 deaths were expected, representing 24.1% of the total. The colon and rectum rank first among the primary sites with 146,970 new cases, followed by the pancreas, liver and intrahepatic bile ducts, stomach and esophagus. Both the incidence and mortality rate of colorectal cancer have declined over the past two decades, thanks to improved early detection and treatments. On the other hand, the incidence of pancreatic cancer has been slightly increasing over the past 15 years to reach an estimated 42,470 new cases in 2009, and no improvement in survival rates has been achieved over the same period. Survival rates for esophageal, gastric and liver cancers have all improved over the past two decades.

Although PET-CT is now fully integrated into the management algorithms of several of these tumors, the field is still rapidly evolving. New clinical indications for FDG imaging are actively investigated, such as the systematic follow-up of colorectal cancer with FDG-PET-CT. Innovative tracers are also emerging in the clinical field, with very specific indications. This is well illustrated by somatostatin analogs labeled with the positron-emitter ^{68}Ga. Technological improvements, in particular combined PET-MRI, will not only offer new applications but also raise new questions.

3 PET-CT Protocols

It has now been several years since manufacturers have retired PET only scanners from their catalogs. All devices are thus PET-CT scanners combining the anatomic and metabolic information in a single imaging session. There are no major differences in the operation of the various PET systems that are currently available. The injected dose and duration of acquisition may vary depending on the crystal material, and various reconstruction algorithms may be used, but these parameters do not affect in a major way the day-to-day practice. Standard PET protocols are favored, with patients being asked to fast for 6 h and verification of the blood glucose level before injecting FDG. The uptake period is usually 60–90 min. On the other hand, most current PET-CT systems are equipped with multidetector CT scans, allowing a wide range of CT acquisitions with very different results in terms of diagnostic yield. In short, CT may be used solely for attenuation correction and gross anatomic localization of the metabolic activity, or it may be used as a full diagnostic procedure, which might be as complex as combining FDG-PET and CT colonography in a single procedure (Kinner et al. 2007). Between these two extreme options, exist multiple choices regarding the CT dose, rotation speed and collimation, the use of oral or intravenous contrast agents and the number of acquisition phases for the CT. The choice of the CT protocol will depend

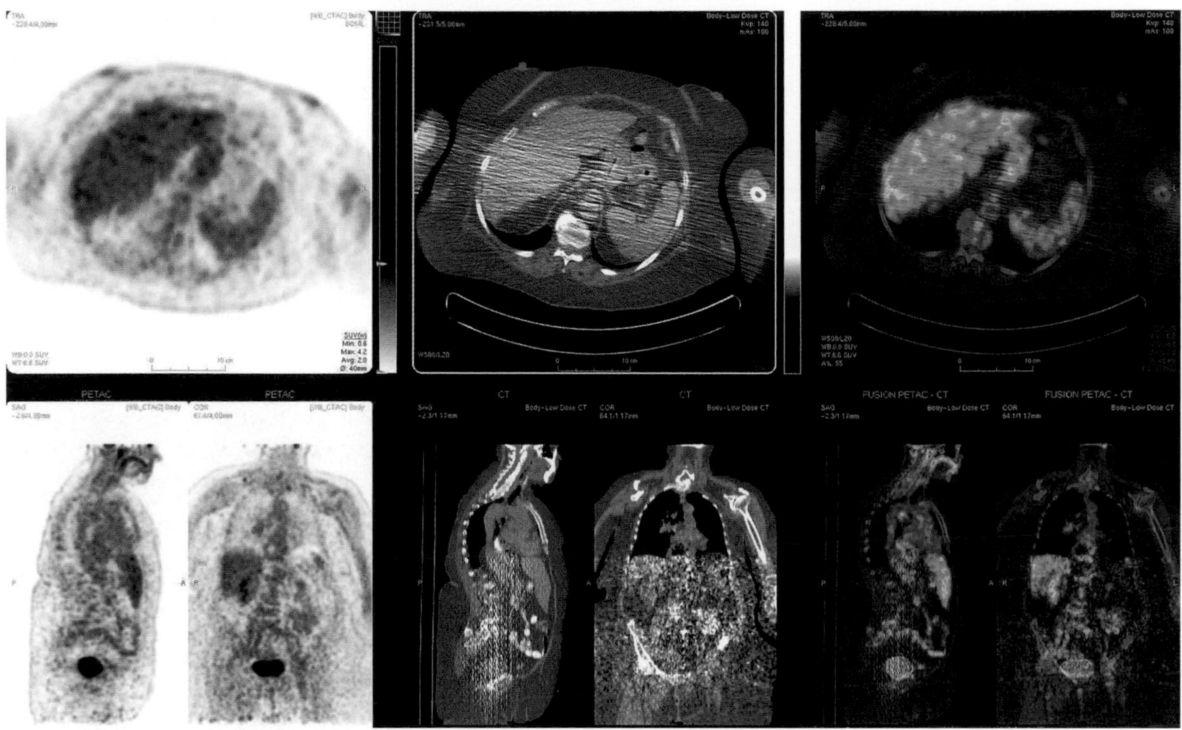

Fig. 1 Example showing the limitations of low-dose CT (100 mAs, 140 kV). This patient's weight was 126 kg for 157 cm (BMI 52) and the CT is not interpretable

on the clinical indication but mostly on the local set-up and favored diagnostic algorithms, as there is no consensus with regard to the optimal methodology.

3.1 CT Protocols

Tube current is the easiest parameter to adapt depending on the objectives of the CT acquisition. For attenuation correction purposes only, the lowest radiation dose is desired and the tube current is often set to 20–40 mAs for all patients, regardless of their weight and size. Although it may provide useful anatomic information in very slim patients, such protocol cannot be relied upon in every patient. Basically, when choosing this protocol, one renounces to the anatomical part of the PET-CT. Low-dose protocols are favored when children are investigated, as other non-ionizing radiology techniques such as MRI or US are used in place of the full diagnostic CT. Another option is to adapt the tube current to the body habitus of the patient with the aim of obtaining the best trade off between radiation dose, which should be the lowest dose achievable, and anatomic information, which may encompass general anatomic localization, detection and characterization of some structural anomalies such as peritoneal nodules and enlarged lymph nodes, especially when a reconstruction is performed with slices thinner than the 4–5 mm thick slices usually generated by the default reconstruction protocol. While this approach is simple and straight-forward, it is limited in the distinction between bowel and other structures and this CT part is very limited in characterizing liver lesions, except for very crude segment localization. Regardless of the CT settings, the patients are usually freely breathing which may generate artifacts and decrease its diagnostic value especially in the chest and some in the upper abdomen. Overall, however, such approach is used in many centers, in particular those where nuclear medicine and radiology departments are distinct entities. In addition, many patients referred for PET-CT already had a diagnostic CT or MRI, often available through the hospital PACS system. Figures 1 and 2 show two examples of low-dose CT studies.

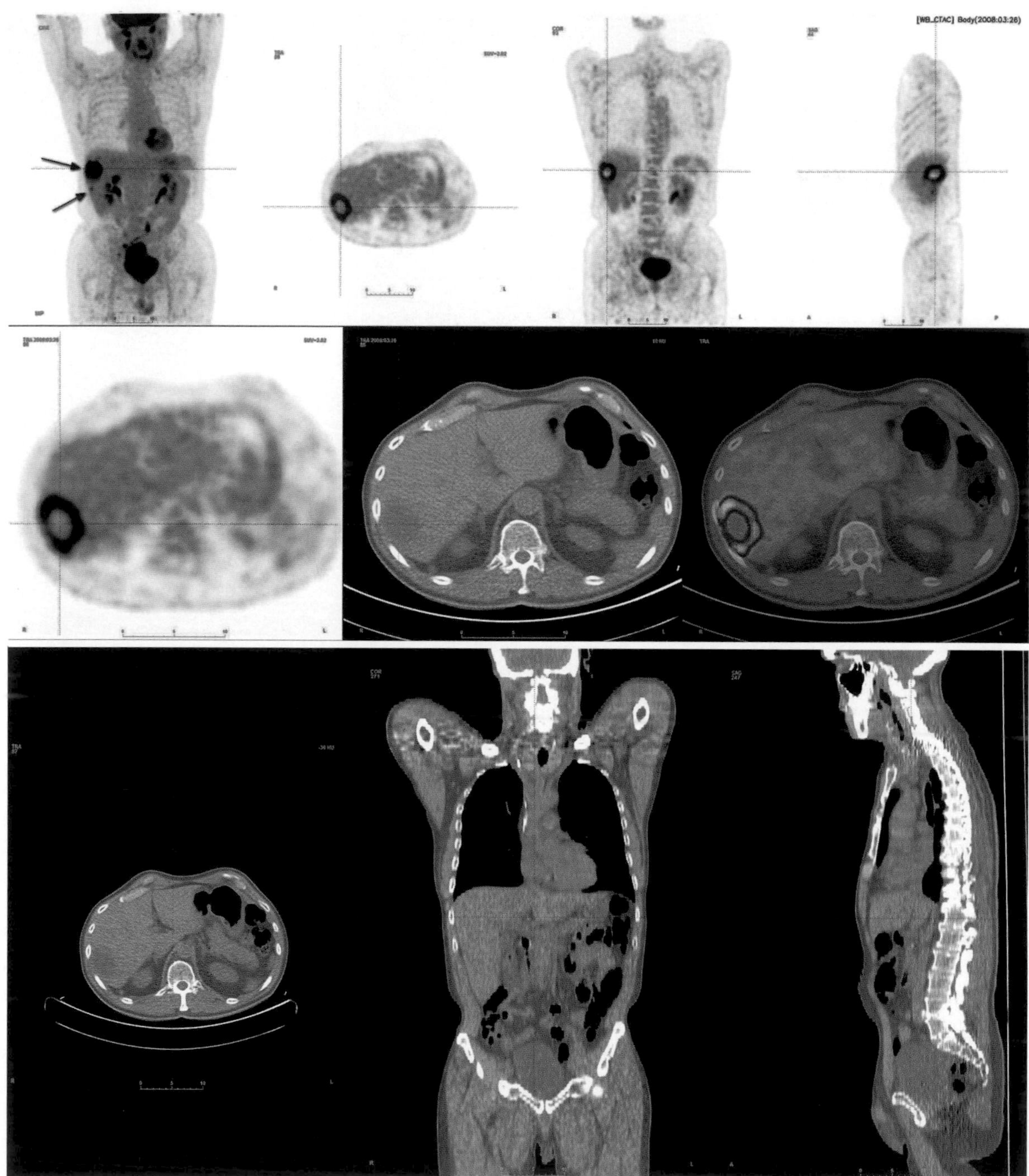

Fig. 2 FDG-PET-CT in a 63-year-old patient with recurrent colon cancer. The body mass index is 24 (73 kg, 172 cm). CT tube current was 50 mAs with 120 kV. The CT is useful for general anatomic localization but it shows several beam hardening artifacts, which makes interpretation of the abdominal cavity difficult. Liver metastases are clearly seen on the PET study (*arrows* on the 3D-projection image), including a large hypodense lesion on the low-dose CT

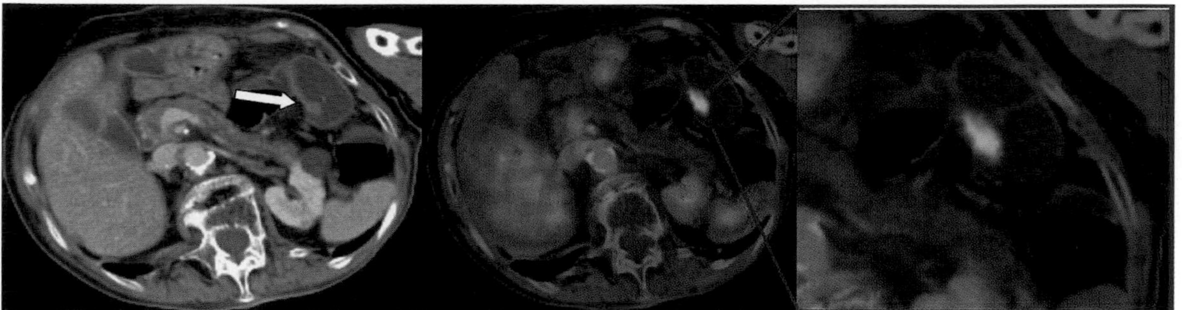

Fig. 3 A cancer of the descending colon is clearly seen on the CT colonography (*arrow*) and as a focus of increased FDG uptake. Both the PET study and the CT colonography were obtained during a single imaging procedure (courtesy Patrick Veit-Haibach, MD)

3.2 Contrast Enhancement

Water may be used as a negative oral contrast agent, easy to use and at the lowest cost. One liter is ingested starting 45 min before the imaging procedure, during 20–40 min. It is helpful in the analysis of the proximal part of the digestive tract, especially the stomach. In this case, a last glass of water should be ingested just before starting the PET-CT so that evaluation of the gastric wall is improved by the water distension. Most often, however, positive oral contrast agents are used for imaging malignancies of the digestive tract. Gastrographin is a neutral iodinated contrast medium that can be used even in patients with possible leakage into the abdominal cavity. Solutions containing barium sulfate are an alternative but they may lead to peritonitis if released into the intraperitoneal cavity. Regardless of the contrast agent, the methodology is similar to the one exposed above, with a volume of approximately 1 liter ingested over a period of 20–40 min, starting 45 min before the PET-CT acquisition.

While oral contrast agents may be used on systematically without altering a PET center's practice, modifying the throughput and introducing additional risks for the patient, the same does not hold true for IV contrast. Intravenous contrast is necessary whenever a diagnostic-quality CT of the GI tract is needed, and the CT scanner acquisition settings have to be adapted in consequence. It is nevertheless feasible, using two different approaches: in the simplest approach, IV contrast is given before the initial CT acquisition is performed, which is thus used as a whole-body venous/portal phase CT investigation and for attenuation correction of the PET data (Antoch et al. 2004a, b). Another approach combines a low-dose CT for attenuation correction followed by the PET acquisition and, if needed, a dual or even triple-phase CT over a region of interest, for instance the liver (Pfannenberg et al. 2007). This approach probably yields the highest diagnostic information but requires a tight collaboration between radiologists and nuclear medicine physicians. Finally, it is even possible to combine PET and CT colonography as shown in Fig. 3. The clinical value of the various imaging approaches, with and without IV contrast, will be addressed for each specific concern in the following sections.

4 Esophageal and Gastric Cancers

4.1 Esophageal Cancer

Tumors arising from the upper two-thirds of the esophagus are usually squamous cell carcinomas, whereas those arising from the lower third and gastroesophageal junction are more often adenocarcinomas. The incidence and prevalence of the adenocarcinomas has increased over the past decades (Blot and Mclaughlin 1999). Regardless of the histopathology, the prognosis remains very dire, with 5 year survival rates ranging from 15 to 39%. Surgery is the major treatment, and increasingly it is performed after neo-adjuvant therapies such as chemotherapy or chemoradiotherapy.

4.1.1 Diagnosis and Staging

Overall, the detection rate of esophageal carcinomas by FDG-PET/CT is not only high, but it is also directly related to the local stage of the tumor at presentation. In a study of 149 patients, PET was positive in 80% of the cases, with a distribution

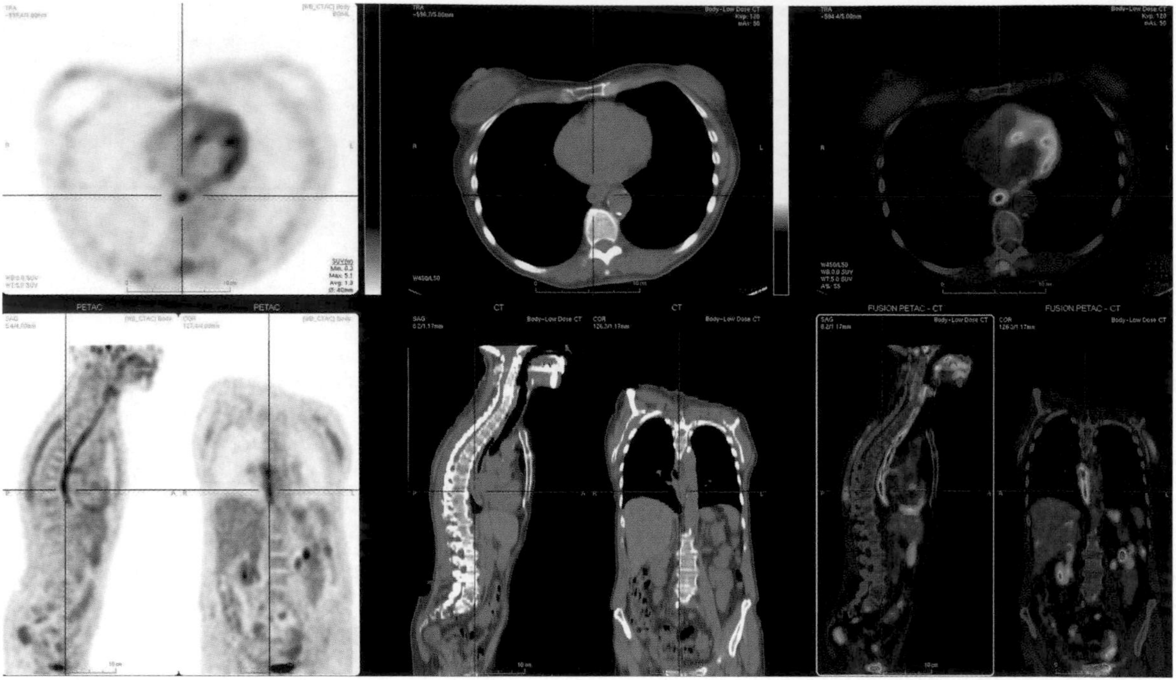

Fig. 4 Diffuse FDG uptake by the entire esophagus. Endoscopy only showed moderate esophagitis

reflecting the T stage: only 43% of the T1 tumors were detected, 83% of T2 tumors, 97% of T3 tumors and all T4 tumors (Kato et al. 2005). On the other hand, benign conditions such as esophagitis may display locally increased FDG uptake. Although usually recognizable when the uptake is linear and mild, foci at the gastroesophageal junction are not infrequent and may require endoscopic evaluation. An example of diffuse esophagitis is shown in Fig. 4.

Staging of esophageal cancer is performed according to the TNM system, which considers two possibilities regarding the nodal status: N0, no regional lymph nodes, and N1, regional lymph node metastasis. The M stage depends on the location of the primary: M1a refers to metastases in celiac nodes for tumors of the lower esophagus and to metastases in cervical nodes in tumors of the upper esophagus. M0 refers to no distant metastases and M1b to other distant metastases. For tumors of the mid-esophagus, M1a is not applicable as non-regional nodes and distant metastases are associated with an equally poor prognosis and both categorized as M1b. Overall, both CT and FDG-PET-CT are less effective for T and N staging, compared to results achieved using endoscopic ultrasonography (EUS). A meta-analysis of 12 publications dealing with FDG-PET in the nodal staging showed a pooled sensitivity of 51% with a specificity of 84% (Van Westreenen et al. 2004). Recent data suggest an added clinical value of integrated FDG-PET-CT over PET or CT alone (Kato et al. 2008; Okada et al. 2009) but the sensitivity remains low compared to EUS with a limited impact on the locoregional staging (Keswani et al. 2009). FDG-PET/CT contributes more significantly to the M staging, although reports are conflicting regarding its real clinical impact. Unsuspected distant metastases were found in 14% of the patients in a prospective multicenter trial, of which 5% were pathologically confirmed (Meyers et al. 2007). On the other hand, a recent Australian multicenter study report changes in management in 38% of the patients (Chatterton et al. 2009). One hundred twenty-nine patients considered for curative treatment after conventional methods were included and PET detected additional lesions in 53 patients (41%). Unfortunately, this study does not report whether EUS was systematically performed in all patients. Nevertheless, in a series of 50 patients who were selected for curative surgery by a multidisciplinary team after reviewing CT and EUS data, PET-CT changed the management in 12% by

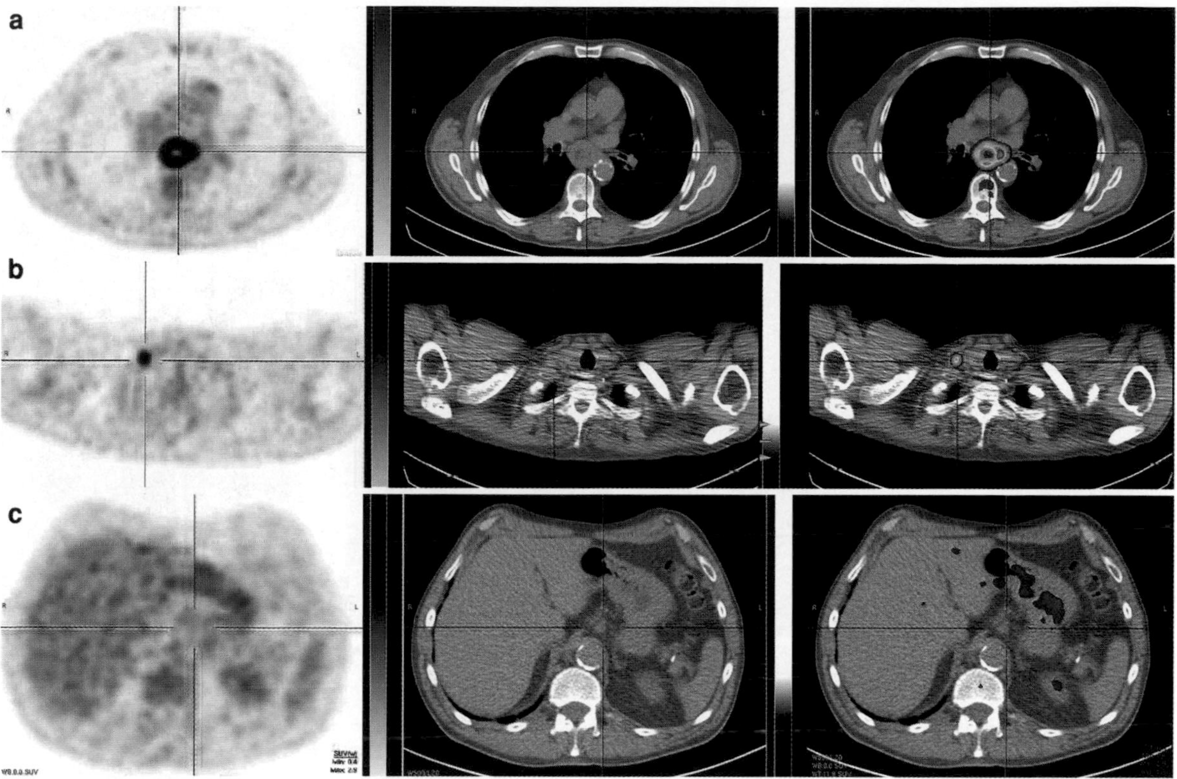

Fig. 5 Initial staging of a squamous cell carcinoma of the lower esophagus. The large tumor is highly hypermetabolic (**a**) and PET-CT reveals a nodal metastasis in the right supraclavicular area (**b**). On the other hand, an equivocal lymph node seen on CT and EUS in the celiac area is not hypermetabolic on FDG-PET (**c**)

detecting unknown distant metastases, thus avoiding futile surgery in these patients (Berrisford et al. 2008). Overall, the combination of EUS, chest CT and FDG-PET-CT is generally considered as the best pretherapeutic staging strategy. Figure 5 shows an example of PET/CT for initial staging.

4.1.2 Prognosis and Assessment of Response to Treatment

A recent meta-analysis of studies evaluating the prognostic value of the tumor SUV prognosis before treatment found a high metabolic activity to be an indicator of poor outcome, with combined hazard ratios of 1.86 with regard to the survival and of 2.52 with regard to recurrence (Pan et al. 2009). Although higher metabolic activities have been consistently associated with poor outcome, the molecular rationale behind these clinical observations remains unknown, as SUV does not seem to correlate with any of the known molecular markers such as p53, EGFR or VEGF assessed by immunohistochemistry (Taylor et al. 2009). Despite these observations, the initial SUV is not currently included in the parameters directing the treatment strategy.

The situation is quite different in the evaluation of response to treatment, as numerous articles are available showing the capability of PET to predict the pathological response after neo-adjuvant treatments. Of these, the MINICON phase II trial demonstrated the feasibility of a PET-guided treatment algorithm (Lordick et al. 2007). In this study, the metabolic response was evaluated after 2 weeks of platinum-based chemotherapy. Metabolic responders were further treated with chemotherapy, while nonresponders proceeded directly to surgery. After a median follow-up of 2–3 years, the median overall survival was not reached in the responders while it was 25.8 months in the nonresponders. Major histological remissions were observed in 58% of the responders and in none of the nonresponders. Several major methodological issues remain unsettled; however, in particular the method for measuring the

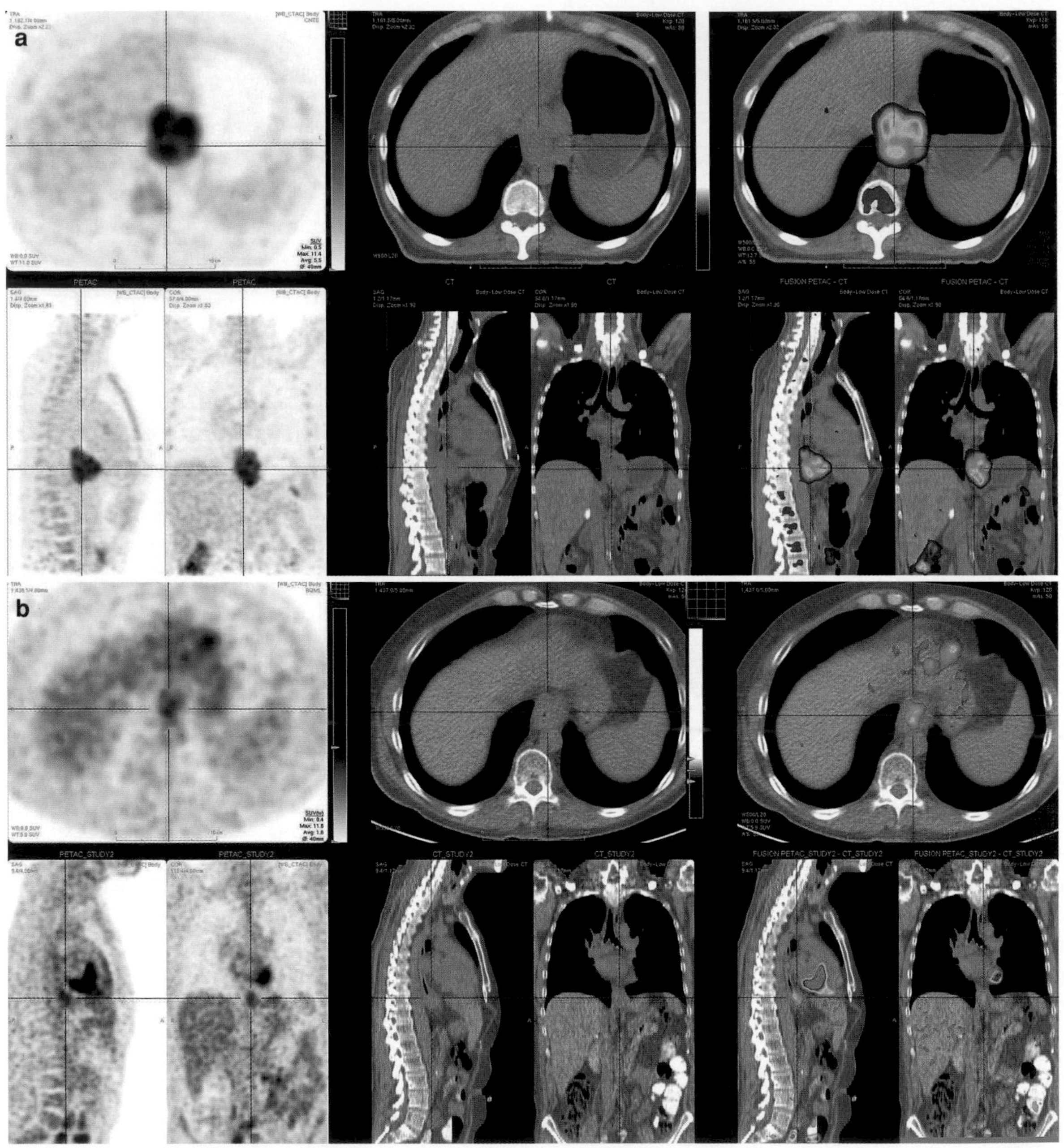

Fig. 6 Poorly differentiated adenocarcinoma of the distal esophagus, before (**a**) and 2 weeks after completion of concomitant chemoradiotherapy (**b**). The initial stage was T3N0M0. There is an excellent metabolic response and a surgery with curative intent was performed

metabolic response and the optimal timing of the interim PET study. In the MUNICON trial, a 35% decrease in SUVmean was used as a cut-off value determining a metabolic response but other thresholds have been proposed, including more complex indices combining tumor diameter and SUV (Krause et al. 2009; Roedl et al. 2009). A good metabolic response on PET-CT is illustrated in Fig. 6.

4.2 Gastric Cancer

Unlike esophageal cancer, data is rather scarce regarding the clinical value of FDG-PET-CT in gastric cancer. It appears that the sensitivity is too low to reliably assess the T and N stages of the disease (Stahl et al. 2003; Yun et al. 2005). PET/CT may detect additional distant metastases in patients selected for surgery (Chen et al. 2005a), but it is not currently validated as a part of the routine workup of patients with gastric cancer. An alternative tracer might be 3′-deoxy-3′-(18)F-fluorothymidine (FLT), which explores tumor proliferation rather than metabolism. Recent data suggest that FLT PET/CT is significantly more sensitive than FDG in detecting gastric cancer and that it might be of use in the evaluation of the response to treatment (Herrmann et al. 2007; Kameyama et al. 2009).

5 Pancreatic Cancer

Pancreatic cancer is the second most common malignancy of the digestive tracts representing 3% of all cancers and 6% of all cancer-related deaths (American_Cancer_Society 2009). The incidence has slightly increased and the mortality rate has been relatively stable over the past two decades. Pancreatic cancer remains a deadly disease, with 1 and 5 years survival rates of only 24 and 5%, respectively. This is mainly related to the paucity of initial symptoms. As a result, >10% of the patients are diagnosed at an early stage. Regardless, pancreatic cancers are aggressive, and even localized diseases are associated with a 5 year survival rate of only 20%. The most common pathological type by far is the ductal adenocarcinoma, with acinar cell carcinomas accounting for only 1–2% of all pancreatic cancer. Neuroendocrine tumors are discussed in a separate section of this chapter. Surgery is the only treatment capable of achieving long-term survival, often combined with adjuvant chemotherapy. Only a minority of patients are eligible for curative surgery, due to frequent extensive local disease, nodal spread or the presence of liver metastases.

5.1 Diagnosis

CT is the first-line imaging modality for diagnosing pancreatic cancer. According to a meta-analysis published in 2005, the sensitivity and specificity of CT was 91 and 85%, respectively compared with 84 and 82% for MRI (Bipat et al. 2005a, b). In this analysis, US had a sensitivity of 76% and a specificity of 75%. In this setting, FDG-PET is often performed to characterize a mass detected on CT and for which the malignant nature remains equivocal. A meta-analysis of 17 studies performed before the advent of PET-CT reports an overall summary estimate for sensitivity and specificity of 81 and 66%, respectively (Orlando et al. 2004). Interestingly, the sensitivity of PET increased to 100% when performed after an indeterminate result for CT, with a specificity unchanged at 68%. The specificity may be limited by significant uptake by inflammatory masses, such as encountered in acute or even chronic pancreatitis (Shreve 1998). A very recent meta-analysis compared PET, PET/CT and endoscopic ultrasonography (EUS) in diagnosing pancreatic carcinoma (Tang et al. 2009). Such evaluation is highly relevant from a clinical standpoint, as EUS is widely used for detecting and characterizing clinically suspected pancreatic masses, in spite of very large variations in the diagnostic accuracies reported in the literature. It appears that PET/CT is significantly more sensitive (90 vs. 81%) but less specific (80 vs. 93%) than EUS. In terms of accuracy, both PET/CT and EUS performed slightly better than PET alone. From these data, PET-CT emerges as a very valuable tool for ruling out malignancy in presence of indeterminate lesions on CT, thanks to its high sensitivity and negative predictive value. Furthermore, as discussed below, PET/CT helps staging the tumor once the diagnosis has been made and significantly contributes to determining its surgical resectability. On the other hand, EUS has the advantage of providing cytological samples by fine needle aspiration with very limited associated morbidity. However, EUS lacks sensitivity in diagnosing cancer in patients with chronic pancreatitis. Additionally, and quite importantly, the meta-analysis by Tang et al. observed a significant heterogeneity in the results available for EUS, which somewhat questions the validity of projecting the pooled sensitivity and specificity figures into the routine clinical practice. A pancreatic cancer evaluated by PET-CT is shown in Fig. 7.

5.2 Staging

As surgery is the only potentially curative treatment, all staging imaging procedures aim at assessing the

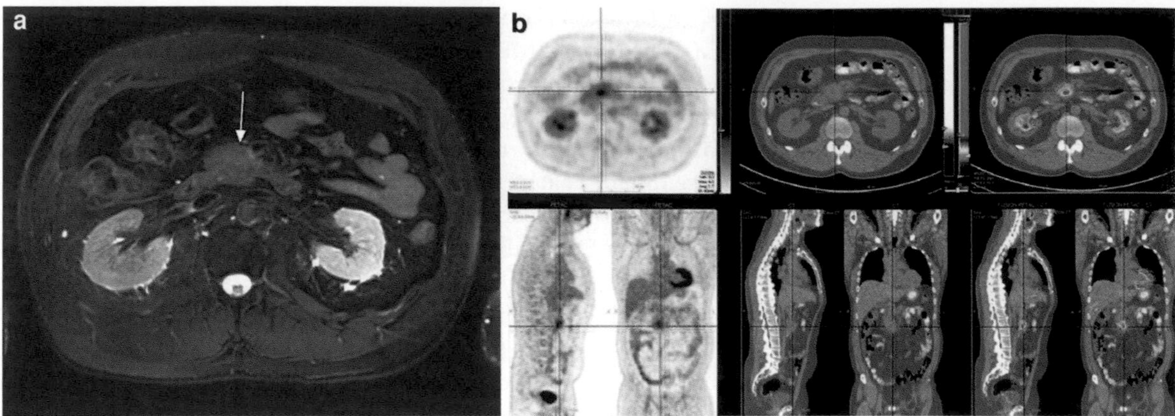

Fig. 7 This 46-year-old patient was hospitalized with a clinical syndrome consistent with acute pancreatitis. The exploration performed after resolution of the acute phase showed a mass in the head of the pancreas. The MRI suggested an autoimmune pancreatitis (**a**, transaxial T2w-image), but could not rule out cancer. EUS was consistent with a neoplastic process and also showed 2 suspicious nodes in the liver hilum and a suspicious liver lesion. PET-CT showed heterogeneously increased FDG uptake in the pancreatic mass, without any other abnormality (**b**). Surgery was carried out and revealed a 3 cm adenocarcinoma, N0M0

resectability of the tumor. The decision to operate depends on many factors and is usually taken after a multidisciplinary discussion of every case. The extent of the locoregional regional invasion, in particular the relationship of the tumor with the neighboring vessels is of primary importance. Unresectable locally advanced disease is usually treated by chemoradiotherapy. Nodal metastases are a contraindication to surgery only when they are located beyond the field of resection. Distant metastases preclude any attempt at curative surgery.

Similar to diagnosis, CT and EUS are the primary tools for staging pancreatic cancers, sometimes complemented by MR cholangiopancreatography, which provides excellent depiction of the extra-hepatic biliary tract and pancreatic ducts. FDG-PET-CT also plays a complementary role, with a very high positive predictive value for determining resectability. A clinical impact was found in 16% of patients selected for surgery following conventional methods, by detecting distant lesions, either primary or secondary (Heinrich et al. 2005). A protocol combining PET and triple-phase CT (non-enhanced low dose, arterial phase, portal phase) was recently proposed by the group in Zürich, with excellent clinical results (Strobel et al. 2008). Resectability status was assessed using this protocol with a positive predictive value of 82% and a negative predictive value of 96%. This was significantly more accurate than PET alone (Fig. 8).

6 Colorectal Cancer

Colorectal cancer is the third most common cancer in both women and men (American_Cancer_Society 2009). As mentioned earlier, both the incidence and mortality rate are significantly decreasing. The 5 year survival rate is currently 64%. It increases to 90% when the disease is diagnosed at an early stage, which fortunately happens in about 40% of all colorectal cancer patients. Surgery is curative without any further treatment in localized disease. Neo-adjuvant or adjuvant chemotherapy is given in case of locally advanced colon cancer or nodal spread. For rectal cancer, combined chemoradiotherapy followed by surgery is highly effective. Several lines of chemotherapy are available in case of metastatic disease, including anti-angiogenesis monoclonal antibodies such as Bevacizumab (Avastin). A variety of treatments targeted toward liver or lung metastases may also be applied in selected case, possibly in combination. This includes surgical metastasectomy, CT or US-guided radiofrequency ablation and selective internal radiation therapy (SIRT), among others. Considering the wide array of efficient therapeutic options, accurate staging is of primary importance in order to select the most appropriate strategy for each individual patient.

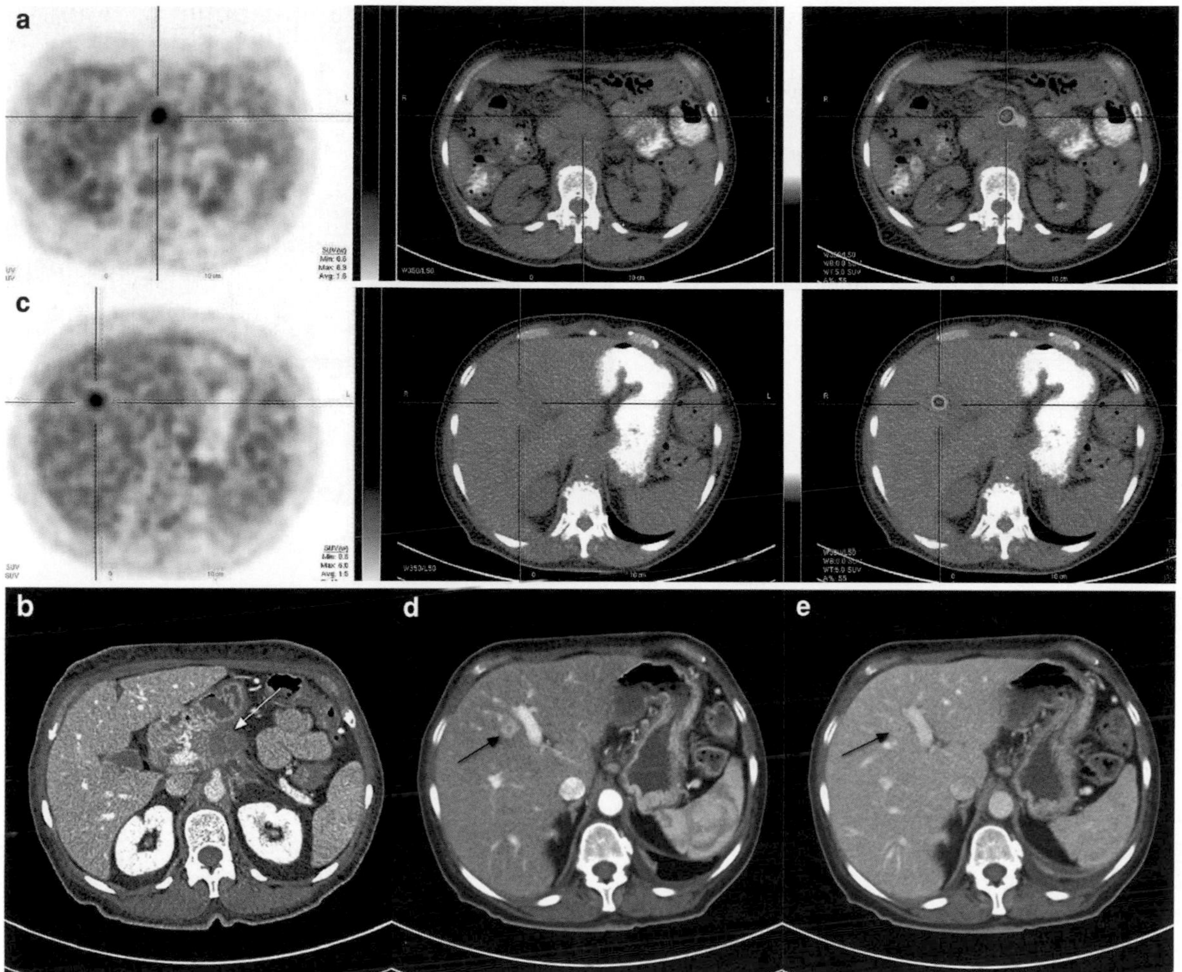

Fig. 8 Initial staging of an adenocarcinoma of the pancreatic body. The PET-CT shows a focus of highly increased activity within the lesion (**a**), which is larger on the diagnostic CT performed separately (**b**). There is also a 15 mm liver metastasis in the segment IV, clearly seen on the PET-CT (**c**) and the arterial phase of the CT (**d**) and barely identified on the portal phase of the CT (**e**)

6.1 Initial Staging

For colon cancer, the current consensus is that PET/CT is not routinely indicated at baseline in the absence of evidence of synchronous metastases. Although some studies found a positive clinical impact of PET in the initial staging (Llamas-Elvira et al. 2007), others failed to show any additional value over CT (Furukawa et al. 2006). The conventional workup thus mainly relies upon CT of the chest, abdomen and pelvis. PET-CT may however be useful for characterizing equivocal lesions seen on CT (Van Cutsem and Oliveira 2008). An example is shown in Fig. 9. On the other hand, initial results published with PET/CT colonography are highly encouraging and suggest that such integrated approach is more accurate than either CT alone or CT plus PET acquired separately (Veit-Haibach et al. 2006; Nagata et al. 2008). Although PET/CT colonography is methodologically more demanding and requires specific patient preparation including bowel cleansing, the combination of a highly accurate local assessment of tumor spread with a distant staging in a single imaging session appears quite attractive. Few clinical centers currently use such strategy, but the concept clearly warrants further evaluation.

The situation is quite different regarding rectal cancer, for which MRI is the key imaging procedure for determining the local invasion of the tumor. Such

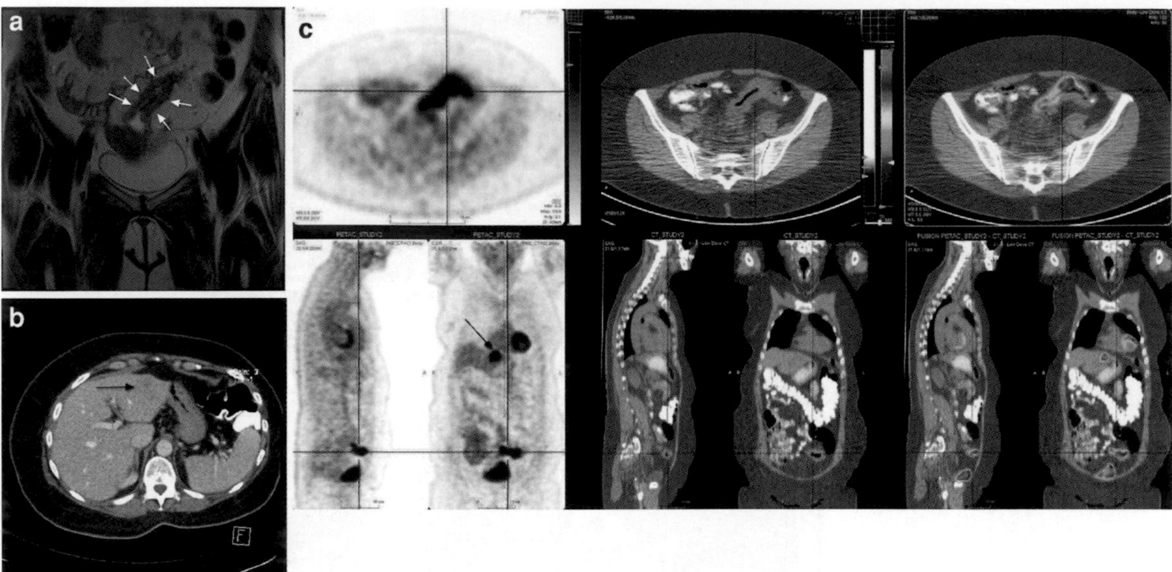

Fig. 9 Initial staging of a large adenocarcinoma of the sigmoid colon. This circumferential lesion is clearly seen on the MRI (**a**, coronal slice). Abdominal ceCT identifies a poorly hypodense lesion in the segment III of the liver (**b**). PET CT shows the hypermetabolic primary tumor and confirms the presence of a liver metastasis (**c**). However all three techniques (MR, CT and PET-CT) failed to recognized the 5 invaded perirectal nodes that 5 were revealed at surgery

information is important as early-stage disease is usually treated by surgery followed by adjuvant treatments, whereas locally advanced disease (T3–4 or positive nodes) benefits from neo-adjuvant radiation therapy or combined chemoradiotherapy before surgery is carried out. All the available conventional imaging techniques, including MRI and EUS, lack sensitivity and specificity in the nodal staging, with values in the range of 55–67 and 74–78%, respectively (Bipat et al. 2004). In this setting, PET has proved valuable in detecting additional lymph nodes or distant metastases, with a clinical impact in up to 27% of the cases (Gearhart et al. 2006; Davey et al. 2008). Furthermore, FDG-PET-CT increasingly contributes defining the irradiation target volume, according to the concept of "biological target volume" that takes into the metabolic activity of the tumor, otherwise identified with anatomical imaging methods. Such information is of great value when highly conformal radiation techniques are to be deployed or when the dose is finely adapted to local variations in tumor biology ("dose painting"). Significant differences in tumor volumes are observed, depending on the technique for delineating the lesions (Bassi et al. 2008). Integrated PET-MR imaging may be of significant value in staging rectal cancer.

6.2 Recurrence: Detection and Staging

Colorectal cancer recurrence occurs with a frequency of 30–50%, even after treatment with curative intent. Frequent sites of recurrence are the liver and lung, often in asymptomatic patients. Early diagnosis may lead to subsequent surgical resection of liver or lung metastases yielding improved 5 year survival rates of 35–40%. PET/CT plays a key role in both the detection and staging of recurrent disease. A recently published meta-analysis reviewed 27 studies evaluating the performance of FDG-PET in detecting recurrent colorectal cancer (Zhang et al. 2009). The pooled sensitivity and specificity was 91 and 83%, respectively. PET appears particularly accurate for detecting pelvic or local recurrence (sensitivity and specificity of 94%) and liver metastases (sensitivity of 97% and specificity of 98%). Various surveillance strategies have been proposed in patients treated with curative intent. When increased CEA levels are the initial sign, imaging studies aim at localizing the site of recurrence. PET is highly sensitive in this setting, with a detection rate of 79% in a series of 50 patients, of whom 28% were treated with curative intent (Flamen et al. 2001) (Fig. 10). Building upon the observation that intensive surveillance after initial

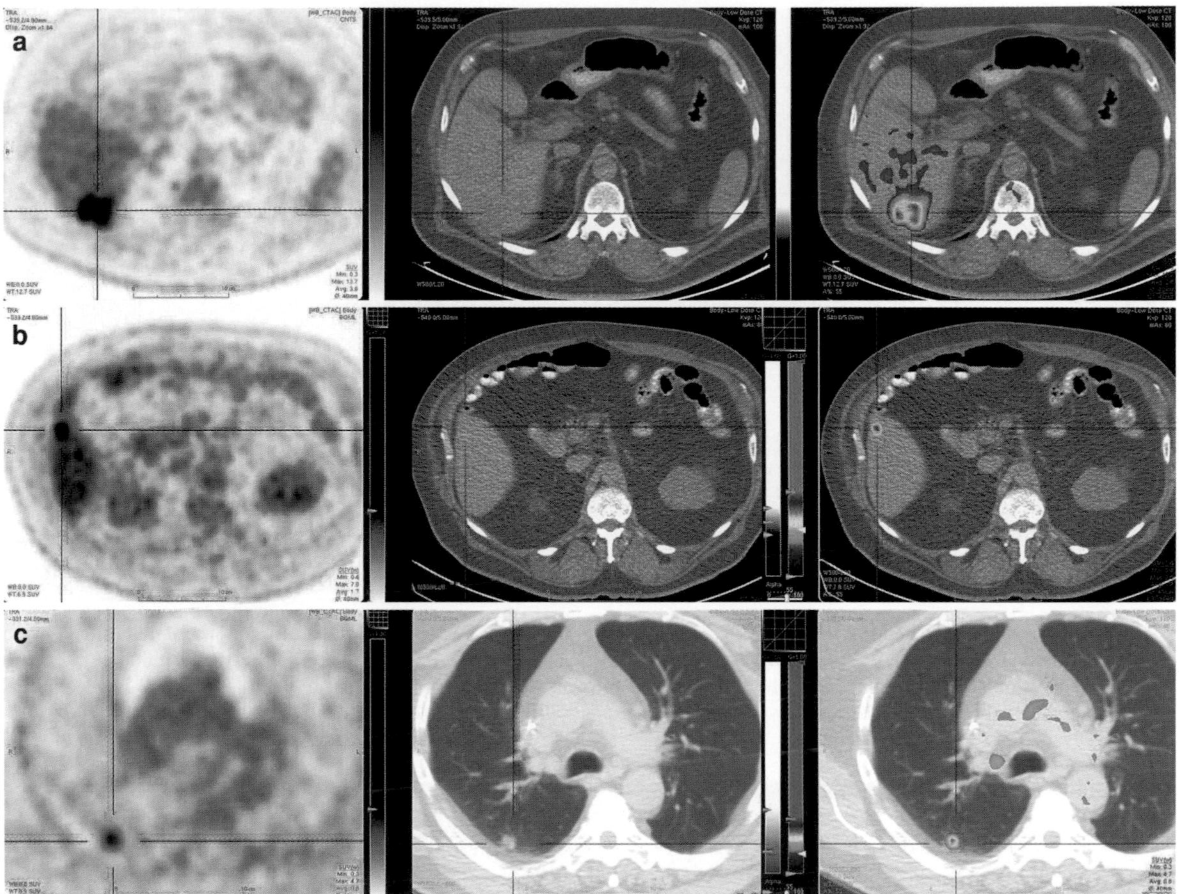

Fig. 10 This patient had surgery for a colon cancer 10 months ago. The PET-CT is performed, as a first line exam, for investigating increased CEA levels. It reveals multifocal recurrence, with 2 liver metastases (**a** and **b**) and 1 lung metastasis (**c**)

curative surgery does improve survival (Rodriguez-Moranta et al. 2006), recent studies evaluated the clinical impact of surveillance strategies utilizing whole-body PET-CT. Sobhani et al. performed a prospective randomized trial comparing a strategy based upon conventional methods (tumor markers, US, chest X-ray and abdominal CT) with a strategy including PET at 9 and 15 months post treatment (Sobhani et al. 2008). In the PET group, recurrences were detected after 12.1 months (versus 15.4 months in the control group) and complete (R0) resections were more frequently achieved than in the control group. Another recent study of 132 patients equally supported applying an aggressive strategy, which in this case used integrated PET/CT 6, 12 and 24 months after surgery (Sorensen et al. 2010). Although the current clinical guidelines do not recommend the systematic use of FDG-PET-CT in the monitoring of colorectal cancer, there is a strong possibility that it will change in the near future. A PET/CT scan identifying recurrent disease is shown in Fig. 11.

PET/CT is on the other hand fully recommended in the preoperative workup of known recurrent disease. The liver is the primary site of distant recurrence and limited disease is amenable to surgical resection with curative intent. PET has shown a major impact in the management either by more accurately depicting the extent of the liver involvement or by detecting unknown distant lesions. In a randomized trial including 150 patients with liver metastases from colorectal cancer selected for surgery by CT (Ruers et al. 2009), half the patients had a FDG-PET in addition to the conventional workup. The endpoint was futile surgery, defined as any laparotomy that did not result in an R0 resection that revealed benign disease or resulted in a disease-free survival

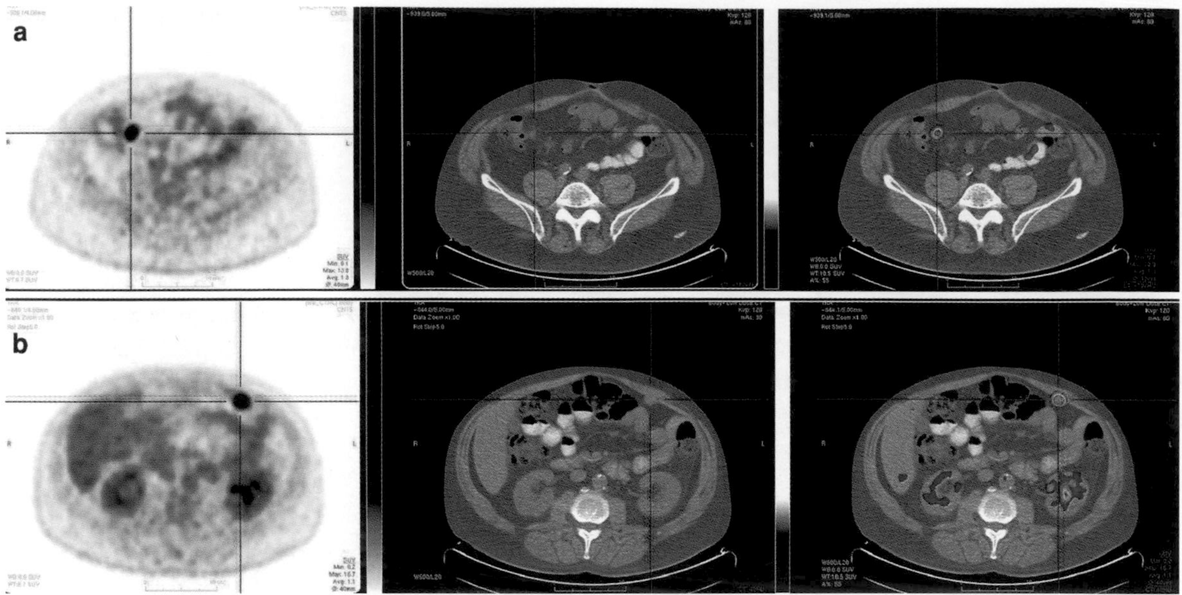

Fig. 11 Peritoneal recurrence in a patient with a history of sigmoid colon cancer treated by surgery and adjuvant chemotherapy 3 years ago. Routine follow-up CT showed a small soft tissue nodule next to the cecum. The lesion was clearly seen on the PET-CT study (**a**), which also showed an additional lesion in the left abdominal wall (**b**). Surgery with curative intent was carried out. Both lesions were pathologically confirmed and no additional lesions were found

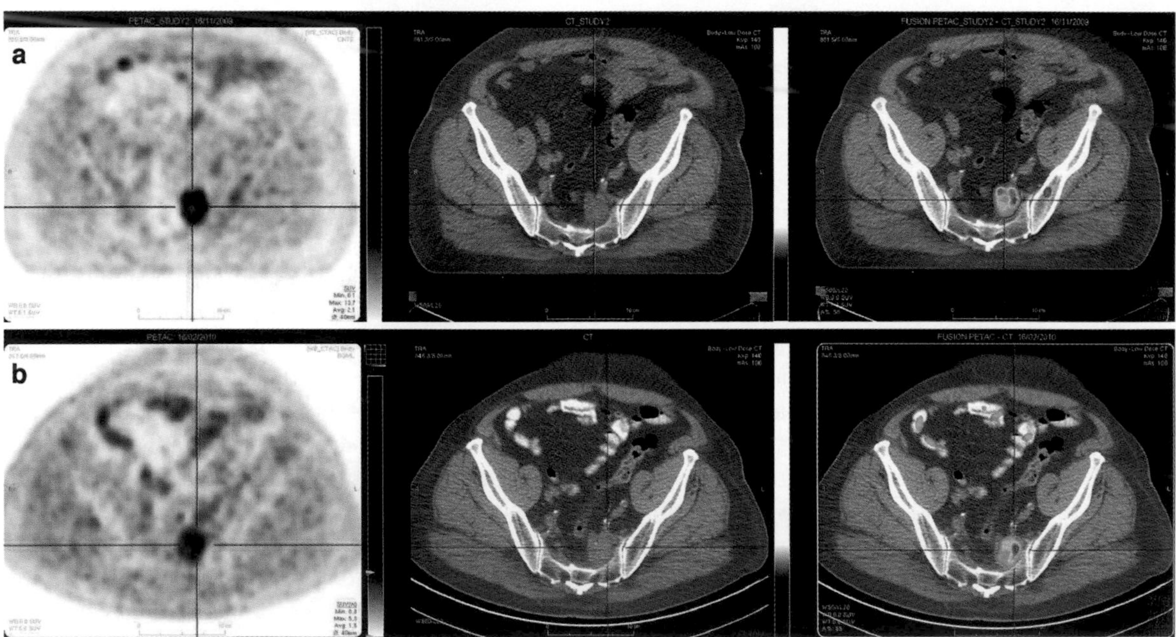

Fig. 12 Pelvic recurrence of colon adenocarninoma. PET-CT was performed before (**a**) and after (**b**) neoadjuvant chemoradiotherapy and showed a poor metabolic response. Pathology confirmed the persistence of extensive disease in the surgical sample

shorter than 6 months. The number of such futile surgeries was reduced by 38% in the PET group, from 34 (45)–21(28%). Overall, the addition of FDG-PET to the conventional workup prevented unnecessary surgery in 1 of 6 patients. This study was performed using a standalone PET scanner and several methodological issues remain to be clarified. Regarding the CT acquisition protocol, it appears that the major advantage of contrast-enhanced PET-CT (PET/ceCT) over PET/CT lays in a better segmental localization of liver metastases while non-enhanced PET/CT seems to perform equally well for detecting and localizing all other lesions (Soyka et al. 2008).

6.3 Assessment of Response to Treatment

Limited data is available regarding FDG in the chemotherapy monitoring of advanced colorectal cancer and the two largest studies yielded contradictory results. de Geus-Oei et al. reported in 2008 that the PET response measured at 2 months after the start of treatment predicted the overall survival and disease-free survival rates in a series of 50 patients (de Geus-oei et al. 2008). Conversely, 1 year later, Bystrom et al. did not find any correlation between metabolic response after 2 cycles of chemotherapy and time to progression or overall survival in a population of 51 patients (Bystrom et al. 2009). In any case, there is insufficient data to support using PET in the routine clinical setting. Much more convincing data are available concerning the neoadjuvant treatment of rectal cancer. In this situation, the metabolic response is generally well correlated with the pathology response, and is superior to conventional imaging techniques in this regard (de Geus-Oei et al. 2009). Whether the post-treatment evaluation could significantly affect the management, possibly through altering the surgical approach, is not known (Fig. 12). Finally, encouraging results were obtained for assessing the result of local ablative therapy of liver metastases (de Geus-Oei et al. 2009), but the available data suggests that it is premature to recommend using PET routinely in this indication.

7 Primary and Secondary Tumors of the Liver

Primary cancers of the liver and intrahepatic bile ducts represent only 1.5% of the total number of estimated new cases in 2009 in the US, yet the mortality represents 3.2% of all cancer-related deaths for the same period (American_Cancer_Society 2009). Over 85% of these tumors are hepatocellular carcinomas (HCC), whose incidence is increasing worldwide. Cholangiocarcinoma is less frequent, representing 10–15% of all hepatobiliary malignancies. These tumors originate from the intra- or extra-hepatic bile ducts, most often at the bifurcation of the hepatic ducts in the hilar region. Hepatic metastases are much more frequent than primary tumors, as liver is a common site of hematogenous metastatic spread. Cancers of the digestive tract and singularly colorectal cancers are the primary sources of liver metastases although breast and lung cancers are also associated with a high prevalence of liver spread.

7.1 Hepatocarcinoma

The sensitivity of FDG-PET and PET-CT is very low for detecting HCC. These tumors may appear as areas of decreased activity, increased activity or normal activity and the pattern of uptake seems fairly well correlated with the differentiation and aggressiveness of the tumor (Fig. 13). Increased uptake is usually seen in high-grade HCC and has been associated with gene expression profiles related with poor prognosis indicators (Lee et al. 2004). As a result, FDG-PET may be used as a predictor of outcome. Patients with hypermetabolic tumors tend to have shorter survival rates and higher recurrence rates after surgical resection (Shiomi et al. 2001; Seo et al. 2007). Similar observations were recently made in patients who had liver transplantation for treating their HCC. Increased FDG uptake by the tumor was an independent predictor of recurrence in these patients and it was associated with microvascular invasion in the pathological samples (Kornberg et al. 2009; Lee et al. 2009). Methodological questions exist as to the optimal way for quantifying the tumor metabolism, but it appears that the tumor to normal liver activity ratios might be the best predictor, rather than the SUV alone (Seo et al. 2007; Lee et al. 2009). In addition to tumor grade, the size of the lesion is also a factor affecting the sensitivity of FDG-PET-CT. In a series of 99 HCCs, the sensitivities according to tumor size (1–2, 2–5, and >/=5 cm) were 27.2, 47.8, and 92.8%, respectively (Park et al. 2008). In addition to characterizing the primary tumor, PET may be useful in the preoperative setting in detecting metastatic disease. The sensitivity of PET for distant lesions is usually higher than for the

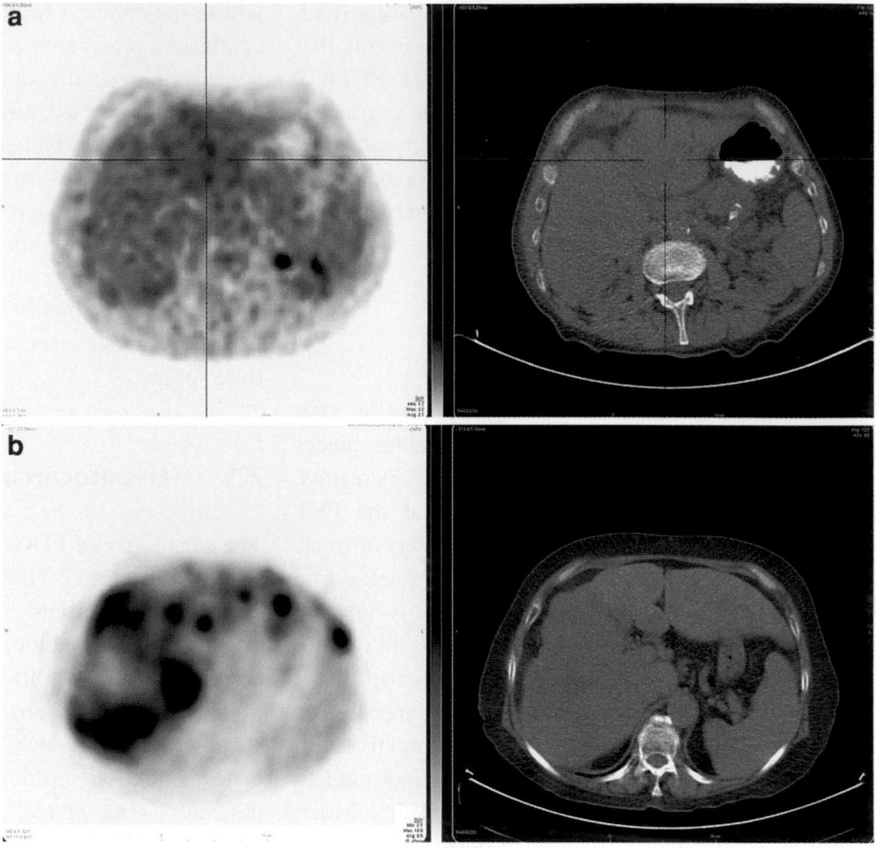

Fig. 13 Two examples of hepatocarcinomas. **a** shows a large lesion in left liver lobe, with only mild FDG uptake. **b** shows a highly hypermetabolic multifocal disease

primary, and for whole-body staging it was found superior to CT (Park et al. 2008; Kawaoka et al. 2009). Finally, FDG-PET-CT has been proposed for assessing disease activity after non-operative therapies such as transcatheter arterial chemoembolization or radiofrequency ablation (Higashi et al. 2010) and for locating suspected recurrence based upon elevated alfa-fetoprotein levels (Chen et al. 2005b; Han et al. 2009). Due to the low sensitivity of FDG-PET for detecting HCC, alternative tracers have been proposed, in particular ^{11}C-acetate. This tracer enters the Krebs cycle as a substrate for beta-oxidation in fatty acid synthesis and cholesterol synthesis. Fatty acid synthesis is believed to be the major reason for uptake of ^{11}C-acetate by liver tumors. The largest study to date was published by Park et al. who found that ^{11}C-acetate PET/CT improved the overall sensitivity, although it remained low for small HCCs (Park et al. 2008). In addition the extrahepatic staging was not improved compared to FDG-PET/CT.

7.2 Cholangiocarcinoma

The sensitivity of FDG-PET for detecting cholangiocarcinomas depends on the location and morphological type of the tumor. It is in the range of 85–95% for intrahepatic mass-forming lesions, but much lower for the hilar or extrahepatic periductal infiltrating lesions, where sensitivity values as low as 18% have been reported in the literature (Kato et al. 2002; Anderson et al. 2004; Corvera et al. 2008). Lymph node spread and dissemination to distant organs are frequent at the time of diagnosis, and PET has proved valuable for detecting such metastases, changing the management in up to 24% of the patients (Petrowsky et al. 2006; Corvera et al. 2008).

7.3 Liver Metastases

Three meta-analyses comparing the relative diagnostic performances of various imaging modalities for detecting liver metastases are available. The first one

Table 1 Meta-analysis of the diagnostic performances of US, CT, MRI and PET for detecting liver metastases from colorectal cancers (Floriani et al. 2010)

	Patients				Lesions			
	Sens. (%)	Spec. (%)	LR−	LR+	Sens. (%)	Spec. (%)	LR−	LR+
US	63	97.6	0.34	16.88	NA	NA	NA	NA
CT	74.8	95.6	0.38	11.66	82.6	56.6	0.41	1.77
MRI	81.1	97.2	0.35	29.16	86.3	87.2	0.2	6.53
PET	93.8	98.7	0.008	51.53	86	97.2	0.48	13.43

Sens. = sensitivity, spec. = specificity, LR− = negative likelihood ratio, LR+ = positive likelihood ratio

was published in 2002 and included studies published until 1996 for US and 2000 for CT, MRI and PET (Kinkel et al. 2002). The mean weighted sensitivity was 66% for US, 70% for CT, 71% for MRI and 90% for PET. The second meta-analysis included studies published until December 2003 and focused on liver metastases from colorectal cancer (Bipat et al. 2005b). Again, PET was the most sensitive technique for both identifying patients with liver metastases and for detecting individual lesions. In the patients-based analysis, the sensitivities were 94.6, 64.7 and 75.8% for PET, spiral CT and 1,5T MRI, respectively. In the per-lesion analysis, these values were 75.9, 63.8 and 64.4%, respectively. A third meta-analysis was very recently published, with different selection criteria, as only series comparing at least 2 different imaging modalities in CRC patients were retained (Floriani et al. 2010). The results are summarized in Table 1 and confirm PET as the technique with the highest differential in likelihood ratios for identifying metastatic patients, whereas the results are fairly similar for PET and MRI in terms of individual lesion analysis. The results of these meta-analyses should be pondered taking into account several factors. In general, MRI with liver-specific contrast agent such as mangafodipir disodium (MnDPDP) or with superparamagnetic iron oxide (SPIO) performs better than the conventional gadolinium-based agents. The routine clinical results will thus vary depending on the MR methodology that is used. The size of the lesions also intervenes, and MRI is considered more sensitive than FDG-PET/CT for detecting small lesions (Kong et al. 2008). The PET/CT procedure may also integrate a diagnostic contrast-enhanced CT study. The usefulness of such combined PET-ceCT appears quite clearly in patients scheduled to undergo surgical resection of liver metastases, as the ceCT component is crucial for a precise segmental localization the hypermetabolic metastases, but seems otherwise limited (Chua et al. 2007; Soyka et al. 2008). Overall, it appears that FDG-PET-CT is highly sensitive and specific for identifying patients with liver metastases. It is strongly recommended in patients selected for liver surgery with curative intent. In addition to improving the liver staging, PET/CT has a determinant impact on patients' management by detecting extrahepatic lesions, thus preventing or modifying the surgical approach (Wiering et al. 2005). In this indication, the combination of whole-body PET/CT and MRI with tissue-specific contrast contrast agents is undoubtedly the most powerful for accurately selecting surgical patients. In the post-therapeutic setting, a growing body of evidence supports using PET for assessing the response to non-surgical treatments such as selective radio-embolization with 90Y-labeled microspheres or radiofrequency ablation, although it is too early to consider PET as the sole imaging gold standard (Lin et al. 2007; Kuehl et al. 2008). Figure 14 illustrates the metabolic appearance of 2 different liver lesions.

8 GIST

Gastrointestinal stromal tumors (GIST) are mesenchymal tumors derived from interstitial cell of Cajal in the myenteric plexus. They account for >3% of all gastrointestinal tumors and they mostly arise from the stomach and small bowel (Miettinen and Lasota 2001). The primary treatment is surgery, as these tumors are resistant to chemotherapy and irradiation. Approximately 80–85% of GISTs harbor activating mutations of the KIT tyrosine kinase (Corless et al. 2004). As a result, they tend to show a high response rate to the kinase inhibitor Imatinib. The evaluation of the response to such treatment cannot be performed using the conventional criteria of target lesion size as

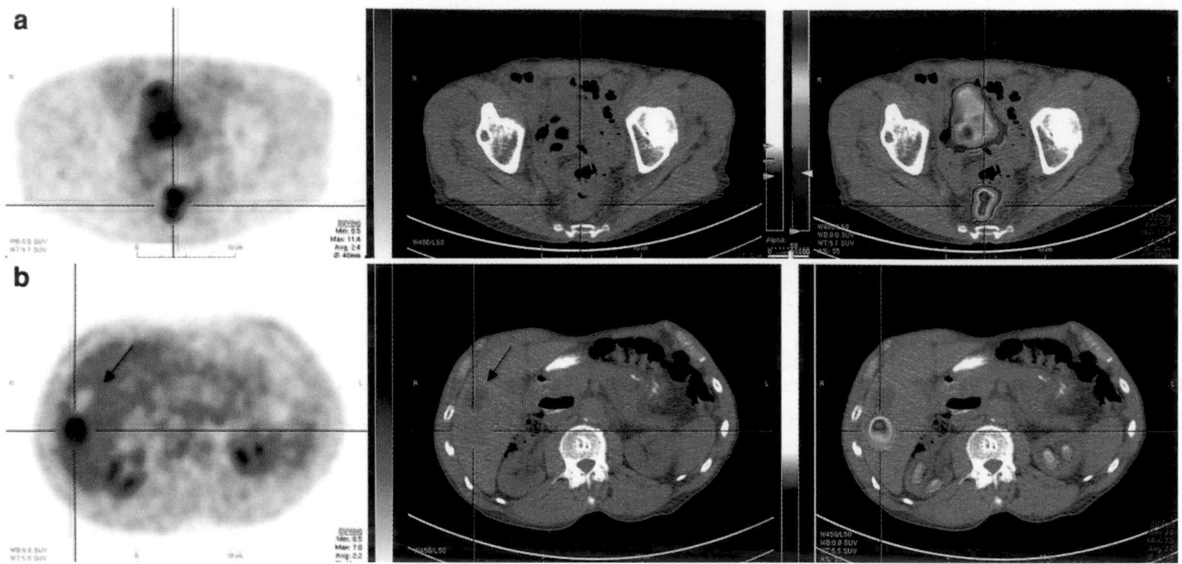

Fig. 14 Known rectal cancer (**a**) with equivocal liver lesions on CT. A metastasis is clearly seen as a hyperactive focus, next to a cold cystic lesion (*arrow* on **b**)

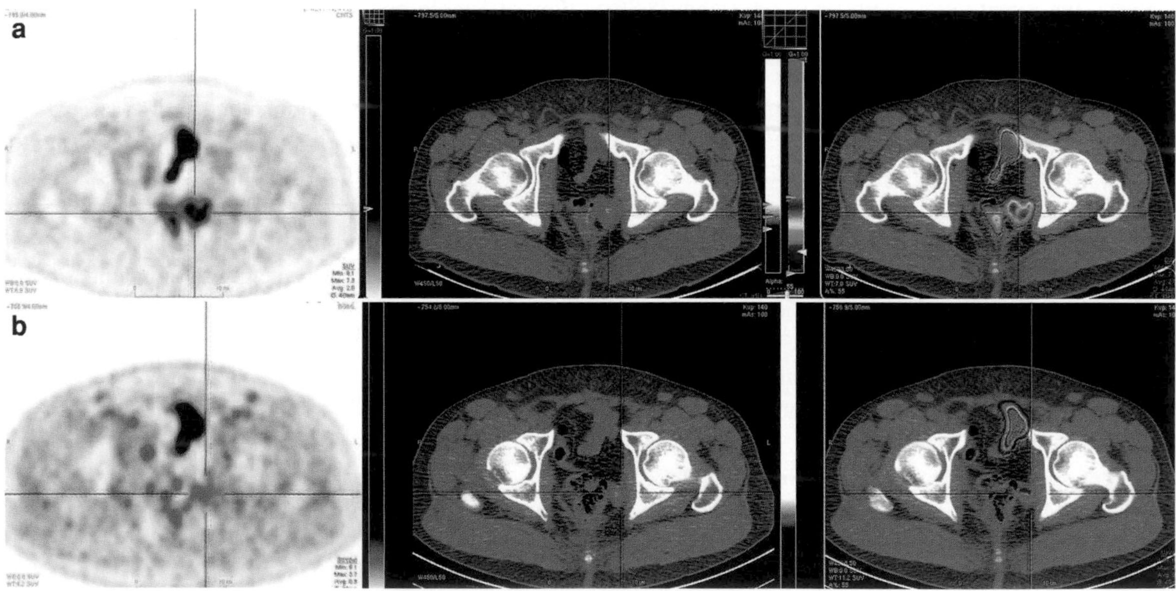

Fig. 15 Rectal GIST before (**a**) and after (**b**) a treatment by imagine was initiated. The mass has not significantly changed on CT, whereas there is markedly decrease in metabolic activity

measured with cross-sectional imaging (RECIST criteria). Indeed, unlike conventional cytotoxic drugs, tyrosine kinase inhibitors may be very effective at shutting down the tumor without any observable reduction in size for a prolonged period of time. It has been observed that the glucose metabolism is a very early indicator of the response to tyrosine kinase inhibitors: Stroobants et al. described a metabolic response in 13/17 GIST as early as 8 days after the Imatininb treatment was initiated, and such response was associated with a longer progression-free survival (Stroobants et al. 2003) (Fig. 15). Furthermore the early metabolic response is a better predictor of long-term outcome than the radiological response at 8 weeks, as measured using conventional criteria (Jager et al. 2004). CT imaging provides nonetheless valuable information, as PET/CT has proved superior to either PET or CT alone for both staging and assessing the therapeutic response (Antoch et al. 2004a, b; Goerres et al. 2005). Original CT response indicators were developed based upon a combination of tumor density and size criteria (Choi et al. 2004), or changes in the enhancement pattern (Mabille et al. 2009) so that the combination of PET and ceCT appears to be the most powerful for guiding the clinicians in their management of GIST patients, not only for evaluating early on the response to treatment but also to detect development of resistance to Imatininb (Van den Abbeele 2008).

9 Neuroendocrine Tumors

Neuroendocrine tumors (NETs) are a heterogeneous group of tumors characterized by distinct histopathology pattern and endocrinology metabolism. The most common locations are the respiratory and gastroenteropancreatic tracts. One-third to half of these tumors are deemed functional, i.e. secreting hormones responsible for symptoms such as carcinoid syndrome or severe hypoglycemia, depending on the tumor type. NETs are most often well-differentiated tumors with low proliferation index but a minority present as more aggressive tumors with a tendency to metastasize, typically to the liver. The initial step in the diagnosis of NETs relies upon biological measurement of markers such as chromogranin A, gastrin, insulin or metanephrines. Locating the primary is the next step and may be difficult as NETs are often small tumors in highly variable locations. In addition to their histopathologic features, NETs are also often classified according to their location, i.e. foregut (pancreas, stomach and duodenum), midgut (small bowel and appendix) and hindgut (colon and rectum). As conventional imaging methods often fail to identify and localize NETs, functional imaging techniques play a major role in this setting.

9.1 FDG-PET/CT

FDG is not the most effective tracer for diagnosing and staging NETs. In fact, the overall detection rate of FDG-PET in NETs is low, due to the fact that most of these tumors are well differentiated and display near-normal glucose metabolism (Adams et al. 1998; Belhocine et al. 2002). The sensitivity of FDG-PET appears directly related to the degree of differentiation of the tumor, with a significantly higher detection rate for lesions with a high proliferation index (Pasquali et al. 1998). FDG-PET may complement somatostatin receptor scintigraphy (SRS) as it may pick up additional undifferentiated tumors that are negative with SRS. Nonetheless, the clinical value of FDG-PET in NETs mainly relies on its biological characterization of the tumor. Indeed, increased FDG uptake is strongly associated with shorter progression-free survival and overall survival, including in patients with low-grade NETs (Garin et al. 2009). In a prospective study of 98 patients with NET, FDG-PET showed a strong prognostic value, actually higher than the prognostic value of traditional markers such as Ki67, chromogranin A, and liver metastases (Binderup et al. 2010). This recent information is not yet integrated in the current clinical management algorithms but there may be an important role for FDG-PET in the future.

9.2 PET/CT with Alternative Tracers

The poor diagnostic performances of conventional radiological methods and FDG-PET, combined with specific biological properties of NETs, set the stage for alternative PET tracers. First, most NET cells highly express somatostatin receptors, in particular the subtype 2 (SSTR2). Radiolabeled somatostatin analogs are therefore particularly well suited for imaging these tumors. In recent years, several such tracers have been developed, labeled with ^{68}Ga. These include DOTA-TOC, DOTA-TATE and DOTA-NOC (Antunes et al. 2007). PET-CT imaging with these tracers combine the high specificity of SRS with high spatial resolution and overall sensitivity. A second interesting biological property of NET is their

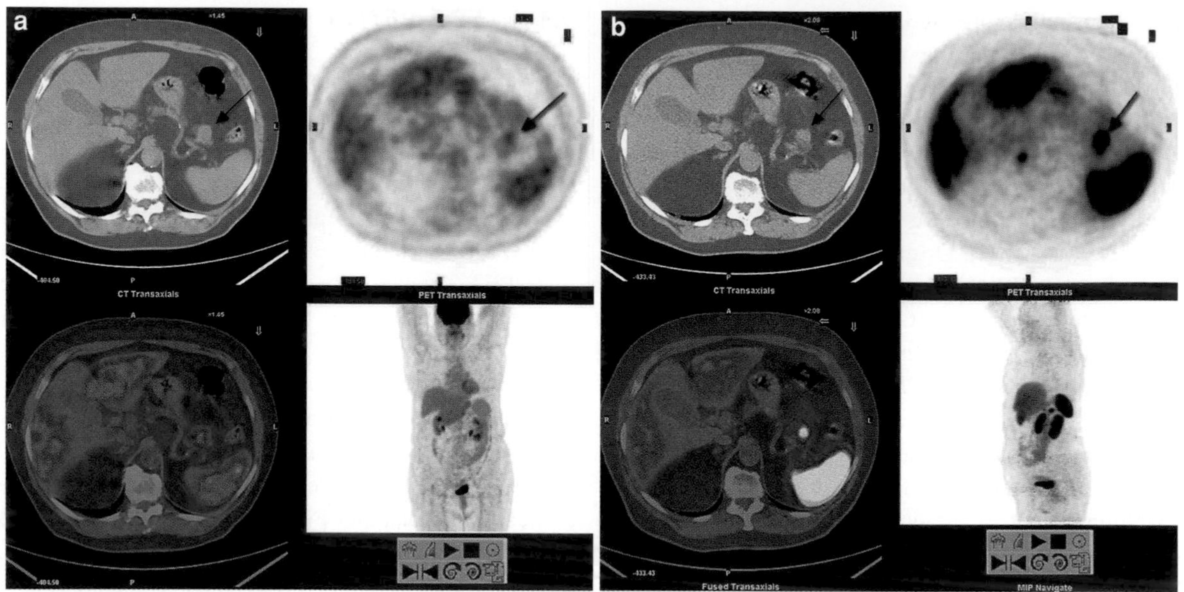

Fig. 16 FDG-PET-CT is performed for characterizing a mass in the tail of the pancreas. It only shows a very faint uptake (*arrow*, **a**). A DOTA-NOC PET-CT is performed 2 weeks later, showing a highly increased uptake, consistent with a tumor expressing SSTR (*arrow*, **b**). Surgery confirmed a neuroendocrine tumor. Images courtesy of Paolo CASTELLUCCI, MD

biogenic amine production and storage mechanism. F-DOPA is a ^{18}F-labeled aromatic amino acid that is avidly taken up by NETs trough this mechanism. Both tracers are being extensively studied, with highly encouraging results. Somatostatin analogs labeled with ^{68}Ga are consistently more sensitive than SRS while maintaining a high specificity (Gabriel et al. 2007; Kwekkeboom et al. 2010). The radioisotope ^{68}Ga is available from a generator and has a physical half-life of 68 min, which is well suited for PET imaging. In addition, the synthesis process is rather straightforward, fast and generates high yields (Zhernosekov et al. 2007). As radioisotope therapy with somatostatin analogs labeled with beta-emitters (^{177}Lu-DOTA-TATE or ^{90}Y-DOTA-TOC) have become increasingly proposed in progressive metastasized NETs, their positron-emitter counterparts can also be extremely useful in selecting the patients who are susceptible to benefit from such treatment (SR mapping) and in determining the optimal dosimetry (Kwekkeboom et al. 2010). PET with F-DOPA has also shown promising results in terms of diagnostic accuracy (Becherer et al. 2004). Regarding the NETS of the digestive tract; however, F-DOPA is likely to be of limited value, as the most significant clinical impact was observed in other tumor subtypes, in particular medullary thyroid carcinomas. Overall, and even though direct comparative studies of F-DOPA and ^{68}Ga-labelled compounds remain scarce, the available results suggest better diagnostic performances for the later (Ambrosini et al. 2008; Haug et al. 2009; Putzer et al. 2010). An example of PNET diagnosed with DOTA-NOC is shown in Fig. 16.

10 Perspectives

The development of molecular imaging in gastrointestinal malignancies, just as in oncology in general, is likely to follow two major pathways. The first one relates to innovative radiotracers exploring original biological targets. A highly attractive example is angiogenesis, which plays a major role in tumor growth and dissemination. Several compounds derived from the RGB peptide are being actively investigated, labeled either with ^{68}Ga or with ^{18}F (Schottelius et al. 2009). These tracers specifically bind to the alpha(v)beta(3) integrin, which is key in the angiogenesis process. Several reports indicate the feasibility of angiogenesis imaging in humans with PET, although there is no series dedicated to gastrointestinal tumors yet (Beer et al. 2006; Schnell et al. 2009). Hypoxia is another attractive target, especially in tumors for which radiation therapy is involved.

Although progresses have been somewhat slower than initially expected, the interest of the scientific community toward hypoxia imaging with PET remains sustained (Mees et al. 2009; Dalah et al. 2010). Technology is a second major research avenue with the development of hybrid PET-MR devices. PET-CT has been a tremendous step forward, and it has been very rapidly adopted by the nuclear medicine community. PET-CT has considerably reduced the image acquisition time, as the attenuation map is now obtained with a very fast CT study instead of a lengthy transmission scan. Furthermore and more importantly, the addition of anatomical information to the metabolic survey has significantly improved the diagnostic accuracy. PET-MR will face very different challenges, as the overall length of the imaging procedure will actually increase compared to current PET-CT procedures, leading to important questions regarding the throughput. The cost-effectiveness will have to be carefully studied, considering that both the investment and the operating costs will be driven up with PET-MR compared with PET-CT. It is also not clear whether performing simultaneously or near simultaneously the PET and the MR studies will be of significant clinical value compared to the two studies performed separately as in the current practice. Nevertheless, considering gastrointestinal tumors, the perspective of a one stop PET-MR for the preoperative evaluation of liver metastases or for the pretherapeutic assessment of rectal cancer appears quite attractive and warrants clinical investigation.

References

Adams S, Baum R, Rink T, Schumm-Drager PM, Usadel KH, Hor G (1998) Limited value of fluorine-18 fluorodeoxyglucose positron emission tomography for the imaging of neuroendocrine tumours. Eur J Nucl Med 25(1): 79–83

Ambrosini V, Tomassetti P, Castellucci P, Campana D, Montini G, Rubello D, Nanni C, Rizzello A, Franchi R, Fanti S (2008) Comparison between 68Ga-DOTA-NOC and 18F-DOPA PET for the detection of gastro-entero-pancreatic and lung neuro-endocrine tumours. Eur J Nucl Med Mol Imaging 35(8):1431–1438

American_Cancer_Society (2009) Cancer Facts & Figures. American Cancer Society, Atlanta

Anderson CD, Rice MH, Pinson CW, Chapman WC, Chari RS, Delbeke D (2004) Fluorodeoxyglucose PET imaging in the evaluation of gallbladder carcinoma and cholangiocarcinoma. J Gastrointest Surg 8(1):90–97

Antoch G, Kanja J, Bauer S, Kuehl H, Renzing-Koehler K, Schuette J, Bockisch A, Debatin JF, Freudenberg LS (2004a) Comparison of PET, CT, and dual-modality PET/CT imaging for monitoring of imatinib (STI571) therapy in patients with gastrointestinal stromal tumors. J Nucl Med 45(3):357–365

Antoch G, Saoudi N, Kuehl H, Dahmen G, Mueller SP, Beyer T, Bockisch A, Debatin JF, Freudenberg LS (2004b) Accuracy of whole-body dual-modality fluorine-18–2-fluoro-2-deoxy-D-glucose positron emission tomography and computed tomography (FDG-PET/CT) for tumor staging in solid tumors: comparison with CT and PET. J Clin Oncol 22(21):4357–4368

Antunes P, Ginj M, Zhang H, Waser B, Baum RP, Reubi JC, Maecke H (2007) Are radiogallium-labelled DOTA-conjugated somatostatin analogues superior to those labelled with other radiometals? Eur J Nucl Med Mol Imaging 34(7):982–993

Bassi MC, Turri L, Sacchetti G, Loi G, Cannillo B, La Mattina P, Brambilla M, Inglese E, Krengli M (2008) FDG-PET/CT imaging for staging and target volume delineation in preoperative conformal radiotherapy of rectal cancer. Int J Radiat Oncol Biol Phys 70(5):1423–1426

Becherer A, Szabo M, Karanikas G, Wunderbaldinger P, Angelberger P, Raderer M, Kurtaran A, Dudczak R, Kletter K (2004) Imaging of advanced neuroendocrine tumors with (18)F-FDOPA PET. J Nucl Med 45(7):1161–1167

Beer AJ, Haubner R, Sarbia M, Goebel M, Luderschmidt S, Grosu AL, Schnell O, Niemeyer M, Kessler H, Wester HJ, Weber WA, Schwaiger M (2006) Positron emission tomography using [18F]Galacto-RGD identifies the level of integrin alpha(v)beta3 expression in man. Clin Cancer Res 12(13):3942–39429

Belhocine T, Foidart J, Rigo P, Najjar F, Thiry A, Quatresooz P, Hustinx R (2002) Fluorodeoxyglucose positron emission tomography and somatostatin receptor scintigraphy for diagnosing and staging carcinoid tumours: correlations with the pathological indexes p53 and Ki-67. Nucl Med Commun 23(8):727–734

Berrisford RG, Wong WL, Day D, Toy E, Napier M, Mitchell K, Wajed S (2008) The decision to operate: role of integrated computed tomography positron emission tomography in staging oesophageal and oesophagogastric junction cancer by the multidisciplinary team. Eur J Cardiothorac Surg 33(6):1112–1116

Binderup T, Knigge U, Loft A, Federspiel B, Kjaer A (2010) 18F-fluorodeoxyglucose positron emission tomography predicts survival of patients with neuroendocrine tumors. Clin Cancer Res 16(3):978–985

Bipat S, Glas AS, Slors FJ, Zwinderman AH, Bossuyt PM, Stoker J (2004) Rectal cancer: local staging and assessment of lymph node involvement with endoluminal US, CT, and MR imaging–a meta-analysis. Radiology 232(3): 773–783

Bipat S, Phoa SS, van Delden OM, Bossuyt PM, Gouma DJ, Lameris JS, Stoker J (2005a) Ultrasonography, computed tomography and magnetic resonance imaging for diagnosis and determining resectability of pancreatic adenocarcinoma: a meta-analysis. J Comput Assist Tomogr 29(4):438–445

Bipat S, van Leeuwen MS, Comans EF, Pijl ME, Bossuyt PM, Zwinderman AH, Stoker J (2005b) Colorectal liver metastases: CT, MR imaging, and PET for diagnosis–meta-analysis. Radiology 237(1):123–131

Blot WJ, McLaughlin JK (1999) The changing epidemiology of esophageal cancer. Semin Oncol 26 (5 Suppl 15):2–8

Bystrom P, Berglund A, Garske U, Jacobsson H, Sundin A, Nygren P, Frodin JE, Glimelius B (2009) Early prediction of response to first-line chemotherapy by sequential [18F]-2-fluoro-2-deoxy-D-glucose positron emission tomography in patients with advanced colorectal cancer. Ann Oncol 20(6):1057–1061

Chatterton BE, Ho Shon I, Baldey A, Lenzo N, Patrikeos A, Kelley B, Wong D, Ramshaw JE, Scott AM (2009) Positron emission tomography changes management and prognostic stratification in patients with oesophageal cancer: results of a multicentre prospective study. Eur J Nucl Med Mol Imaging 36(3):354–361

Chen J, Cheong JH, Yun MJ, Kim J, Lim JS, Hyung WJ, Noh SH (2005a) Improvement in preoperative staging of gastric adenocarcinoma with positron emission tomography. Cancer 103(11):2383–2390

Chen YK, Hsieh DS, Liao CS, Bai CH, Su CT, Shen YY, Hsieh JF, Liao AC, Kao CH (2005b) Utility of FDG-PET for investigating unexplained serum AFP elevation in patients with suspected hepatocellular carcinoma recurrence. Anticancer Res 25(6C):4719–4725

Choi H, Charnsangavej C, de Castro Faria S, Tamm EP, Benjamin RS, Johnson MM, Macapinlac HA, Podoloff DA (2004) CT evaluation of the response of gastrointestinal stromal tumors after imatinib mesylate treatment: a quantitative analysis correlated with FDG PET findings. Am J Roentgenol 183(6):1619–1628

Chua SC, Groves AM, Kayani I, Menezes L, Gacinovic S, Du Y, Bomanji JB, Ell PJ (2007) The impact of 18F-FDG PET/CT in patients with liver metastases. Eur J Nucl Med Mol Imaging 34(12):1906–1914

Corless CL, Fletcher JA, Heinrich MC (2004) Biology of gastrointestinal stromal tumors. J Clin Oncol 22(18): 3813–3825

Corvera CU, Blumgart LH, Akhurst T, DeMatteo RP, D'Angelica M, Fong Y, Jarnagin WR (2008) 18F-fluorodeoxyglucose positron emission tomography influences management decisions in patients with biliary cancer. J Am Coll Surg 206(1):57–65

Dalah E, Bradley D, Nisbet A (2010) Simulation of tissue activity curves of (64)Cu-ATSM for sub-target volume delineation in radiotherapy. Phys Med Biol 55(3):681–694

Davey K, Heriot AG, Mackay J, Drummond E, Hogg A, Ngan S, Milner AD, Hicks RJ (2008) The impact of 18-fluorodeoxyglucose positron emission tomography-computed tomography on the staging and management of primary rectal cancer. Dis Colon Rectum 51(7): 997–1003

de Geus-Oei LF, van Laarhoven HW, Visser EP, Hermsen R, van Hoorn BA, Kamm YJ, Krabbe PF, Corstens FH, Punt CJ, Oyen WJ (2008) Chemotherapy response evaluation with FDG-PET in patients with colorectal cancer. Ann Oncol 19(2):348–352

de Geus-Oei LF, Vriens D, van Laarhoven HW, van der Graaf WT, Oyen, WJ (2009) Monitoring and predicting response to therapy with 18F-FDG PET in colorectal cancer: a systematic review. J Nucl Med 50 (Suppl 1): 43S–54S

Flamen P, Hoekstra OS, Homans F, Van Cutsem E, Maes A, Stroobants S, Peeters M, Penninckx F, Filez L, Bleichrodt RP, Mortelmans L (2001) Unexplained rising carcinoembryonic antigen (CEA) in the postoperative surveillance of colorectal cancer: the utility of positron emission tomography (PET). Eur J Cancer 37(7):862–869

Floriani I, Torri V, Rulli E, Garavaglia D, Compagnoni A, Salvolini L, Giovagnoni A (2010) Performance of imaging modalities in diagnosis of liver metastases from colorectal cancer: a systematic review and meta-analysis. J Magn Reson Imaging 31(1):19–31

Furukawa H, Ikuma H, Seki A, Yokoe K, Yuen S, Aramaki T, Yamagushi S (2006) Positron emission tomography scanning is not superior to whole body multidetector helical computed tomography in the preoperative staging of colorectal cancer. Gut 55(7):1007–1111

Gabriel M, Decristoforo C, Kendler D, Dobrozemsky G, Heute D, Uprimny C, Kovacs P, Von Guggenberg E, Bale R, Virgolini IJ (2007) 68Ga-DOTA-Tyr3-octreotide PET in neuroendocrine tumors: comparison with somatostatin receptor scintigraphy and CT. J Nucl Med 48(4):508–518

Garin E, Le Jeune F, Devillers A, Cuggia M, de Lajarte-Thirouard AS, Bouriel C, Boucher E, Raoul JL (2009) Predictive value of 18F-FDG PET and somatostatin receptor scintigraphy in patients with metastatic endocrine tumors. J Nucl Med 50(6):858–864

Gearhart SL, Frassica D, Rosen R, Choti M, Schulick R, Wahl R (2006) Improved staging with pretreatment positron emission tomography/computed tomography in low rectal cancer. Ann Surg Oncol 13(3):397–404

Goerres GW, Stupp R, Barghouth G, Hany TF, Pestalozzi B, Dizendorf E, Schnyder P, Luthi F, von Schulthess GK, Leyvraz S (2005) The value of PET, CT and in-line PET/CT in patients with gastrointestinal stromal tumours: long-term outcome of treatment with imatinib mesylate. Eur J Nucl Med Mol Imaging 32(2):153–162

Han AR, Gwak GY, Choi MS, Lee JH, Koh KC, Paik SW, Yoo BC (2009) The clinical value of 18F-FDG PET/CT for investigating unexplained serum AFP elevation following interventional therapy for hepatocellular carcinom. Hepatogastroenterology 56(93):1111–1116

Haug A, Auernhammer CJ, Wangler B, Tiling R, Schmidt G, Goke B, Bartenstein P, Popperl G (2009) Intraindividual comparison of 68Ga-DOTA-TATE and 18F-DOPA PET in patients with well-differentiated metastatic neuroendocrine tumours. Eur J Nucl Med Mol Imaging 36(5):765–770

Heinrich S, Goerres GW, Schafer M, Sagmeister M, Bauerfeind P, Pestalozzi BC, Hany TF, von Schulthess GK, Clavien PA (2005) Positron emission tomography/computed tomography influences on the management of resectable pancreatic cancer and its cost-effectiveness. Ann Surg 242(2):235–243

Herrmann K, Ott K, Buck AK, Lordick F, Wilhelm D, Souvatzoglou M, Becker K, Schuster T, Wester HJ, Siewert JR, Schwaiger M, Krause BJ (2007) Imaging gastric cancer with PET and the radiotracers 18F-FLT and 18F-FDG: a comparative analysis. J Nucl Med 48(12):1945–1950

Higashi T, Hatano E, Ikai I, Nishii R, Nakamoto Y, Ishizu K, Suga T, Kawashima H, Togashi K, Seo S, Kitamura K, Takada Y, Kamimoto S (2010) FDG PET as a prognostic predictor in the early post-therapeutic evaluation for unresectable hepatocellular carcinoma. Eur J Nucl Med Mol Imaging 37(3):468–482

Jager PL, Gietema JA, van der Graaf WT (2004) Imatinib mesylate for the treatment of gastrointestinal stromal tumours: best monitored with FDG PET. Nucl Med Commun 25(5):433–438

Kameyama R, Yamamoto Y, Izuishi K, Takebayashi R, Hagiike M, Murota M, Kaji M, Haba R, Nishiyama Y (2009) Detection of gastric cancer using 18F-FLT PET: comparison with 18F-FDG PET. Eur J Nucl Med Mol Imaging 36(3):382–388

Kato H, Kimura H, Nakajima M, Sakai M, Sano A, Tanaka N, Inose T, Faried A, Saito K, Ieta K, Sohda M, Fukai Y, Miyazaki T, Masuda N, Fukuchi M, Ojima H, Tsukada K, Oriuchi N, Endo K, Kuwano H (2008) The additional value of integrated PET/CT over PET in initial lymph node staging of esophageal cancer. Oncol Rep 20(4): 857–862

Kato H, Miyazaki T, Nakajima M, Takita J, Kimura H, Faried A, Sohda M, Fukai Y, Masuda N, Fukuchi M, Manda R, Ojima H, Tsukada K, Kuwano H, Oriuchi N, Endo K (2005) The incremental effect of positron emission tomography on diagnostic accuracy in the initial staging of esophageal carcinoma. Cancer 103(1):148–156

Kato T, Tsukamoto E, Kuge Y, Katoh C, Nambu T, Nobuta A, Kondo S, Asaka M, Tamaki N (2002) Clinical role of (18) F-FDG PET for initial staging of patients with extrahepatic bile duct cancer. Eur J Nucl Med Mol Imaging 29(8):1047–1054

Kawaoka T, Aikata H, Takaki S, Uka K, Azakami T, Saneto H, Jeong SC, Kawakami Y, Takahashi S, Toyota N, Ito K, Hirokawa Y, Chayama K (2009) FDG positron emission tomography/computed tomography for the detection of extrahepatic metastases from hepatocellular carcinoma. Hepatol Res 39(2):134–142

Keswani RN, Early DS, Edmundowicz SA, Meyers BF, Sharma A, Govindan R, Chen J, Kohlmeier C, Azar RR (2009) Routine positron emission tomography does not alter nodal staging in patients undergoing EUS-guided FNA for esophageal cancer. Gastrointest Endosc 69(7):1210–1217

Kinkel K, Lu Y, Both M, Warren RS, Thoeni RF (2002) Detection of hepatic metastases from cancers of the gastrointestinal tract by using noninvasive imaging methods (US, CT, MR imaging, PET): a meta-analysis. Radiology 224(3):748–756

Kinner S, Antoch G, Bockisch A, Veit-Haibach P (2007) Whole-body PET/CT-colonography: a possible new concept for colorectal cancer staging. Abdom Imaging 32(5): 606–612

Kong G, Jackson C, Koh DM, Lewington V, Sharma B, Brown G, Cunningham D, Cook GJ (2008) The use of 18F-FDG PET/CT in colorectal liver metastases–comparison with CT and liver MRI. Eur J Nucl Med Mol Imaging 35(7):1323–1329

Kornberg A, Kupper B, Thrum K, Katenkamp K, Steenbeck J, Sappler A, Habrecht O, Gottschild D (2009) Increased 18F-FDG uptake of hepatocellular carcinoma on positron emission tomography independently predicts tumor recurrence in liver transplant patients. Transplant Proc 41(6):2561–2563

Krause BJ, Herrmann K, Wieder H, zum Buschenfelde CM (2009) 18F-FDG PET and 18F-FDG PET/CT for assessing response to therapy in esophageal cancer. J Nucl Med 50 (Suppl 1):89S–96S

Kuehl H, Antoch G, Stergar H, Veit-Haibach P, Rosenbaum-Krumme S, Vogt F, Frilling A, Barkhausen J, Bockisch A (2008) Comparison of FDG-PET, PET/CT and MRI for follow-up of colorectal liver metastases treated with radiofrequency ablation: initial results. Eur J Radiol 67(2): 362–371

Kwekkeboom DJ, Kam BL, van Essen M, Teunissen JJ, van Eijck CH, Valkema R, de Jong M, de Herder WW, Krenning EP (2010) Somatostatin receptor-based imaging and therapy of gastroenteropancreatic neuroendocrine tumors. Endocr Relat Cancer 17(1):R53–73

Lee JD, Yun M, Lee JM, Choi Y, Choi YH, Kim JS, Kim SJ, Kim KS, Yang WI, Park YN, Han KH, Lee WJ, Yoo N, Lim SM, Park JH (2004) Analysis of gene expression profiles of hepatocellular carcinomas with regard to 18F-fluorodeoxyglucose uptake pattern on positron emission tomography. Eur J Nucl Med Mol Imaging 31(12): 1621–1630

Lee JW, Paeng JC, Kang KW, Kwon HW, Suh KS, Chung JK, Lee MC, Lee DS (2009) Prediction of tumor recurrence by 18F-FDG PET in liver transplantation for hepatocellular carcinoma. J Nucl Med 50(5):682–7

Lin M, Shon IH, Wilson R, D'Amours SK, Schlaphoff G, Lin P (2007) Treatment response in liver metastases following 90Y SIR-spheres: an evaluation with PET. Hepatogastroenterology 54(75):910–912

Llamas-Elvira JM, Rodriguez-Fernandez A, Gutierrez-Sainz J, Gomez-Rio M, Bellon-Guardia M, Ramos-Font C, Rebollo-Aguirre AC, Cabello-Garcia D, Ferron-Orihuela A (2007) Fluorine-18 fluorodeoxyglucose PET in the preoperative staging of colorectal cancer. Eur J Nucl Med Mol Imaging 34(6):859–867

Lordick F, Ott K, Krause BJ, Weber WA, Becker K, Stein HJ, Lorenzen S, Schuster T, Wieder H, Herrmann K, Bredenkamp R, Hofler H, Fink U, Peschel C, Schwaiger M, Siewert JR (2007) PET to assess early metabolic response and to guide treatment of adenocarcinoma of the oesophagogastric junction: the MUNICON phase II trial. Lancet Oncol 8(9):797–805

Mabille M, Vanel D, Albiter M, Le Cesne A, Bonvalot S, Le Pechoux C, Terrier P, Shapeero LG, Dromain C (2009) Follow-up of hepatic and peritoneal metastases of gastrointestinal tumors (GIST) under Imatinib therapy requires different criteria of radiological evaluation (size is not everything!!!). Eur J Radiol 69(2):204–208

Mees G, Dierckx R, Vangestel C, Van de Wiele C (2009) Molecular imaging of hypoxia with radiolabelled agents. Eur J Nucl Med Mol Imaging 36(10):1674–1686

Meyers BF, Downey RJ, Decker PA, Keenan RJ, Siegel BA, Cerfolio RJ, Landreneau RJ, Reed CE, Balfe DM, Dehdashti F, Ballman KV, Rusch VW, Putnam JB Jr (2007) The utility of positron emission tomography in staging of potentially operable carcinoma of the thoracic esophagus: results of the American College of Surgeons Oncology Group Z0060 trial. J Thorac Cardiovasc Surg 133(3):738–745

Miettinen M, Lasota J (2001) Gastrointestinal stromal tumors–definition, clinical, histological, immunohistochemical, and molecular genetic features and differential diagnosis. Virchows Arch 438(1):1–12

Nagata K, Ota Y, Okawa T, Endo S, Kudo SE (2008) PET/CT colonography for the preoperative evaluation of the colon proximal to the obstructive colorectal cancer. Dis Colon Rectum 51(6):882–890

Okada M, Murakami T, Kumano S, Kuwabara M, Shimono T, Hosono M, Shiozaki H (2009) Integrated FDG-PET/CT compared with intravenous contrast-enhanced CT for evaluation of metastatic regional lymph nodes in patients with resectable early stage esophageal cancer. Ann Nucl Med 23(1):73–80

Orlando LA, Kulasingam SL, Matchar DB (2004) Meta-analysis: the detection of pancreatic malignancy with positron emission tomography. Aliment Pharmacol Ther 20(10):1063–1070

Pan L, Gu P, Huang G, Xue H, Wu S (2009) Prognostic significance of SUV on PET/CT in patients with esophageal cancer: a systematic review and meta-analysis. Eur J Gastroenterol Hepatol 21(9):1008–1015

Park JW, Kim JH, Kim SK, Kang KW, Park KW, Choi JI, Lee WJ, Kim CM, Nam BH (2008) A prospective evaluation of 18F-FDG and 11C-acetate PET/CT for detection of primary and metastatic hepatocellular carcinoma. J Nucl Med 49(12):1912–1921

Pasquali C, Rubello D, Sperti C, Gasparoni P, Liessi G, Chierichetti F, Ferlin G, Pedrazzoli S (1998) Neuroendocrine tumor imaging: can 18F-fluorodeoxyglucose positron emission tomography detect tumors with poor prognosis and aggressive behavior? World J Surg 22(6):588–592

Petrowsky H, Wildbrett P, Husarik DB, Hany TF, Tam S, Jochum W, Clavien PA (2006) Impact of integrated positron emission tomography and computed tomography on staging and management of gallbladder cancer and cholangiocarcinoma. J Hepatol 45(1):43–50

Pfannenberg AC, Aschoff P, Brechtel K, Muller M, Klein M, Bares R, Claussen CD, Eschmann SM (2007) Value of contrast-enhanced multiphase CT in combined PET/CT protocols for oncological imaging. Br J Radiol 80(954):437–445

Putzer D, Gabriel M, Kendler D, Henninger B, Knoflach M, Kroiss A, Vonguggenberg E, Warwitz B, Virgolini IJ (2010) Comparison of 68Ga-DOTA-Tyr3-octreotide and 18F-fluoro-L-dihydroxyphenylalanine positron emission tomography in neuroendocrine tumor patients. Q J Nucl Med Mol Imaging 54(1):68–75

Rodriguez-Moranta F, Salo J, Arcusa A, Boadas J, Pinol V, Bessa X, Batiste-Alentorn E, Lacy AM, Delgado S, Maurel J, Pique JM, Castells A (2006) Postoperative surveillance in patients with colorectal cancer who have undergone curative resection: a prospective, multicenter, randomized, controlled trial. J Clin Oncol 24(3):386–393

Roedl JB, Halpern EF, Colen RR, Sahani DV, Fischman AJ, Blake MA (2009) Metabolic tumor width parameters as determined on PET/CT predict disease-free survival and treatment response in squamous cell carcinoma of the esophagus. Mol Imaging Biol 11(1):54–60

Ruers TJ, Wiering B, van der Sijp JR, Roumen RM, de Jong KP, Comans EF, Pruim J, Dekker HM, Krabbe PF, Oyen WJ (2009) Improved selection of patients for hepatic surgery of colorectal liver metastases with (18)F-FDG PET: a randomized study. J Nucl Med 50(7):1036–1041

Schnell O, Krebs B, Carlsen J, Miederer I, Goetz C, Goldbrunner RH, Wester HJ, Haubner R, Popperl G, Holtmannspotter M, Kretzschmar HA, Kessler H, Tonn JC, Schwaiger M, Beer AJ (2009) Imaging of integrin alpha(v)beta(3) expression in patients with malignant glioma by [18F] Galacto-RGD positron emission tomography. Neuro Oncol 11(6):861–870

Schottelius M, Laufer B, Kessler H, Wester HJ (2009) Ligands for mapping alphavbeta3-integrin expression in vivo. Acc Chem Res 42(7):969–980

Seo S, Hatano E, Higashi T, Hara T, Tada M, Tamaki N, Iwaisako K, Ikai I, Uemoto S (2007) Fluorine-18 fluorodeoxyglucose positron emission tomography predicts tumor differentiation, P-glycoprotein expression, and outcome after resection in hepatocellular carcinoma. Clin Cancer Res 13(2 Pt 1):427–433

Shiomi S, Nishiguchi S, Ishizu H, Iwata Y, Sasaki N, Tamori A, Habu D, Takeda T, Kubo S, Ochi H (2001) Usefulness of positron emission tomography with fluorine-18-fluorodeoxyglucose for predicting outcome in patients with hepatocellular carcinoma. Am J Gastroenterol 96(6):1877–1880

Shreve PD (1998) Focal fluorine-18 fluorodeoxyglucose accumulation in inflammatory pancreatic disease. Eur J Nucl Med 25(3):259–264

Sobhani I, Tiret E, Lebtahi R, Aparicio T, Itti E, Montravers F, Vaylet C, Rougier P, Andre T, Gornet JM, Cherqui D, Delbaldo C, Panis Y, Talbot JN, Meignan M, Le Guludec D (2008) Early detection of recurrence by 18FDG-PET in the follow-up of patients with colorectal cancer. Br J Cancer 98(5):875–880

Sorensen N, Jensen A, Wille-Jorgensen P, Friberg L, Rordam L, Ingeman L, Hennild V (2010) Strict follow-up programme including CT and F-FDG-PET after curative surgery for colorectal cancer. Colorectal Dis 12(10):e224–e228

Soyka JD, Veit-Haibach P, Strobel K, Breitenstein S, Tschopp A, Mende KA, Lago MP, Hany TF (2008) Staging pathways in recurrent colorectal carcinoma: is contrast-enhanced 18F-FDG PET/CT the diagnostic tool of choice? J Nucl Med 49(3):354–361

Stahl A, Ott K, Weber WA, Becker K, Link T, Siewert JR, Schwaiger M, Fink U (2003) FDG PET imaging of locally advanced gastric carcinomas: correlation with endoscopic and histopathological findings. Eur J Nucl Med Mol Imaging 30(2):288–295

Strobel K, Heinrich S, Bhure U, Soyka J, Veit-Haibach P, Pestalozzi BC, Clavien PA, Hany TF (2008) Contrast-enhanced 18F-FDG PET/CT: 1-stop-shop imaging for assessing the resectability of pancreatic cancer. J Nucl Med 49(9):1408–1413

Stroobants S, Goeminne J, Seegers M, Dimitrijevic S, Dupont P, Nuyts J, Martens M, van den Borne B, Cole P, Sciot R, Dumez H, Silberman S, Mortelmans L, van Oosterom A (2003) 18FDG-Positron emission tomography for the early prediction of response in advanced soft tissue sarcoma treated with imatinib mesylate (Glivec). Eur J Cancer 39(14):2012–2020

Tang S, Huang G, Liu J, Liu T, Treven L, Song S, Zhang C, Pan L, Zhang T (2009) Usefulness of (18)F-FDG PET, combined

FDG-PET/CT and EUS in diagnosing primary pancreatic carcinoma: A meta-analysis. Eur J Radiol

Taylor MD, Smith PW, Brix WK, Wick MR, Theodosakis N, Swenson BR, Kozower BD, Jones DR (2009) Correlations between selected tumor markers and fluorodeoxyglucose maximal standardized uptake values in esophageal cancer. Eur J Cardiothorac Surg 35(4):699–705

Van Cutsem EJ, Oliveira J (2008) Colon cancer: ESMO clinical recommendations for diagnosis, adjuvant treatment and follow-up. Ann Oncol 19 (Suppl 2):ii29–30

Van den Abbeele AD (2008) The lessons of GIST–PET and PET/CT: a new paradigm for imaging. Oncologist 13 (Suppl 2):8–13

van Westreenen HL, Westerterp M, Bossuyt PM, Pruim J, Sloof GW, van Lanschot JJ, Groen H, Plukker JT (2004) Systematic review of the staging performance of 18F-fluorodeoxyglucose positron emission tomography in esophageal cancer. J Clin Oncol 22(18):3805–3812

Veit-Haibach P, Kuehle CA, Beyer T, Stergar H, Kuehl H, Schmidt J, Borsch G, Dahmen G, Barkhausen J, Bockisch A, Antoch G (2006) Diagnostic accuracy of colorectal cancer staging with whole-body PET/CT colonography. JAMA 296(21):2590–2600

Wiering B, Krabbe PF, Jager GJ, Oyen WJ, Ruers TJ (2005) The impact of fluor-18-deoxyglucose-positron emission tomography in the management of colorectal liver metastases. Cancer 104(12):2658–2670

Yun M, Lim JS, Noh SH, Hyung WJ, Cheong JH, Bong JK, Cho A, Lee JD (2005) Lymph node staging of gastric cancer using (18)F-FDG PET: a comparison study with CT. J Nucl Med 46(10):1582–1588

Zhang C, Chen Y, Xue H, Zheng P, Tong J, Liu J, Sun X, Huang G (2009) Diagnostic value of FDG-PET in recurrent colorectal carcinoma: a meta-analysis. Int J Cancer 124(1):167–173

Zhernosekov KP, Filosofov DV, Baum RP, Aschoff P, Bihl H, Razbash AA, Jahn M, Jennewein M, Rosch F (2007) Processing of generator-produced 68Ga for medical application. J Nucl Med 48(10):1741–1748

Genitourinary

Jacqueline Brunetti and Patrick J. Peller

Contents

J. Brunetti (✉)
Department of Radiology,
Holy Name Medical Center,
718 Teaneck Road,
Teaneck, NJ 07666, USA
e-mail: brunetti@mail.holyname.org

P. J. Peller
Department of Radiology,
Mayo Clinic, 200, 1st Street, SW,
Rochester, MN 55905, USA

Abstract

The utility of FDG PET/CT in malignancies of the genitourinary tract varies significantly with tumor type, stage, and location. To best implement FDG PET/CT into the clinical care of patients with urologic malignancies, it is critical to understand the differences in tumor metabolism at diagnosis as well as the changes in advanced disease. With increasing economic restrictions in healthcare, it is critical for the nuclear physician to have a clear understanding of what modalities can provide the most accurate information for best therapy choice. GU tract cancers differ in glycolytic activity and therefore the indications for FDG PET/CT are specific to each tumor type. Within this category of neoplasm, FDG PET/CT is best suited to restaging and problem solving. 18F-fluoride PET/CT and non-commercially available positron choline analogs provide improved accuracy in restaging select patients with treated prostate cancer.

1 Key Points

Genitourinary malignancies account for about 25% of all cancers in the US each year. FDG uptake in genitourinary cancers is quite variable, both within and between the different histologic types. FDG PET has a limited role in diagnosis and staging of most genitourinary cancers. Detection of malignancy in the genitourinary tract can be hampered by FDG excretion in the urine. The clinical utility of FDG PET/CT is primarily in restaging genitourinary cancers. Problem solving with PET/CT is employed when other imaging

P. Peller et al. (eds.), *PET-CT and PET-MRI in Oncology*, Medical Radiology. Diagnostic Imaging,
DOI: 10.1007/174_2012_604,

studies are equivocal and especially in discriminating postradiation or postsurgical changes from metastasis. Physicians interpreting PET/CT scans must be alert for genitourinary malignancies only visible on the CT component of the examination and incidental FDG-avid tumors. Although this chapter emphasizes the applications of FDG PET/CT, a growing body of published data is demonstrating that radiolabeled choline PET/CT is quite useful in identifying recurrent and metastatic prostate cancer.

2 Introduction

Evolving trends in cancer management utilizing molecular targeted therapies, minimally invasive surgical and interventional techniques and focused radiotherapy require highly accurate staging and tumor surveillance methods. For many cancers, FDG PET/CT has been shown to provide improved accuracy over conventional anatomic cross-sectional imaging. As a result of the National Oncologic PET Registry (NOPR), there is increasing published data on the utility of PET/CT in previously nonreimbursed diagnostic categories. Prostate, bladder, and renal malignancies were among the top 10 cancer indications for PET imaging under NOPR guidelines. (Hillner et al. 2008) Consequently, as a result of collated data, urologic tumors, except for prostate cancer (PCA), are now covered under initial treatment strategy, but all subsequent PET/CT scans still require enrollment in the NOPR. Continuing research and development of other positron agents that target other cellular processes including cellular membrane synthesis, proliferation, acetate, choline, and potentially other agents that target hypoxia or endothelial growth factors, may further improve imaging in this patient population.

3 Renal Cell Cancer

3.1 Diagnosis

Eighty-five percent of renal cell malignancies are of the adenocarcinoma cell type, with transitional cell carcinoma comprising most of the remainder (National Cancer Institute statistics). As a result of the increasing use of cross-sectional imaging and the improved resolution of these modalities, renal cell adenocarcinoma is frequently an incidental finding. The National Cancer Data Base reports that in 2006, 48.5% of all renal cancers were diagnosed at Stage I.

There is little data to support the use of FDG PET in renal cell carcinoma diagnosis. Early reports suggested value for differentiating benign from malignant renal cortical lesions (Goldberg et al. 1997) (Fig. 1). This is not supported by published data of other authors. Ramdave et al. (2001) in a series of 25 patients with biopsy-confirmed renal carcinoma describe uptake patterns that include photopenia, isometabolic, and hypermetabolic uptake in tumors greater than 2 cm in size. Kang et al. (2004) reports a sensitivity of only 60% in detection of primary renal cell carcinomas. Detection of primary renal cell cancer is hampered by renal excretion of FDG, lesion size, and the presence of cystic or necrotic components and variable uptake of FDG (Figs. 2, 3 and 4). Expression of GLUT 1 transporter is not uniformly increased in RCC and therefore FDG lesion uptake is variable. Miyakita et al. (2002) report increased FDG uptake in only 31.5% of patients with histologically confirmed RCC. Despite the limitations, it is worthwhile to carefully evaluate PET/CT fusion images with respect to the distribution of FDG as incidental cancers may be found (Osman et al. 2005). An interesting potential role for FDG PET has been suggested by Sun et al. (2009) as a method for detecting renal malignancy in patients with end-stage renal disease. Although the reported sensitivity was only 67%, positive predictive value was 90% and the modality might be helpful in this group of patients in whom imaging is frequently difficult. Continuing technical improvements in PET/CT including gains in resolution, utilization of gated acquisition, and contrast-enhanced PET/CT techniques may result in improved lesion detection. As it is accepted routine to monitor incidental small renal masses, new generation PET/CT might provide a non-invasive method of characterizing these slow growing lesions.

3.2 Metastatic Disease

The probability of synchronous metastasis at the time of diagnosis of renal cell carcinoma is directly related to tumor size, and the incidence rises dramatically in

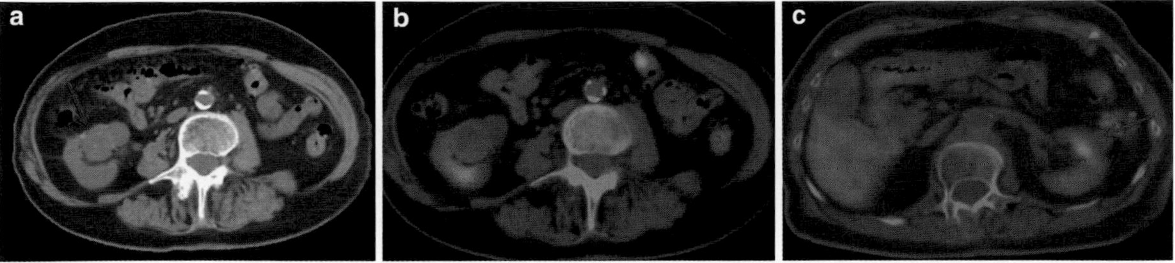

Fig. 1 An 85-year-old woman with renal cell carcinoma in the lower pole of the right kidney and a cyst in the upper pole of the left kidney. Images include a non-contrast axial CT image (**a**) and an axial fused PET/CT image (**b**) and axial fused PET/CT image of the left renal lesion. The metabolic activity in the solid component of the right renal lesion (*arrow*) is less that normal renal cortical activity. There is no uptake in the more medial cystic component. A cortical lesion in the left kidney (*arrow*) of the same patient displays no activity on PET/CT (**c**) and is confirmed as an anechoic cyst on ultrasound

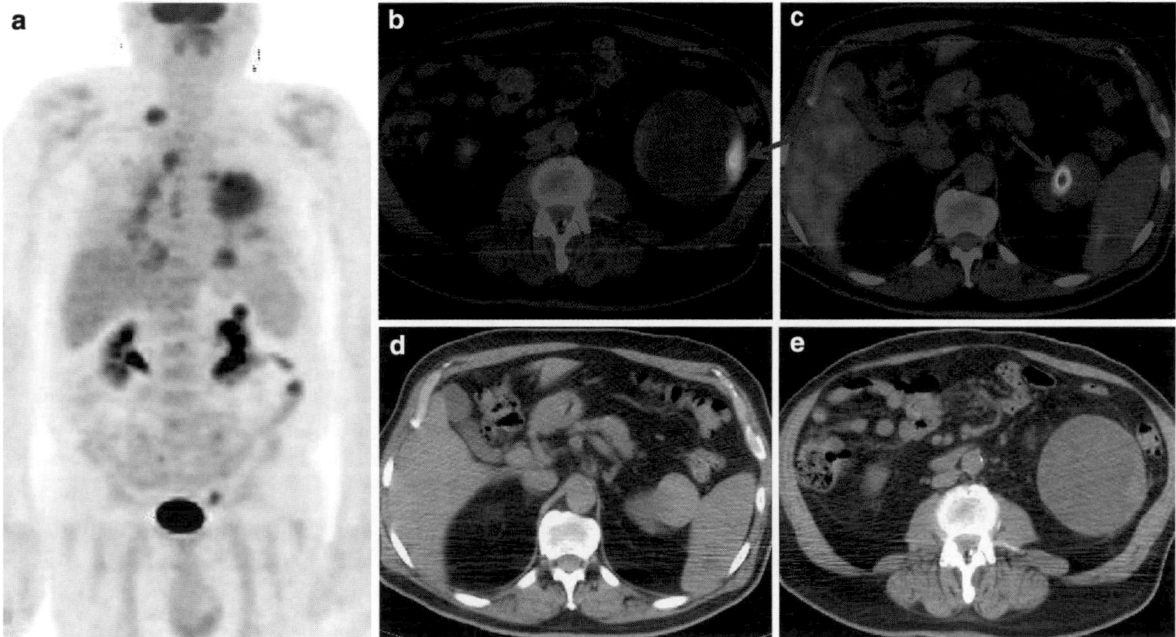

Fig. 2 A 75-year-old-man, imaged for initial staging of non-small cell lung cancer. Images include a MIP scan (**a**), axial fused PET/CT images (**b, c**) and axial non-contrast CT images (**d, e**). The MIP scan demonstrates extensive thoracic malignancy but also exophytic, metabolically active lesions in the upper and lower pole regions of the left kidney. Fused PET/CT images demonstrate intense metabolic activity only in the periphery of the left renal lesions (*arrows*), subsequently biopsy proven to be renal cell carcinomas

lesions greater than 4 cm in size. Ten to twenty percent of patients with organ-confined disease at diagnosis will develop metastases (Crispen et al. 2008). Most of the published data regarding the use of FDG PET in metastatic renal cell cancer report results of conventional PET and not PET/CT. Sensitivity in detection of metastasis ranges from 63.6 to 87% and therapy change as a result of PET findings occurs in 40 to 50% of patients (Majhail et al. 2003; Safaei et al. 2002). More recently, FDG PET/CT has been shown to be as accurate as conventional imaging in detection of metastatic disease (Fig. 5). Park et al. (2009) compared the results of PET/CT in 63 patients at high risk for recurrent renal cell cancer, and report

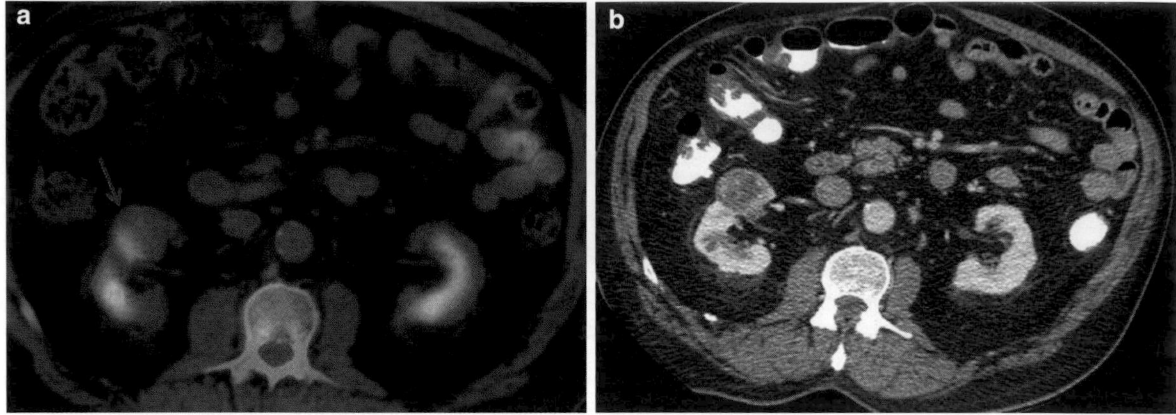

Fig. 3 A 66-year-old man with a right renal mass discovered on a CT scan performed for recurrent GI bleed. Images include axial fused PET/CT (**a**) and axial contrast-enhanced CT (**b**). Variable activity is demonstrated in the right renal mass (*arrow*) that does not appear to correspond to regional abnormalities on the CT, possibly induced by respiratory motion

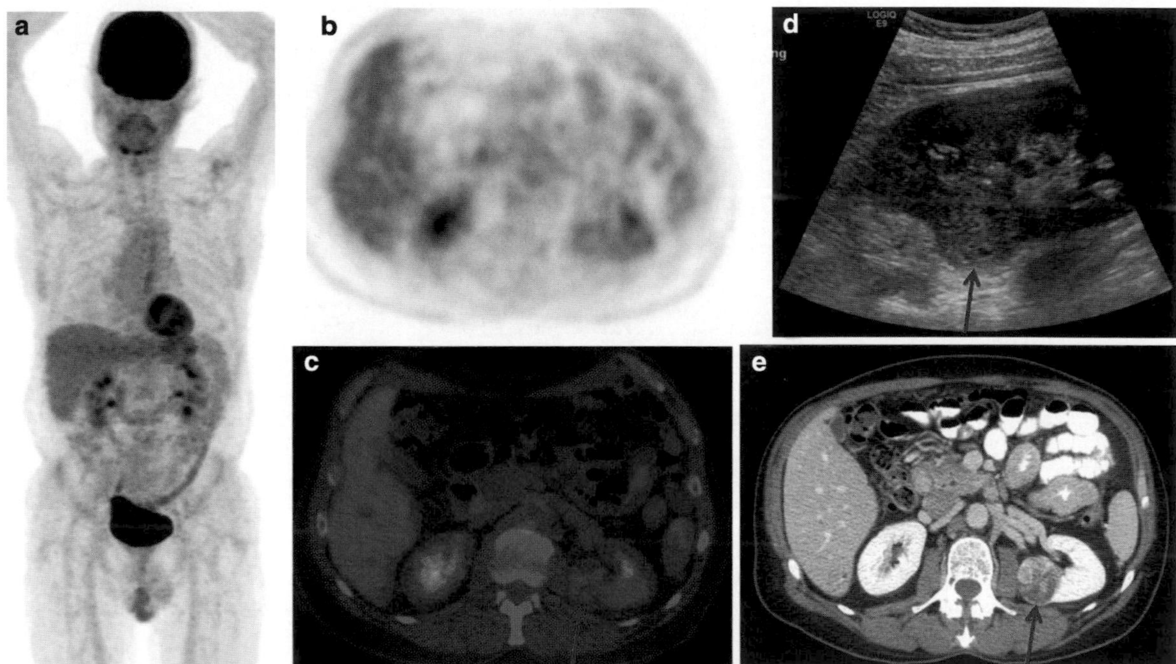

Fig. 4 A 61-year-old man with a history of a Clark level IV melanoma underwent a PET/CT (**a** MIP, **b** axial PET, **c** fused, **d** long axis left kidney US, **e** axial CT), which demonstrates an exophytic left renal mass with mild FDG uptake (*arrow*). Ultrasound demonstrates an isoechoic solid-appearing mass in the mid left kidney. Contrast-enhanced CT demonstrates heterogeneous enhancing mass in the medial left kidney. Surgical resection yielded a 4.1 cm grade 2 renal cell carcinoma

an accuracy of 85.7% for PET/CT in detection of lymph node or distant metastatic sites, with a sensitivity of 89.5%, specificity of 83.3%, positive predictive value of 77.3%, and negative predictive value of 92.6% (Fig. 6). The authors also suggest that the whole body capability of PET/CT allows imaging of all organs without the possible damaging effects of intravenous contrast.

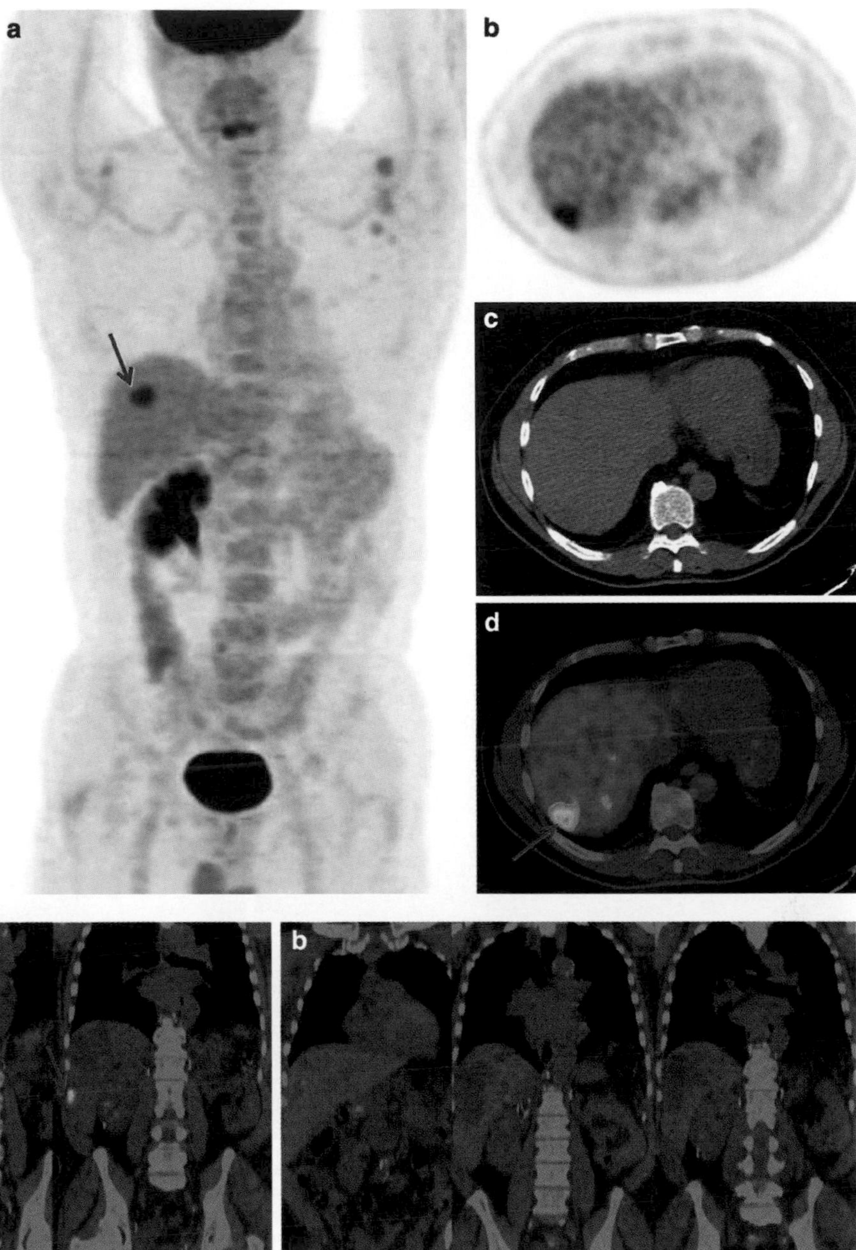

Fig. 5 A 48-year-old man with a history of left renal cell carcinoma presents for restaging PET/CT (**a** MIP, **b** axial PET, **c** axial CT, **d** axial fused). There is a 2.3 cm right hepatic mass with intense FDG uptake (*arrow*). The mildly hypermetabolic left axillary lymph nodes are noted and were found to be inflammatory. The wedge resection of the liver demonstrated a grade 3 renal cell carcinoma metastasis

Fig. 6 A 72-year-old man with papillary renal cell carcinoma metastasis to liver. Images include pretherapy coronal fused PET/CT (**a**) and postchemotherapy coronal fused PET/CT (**b**). Postchemotherapy PET/CT reveals a reduction in metabolic activity in the hepatic metastases

4 Urothelial Carcinomas

4.1 Diagnosis

Ninety percent of urothelial cancers originate in the bladder with the remaining 10% occurring in the renal pelvis and ureter. Transitional cell cancer is the most common histologic cell type, with squamous cell lesions occurring in the distal third of the ureters and accounting for 3% of urinary tumors. TCC is typically multifocal and recurrence rate after therapy is high. For bladder cancers, prognosis is dependent on depth of invasion, tumor grade, and presence of vascular or lymphatic invasion. Cystoscopy and biopsy determine cell type, grade,

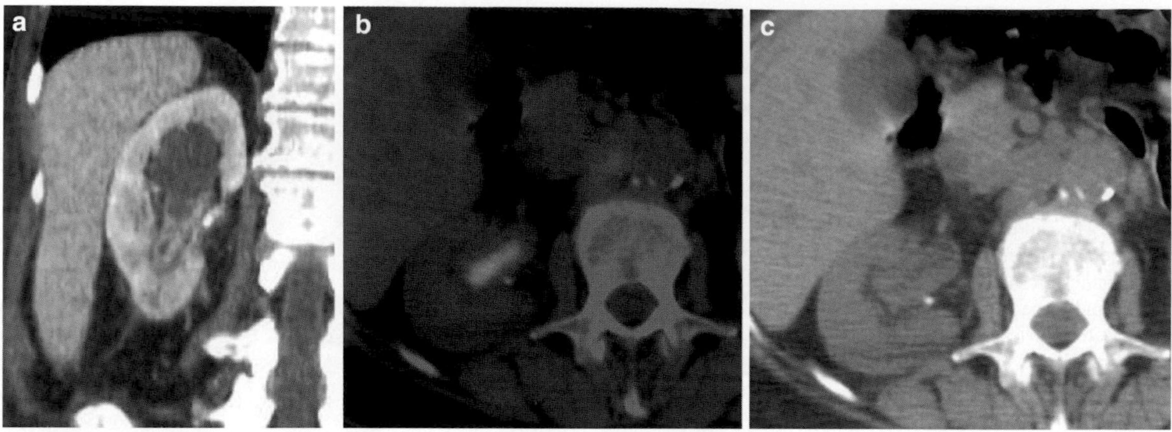

Fig. 7 A 71-year-old woman diagnosed with right renal TCC. Images include coronal contrast-enhanced CT (**a**), axial fused PET/CT (**b**) and axial non-contrast CT (**c**) of the right kidney. PET/CT image displays intense activity in the right renal collecting system that prevents detection of possible metabolic activity within the urothelial malignancy. There is, however, metabolic activity identified on PET/CT within a metastatic aorto-caval lymph node (*arrow*)

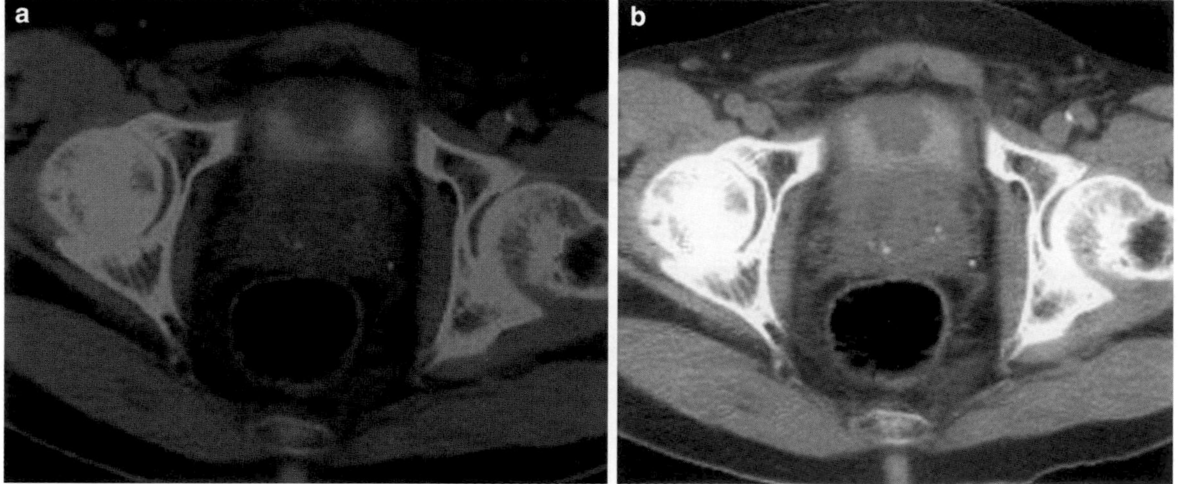

Fig. 8 A 67-year-old man has a low-grade papillary urothelial carcinoma. Images include axial fused PET/CT (**a**) and axial contrast-enhanced CT (**b**). The bladder malignancy displays no glycolytic activity and can be indentified only due to its size and with reduction of image intensity on the PET/CT image

and depth of invasion. Conventional imaging with CT or MRI provides gross assessment of the status of the perivesicular tissues, but is limited in specificity. Tumors of the renal pelvis and ureter are best imaged by excretory or retrograde urography or CT urography. CT urography provides superior imaging of the renal collecting system allowing assessment of the lumen, wall, periureteral soft tissues, and determination of nodal disease.

FDG PET is severely limited in detection of primary bladder cancers and lesions of the upper tracts as evaluation of the collecting system elements, bladder wall, periureteral, and perivesicular soft tissues is hampered by the urinary excretion of FDG (Figs. 7, 8). Several authors have suggested hydration and diuresis with delayed imaging to improve detection of primary and recurrent lesions (Anjos et al. 2007; Chen et al. 2009). The utility, however, of such methods is questionable.

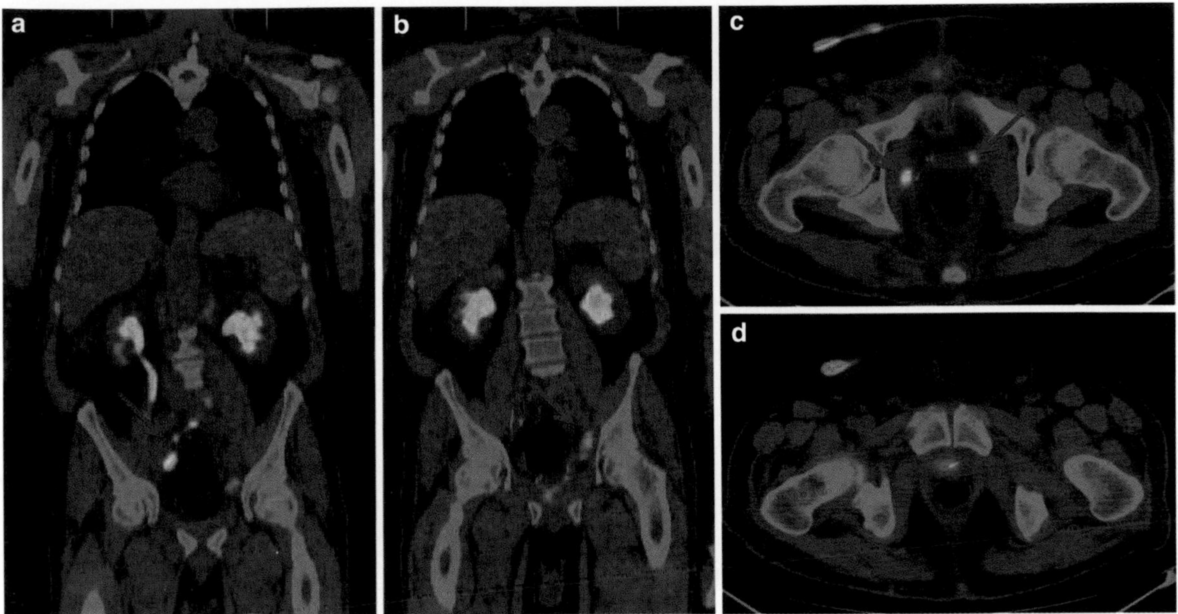

Fig. 9 A 78-year-old man with metastatic bladder cancer. PET/CT is performed for restaging prior to initiating chemotherapy. Images include coronal fused PET/CT (**a, b**) and axial fused PET/CT of the pelvis (**c, d**) Coronal images demonstrate extensive pelvic and retroperitoneal metastatic adenopathy (*arrows*). Axial images reveal foci of metastatic disease in the bladder bed (*arrows*)

4.2 Metastatic Disease

There is conflicting evidence concerning the utility of PET and PET/CT in detection of locoregional nodal metastatic disease at initial presentation of bladder cancer. Early reports utilizing conventional FDG PET indicated a poor sensitivity of 67% in detection of regional lymph node metastases and moderate specificity and accuracy of 86 and 80%, respectively (Bachor et al. 1999). More recent studies utilizing PET/CT demonstrate no significant gains in sensitivity and specificity over conventional PET or over CT alone (Drieskens et al. 2005; Kibel et al. 2009; Swinnen et al. 2009). However, there may be prognostic value in preoperative PET findings. Drieskens et al. compared pathology results with preoperative PET and CT findings in 55 patients with bladder cancer. For detection of nodal metastases, the sensitivity, specificity, and accuracy is reported to be 60, 88, and 78%, respectively. The median survival time in patients with PET-positive nodal disease was only 13.5 months compared to 32 months in those patients with PET-negative nodes. Similar findings are published by Kibel et al. (2009). The authors imaged 43 patients with negative CT and bone scintigraphy with PET/CT prior to cystectomy and lymphadenectomy. PET/CT findings were compared to surgical pathology results as well as survival. A sensitivity of 70% and specificity of 94% in detection of occult metastasis is reported. A positive PET/CT correlated with poorer disease-free and overall survival compared to patients with negative PET/CT.

There is scant data on the value of PET and PET/CT in detection of recurrent or residual disease in bladder cancer. (Fig. 9). Jadvar et al. (2008) published a series of 35 patients with treated bladder cancer who were imaged with PET and PET/CT. Unsuspected metastases were identified in 3 patients. In 1 patient, PET accurately excluded metastatic disease in a region of postradiation and postsurgical soft tissue density. In 17% of patients, PET/CT findings resulted in a management change.

5 Prostate

5.1 Diagnosis

Prostate cancer (PCA) has surpassed lung cancer as the most frequently diagnosed malignancy in men in the US, and this is likely the result of widespread use of screening with prostate specific antigen (PSA)

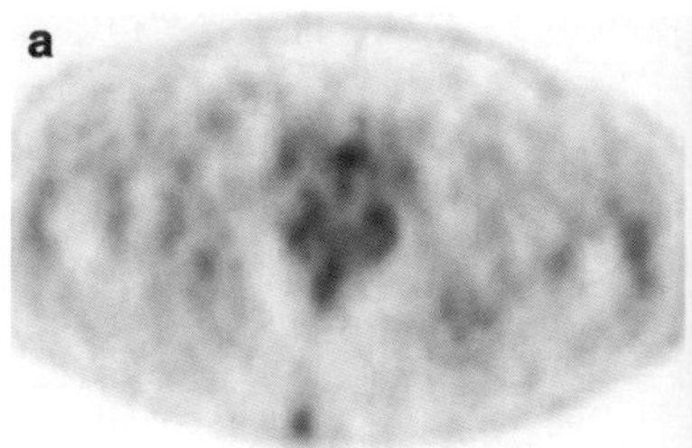

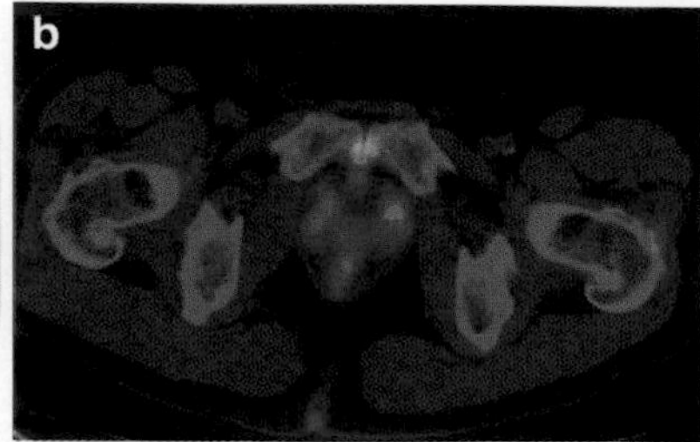

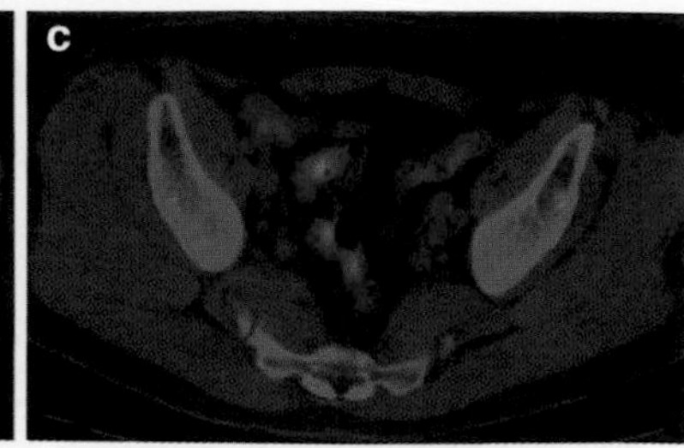

Fig. 10 A 68-year-old man with PCA, Gleason score 7, PSA 10.2. Images include axial PET (**a**) and axial fused FDG PET/CT of the prostate (**b**), and axial fused PET/CT of the pelvis (**c**). Low-level heterogeneous metabolic activity is present in the prostate gland. A metastatic left external iliac lymph node is negative on PET/CT

(American Cancer Society 2006). The success of PSA screening is reflected in the fact that PCAs are most frequently diagnosed while still organ-confined. PCA is a heterogeneous disease with variable aggressiveness and treatment decisions are based on multiple factors that include Gleason score, PSA level, stage, patient life expectancy, and comorbidites. Initial tumor staging is based on PSA level, digital rectal examination (DRE), multi-quadrant transrectal sonographic biopsy, and Gleason score. MRI is useful for determination of capsular and seminal vesicle involvement. MRI spectroscopy, diffusion imaging, nanoparticle contrast agents, and sonographic contrast agents are areas of continuing research.

FDG uptake in normal prostate parenchyma is low with SUV levels ranging from 1.1 to 3.7 (Jadvar et al. 2008). In PCA, overexpression of GLUT 1 transporters, as determined in vitro, is greater in hormone-resistant, poorly differentiated cell types than in well-differentiated, androgen-sensitive cell lines and this is reflected in higher FDG uptake in these cancers (Effert et al. 2004). Higher levels of GLUT 1 gene expression are found in PCA in comparison to benign prostatic hypertrophy and correlate with Gleason score and a hypoxia marker, lysyl oxidase (Stewart et al. 2008). It is not surprising therefore that higher FDG PET SUV values resulting from these altered cellular factors in primary PCA are associated with increasing aggressiveness and poorer prognosis (Oyama et al. 2002). There is, however, significant overlap in FDG uptake within normal prostate parenchyma, benign prostatic hypertrophy, and PCA, and therefore, there is no role for FDG PET in initial diagnosis (Figs. 10, 11), (Effert et al. 1996; Hofer et al. 1999; Liu et al. 2001). Proximity of the prostate to the intense activity in the urinary bladder, cited as a pitfall in PCA detection, is less an issue with PET/CT and new iterative reconstruction techniques as it was with conventional PET.

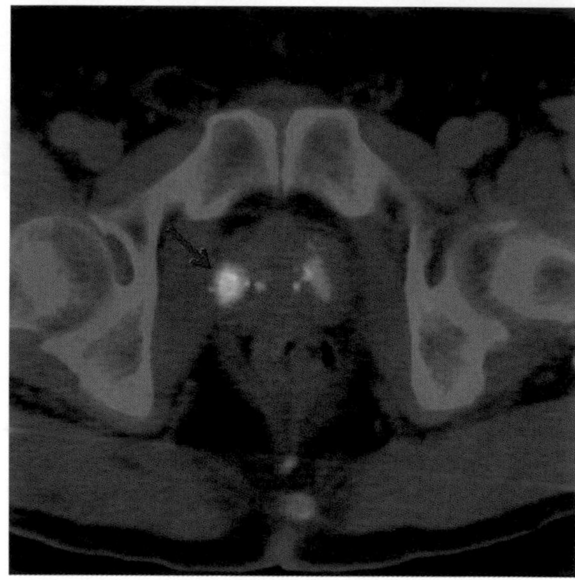

Fig. 11 Axial fused FDG PET/CT image of the prostate demonstrates foci of hypermetabolic activity in the peripheral zone of the gland (*arrow*). Biopsy, performed to investigate an elevated PSA revealed prostatitis and no evidence of neoplasm

5.2 Metastatic Disease

The incidence of metastatic disease at initial diagnosis of PCA is approximately 5% (SEER 2008). The accuracy of both CT and MRI in detection of pelvic nodal metastases is limited and pelvic lymphadenectomy remains the gold standard for determination of N stage. Recurrence following radical prostatectomy in patients with organ-confined, Gleason score of 6 or less is extremely low with recurrence rates of 0.5% (Hernandez et al. 2008). Despite radical prostatectomy, however, 15 to 40% of patients will develop tumor recurrence within 5 years (Han et al. 2001; Ward and Moul 2005). Some patients will suffer biochemical relapse, i.e., rising PSA level without anatomic imaging findings. As there are limited treatment options, i.e., salvage prostatectomy, radiotherapy, and chemical castration, it is critical that precise restaging strategies be employed. Bone metastases present additional dilemmas as findings on conventional bone scan do not accurately represent tumor activity. It is in these patient populations that improved imaging may significantly impact therapy decision making as a posttreatment rise in serum PSA can be due to local and/or distant metastasis. There is a subset of patients with "clinically insignificant" PCA, defined as Gleason score less than 8, less than 50% of biopsy positive for cancer and PSA below 10–15 ng/dl in whom treatment may be delayed until there is clinical evidence of progression. Active surveillance of these patients is accomplished by serial PSA and DRE but, there is currently no method to predetermine which patients are at higher risk and improved strategies to detect tumor progression may be beneficial in this group.

Early reports on the utility of FDG PET in detecting prostate metastatic disease provided conflicting data regarding sensitivity in detection that is at least in part the result of the heterogeneous nature of the disease (Shreve et al. 1996; Sanz et al. 1999; Heicappell et al. 1999). Despite the lack of supportive data, PCA was the most frequent cancer type imaged under the National Oncologic PET Guidelines (Hillner et al. 2008). Although, the higher number of PCAs submitted is a reflection of the high frequency of this disease, it is also an indication of a need for better determination of disease extent and activity. There is accumulating data that indicates that metastatic PCA displays genotypic and phenotypic variability from patient to patient but also within the same patient and novel molecular imaging agents may help to better stratify risk and therapy decisions. (Chou and Figg 2005). Several positron ligands have been proposed for imaging metastatic prostate cancer. These include C-11 and F-18 labeled choline and C-11 acetate, and of these F-18 fluorocholine, due to the possibility of commercial production, may be the most promising for detection of metastatic disease. (Oyama et al. 2003; Schmid et al. 2005; Giovacchini et al. 2008; Pelosi et al. 2008).

There is evidence, however, to support the use of FDG PET in selected patients with metastatic disease. Schoder et al. (2005), identified sites of recurrent tumor with FDG PET in 31% of a group of 91 patients with biochemical relapse. The likelihood of a positive FDG PET scan in this patient series increased with increasing serum PSA and PSA velocity. With a PSA of at least 2.4 ng/mL the sensitivity and specificity of FDG PET for metastatic tumor detection was 80 and 73% respectively. Using a PSA velocity of 1.3 ng/mL/y as an indicator of disease, a sensitivity of 71% and specificity of 77% was demonstrated. In this group, 21 patients had recurrent disease in the prostate bed. PET identified only 5 while 7 were detected by MRI, and in no instance was disease detected by CT. Chang et al. (2003) report FDG PET results in a group of 24 patients with PSA-relapse after treatment for localized PCA. All patients had negative bone scan and equivocal CT scan findings and all underwent pelvic lymphadenectomy. For the detection of pelvic lymph nodes, the sensitivity, specificity, and accuracy of FDG PET was 75, 83, and 100% respectively. FDG PET may provide improved lesion detection in patients with advanced PCA who demonstrate persistent detectable PSA or rising PSA despite therapy (Fig. 12), (Sung et al. 2003). As glucose metabolism has been shown to be modulated by androgens, FDG PET may provide a non-invasive measure of response to androgen therapy. (Jadvar et al. 2005).

Detection and assessment of biologic activity of bone metastases is an evolving area of research (Logothetis et al. 2008; Rentsch et al. 2009). It is increasingly apparent that FDG PET can discriminate between quiescent and progressive osseous metastases. Morris, et al. (2002) compared FDG PET, bone scan, CT, and MRI in 17 patients with rising PSA and conventional imaging findings of progressive disease. All bone lesions detected on FDG PET were proven to represent active disease on subsequent imaging. Furthermore, changes in SUV correlated with changes in PSA, suggesting a role

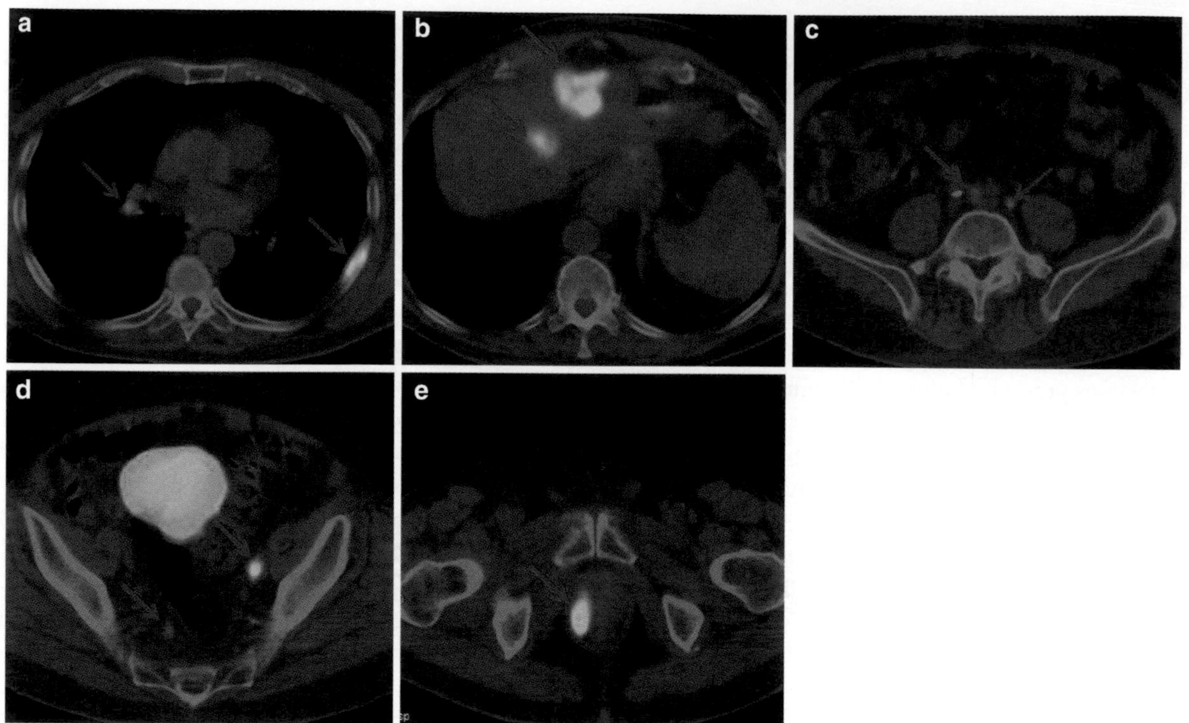

Fig. 12 An 85-year-old man with metastatic PCA, Gleason 9. Treated with hormone therapy in 2007–2008, with rising PSA, now 207 while on Nilandron. Images include axial fused FDG PET/CT of the thorax, (**a**), liver (**b**), retroperitoneum (**c**), pelvis (**d**), and prostate (**e**). Intense metabolic activity is evident in right hilar, rib, hepatic, and nodal metastases, as well as local tumor recurrence in the right neurovascular bundle

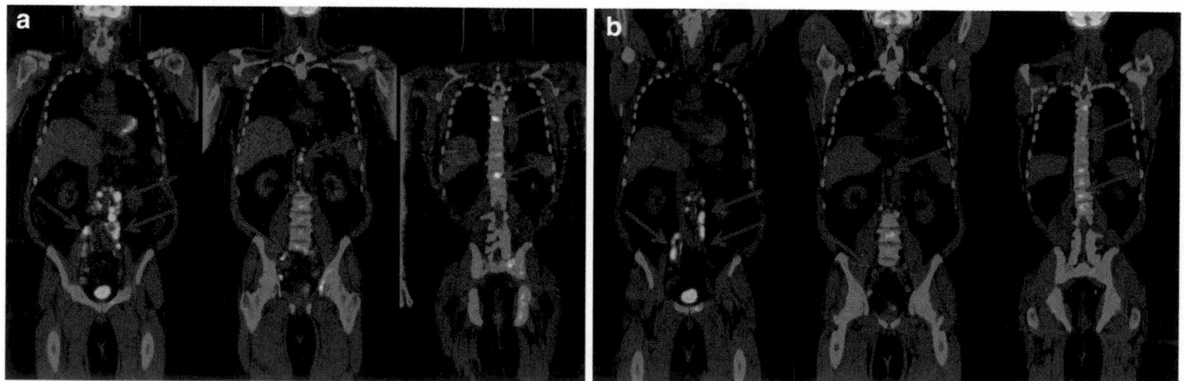

Fig. 13 A 64-year-old man with metastatic PCA. FDG PET/CT scans are performed for restaging and following therapy with Lupron, Casodex, and Taxotere. Images include pretreatment coronal fused PET/CT (**a**) and postchemotherapy coronal fused PET/CT scans (**b**). Posttherapy scans demonstrate partial response with reduction in size and metabolic activity in metastatic adenopathy and osseous metastases (*arrows*)

for FDG in therapy monitoring. Oyama et al. (2001) imaged 10 PCA patients prior to and after initiation of endocrine therapy and compared the changes in lesion FDG, SUV, and PSA. A decrease in FDG uptake paralleled decreasing PSA levels and prostate size (Figs. 13, 14 and 15). Further investigation is necessary to determine the appropriate role of FDG in this application.

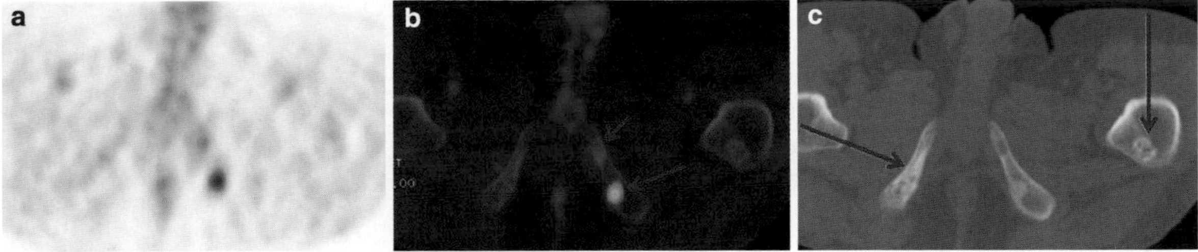

Fig. 14 An 82-year-old man with metastatic PCA and rising PSA. Images include: axial FDG PET (**a**), axial fused FDG PET/CT (**b**) and non-contrast CT images. Osseous metastases display varying metabolic activity. Intense uptake is seen in a metabolically active lesion in the posterior left ischial bone (*arrow*) and low-level uptake is present in a lytic lesion in the anterior left ischial bone (*arrow head*). Blastic metastases in the *right* ischial bone and left femur are negative on FDG PET (*long arrows*) (**c**)

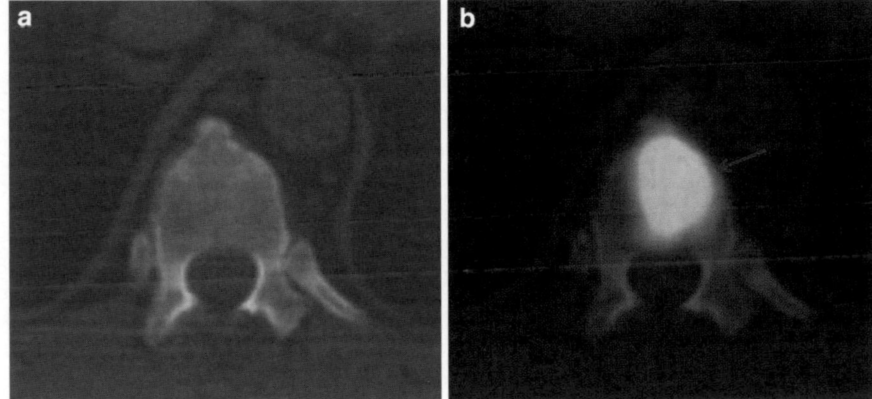

Fig. 15 Intensely metabolically active prostate metastasis without bone changes on CT (*arrow*). Images are axial CT (**a**) and axial fused FDG PET/CT (**b**)

6 Testicular

6.1 Diagnosis

Germ cell tumor (GCT), which comprises 95% of testicular neoplasms, accounts for only 2% of all human malignancies, but is the most common solid tumor in men aged 15–34 years (Garner et al. 2005; Manecksha and Fitzpatrick 2009). Although the incidence of this disease is rising, the mortality rate is declining due to effective surgical, chemotherapy, and radiotherapy regimens. Several risk factors have been identified: a positive family history, i.e., a brother or father with testicular cancer, undescended testis, infertility or subfertility, prior testicular malignancy, and Klinefelter syndrome (Ulbright et al. 1997). The classification of GCTs is based on the embryologic origin and divides seminomatous from non-seminomatous lesions. Non-seminomatous germ cell tumors (NSGCT) tend to be more aggressive and include yolk sac, embryonal, trophoblastic, teratoma, and mixed cell types. At the time of diagnosis, prognosis is established by histologic assessment of vascular invasion and the status of serum tumor markers (alpha fetoprotein, beta-human gonadotropin, and lactate dehydrogenase), the location of the primary tumor, i.e., testicular or extragonadal, and the presence of distant metastases.

Tumors come to diagnosis as a result of a palpable testicular mass, a presentation similar to orchitis, or, in cases of extragonadal GCT, symptoms referable to the site of occurrence. The presence of a testicular mass is confirmed with high-resolution sonography and followed by orchiectomy. MRI has been advocated as a modality to better characterize lesions, but, as orchiectomy is the indicated management, the added information provided by MRI is of questionable value.

There is no role for FDG PET in diagnosis of testicular cancer. Normal testes will display homogeneous physiologic FDG uptake with SUVs ranging from 1.23 to 3.85, declining with age (Kitajima et al. 2007; Kosida et al. 1997). Although seminomas are more FDG avid than NSCGT, there is significant overlap of SUV values (Cremerius et al. 1998). Inflammatory lesions, primary lymphoma, and metastatic disease may also result in foci of testicular hypermetabolism (Morgan et al. 2004; Scalcione et al. 2009; Ulbright et al. 1997).

6.2 Metastatic Disease

Seminomatous neoplasms initially metastasize via lymphatics with blood borne metastases occurring late in the disease. NSGCT may disseminate early via both lymphatic and hematogenous routes. The initial pattern of nodal spread differs depending on the side of origin. Nodal metastases from right side lesions will first involve aortocaval retroperitoneal nodes below the renal vessels. Left sided lesions will metastasize to left paraortic nodes and may involve retroperitoneal nodes above the left renal hilum (Donahue 1984; Sohaib et al. 2008, Figs. 16, 17). Chemotherapy results in complete remission in over 90% of patients. Approximately 60% of patients have postchemotherapy residual masses consisting of viable tumor or necrosis, and 10 to 15% of these will relapse (Fossa et al. 1997). Patients with advanced disease or relapsed disease are treated with chemotherapy, with surgical resection reserved for patients with a solitary site of disease and palliative radiation therapy for those patients unresponsive to other measures.

The inadequacy of CT for differentiating tumor from fibrosis or necrosis led to anticipation that imaging with FDG PET might provide a more accurate method of determining management. Early data regarding the utility of FDG PET in staging and posttherapy assessment of residual masses was conflicting due to study design and patient selection (Ganjoo et al. 1999; De Santis et al. 2004). When evaluating residual seminomatous masses greater than 3 cm, Becherer et al. (2005) report a sensitivity of 80% and specificity of 100% for FDG PET that was better than the 73% achieved for both CT sensitivity and specificity. For lesions less that 3 cm size, 3 of 47 lesions had a false negative result on PET. The authors report no false positives in this series and conclude that for lesions greater than or equal to 3 cm size, a positive scan is highly predictive of the presence of viable tumor. FDG PET is recommended as a primary staging tool for use in patients with Stage I and II NSGCT with questionable CT findings by de Wit et al. (2008). Seventy-two patients were imaged

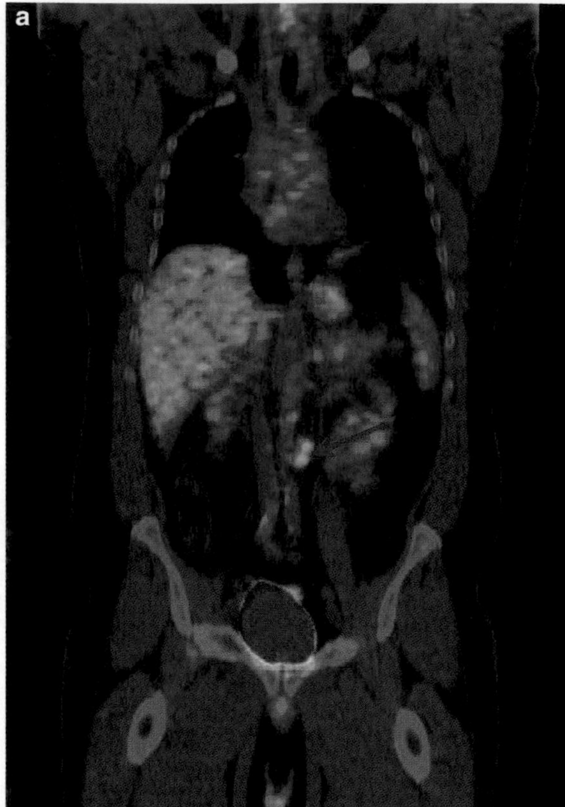

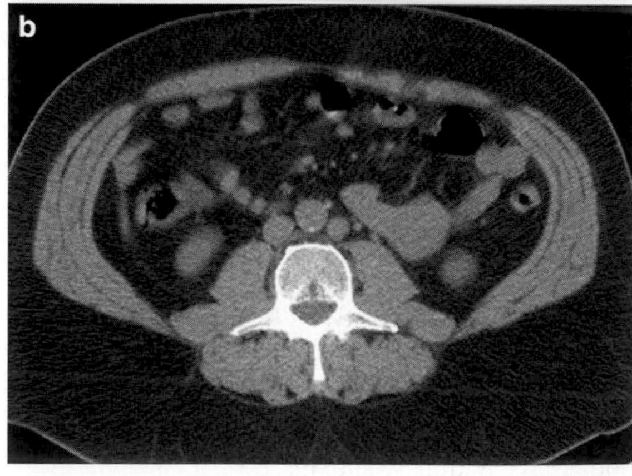

Fig. 16 A 41-year-old man, status post right orchiectomy for seminoma in 1997 and left for new diagnosis of seminoma in 2009. PET/CT is performed for staging. Images include coronal fused PET/CT (**a**) and axial non-contrast CT (**b**). The PET/CT scan revealed two metabolically active left paraortic lymph nodes (*arrow*), subsequently biopsy proven to be metastatic seminoma

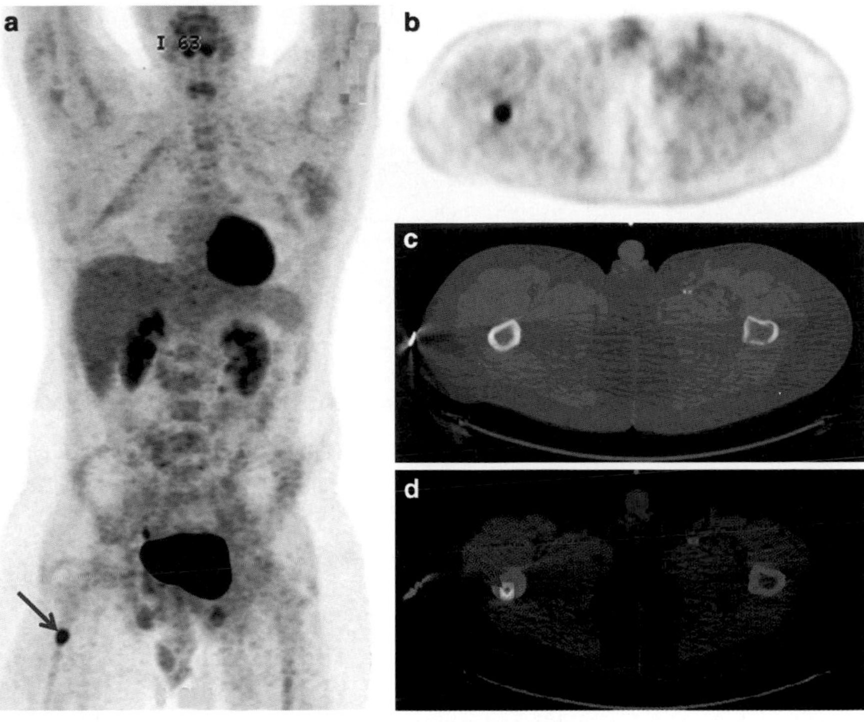

Fig. 17 A 31-year-old man with mixed germ cell tumor of testis status postchemotherapy, surgery, and tandem stem cell transplant, presents with biochemical recurrence. A single metastatic focus identified in the proximal right femur on FDG PET/CT (**a** MIP, **b** axial PET, **c** axial CT, **d** axial fused), which responded well to radiation therapy

with FDG PET and CT and results validated by retroperitoneal nodal dissection. The authors report a positive predictive value for FDG PET of 95 versus 87% for CT. The sensitivity and specificity of PET was 66 and 98% respectively, whereas these values for CT were 41 and 95%. The negative predictive value of PET was 78%, reflecting the inability of this modality to detect microscopic disease. Clinical Stage I patients with lymphovascular invasion-positive NSGCT are at high risk for relapse. Huddart et al. imaged 111 patients with diagnosed NSGCT, positive for lymphovascular invasion with FDG PET or PET/CT. Eighty-eight patients had negative PET scans and 23 were positive. Of these, 87 underwent surveillance rather than adjuvant chemotherapy. Within 12 months, 33 patients with negative PET scans relapsed. These authors site inability of FDG PET to detect microscopic disease as a limiting factor.

More recently published data does not support the routine use of FDG PET for either initial staging or the assessment of postchemotherapy masses due to the high frequency of false positive PET results. The results of a prospective multicenter trial of 20 patients with residual or recurrent seminoma are presented by Hinz et al. (2008). Patients were imaged with FDG PET and CT prior to surgical excision to determine the accuracy of FDG PET in detecting viable tumor. Scan findings were compared to surgical histopathology. FDG PET was considered abnormal in masses with an SUV greater than 2. Of the 20 patients, 18 had residual masses, 3 of which were determined to be viable tumor and 17 were benign. There were no false negative FDG PET findings and all of the lesions with viable tumor were identified and PET positive. Nine patients, however, had false positive PET results, yielding a positive predictive value of only 25%. The sensitivity of FDG PET in this series was 100%, but the specificity was only 47%. The authors conclude that although FDG PET can exclude residual disease in recurrent masses the modality is not sufficiently specific to be the sole determinant of surgical excision in patients with residual postchemotherapy masses (Fig. 18). Similar results have been published regarding accuracy in prediction of tumor viability in patients with NSGCT. Oechsle et al. (2008) report the results of a multicenter prospective trial of 121 patients with Stage IIC or Stage III NSGCT scheduled for resection after completion of chemotherapy. FDG PET results were compared to CT, serum tumor markers and histopathology. For PET imaging, the sensitivity was 70%, which was significantly greater than the sensitivity of 40% for tumor markers. The positive predictive value for PET was

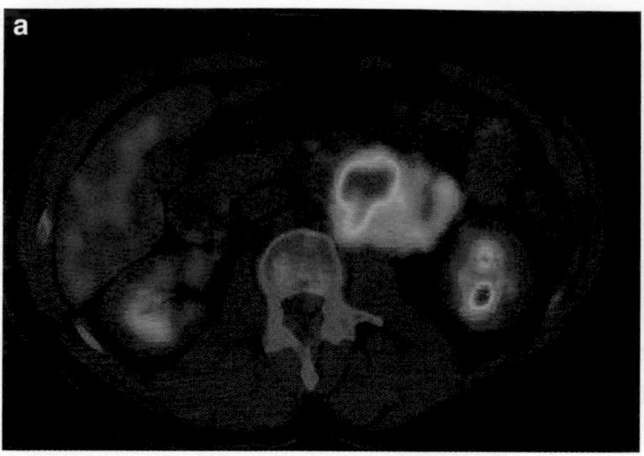

Fig. 18 A 52-year-old man with primary retroperitoneal seminoma. FDG PET/CT scans are performed for initial staging and after initial course of chemotherapy with bleomycin. Images are pretreatment axial fused FDG PET/CT (**a**) and postchemotherapy axial fused FDG PET/CT (**b**). Pretreatment image demonstrates intense metabolic activity within the retroperitoneal seminoma (*arrow*). After treatment there is a marked reduction in lesion size and complete resolution of metabolic activity

59%, not significantly different from 55% for CT and 61% for tumor markers.

Although there are no published reports, it may be possible that dual-time point imaging of postchemotherapy masses might improve the accuracy of FDG PET by better detection of inflammatory lesions. Interesting autopsy data on metastatic GCT identifies differing histology in metastatic lesions when compared to the primary lesion (Dixon 1953). It is conceivable that some metastatic lesions may be false negative on FDG PET due to different histology.

7 Additional PET Radiopharmaceuticals

7.1 ^{18}F-fluoride

Tc-99 MDP or HDP bone scans are commonly used to detect bony metastases in high risk or symptomatic patients with genitourinary malignancies, especially those with PCA. However, ^{18}F-fluoride PET/CT has been shown to be more sensitive than bone scintigraphy for the detection of osseous metastases in cancer patients. A prospective study of PCA cancer patients showed that ^{18}F-fluoride PET had a sensitivity of 100% for the detection of bone metastases, compared to 70% for conventional bone scan (Even-Sapir E et al. 2006). ^{18}F-fluoride PET/CT in another study for the detection of bone metastases yielded a sensitivity of 81%, and a specificity of 93% (Apolo AB et al. 2008). Unfortunately, ^{18}F-fluoride is not tumor specific and abnormal tracer uptake can also be seen in benign bone lesions. The specificity of ^{18}F-fluoride PET imaging is greatly improved with integrated PET/CT. Coregistered CT images allow more accurate characterization of areas of benign tracer uptake. The addition of CT and fused PET/CT images improves diagnostic confidence and limits false positives (Even-Sapir E et al. 2006).

7.2 C-11 and F-18 Choline

Choline is an essential building block for the construction of the phospholipid cell membrane. The rapid cellular proliferation of tumors requires increased metabolism of cell membrane components and therefore increased utilization of choline. Choline, like FDG, is phosphorylated upon entry into the cell and prevents diffusion out of the cell. Choline kinase is the initial enzyme resulting in the conversion of choline into phosphatidylcholine for membrane construction (Podo 1999). The choline molecule can be labeled with either Carbon-11 or Fluorine-18. Radiolabeled choline has high accumulation in salivary glands, liver, pancreas, bowel, and renal parenchyma (Murphy et al. 2011).

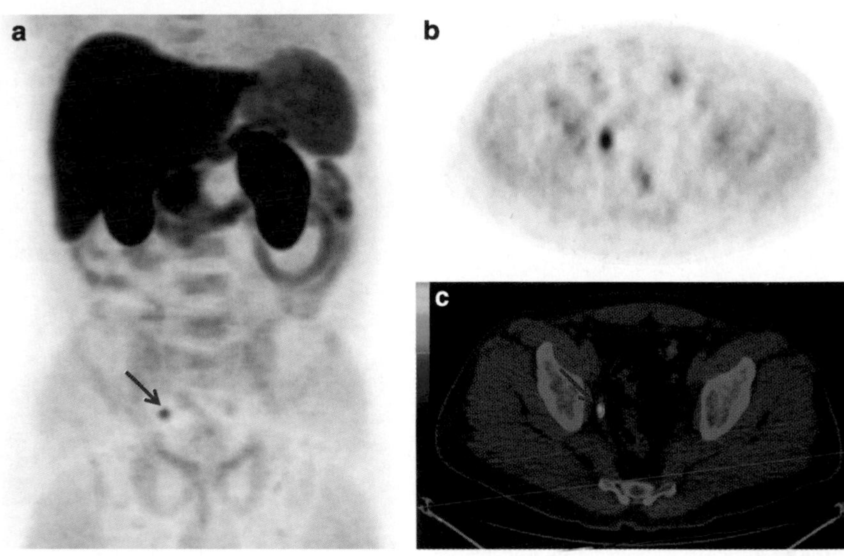

Fig. 19 A 57-year-old man with PCA treated with radical prostatectomy 2 years prior, now presents with a PSA of 1.0. C-11 Choline PET/CT (**a** MIP, **b** axial PET, **c** fused) demonstrates a 6 mm nodal focus in the right pelvis. No abnormality was demonstrated on pelvic MRI. Surgical lymph node resection confirmed a single right pelvic lymph node positive for PCA

Radiolabeled choline PET/CT can readily identify malignant foci in the prostate gland with a sensitivity of 66–81% and a specificity of 43–87% compared to pathology (Farsad et al. 2005; Martorana et al. 2006; Giovacchini et al. 2008; Reske et al. 2006). In one study ^{11}C-choline PET/CT yielded similar accuracy as unenhanced MRI with an endorectal coil, 67 versus 61% respectively compared with sextant-based pathologic verification (Testa et al. 2007). Choline PET/CT aids MRI prostate gland evaluation following biopsy in the presence of hemorrhage, as the signal from the blood can be similar to PCA. Choline PET/CT suffers several limitations: limited resolution for tumor foci of less than 5 mm, focal inflammatory and high-grade prostatic intraepithelial neoplasia uptake mimics malignancy, and normal adjacent urine and rectal activity overlaps the prostate bed. Accurate coregistration of PET/CT fusion images, use of a three-way flushing urinary catheter, and repeat prone images of the pelvis can aid assessment of the prostate bed. MRI with an endorectal coil and diffusion-weighted and dynamic contrast-enhanced sequences offers excellent depiction of PCA within the gland and immediately adjacent tissues. In practice, choline PET/CT is generally focused on identifying nodal and bony metastases (Igerc et al. 2008; Reske et al. 2008, Breeuwsma et al. 2010).

C-11 or F-18 labeled choline PET/CT frequently detects lymph node metastases that are below the size criteria used by CT or MRI (Fig. 19). The sensitivity of choline PET/CT is 60–100% for the detection of pathologically confirmed nodal metastases, which is significantly higher than CT (26–56%) and MRI (22–56%) with superior specificity, 86–98% versus 79–83% (Scattoni et al. 2007; Schiavina et al. 2008; Hovels et al. 2008). Radiocholine uptake in the mid external iliac, common iliac, and retroperitoneal nodes has a positive predictive value of more than 90% for metastatic disease. Choline PET/CT frequently identifies nodal disease in the mediastinum and supraclavicular regions. Low-level choline activity is common seen in the inguinal and hilar lymph nodes, typically symmetric, usually decreases with delayed images and is considered to be benign (Eschmann et al. 2007; Rinnab et al. 2007; Giovacchini et al. 2010; Rinnab et al. 2009; Husarik et al. 2008). False positive choline uptake is seen in nodal inflammation, especially induced by active granulomatous disease (Schillaci et al. 2010).

Osseous metastases are commonly detected by choline PET/CT and most are not sclerotic (Fig. 20). These nonsclerotic bony lesions due to PCA cannot be detected by traditional bone scintigraphy and diagnostic CT. The choline uptake in osseous metastases is generally inversely proportional to the degree of sclerosis. With hormonal therapy lesions became more sclerotic over time and radiolabeled choline uptake declines. Initial data suggests that PCA skeletal metastases start out as choline-avid marrow lesions and become sclerotic, with less activity on choline PET/CT as healing occurs in response to therapy (Fuccio et al. 2010; Beheshti et al. 2009; Tuncel et al. 2008).

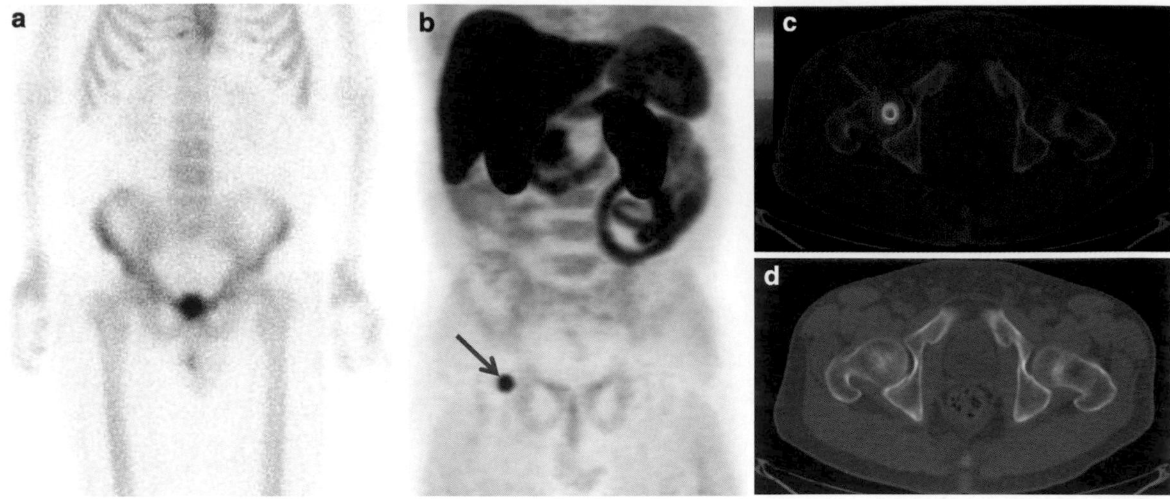

Fig. 20 A 62-year-old man with a history of Gleason 7 PCA status post radical prostatectomy, presents for biochemical recurrence (PSA 0.8). Bone scintigraphy was negative. C-11 Choline PET/CT (**a** bone scan, **b** MIP, **c** fused, **d** axial CT) demonstrates a single focus of intense choline uptake in the right femoral head with no abnormality on corresponding CT images

C-11and F-18-labeled choline PET/CT is primarily used for patients with biochemical recurrence after earlier definitive therapies, prostatectomy and/or external beam radiation. The largest patient population studied to date ($n = 1200$ men) showed ^{11}C-choline PET/CT to have a sensitivity of 89%, specificity of 100%, for the overall detection of recurrent PCA in patients with low (mean 1.6 ng/ml) but rising PSA levels (Sciuto et al. 2011).

8 PET/MR

MRI of the genitourinary tract often aids in many aspects of cancer management, from initial detection to treatment planning and follow-up. With the exception of PCA, contrast-enhanced CT remains the major cross-sectional imaging tool for most cancers in the abdomen and pelvis. Development of integrated PET/CT scanners was a tremendous step forward with rapid CT as the transmission scan and the ability to merge contrast-enhanced CT and FDG PET. Currently, the utilization of PET/CT in genitourinary cancers is still evolving.

Hybrid PET/MRI will face significant technical challenges. The largest logistical problem is the length of MRI procedures, which range from 30 to 60 min. MRI time currently exceeds PET/CT by 50–100%. It is not clear whether simultaneous PET and MRI studies will be more useful than the 2 performed separately. For PCA evaluation, the possibility of one-stop radiolabeled choline PET/MRI for biochemical recurrence is quite attractive. Significant clinical investigation is required.

References

American Cancer Society (2006) Cancer facts and figures 2007. Publication no. 500807. American Cancer Society, Atlanta

Anjos DA, Etchebehere EC, Ramos CD, Santos AO, Albertotti C, Camargo EE (2007) 18F-FDG PET/CT delayed images after diuretic for restaging invasive bladder cancer. J Nucl Med 48:764–770

Apolo AB, Pandit-Taskar N, Morris MJ (2008) Novel tracers and their development for the imaging of metastatic prostate cancer. J Nucl Med 49:2031–2041

Bachor R, Kotzerke J, Reske SN, Hautmann R (1999) Lymph node staging of bladder neck carcinoma with positron emission tomography. Urol A 38:46–50

Becherer A, De Sants M, Karanikas G, Szabo M, Bokemeyer C, Dohmen BM, Pont J, Dudczak R, Dittrich C, Kletter K (2005) FDG PET is superior to CT in the prediction of viable tumor in post-chemotherapy seminoma residuals. Eur J Radiol 54:284–288

Beheshti M, Vali R, Waldenberger P et al (2009) The use of F-18 choline PET in the assessment of bone metastases in prostate cancer: correlation with morphological changes on CT. Mol Imaging Biol 11:446–454

Breeuwsma AJ, Pruim J, van den Bergh AC, Leliveld AM, Nijman RJ, Dierckx RA, de Jong IJ (2010) Detection of local, regional, and distant recurrence in patients with psa relapse after external-beam radiotherapy using (11)C-choline positron emission tomography. Int J Radiat Oncol Biol Phys 77:160–164

Chang CH, Wu HC, Tsai JJ, Shen YY, Changlai SP, Kao A (2003) Detecting metastatic pelvic lymph nodes by 18F-2-deoxyglucose positron emission tomgraphy in patients with prostate-specific antigen relapse after treatment for localized prostate cancer. Urol Int 70:311–315

Chen YW, Huang MY, Hou PN, Chang CC, Lee CS, Lian SL (2009) FDG PET/CT diuretic imaging techniques for differentiating invasive pelvic cancer. Clin Nucl Med 34: 233–235

Chou CH, Figg WD (2005) Molecular and Phenotypic Heterogeneity of metastatic prostate cancer. Cancer Biol Ther 4: 166–167

Cremerius U, Effert PJ, Adam G, Sabri O, Zimny M, Wagenknecht G, Jakse G, Buell U (1998) FDG PET for detection and therapy control of metastatic germ cell tumor. J Nucl Med 39:815–822

Crispen PL, Boorjian SA, Lohse CM, Leibovich BC, Kwon ED (2008) Predicting disease progression after nephrectomy for localized renal cell carcinoma: the utility of prognostic models and biomarkers. Cancer 113:450–460

De Santis M, Becherer A, Bokemeyer C, Stoiber F, Oechsle K, Sellner F, Lang A, Kletter K, Dohmen BM, Dittrich C, Pont J (2004) 2-^{18} fluoro-deoxy-D-glucose positron emission tomography is a reliable predictor for viable tumor in postchemotherapy seminoma: an update of the prospective multicentric SEMPET trial. J Clin Oncol 22:1034–1039

de Wit M, Brenner W, Hartmann M, Kotzerke J, Hellwig D, Lehmann J, Franzius C, Kliesch S, Schlemmer M, Tatsch K, Heicappoll R, Geworski L, Amthauer H, Dohmen BM, Schirrmeister H, Cremerius U, Bokemeyer C, Bares R (2008) [18F]-FDG-PET in clinical stage I/II non-seminomatous germ cell tumours: results of the german multicenter trial. Ann Oncol 19:1619–1623

Dixon FJ, Moore RA (1953) Testicular tumors; a clinicopathological study. Cancer 6:427–454

Donahue JP (1984) Metastatic pathways of nonseminomatous germ cell tumors. Semin Urol 2:217–229

Drieskens O, Oyen R, Van Poppel H, Vankan Y, Flamen P, Mortelmans L (2005) FDG-PET for pre-operative staging of bladder cancer. Eur J Nucl Med Mol Imaging 32:1412–1417

Effert P, Beniers AJ, Tamimi Y, Handt S (2004) Jakse G Expression of glucose transporter 1 (Glut-1) in cell lines and clinical specimens from human prostate carcinoma. Anticancer Res 24:2057–2063

Effert PJ, Bares R, Handt S, Wolff JM, Bull U, Jakse G (1996) Metabolic imaging of untreated prostate cancer by positron emission tomography with 18fluorine-labeled deoxyglucose. J Urol 155:994–998

Eschmann SM, Pfannenberg AC, Rieger A et al (2007) Comparison of ^{11}C-choline-PET/CT and whole body-MRI for staging of prostate cancer. Nuklearmedizin 46:161–168

Even-Sapir E, Metser U, Mishani E, Lievshitz G, Lerman H, Leibovitch I (2006) The detection of bone metastases in patients with high -risk prostate cancer: 99mTc-MDP Planar bone scintigraphy, single- and multifield- of-view SPECT, 18F-fluoride PET, and 18F-fluoride PET/CT. J Nucl Med 47:287–297

Farsad M, Schiavina R, Castellucci P, Nanni C, Corti B, Martorana G, Canini R, Grigioni W, Boschi S, Marengo M, Pettinato C, Salizzoni E, Monetti N, Franchi R, Fanti S (2005) Detection and localization of prostate cancer: correlation of (11)C-choline PET/CT histopathologic step-section analysis. J Nucl Med 46:1642–1649

Fossa SD, Oliver RT, Stenning SP, Horwich A, Wilkinson P, Read G, Mead GM, Roberts JT, Rustin G, Cullen MH, Kaye SB, Harland SJ, Cook P (1997) Prognostic factors for patients with advanced seminoma treated with platinum-based chemotherapy. Eur J Cancer 33:1380–1387

Fuccio C, Castellucci P, Schiavina R et al (2010) Role of ^{11}C-choline PET/CT in the restaging of prostate cancer patients showing a single lesion on bone scintigraphy. Ann Nucl Med 24:485–492

Ganjoo KN, Chan R, Sharma M, Einhorn LH (1999) Positron emission tomography scans in the evaluation of postchemotherapy residual masses in patients with seminoma. J Clin Oncol 17:3457–3460

Garner MJ, Turner MC, Ghadirian P, Krewski D (2005) Epidemiology of testicular cancer: an overview. Int J Cancer 116:331–339

Giovacchini G, Picchio M, Coradeschi E et al (2010) Predictive factors of [(^{11})C]choline PET/CT in patients with biochemical failure after radical prostatectomy. Eur J Nucl Med Mol Imaging 37:301–309

Giovacchini G, Picchio M, Coradeschi E, Scattoni V, Bettinardi V, Cozzarini C, Feschi M, Fazio F, Messa C (2008) [(11)C]choline uptake with PET/CT for the initial diagnosis of prostate cancer: relation to PSA levels, tumor stage and anti-androgenic therapy. Eur J Nucl Med Mol Imaging 35:1065–1073

Goldberg MA, Mayo-Smith WW, Papanicolaou N, Fischman AJ, Lee MJ (1997) FDG PET characterization of renal masses: preliminary experience. Clin Radiol 52:510–515

Han M, Partin AW, Pound CR, Epstein JI, Walsh PC (2001) Long-term biochemical disease-free and cancer –specific survival following anatomic radical retropubic prostatectomy: the 15-year Johns Hopkins experience. Urol Clin North Am 28:555–565

Heicappell R, Muller-Matheis V, Reinhardt M, Vosberg H, Gerharz CD, Muller-Gartner H, Ackermann R (1999) Staging of pelvic lymph nodes in neoplasms of the bladder and prostate by positron emission tomography with 2-[(18)F]-2-deoxy-D-glucose. Eur Urol 36:582–587

Hernandez DJ, Nielson ME, Han M, Trock BJ, Partin AW, Walsh PC, Epstein JI (2008) Natural History of pathologically organ-confined (pT2), Gleason score 6 or less, prostate cancer after radical prostatectomy. Urology 72: 172–6

Hillner BE, Siegel BA, Shields AF, Liu D, Gareen IF, Hunt E, Coleman RE (2008) Relationship between cancer type and impact of PET and PET/CT on intended patient management: findings of the national oncologic PET registry. J Nucl Med 49:1928–1935

Hinz S, Schrader M, Kempkensteffen C, Bare R, Brenner W, Krege S, Franzius C, Kliesch S, Heicappel R, Miller K, de Wit M (2008) The role of positron emission tomography in the evaluation of residual masses after chemotherapy for advanced stage seminoma. J Urol 179:936–940

Hofer C, Laubenbachner C, Block T, Breul J, Hartung R, Schwaiger M (1999) Fluorine-18-fluorodeoxyglucose positron emission tomography is useless for the detection of local recurrence after radical prostatectomy. Eur Urol 36:31–35

Hovels AM, Heesakkers RA, Adang EM, Jager GJ, Strum S, Hoogeveen YL, Severens JL, Barentsz JO (2008) The diagnostic accuracy of CT and MRI in staging of pelvic lymph nodes in patients with prostate cancer: a meta-analysis. Clin Radiol 63:387–395

Husarik DB, Miralbell R, Dubs M et al (2008) Evaluation of [(18)F]-choline PET/CT for staging and restaging of prostate cancer. Eur J Nucl Med Mol Imaging 35:253–263

Igerc I, Kohlfurst S, Gallowitsch HJ, Matschnig S, Kresnik E, Gomez-Segovia I, Lind P (2008) The value of 18F-choline PET/CT in patient with elevated PSA-level and negative prostate needle biopsyfor localization of prostate cancer. Eur J Nucl Med Mol Imaging 35:976–983

Jadvar H, Quan V, Henderson RW, Conti PS (2008) [F-18]-Fluorodeoxyglucose PET and PET-CT in diagnostic imaging evaluation of locally recurrent metastatic bladder transitional cell carcinoma. Int J Clin Oncol 13:42–47

Jadvar H, Xiankui L, Shahanian A, Park R, Tohme M, Pinski J, Conti PS (2005) Glucose metabolism of human prostate cancer mouse xenografts. Mol Imaging 4:91–97

Kang DE, White RL Jr, Zuger JH, Sasser HC, Teigland CM (2004) Clinical use of fluorodeoxyglucose F 18 positron emission tomography for detection of renal cell carcinoma. J Urol 171:1806–1809

Kibel AS, Dehdashti F, Katz MD, Klim AP, Grubb RL, Humphrey PA, Siegel C, Cao D, Gao F, Siegel BA (2009) Prospective study of [18F] fluorodeoxyglucose positron emission tomography/computed tomography for staging of muscle-invasive bladder cancer. J Clin Oncol 27:4314–4320

Kitajima K, Nakamoto Y, Send M, Onishi Y, Okizuka H, Sugimura K (2007) Normal uptake of 18-F FDG in the testes: an assessment by PET/CT. Ann Nucl Med 21: 405–410

Kosida S, Fisher S, Kison PV, Wahl RL, Grossman HB (1997) Uptake of 2-doxy-2[18F] fluoro-D-glucose in the normal testis: retrospective PET study and animal experiment. Ann Nucl Med 11:195–199

Liu IJ, Zafar MB, Lai YH, Segall GM, Terris MK (2001) Fluorodeoxyglucose positron emission tomography studies in clinically organ-confined prostate cancer. Urology 57: 108–111

Logothetis CJ, Navone NM, Lin SH (2008) Understanding the biology of bone metastases: key to the effective treatment of prostate cancer. Clin Cancer Res 14:1599–1602

Majhail NS, Urbain JL, Albani JM, Kanvinde MH, Rice TW, Novick AC, Mekhail TM, Olencki TE, Elson P, Bukowski RM (2003) F-18 fluorodeoxyglucose positron emission tomography in the evaluation of distant metastases from renal cell carcinoma. J Clin Oncol 21:3995–4000

Manecksha RP, Fitzpatrick JM (2009) Epidemiology of testicular cancer. BJU 104:1329–1333

Martorana G, Schiavina R, Corti B, Farsad M, Salizzoni E, Brunocilla E, Bertaccini A, Manferrari F, Castellucci P, Fanti S, Canini R, Grigioni WF, D'Errico Grigioni A (2006) 11C-choline postron emission tomography/computerized tomography for tumor localization of primary prostate cancer in comparison with 12- core biopsy. J Urol 176: 954–960

Miyakita H, Tokunaga M, Onda H, Usui Y, Kinoshita H, Kawamura N, Yasuda S (2002) Significance of 18F-fuorodeoxyglucose positron emission tomography (FDG-PET) for detection of renal cell carcinoma and immunohistochemical glucose transporter 1 (GLUT-1) expression in the cancer. Int J Urol 9:15–18

Morgan K, Srinivas S, Freiha F (2004) Synchronous solitary metastasis of transitional cell carcinoma of the bladder to the testis. Urology 64:808–809

Morris MJ, Akhurst T, Osman I, Nunez R, Macapinlac H, Siedlecki K, Verbel D, Schwartz L, Larson SM, Scher HI (2002) Fluorinated deoxyglucose positron emission tomography in progressive metastatic prostate cancer. Urology 59:913–918

Murphy RC, Kawashima A, Peller PJ (2011) The utility of 11C-choline PET/CT for imaging prostate cancer: a pictorial guide. AJR Am J Roentgenol 196(6):1390–1398

Oechsle K, Hartmann M, Brenner W, Venz S, Weissbach L, Franzius C, Kliesch S, Mueller S, Krege S, Heicappell R, Bares R, Bokemeyer C, de Wit M (2008) [18F] Flurodeoxyglucose positron emission tomography in nonseminomatous germ cell tumors after chemotherapy: the German multicenter positron emission tomography study group. J Clin Oncol 26:5930–5935

Osman MM, Cohade C, Fishman EK, Wahl RL (2005) Clinically significant findings in unenhaced CT portion of the PET/CT studies: frequency in 250 patients. J Nucl Med 46:1352–1355

Oyama N, Akino H, Suzuki Y, Kanamaru H, Ishida H, Tanase K, Sadato N, Yonekura Y (2001) FDG PET for evaluating the change of glucose metabolism in prostate cancer after androgen ablation. Nucl Med Commun 22:963–969

Oyama N, Akino H, Suzuki Y, Kanamaru H, Miwa Y, Tsuka H, Sadato N, Yonekura Y, Okada K (2002) Prognostic value of 2-deoxy-2-[F-18]fluoro-D-glucose positron emission tomography imaging for patients with prostate cancer. Mol Imaging Biol 4:99–104

Oyama N, Miller TR, Dehdashti F, Siegel BA, Fischer KC, Michalski JM, Kibel AS, Andriole GL, Picus J, Welch MJ J (2003) ^{11}C- acetate PET imaging of prostate cancer: detection of recurrent disease at PSA relapse. J Nucl Med 44:549–555

Park JW, Jo MK, Lee HM (2009) Significance of 18F-fluorodeoxyglucose positron-emission tomography/computed tomography for the postoperative surveillance of advanced renal cell carcinoma. BJU 103:615–619

Pelosi E, Arnea V, Skanjeti A, Pirro V, Douroukas A, Pupi A, Mancini M (2008) Role of whole-body (18)F-choline PET/CT in disease detrection in patients with biochemical relapse after radical treatment for prostate cancer. Radio Med 113:895–904

Podo F (1999) Tumour phospholipid metabolism. NMR Biomed 12(7):413–439

Ramdave S, Thomas GW, Berlangieri SU, Bolton DM, Davis I, Tochon-Danguy H, Macgregor D, Scott AM (2001) Clinical role of F-18 fluorodeoxyglucose positron emission tomography for detection and management of renal cell carcinoma. J Urol 66:825–830

Rentsch CA, Cecchini MG, Thalmann GN (2009) Loss of inhibition over master pathways of bone mass regulation results in osteosclerotic bone metastases in prostate cancer. Swiss Med Wkly 1339:220–225

Rinnab L, Mottaghy FM, Blumstein NM et al (2007) Evaluation of [^{11}C]-choline positron-emission/computed tomography in patients with increasing prostate-specific antigen levels after primary treatment for prostate cancer. BJU Int 100:786–793

Rinnab L, Simon J, Hautmann RE et al (2009) [(11)C]choline PET/CT in prostate cancer patients with biochemical recurrence after radical prostat ectomy. World J Urol 27: 619–625

Reske SN, Blumstein NM, Neumaier B, Gottfried HW, Finsterbusch F, Kocot D, Moller P (2006) Imaging prostate cancer with 11C-choline PET/CT. J Nucl Med 47:1249–1254

Reske SN, Blumstein NM, Glatting G (2008) [11C]choline PET/CT imaging in occult local relapse of prostate cancer after radical prostatectomy. Eur J Nucl Med Mol Imaging 35:9–17

Safaei A, Figlin R, Hoh CK, Silverman DH, Sletzer M, Phleps ME, Czernin J (2002) The usefulness of F-18 deoxyglucose whole-body positron emission tomography (PET) for re-staging renal cell cancer. Clin Nephrol 57:56–62

Sanz G, Robles JE, Gimenez M, Arocena J, Sanchez D, Rodriguez-Rubio F, Rosell D, Richter JA, Berian JM (1999) BJU 84:1028–1031

Scalcione LR, Katz DS, Santoro MS, Mahboob S, Badler RL, Yung EY (2009) Primary testicular lymphoma involving the spermatic cord and gonadal vein. Clin Nucl Med 34: 222–223

Scattoni V, Picchio M, Suardi N, Messa C, Freschi M, Roscigno M, Da Pozzo L, Bocciardi A (2007) detection of lymph-node metastases with intergrated [11C]choline PET/CT in patiens with PSA failure after radical prostatectomy: results confirmed by open pelvic-retroperitoneal lymphadenectomy. Eur Urol 52:423–429

Schiavina R, Scattoni V, Castellucci P, Picchio M, Corti B, Briganti A, Franceschelli A, Sanguedolce F, Bertaccini A, Farsad M, Giovacchini G, Fanti S, Grigioni WF, Fazio F, Montorsi F, Rigatti P, Martorana G (2008) 11C-choline positron emission tomography/computerized tomography for preoperative lymph-node staging in intermediate-risk and high-risk prostate cancer: comparison with staging nomograms. Eur Urol 54:392–401

Schillaci O, Calabria F, Tavolozza M et al (2010) ^{18}F-choline PET/CT physiological distribution and pitfalls in image interpretation: experience in 80 patients with prostate cancer. Nucl Med Commun 31:39–45

Schmid DT, Zweifel R, Cservenyak T, Westera G, Goerres GW, von Schulthess GK, Hany TF (2005) Fluorochole PET/CT in patients with prostate cancer. Radiology 235:623–628

Schoder H, Herrmann K, Gonen M, Hricak H, Eberhard S, Scardino P, Scher HI, Larson SM (2005) 2- [18F]fluorodeoxuglucose positron emission tomography for detection of disease in patients with prostatespecific antigen relapse after radical prostatectomy. Clin Cancer Res 11: 4761–4769

Sciuto R, Simone G, Romano L et al (2011) Phase III Trial on F-18 Fluorocholine PET/CT efficiency in early detection of prostate cancer recurrence: preliminary results ove 1600 studies. Eur J Nucl Med Mol Imaging 38:S111

SEER (2008) The Surveillance, Epidemiology, and End Results Program: cancer of the prostate statistics http://seer.cancer.gov/statfacts/html/prost.html

Shreve PD, Grossman HB, Gross MD, Wahl RL (1996) Metastatic prosate cancer: intitial findings of PET with 2-deoxy-2-[F-18]fluro-D-glucose. Radiology 199:751–756

Sohaib SA, Koh DM, Husband JE (2008) The role of imaging in the diagnosis, staging and management of testicular cancer. AJR 191:387–395

Stewart GD, Gray K, Pennington CJ, Edwards DR, Riddick AC, Ross JA, Habib FK (2008) Analysis of hypoxia-associated gene expression in prostate cancer: lysyl oxidase and glucose transporter-1 expression correlate with Gleason score. 20:1561–1567

Sun SS, Chang CH, Ding HJ, Kao CH, Wu HC, Hsieh TC (2009) Preliminary study of detecting malignancy in Taiwanese ESRD patients. Anticancer Res 29:3459–3463

Sung J, Espiritu JI, Segall GM, Terris MK (2003) Fluorodeoxyglucose positron emission tomography and staging of clinically advanced prostate cancer. BJU 92:24–27

Swinnen G, Maes A, Pottel H, Vanneste A, Billiet I, Lesage K, Werbrouck P (2009) FDG-PET/CT for the preoperative lymph node staging of invasive bladder cancer. Eur Urol [Epub ahead of print]

Testa C, Schiavina R, Lodi R, Salizzoni E, Corti B, Farsad M, Kurhanewicz J, Manferrari F, Brunocilla E, Tonon C, Monetti N, Castellucci P, Fanti S, Coe M, Grigioni WF, Martorana G, Canini R, Barbiroli B (2007) Prostate cancer: sextant localization with MR imaging, MR spectroscopy and 11C-choline PET/CT. Radiology 244:797–806

Tuncel M, Souvatzoglou M, Herrmann K et al (2008) ^{11}C choline positron emission tomography/computed tomography for staging and restaging of patients with advanced prostate cancer. Nucl Med Biol 35:689–695

Ulbright TM, Amin MB, Young RH (1997) Atlas of Tumor Pathology: tumors of the Testis, Adnexae, Spermatic Cord and Scrotum. Armed Forces Institute of Pahology, Wachington, DC

Ward JF, Moul JW (2005) Rising prostate-specific antigen after primary prostate cancer. Nat Clin Pract Urol 2:174–182

Gynecologic

Patrick J. Peller

Contents

Abstract

This chapter reviews the current and evolving clinical roles of PET/PET in the diagnosis, staging, and restaging of gynecological malignancies. For endometrial and cervical carcinoma, PET has proven useful in both the staging of locally advanced cancer and restaging of the disease. PET plays a unique role assessing response to treatment and prognostication. In advanced ovarian carcinoma PET staging may be of value when chemotherapy is used as the primary treatment prior to surgery. When the serum CA-125 is elevated and conventional imaging is negative or equivocal, previously treated ovarian cancer patients benefit from PET/CT identification of disease. PET/CT aids the management of vulvar and vaginal squamous cell cancer, especially in the detection of nodal metastasis.

1 Key Points

The roles of FDG PET/CT imaging in the management of gynecologic malignancies are evolving and remain an area of active research. PET/CT may be helpful in staging high grade or locally advanced endometrial cancers. In patients receiving neoadjuvant chemotherapy, PET/CT should be used for staging. PET has proven useful in staging of untreated advanced cervical cancer, and in planning radiation therapy. FDG PET uptake in primary cervical cancers has prognostic implications. The limited published data on FDG PET imaging in vulvar and vaginal carcinomas suggests utility in staging and restaging

P. J. Peller (✉)
Department of Radiology,
Mayo Clinic, 200 1st Street SW,
Rochester, MN 55905, USA
e-mail: Peller.patrick@mayo.edu

P. Peller et al. (eds.), *PET-CT and PET-MRI in Oncology*, Medical Radiology. Diagnostic Imaging,
DOI: 10.1007/174_2012_621,

disease and that PET/CT is more effective than conventional diagnostic modalities in detecting nodal and distant metastases. The addition of contrast-enhanced CT in FDG PET/CT improves accuracy of staging and restaging of gynecologic malignancies. PET/CT is useful to assess early treatment response to chemotherapy and in the setting of post-treatment to evaluate patients with elevated tumor markers.

2 Introduction

The data supporting the clinical use of FDG PET/CT in malignant gynecologic tumors has been growing slowly over the past decade. This chapter reviews the clinical roles of PET/CT. The utility of PET/CT in screening and the primary diagnosis of gynecologic cancers are virtually nil, except for those malignancies noted incidentally on scans performed for other indications. Staging with PET/CT varies depending on tumor type, grade, and primary size. Generally PET/CT is considered to be superior to conventional imaging methods in restaging due to diagnostic accuracy for the detection of local recurrence and metastatic lesions. The chapter will illustrate the utility and potential limitations of FDG PET/CT imaging for evaluating gynecologic tumors.

PET/CT imaging of gynecologic malignancies requires meticulous exam technique. The high activity in the urinary bladder from excreted FDG may mask the primary, metastatic, and recurrent gynecologic malignancies. When imaging patients with gynecologic cancer, a Foley catheter and continuous bladder irrigation are useful to clear urinary activity. Oral hydration prior to the PET/CT scan appointment and Lasix can aid in clearing renal collecting system and ureteral activity. A separate one-bed prone pelvic view is useful for separation of the bladder and rectovaginal space (Kumar et al. 2004; Ma et al. 2003; Son et al. 2010).

3 Endometrial Cancer

Endometrial cancer is the most common gynecologic cancer and the fourth most common malignancy among women in the US, affecting 1 in 50 (Jemal et al. 2009). Endometrial cancer affects mainly postmenopausal women; particularly those aged 50–65. Endometrial cancer is more common in developed countries where the diet is high in fat. The major risk factors are obesity, diabetes, hypertension, and unopposed estrogen. Adenocarcinoma accounts for more than 80 % of endometrial cancers. Most (over 90 %) women with endometrial cancer have abnormal uterine bleeding and over 30 % of women with postmenopausal bleeding have endometrial cancer. When cancer is suspected, an endometrial biopsy is done, which is more than 90 % accurate (Irvin et al. 2002).

3.1 Staging Endometrial Cancer

The 5-year survival rate for localized endometrial cancer is 96 % compared to regional (67 %) and metastatic disease (17 %) (Jemal et al. 2009). CT and MRI have failed to demonstrate significant benefits in preoperative staging for endometrial cancer. CT and MRI detection of lymph node metastases are based on size and yield a relatively low sensitivity for detecting nodal metastases in endometrial cancer, ranging from 18 to 66 % (Sugiyama et al. 1995; Manfredi et al. 2004; Rockall et al. 2005). Initial research into FDG PET/CT staging in endometrial cancer also showed limitations in sensitivity. Nodal involvement detected by PET/CT and confirmed at surgery had a patient-based sensitivity of 50 % and specificity 86.7 %. This early study included a wide spectrum of tumors and over a third of patients had low-grade endometrial cancer (Kitajima et al. 2008).

Staging standards have recently undergone changes with greater emphasis on prognostic factors: histologic grade, extent of spread, including invasion depth, cervical involvement (glandular involvement versus stromal invasion), and extrauterine metastases (Pecorelli 2009). FDG uptake in primary endometrial tumors is significantly and directly related with the FIGO grade (Nakamura et al. 2010). Staging of high-grade endometrial cancer with PET/CT showed higher accuracy in detecting lymph node involvement and overall patient-based sensitivity, specificity, and accuracy were 57.1 %, 100 %, and 88.5 %, respectively (Picchio et al. 2010). Signorelli et al. 2009, also focused on high-risk clinical early-stage endometrial cancer (grade 2 with deep myometrial invasion, grade 3 with serous and clear-cell carcinoma) and the diagnostic accuracy of FDG PET/CT in detecting pelvic nodal metastases was 77.8 % sensitivity, 100 % specificity, and 94.4 % accuracy. In all studies PET was more sensitive than either CT or MRI

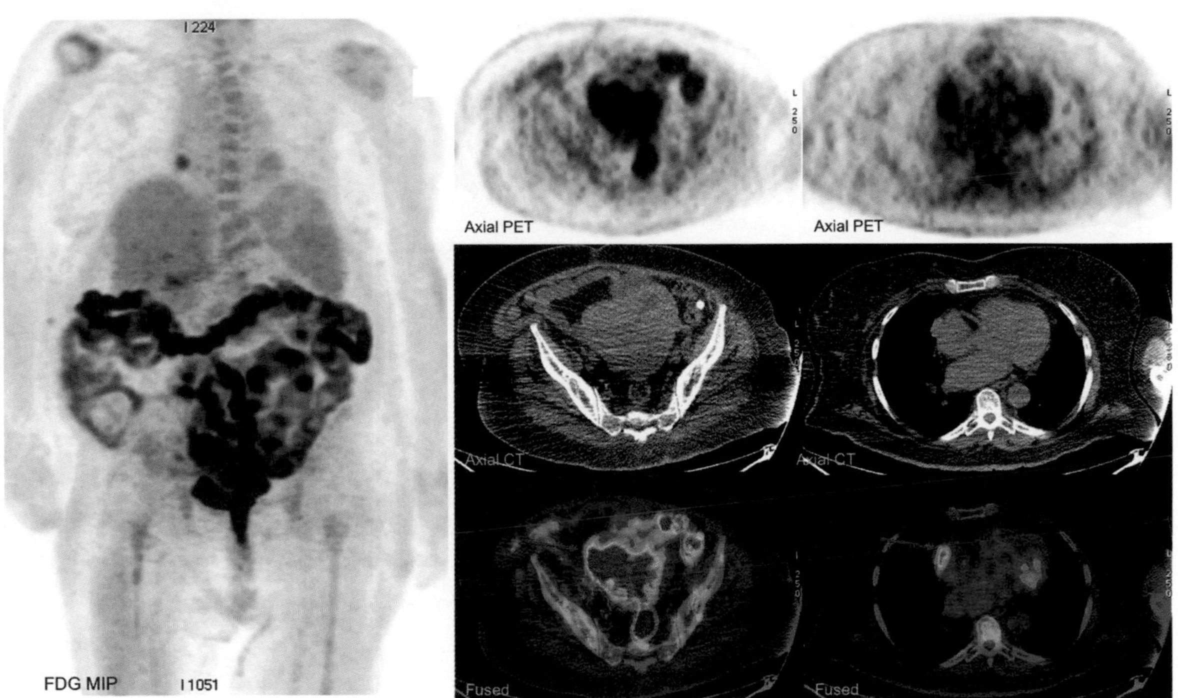

Fig. 1 This 67-year-old woman presented with locally advanced endometrial carcinoma measuring 13 × 12 cm. Biopsy demonstrated a grade 3 malignancy. PET/CT demonstrates intense FDG uptake (SUV_{max} equals 12.1) within the known endometrial cancer (*arrow*). There is an FDG-avid 2.7 cm soft tissue nodule in the medial right middle lobe (*arrow*) with additional multiple subcentimeter nodules within both lungs. Biopsy confirmed the right middle lobe metastasis and the patient underwent chemotherapy

for identifying extranodal metastatic disease (Horowitz et al. 2004). Preoperative imaging with PET and contrast-enhanced CT can aid clinical management in patients with locally aggressive or advanced endometrial cancer to identify metastatic disease, which requires either extensive surgery or systemic chemotherapy (Kitajima et al. 2009), (Fig. 1).

3.2 Restaging Endometrial Cancer

In endometrial cancer treated with chemotherapy, functional imaging with FDG PET provides a tool to assess response. Compared to MRI changes, a substantial decrease in SUV with neoadjuvant chemotherapy was shown to correlate with histologic response at surgery. Patients had an estimated 80 % 5-year survival when there were no residual abnormalities on FDG PET compared to 32 % in patients with residual abnormalities (Ben-Haim et al. 2009).

Fortunately most patients present with early stage endometrial cancer and surgical cure is common, resulting in a 5-year disease-free survival over 90 % (Jemal et al. 2009). As recurrence of endometrial cancer is relatively uncommon, FDG PET is most often used to evaluate patients at high risk for, with suspected or known recurrent disease. In a high-risk patient population, PET/CT detects asymptomatic recurrence with a reported sensitivity of 96 % and specificity of 78 %. Park et al. retrospectively reviewed PET/CT imaging in 66 asymptomatic and 22 symptomatic women who were all clinically disease-free following definitive therapy. They found that PET/CT is highly effective in discriminating true recurrence and resulted in additional treatment in 22 % of patients (Park et al. 2008).

The common sites of endometrial cancer recurrence are the vagina, regional nodes, the peritoneal cavity, and lungs. PET/CT can play an important role in the decision-making process for women with known recurrent endometrial cancer. For patients with an isolated site of recurrence, surgery, and/or radiotherapy may be either curative or provide effective palliation. Vaginal recurrence of endometrial cancer

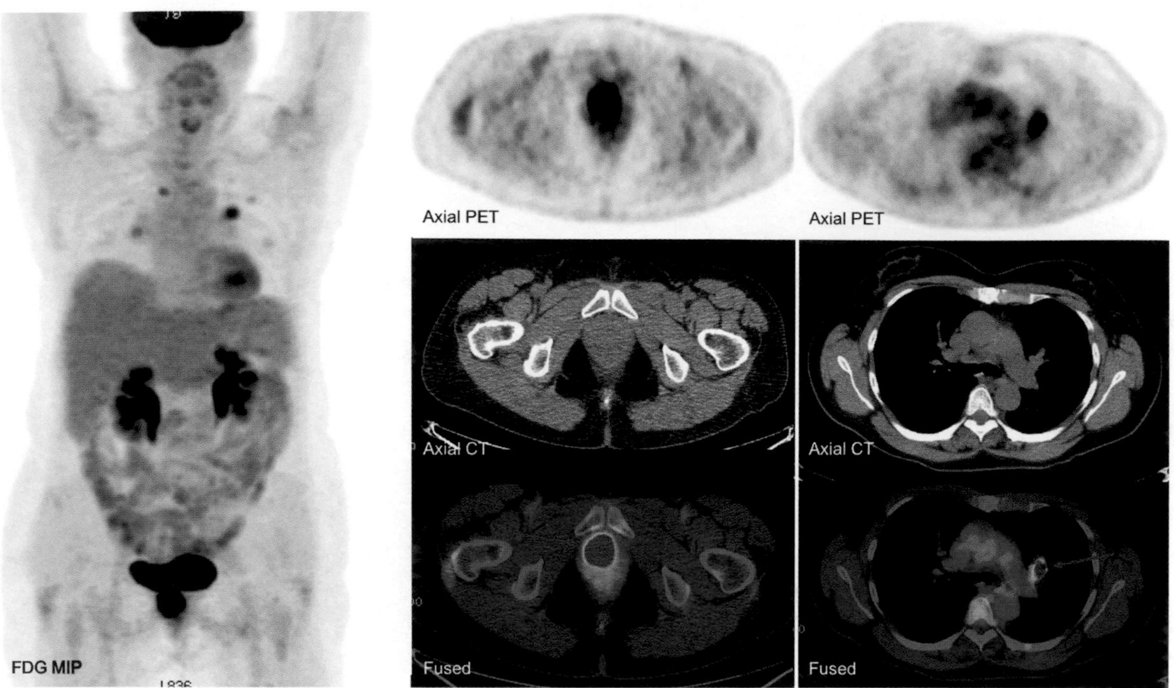

Fig. 2 This 57-year-old woman with a history of stage III serous endometrial cancer treated with hysterectomy and six cycles of chemotherapy 2 years prior now presents with followup CT demonstrating a 2.8 cm perivaginal mass. PET/CT demonstrates intense FDG uptake (SUV_{max} equals 15.3) within the vaginal mass (*arrow*). There are numerous nodular densities scattered throughout both lungs with moderate to intense FDG uptake (*arrow*). CT-guided biopsy confirmed recurrent endometrial cancer in the pelvis and lung; chemotherapy was begun

will present early with vaginal spotting and long-term cure rates are reported to be about 40 %. Using PET/CT to select truly localized disease, Lin et al. reported cure rates of about 90 %. Multifocal recurrence and distant metastasis requires systemic chemotherapy. In women with recurrent endometrial cancer, FDG PET more accurately assesses the disease extent, leading to improved management compared to conventional imaging (Lin et al. 2005), (Fig. 2).

4 Ovarian Cancer

In the US, ovarian cancer is the 2nd most common gynecologic cancer and the deadliest, the 5th leading cause of cancer-related deaths in women (Jemal et al. 2009). Ovarian cancer affects mainly perimenopausal and postmenopausal women. Early cancer is usually asymptomatic; an adnexal mass, often solid, irregular, and fixed, may be discovered incidentally. Symptoms are usually nonspecific in advanced stages (Goff et al. 2004). Ovarian cancer is often fatal because it is usually advanced when diagnosed (Permuth-Wey 2009). Evaluation usually includes ultrasonography, CT or MRI, and measurement of cancer antigen 125. A biopsy is not routinely recommended unless a patient is not a surgical candidate (Roman, et al. 1997; Schutter et al. 1998).

Ovarian cancers are histologically diverse and least 80 % originate in the epithelium. Serous cystadenocarcinomas represent 75 % of epithelial ovarian cancers (Jemal et al. 2009). Ovarian cancer spreads by direct extension, peritoneal seeding, via lymphatic channels to pelvic and retroperitoneal nodes, and hematogenously to the liver and lungs. Staging is traditionally surgical, as treatment usually requires hysterectomy, bilateral salpingo-oophorectomy, and excision of all tumor deposits possible. Prognosis is worse when surgery cannot remove all visibly involved tissue (Petignat et al. 2000; Elit et al. 2002).

The ability of FDG PET to identify a primary ovarian malignancy in patients with an adnexal mass is limited with reported sensitivities of 52–58 % and specificities of 76–78 % (Iyer et al. 2010). Inflammatory adnexal masses, corpus luteum cysts, dermoid cysts, teratoma, and other benign ovarian tumors are common false positives. (Schröder et al. 1999; Kubik-Huch et al. 2000; Fenchel et al. 2002). Low-grade and small ovarian tumors are difficult to detect on PET/CT. Cystic tumors also lead to lower sensitivity because FDG accumulates only in the small solid components (Yoshida et al. 2004). Overall sensitivity for detecting ovarian cancer in an adnexal mass has been reported to be 58 % and the specificity is 76 %, which yields a very low positive predictive value of 25 %, but a high negative predictive value of 93 % (Fenchel et al. 2002).

4.1 Staging Ovarian Cancer

Traditionally staging was performed at the time of definitive surgical treatment. A total hysterectomy, bilateral salpingo-oophorectomy, and infracolic omentectomy is performed with peritoneal biopsies and retroperitoneal lymph node sampling. Patient outcome was highly dependent on tumor stage and optimal surgical debulking. Currently chemotherapy is administered before surgery to reduce the tumor burden and allow more frequent attempts at curative resection (van der Burg et al. 1995; Rose et al. 2004). The use of adjuvant chemotherapy creates the need to image ovarian cancer patients to aid staging. The addition of FDG PET integrated with contrast-enhanced CT in patients with ovarian carcinoma has shown improved staging accuracy. Lesions outside the pelvis are identified better with PET/CT than CT alone, increasing the sensitivity from 24 to 63 % when FDG images were used in conjunction with the CT exam. Integrated PET with CT improves the overall preoperative staging accuracy from 53 to 87 % (Yoshida et al. 2004).

PET/CT also allows measurement of response to chemotherapy. Even a relatively modest 20 % decrease in SUV from baseline after the initial cycle of chemotherapy is associated with improved overall survival. Those patients with an early 20 % decline in FDG tumor uptake have a 38.3 month mean survival versus 23.1 months in patients who demonstrate no metabolic response. FDG PET was more accurate than clinical response criteria and decline CA 125 tumor marker. FDG PET can predict patient outcome after the first cycle of neoadjuvant chemotherapy and has become a tool for early prediction of response (Avril et al. 2005).

4.2 Restaging Ovarian Cancer

Advances in the surgical technique and chemotherapy for ovarian cancer have lengthened survival, but have also increased the incidence of recurrence. The reported relapse rate approaches 75 % in ovarian cancer patients treated with curative intent (Greenlee et al. 2001). Early detection of recurrent disease and exact anatomic localization of metastatic disease are essential for selecting appropriate therapy for each patient. (Fig. 3) CA 125 tumor marker is used extensively to screen for ovarian cancer recurrence. A rising CA 125 level is highly sensitive for recurrent epithelial ovarian cancer, but provides no information about disease extent or location. Unfortunately, CA 125 levels may be falsely negative in 25–50 % of patients with recurrence (Rustin et al. 1996). CT has been the standard imaging technique to evaluate asymptomatic CA 125 elevation and symptoms suggestive of recurrence of ovarian cancer. The ability of CT to diagnose recurrent ovarian cancer has varied widely in the published literature with accuracies of 38–88 % (Sironi et al. 2004). The accuracy of FDG PET/CT has been consistently higher ranging from 68 % to 92 % (Sironi et al. 2004; Chung et al. 2007; Sebastian et al. 2008). The ability to detect recurrence improves with the addition of contrast-enhanced CT to the integrated PET/CT. PET/CT has become the test of choice in patients with a rising CA125 levels and a negative work-up (Sala et al. 2010), (Fig. 4).

When compared to second-look surgeries PET/CT will miss lesions that are less than 5 mm in size, typically considered below the resolution of PET/CT, and likely any imaging technique. The positive predictive value ranges from 89 to 98 % for PET/CT in patients with possible recurrence of ovarian cancer. PET/CT readily identifies extrapelvic lesions; the sensitivity increases as the distance from the primary site increases (Iagaru et al. 2008). PET/CT can be used to select patients with recurrent ovarian cancer for whom cytoreductive surgery is a useful option

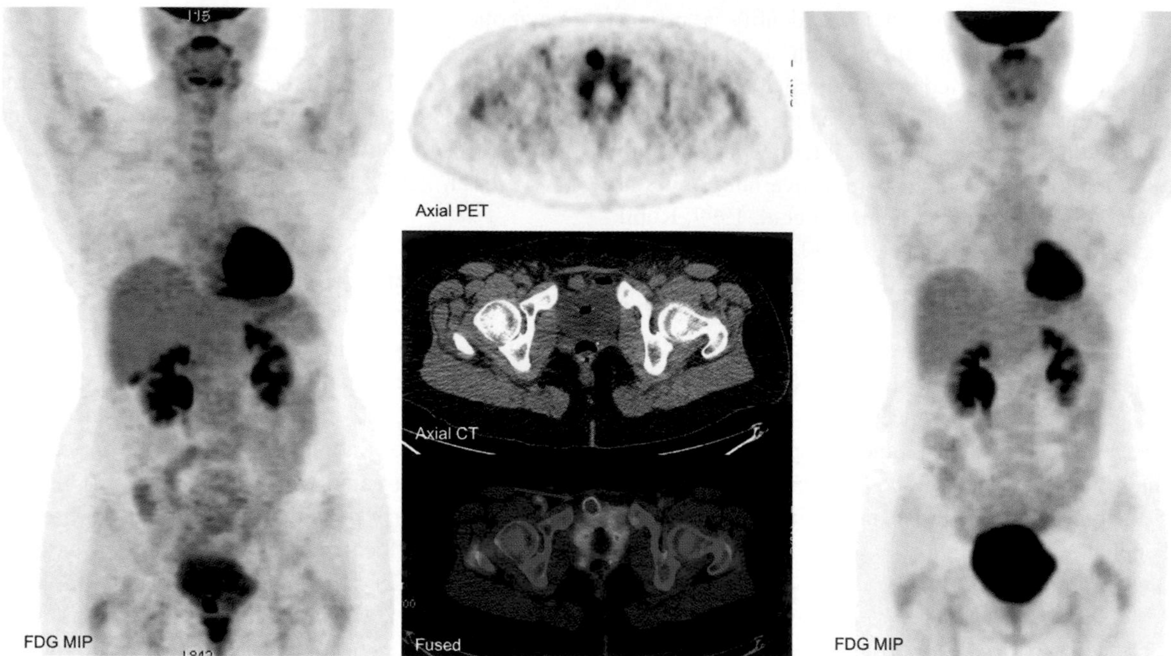

Fig. 3 This patient is a 50-year-old woman with a history of stage III C grade 4 serous papillary ovarian cancer 4 years previously, treated with surgical resection and six cycles of chemotherapy. Second look surgery identified two foci of residual disease and she was treated with intraperitoneal and intravenous chemotherapy. Nearly 3 years following completion of treatment her CA 125 is progressively raising, but the CT scan shows no definite recurrence. PET/CT revealed three FDG avid nodules, the largest of which measured 1.6 cm immediately anterior to the urinary bladder (SUV_{max} 9.1). Repeat cytoreductive surgery removed six macroscopic disease foci, including the three identified by PET/CT. Whole abdominal and pelvic radiation therapy was employed. Follow-up PET/CT (MIP on right) in 6 months was negative for recurrent disease

(Fagotti et al. 2008). The use of PET/CT as a first-line restaging modality in suspected recurrence of ovarian cancer changes the treatment technique for 44–57 % of patients (Simcock et al. 2006; Mangili et al. 2007).

5 Cervical Cancer

Cervical cancer is the third most common gynecologic cancer and the eighth most common cancer among women in the US (Jemal et al. 2009). Mean age at diagnosis is about 50, but nearly half of the cases of invasive cervical cancer occur in patients under the age of 35 years (Pandit-Taskar 2005). Cervical intraepithelial neoplasia caused by human papillomavirus infection typically precedes cervical cancer. Most patients are asymptomatic. The majority of cervical cancer is squamous cell carcinoma; the rest are adenocarcinomas. Diagnosis is by a screening cervical Papanicolaou test and biopsy. Cancers are clinically staged based on biopsy, physical examination, and chest X-ray findings. Since disease extent drives treatment decisions, accurate pretreatment staging is essential. Therapy options include surgery, irradiation, and chemotherapy, singly, in combination or consecutively (Rose et al. 1999; Sedlis et al. 1999; Peters et al. 2000).

Invasive cervical cancer is determined by selected biopsies and the patient's pelvic examination identifies the local extent of the tumor. Tumors confined to the cervix without extension to the vagina, parametrial tissues, bladder, or rectum and less than 4 cm, typically undergo primary surgical resection. If the primary tumor is large ($\geq$2 cm) or adjacent structures are involved, cross-sectional imaging of the abdomen and pelvis is typically performed to identify metastases. Cervical cancer spreads primarily through lymphatic channels toward the pelvic and retroperitoneal lymph nodes and nodal involvement is an important prognostic indicator (Pilleron et al. 1974).

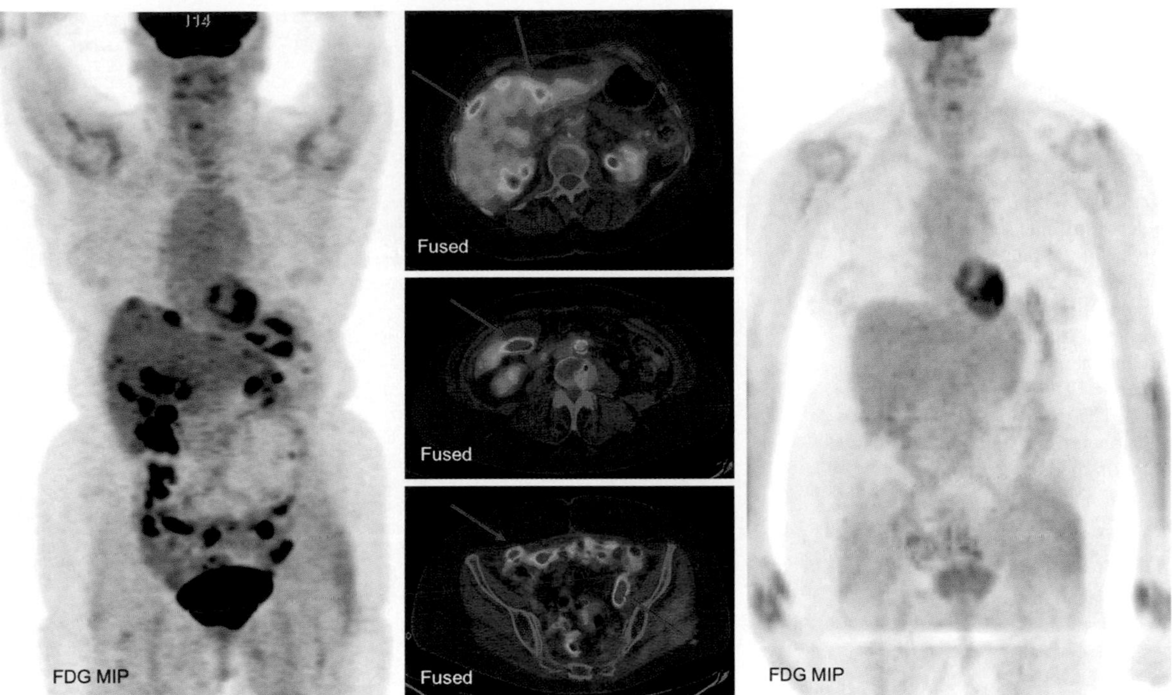

Fig. 4 This patient is a 74-year-old woman with a 5-year history of ovarian cancer with the last cytoreductive surgery 2 years prior. Patient has been receiving chemotherapy with persistent low-level CA 125 levels and nonspecific findings on CT scan. PET/CT reveals numerous intensely FDG-avid abnormalities along the capsule of the liver, colon wall, and peritoneum (*arrows*) highly suspicious for peritoneal spread of ovarian cancer. The patient was placed on a new regimen of chemotherapy and CA 125 levels became negative. The PET/CT (MIP on *right*) at 6 months revealed resolution of FDG-avid lesions (also linear hand movement artifact over thighs)

Hematogenous metastases are uncommon in the early stages of the disease (Kaur et al. 2003).

5.1 Staging Cervical Cancer

Intense FDG uptake is common in primary cervical tumors (Kaur et al. 2003) and primary cervical cancers ≥7 mm will be visible on PET/CT (Son et al. 2010). FDG uptake is correlated with over-expression of the Glut-1 glucose transporter (Yen et al. 2004a, b) and higher SUV_{max} values are associated with an increased risk of nodal metastases (Kitajima et al. 2010). A high SUV_{max} is also an independent risk factor for recurrence after surgical treatment regardless of adjuvant chemotherapy (Son et al. 2010). The SUV_{max} value is also related to overall survival (Patel et al. 2011). Cervical cancer patients with a high SUV_{max} will require more aggressive multimodality treatment (Son et al. 2010). Increased uptake in the endometrium above a cervical tumor should not be confused with tumor extension (Lerman et al. 2004).

Accurate determination of parametrial tumor extension and lymph node metastases is important as therapy is based upon stage (Pandharipande et al. 2009). Cervical cancer cells initially spread through the lymphatics to the parametrial nodes. From the parametrial nodes, there are three routes that tumor cells may travel: laterally to the external iliac nodes, posterior-lateral to the hypogastric nodes along the internal iliac vessels, or posteriorly along the uterosacral ligaments to the lateral sacral and presacral nodes (Kaur et al. 2003; Pandharipande et al. 2009). All three nodal groups then drain into the common iliac nodes and paraaortic nodes (Son et al. 2010). Identification of lymph node status is an important prognostic factor in cervical cancer (Kumar et al. 2004). For IB disease and negative nodes the 5-year survival is 85–95 %, but drops to 45–55 % for those with nodal metastases (Pannu et al. 2001; Kaur et al. 2003), (Fig. 5).

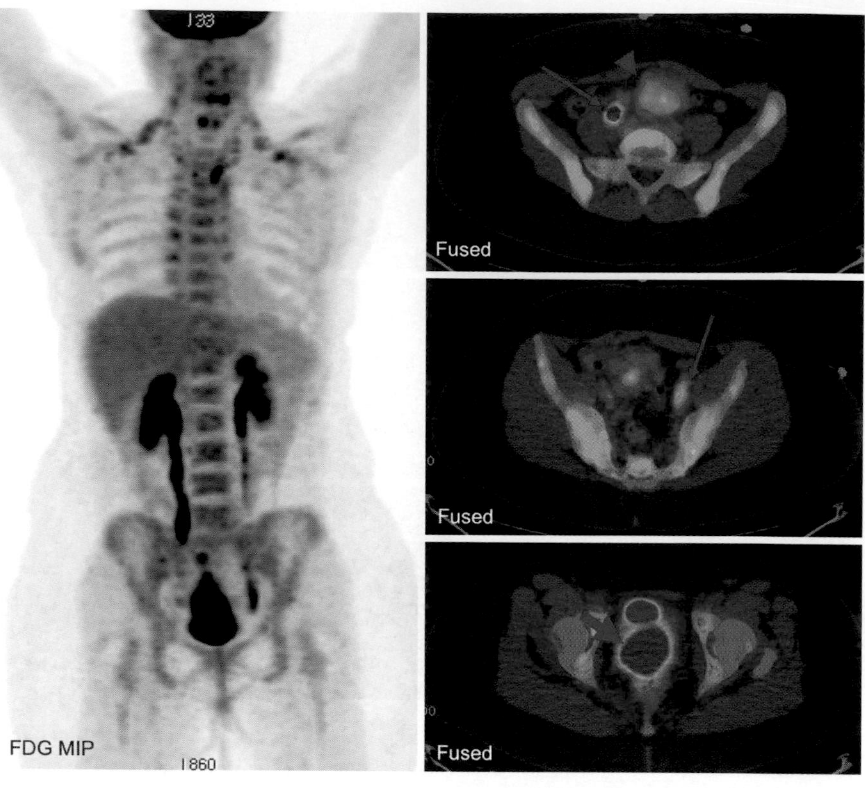

Fig. 5 This 43-year-old woman presented for staging of known cervical cancer. There is intense FDG uptake (SUV_{max} 17.3) in the soft tissue mass producing diffuse enlargement of the cervix (*broad arrow*). There is moderate to intense increased activity in the bilateral enlarged external and common iliac lymph nodes (*arrows*). A uterine fibroid demonstrates mild to moderate FDG uptake (*arrow head*). The patient was treated with concurrent external beam radiation therapy, brachial therapy, and chemotherapy. She remains disease-free at 3 years

In a prospective trial, PET/CT detected 72 % metastatic nodes found at surgery in clinical stage IA or IB cervical cancer patients who underwent radical hysterectomy and pelvic lymph node dissection. The sensitivity rose to 100 % for PET/CT identification of involved nodes larger than 5 mm (Sironi et al. 2006). A meta-analysis has shown that PET/CT has a pooled sensitivity of 79–84 % and a specificity of 95–99 %; compared to 47–50 % and 92–97 % for CT and 56–72 % and 90–96 % for MRI (Son et al. 2010). PET/CT and all imaging cannot detect microscopic metastases, but PET/CT is more accurate than CT or MRI for evaluating lymph node status. PET/CT is highly accurate for the detection of locally recurrent or distant metastatic disease (Patel et al. 2011).

Patients with retroperitoneal nodal metastases consistently have lower overall survival, disease-free survival, and survival after recurrence. The rate of retroperitoneal lymph node metastases is approximately 15–30 % in patients with locally advanced cervical cancer. Routine surgical resection of these nodes results in significant adverse effects and increased morbidity. CT and MRI have low sensitivities, 56 % and 58 %, respectively, for the detection of retroperitoneal nodal disease (Kang et al. 2010). FDG PET identified metastatic retroperitoneal nodes with a sensitivity of 82 % (Ma et al. 2003). This high sensitivity for FDG PET was only found in high-risk patient populations and was far less accurate in patients with early stage disease (sensitivity 34 %) due to the high frequency of microscopic metastases (Kang et al. 2010).

5.2 Radiation Therapy for Cervical Cancer

Radiation therapy is commonly employed in patients with cervical cancer and to destroy the malignant lesions maximal radiation doses must be delivered to the tumor. Avoiding irradiation of healthy tissues minimizes toxicity. Since PET/CT has the best accuracy in detecting disease in lymph nodes and distant lesions, it has become a useful tool for radiation therapy planning. Multiple studies have demonstrated that targeting the hypermetabolic primary cervical tumor and nodal disease yields better results than CT-based planning. The PET/CT images are

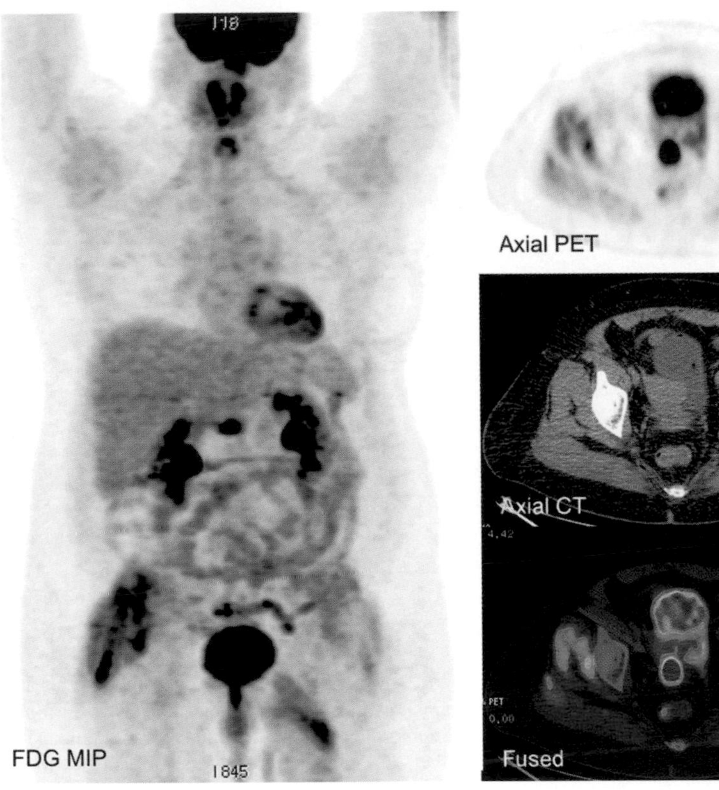

Fig. 6 This 49-year-old woman with known cervical cancer and severe vulvar dysplasia presented for staging. PET/CT demonstrates 2 cm intensely FDG-avid cervical mass consistent with known malignancy (*arrows*). No FDG-avid adenopathy is identified. Wide vulvar and cervix resection revealed stage IB cervical carcinoma and grade 3 in situ carcinoma of the vulva status. The patient received postoperative radiation therapy

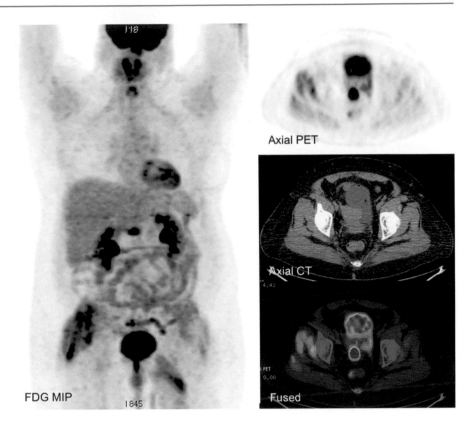

transferred to the therapy planning computers and contouring of normal organs is derived from the CT portion and the active tumor sites are contoured from the FDG PET component. The treatment volume can be planned using the radiotherapy treatment planning software. In many medical centers, PET/CT is now routinely performed for radiation therapy planning in cervical cancer (Esthappan et al. 2008; Lin et al. 2007; MacDonald et al. 2008), (Fig. 6).

5.3 Restaging Cervical Cancer

Approximately 30 % of patients treated for advanced stage cervical cancer develop recurrence and the majority occurs within the first 2 years following completion of therapy. Frequently both local and distant metastases are present at the time of recurrence (Kaur et al. 2003). Early detection of recurrence and institution of aggressive salvage treatment can result in improved patient survival (Schwarz et al. 2007). In a large prospective trial involving asymptomatic cervical cancer patients with no evidence of disease following treatment, FDG PET imaging identified recurrence in 11 % of patients. The sensitivity was 90 % and specificity 76 % for detection of early recurrence (Ryu et al. 2003). PET/CT identifies distant metastases in nearly 70 % of patients with recurrent disease. The most frequent sites are the retroperitoneal nodes, lung, skeleton, and liver (Son et al. 2010), (Fig. 7).

Distinguishing post-radiation changes from recurrent tumor is challenging with CT or MRI. In patients with clinically suspect but equivocal CT or MRI findings, FDG PET has a sensitivity of 92 % and a specificity of 93 % for identifying recurrence. Tumor recurrence identified by PET/CT has prognostic significance; the median overall survival in patients with positive PET exams is 13 months versus 85 % survival at 60 months in the PET negative patients. Restaging with PET changed planned treatment in 60–65 % of cases (van der Veldt et al. 2008). PET/CT can play an important role in clarifying the diagnosis in clinically suspected recurrence (Kaur et al. 2003).

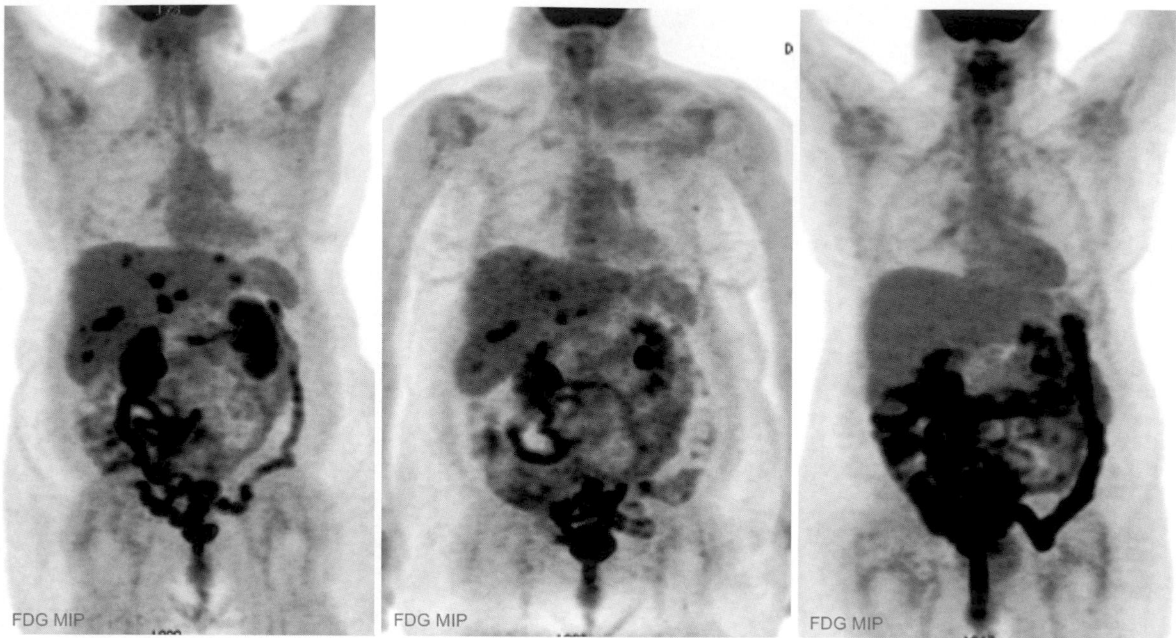

Fig. 7 This 52-year-old woman with a history of cervical cancer 5 years prior treated with radiation therapy now presents for restaging. FDG PET/CT scan demonstrated numerous FDG-avid metastases scattered throughout the liver. CT-guided biopsy confirmed metastatic disease. Chemotherapy was initiated and PET/CT at 3 months (*center image*) showed decrease in number size and intensity of liver metastases and at 6 months resolution of lesions (MIP image on *right*)

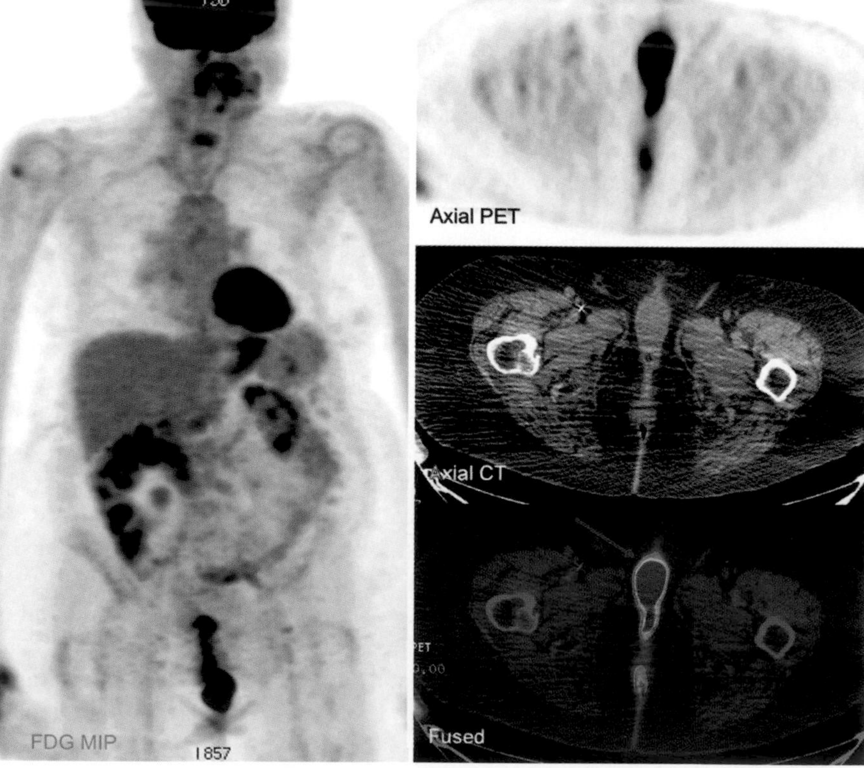

Fig. 8 This 89-year-old woman presented for evaluation of a vulvar mass. PET/CT demonstrates a 4 × 3 × 4 cm intensely FDG-avid (SUV_{max} 10.3) vulvar mass (*arrow*) with the no evidence for nodal or distant metastases. The patient was treated with combined chemotherapy and radiotherapy

6 Vulvar and Vaginal Cancers

Vulvar and vaginal cancers are uncommon and account for about 3–4 % of gynecologic cancers in the US. The cancers are usually a squamous cell skin malignancy and most often occur in elderly women. Human papillomavirus infection is a major risk factor. Vulvar cancer frequently presents as a palpable lesion, whereas the most common symptom of vaginal cancer is abnormal bleeding. Diagnosis is by biopsy. Vulvar and vaginal cancers spread by direct extension into the urethra, bladder, vagina, perineum, anus, or rectum and to locoregional inguinal lymph nodes, similar to most squamous cell malignancies. Staging is based on tumor size and location and on regional lymph node spread (Shah et al. 2009; Woelber et al. 2011; Wu et al. 2008). Treatment traditionally was wide excision and lymph node dissection with a hysterectomy for vaginal cancers. Recently, radiation therapy has become more common to avoid extensive surgery and preserve function (Grigsby 2002; Oonk et al. 2010).

Intense FDG uptake is present in primary vulvar and vaginal cancers and nodal and distant metastases (Fig. 8), but the published data on FDG PET/CT imaging in the management of these two malignancies is limited. In a prospective study comparing FDG PET to surgical pathology, PET demonstrated a sensitivity of 80 %, specificity of 90 %, a positive predictive value of 80 %, and a negative predictive value of 90 % for nodal metastases. PET was more accurate in detecting extranodal than nodal metastases (Cohn et al. 2002). FDG PET was prospectively compared with CT in evaluating 23 patients with vaginal carcinoma. PET visualized the intact primary tumor in 100 % of the patients and abnormal inguinal and pelvic nodes in 35 %, while CT found only 43 % of the primary tumors and 17 % of the inguinal and pelvic nodes (Lamoreaux et al. 2005).

7 PET/MR

Ultrasonography is the major imaging tool for evaluating potential and known malignancies in the pelvis. MRI of the female genital organs is a useful adjunctive imaging technique in newly detected uterine and ovarian masses. MRI's strength is in the depiction of local tumor extent. The role of PET/CT in gynecologic oncology cancers is growing and slowly expanding. Integrated PET/CT with the CT as the transmission scan and contrast-enhanced CT combined with FDG PET plays important clinical roles in identifying distant nodal and hematologic metastases, detecting extent of recurrence, and measuring response to therapy.

Hybrid PET/MR has a number of technical hurdles to clear before clinical use begins. One large clinical problem is throughput. Currently 45–60 min is required for MRI procedures of the pelvis. The MRI time would double the current PET/CT scan duration. It is not clear whether simultaneously performing PET and MRI will be of additive clinical value compared to the two performed separately. The possibility of adding MRI's distinct utility in T staging of gynecologic tumors to FDG PET evaluation of nodal and distant is attractive, but substantial clinical investigation is required.

References

Avril N, Sassen S, Schmalfeldt B et al (2005) Prediction of response to neoadjuvant chemotherapy by sequential F-18-fluorodeoxyglucose positron emission tomography in patients with advanced-stage ovarian cancer. J Clin Oncol 23:7445–7453

Ben-Haim S, Ell P (2009) ^{18}F-FDG PET and PET/CT in the evaluation of cancer treatment response. J Nucl Med 50:88–99

Chung HH, Kang WJ, Kim JW et al (2007) Role of (18F) FDG PET/CT in the assessment of suspected recurrent ovarian cancer: correlation with clinical or histological findings. Eur J Nucl Med Mol Imaging 34:480–486

Cohn DE, Dehdashti F, Gibb RK et al (2002) Prospective evaluation of positron emission tomography for the detection of groin node metastases from vulvar cancer. Gynecol Oncol 85:179–184

Elit L, Bondy SJ, Paszat L et al (2002) Outcomes in surgery for ovarian cancer. Gynecol Oncol 87:260

Esthappan J, Chaudhari S, Santanam L et al (2008) Prospective clinical trial of positron emission tomography/computed tomography image-guided intensity-modulated radiation therapy for cervical carcinoma with positive para-aortic lymph nodes. Int J Radiat Oncol Biol Phys 72:1134–1139

Fagotti A, Fanfani F, Rositto C et al (2008) A treatment selection protocol for recurrent ovarian cancer patients: the role of FDG-PET/CT and staging laparoscopy. Oncology 75:152–158

Fenchel S, Grab D, Nuessle K et al (2002) Asymptomatic adnexal masses: correlation of FDG PET and histopathologic findings. Radiology 223(3):780–788

Goff BA, Mandel LS, Melancon CH et al (2004) Frequency of symptoms of ovarian cancer in women presenting to primary care clinics. JAMA 291:2705–2712

Greenlee RT, Hill Harmon MB, Murray T, Thun M (2001) Cancer statistics, 2001. CA Cancer J Clin 51:15–36

Grigsby PW (2002) Vaginal cancer. Curr Treat Options Oncol 3:125–130

Horowitz NS, Dehdashti F, Herzog TJ et al (2004) Prospective evaluation of FDG-PET for detecting pelvic and para-aortic lymph node metastasis in uterine corpus cancer. Gynecol Oncol 95:546–551

Iagaru AH, Mittra ES, McDougall IR et al (2008) 18F-FDG PET/CT evaluation of patients with ovarian carcinoma. Nucl Med Commun 29:1046–1051

Irvin WP, Rice LW, Berkowitz RS (2002) Advances in the management of endometrial adenocarcinoma. J Reprod Med 47:173–190

Iyer VR, Lee SI (2010) MRI, CT, and PET/CT for ovarian cancer detection and adenexal lesion characterization. Am J Roentgenol 194:311–321

Jemal A, Siegel R, Ward E et al (2009) Cancer statistics, 2009. CA Cancer J Clin 59:225–249

Kang S, Kim SK, Chung DC et al (2010) Diagnostic value of (18)F-FDG PET for evaluation of paraaortic nodal metastasis in patients with cervical carcinoma: a metaanalysis. J Nucl Med 51(3):360–367

Kaur H, Silverman PM, Iyer RB, Verschraegen CF, Eifel PJ, Charnsangavej C (2003) Diagnosis, staging, and surveillance of cervical carcinoma. Am J Roentgenol 180(6):1621–1631

Kitajima K, Murakami K, Yamasaki E et al (2008) Accuracy of 18F-FDG PET/CT in detecting pelvic and paraaortic lymph node metastasis in patients with endometrial cancer. Am J Roentgenol 190(6):1652–1658

Kitajima K, Murakami K, Kaji Y, Sugimura K (2010) Spectrum of FDG PET/CT findings of uterine tumors. Am J Roentgenol 195(3):737–743

Kitajima K, Murakami K, Yamasaki E et al (2009) Accuracy of integrated FDG-PET/contrast-enhanced CT in detecting pelvic and paraaortic lymph node metastasis in patients with uterine cancer. Eur Radiol 19:1529–1536

Kubik-Huch RA, Dörffler W, von Schulthess GK et al (2000) Value of (18F)-FDG positron emission tomography, computed tomography, and magnetic resonance imaging in diagnosing primary and recurrent ovarian carcinoma. Eur Radiol 10(5):761–767

Kumar R, Alavi A (2004) PET imaging in gynecologic malignancies. Radiol Clin North Am 42:1155–1167

Lamoreaux WT, Grigsby PW, Dehdashti F et al (2005) FDG-PET evaluation of vaginal carcinoma. Int J Radiat Oncol Biol Phys 62:733–737

Lerman H, Metser U, Grisaru D, Fishman A, Lievshitz G, Even-Sapir E (2004) Normal and abnormal 18F-FDG endometrial and ovarian uptake in pre- and postmenopausal patients: assessment by PET/CT. J Nucl Med 45:266–271

Lin LL, Grigsby PW, Powell MA, Mutch DG (2005) Definitive radiotherapy in the management of isolated vaginal recurrences of endometrial cancer. Int J Radiat Oncol Biol Phys 63:500–504

Lin LL, Mutic S, Low DA et al (2007) Adaptive brachytherapy treatment planning for cervical cancer using FDG-PET. Int J Radiat Oncol Biol Phys 67:91–96

Ma SY et al (2003) Delayed 18F-FDG PET for detection of paraaortic lymph node metastatses in cervical cancer patients. J Nucl Med 44:1775–1783

Macdonald DM, Lin LL, Biehl K et al (2008) Combined intensity-modulated radiation therapy and brachytherapy in the treatment of cervical cancer. Int J Radiat Oncol Biol Phys 71:618–624

Manfredi R, Mirk P, Maresca G et al (2004) Local-regional staging of endometrial carcinoma: role of MR imaging in surgical planning. Radiology 231(2):372–378

Mangili G, Picchio M, Sironi S (2007) Integrated PET/CT as a first-line re-staging modality in patients with suspected recurrence of ovarian cancer. Eur J Nucl Med Mol Imaging 34:658–666

Nakamura K, Kodama J, Okumura Y et al (2010) The SUVmax of ^{18}F-FDG PET correlates with histological grade in endometrial cancer. Int J Gynecol Cancer 20:110–115

Oonk MH, de Hullu JA, van der Zee AG (2010) Current controversies in the management of patients with early-stage vulvar cancer. Curr Opin Oncol 22:481–486

Pandharipande PV, Choy G, del Carmen MG, Gazelle GS, Russell AH, Lee SI (2009) MRI and PET/CT for triaging stage IB clinically operable cervical cancer to appropriate therapy: decision analysis to assess patient outcomes. Am J Roentgenol 192(3):802–814

Pandit-Taskar N (2005) Oncologic imaging in gynecologic malignancies. J Nucl Med 46:1842–1850

Pannu HK, Corl FM, Fishman EK (2001) CT evaluation of cervical cancer: spectrum of disease. Radiographics 21(5):1155–1168

Park JY, Kim EN, Kim DY et al (2008) Clinical impact of positron emission tomography or positron emission tomography/computed tomography in the posttherapy surveillance of endometrial carcinoma: evaluation of 88 patients. Int J Gynecol Cancer 18(6):1332–1338

Patel CN, Nazir SA, Khan Z, Gleeson FV, Bradley KM (2011) 18F-FDG PET/CT of cervical carcinoma. Am J Roentgenol 196(5):1225–1233

Pecorelli S (2009) Revised FIGO staging for carcinoma of the vulva, cervix, and endometrium. Int J Gynaecol Obstet 105:103–104

Permuth-Wey J, Sellers TA (2009) Epidemiology of ovarian cancer. Methods Mol Biol 472:413–437

Peters WA, Liu PY, Barrett RJ et al (2000) Concurrent chemotherapy and pelvic radiation therapy compared with pelvic radiation therapy alone as adjuvant therapy after radical surgery in high-risk early-stage cancer of the cervix. J Clin Oncol 18:1606–1613

Petignat P, Vajda D, Joris F, Obrist R (2000) Surgical management of epithelial ovarian cancer at community hospitals: a population-based study. J Surg Oncol 75:119

Picchio M, Mangili G, Samanes Gajate AM et al (2010) High-grade endometrial cancer: value of (^{18}F)FDG PET/CT in preoperative staging. Nucl Med Commun 31:506–512

Pilleron JP, Durand JC, Hamelin JP (1974) Prognostic value of node metastasis in cancer of the uterine cervix. Am J Obstet Gynecol 119:458

Rockall AG, Sohaib SA, Harisinghani MG et al (2005) Diagnostic performance of nanoparticle-enhanced magnetic resonance imaging in the diagnosis of lymph node metastases in patients with endometrial and cervical cancer. J Clin Oncol 23:2813–2821

Roman LD, Muderspach LI, Stein SM et al (1997) Pelvic examination, tumor marker level, and gray-scale and Doppler sonography in the prediction of pelvic cancer. Obstet Gynecol 89:493

Rose PG, Bundy BN, Watkins EB et al (1999) Concurrent cisplatin-based radiotherapy and chemotherapy for locally advanced cervical cancer. N Engl J Med 340:1144–1153

Rose PG, Nerenstone S, Brady MF et al (2004) Secondary surgical cytoreduction for advanced ovarian carcinoma. N Engl J Med 351:2489–2497

Rustin GJ, Nelstrop AE, Tuxen MK, Lambert HE (1996) Defining progression of ovarian carcinoma during follow-up according to CA 125: a North Thames Ovary Group study. Ann Oncol 7:361–364

Ryu SY, Kim MH, Choi SC, Choi CW, Lee KH (2003) Detection of early recurrence with 18F-FDG PET in patients with cervical cancer. J Nucl Med 44(3):347–352

Sala E, Kataoka M, Pandit-Taskar N et al (2010) Recurrent ovarian cancer: use of contrast-enhanced CT and PET/CT to accurately localize tumor recurrence and to predict patients' survival. Radiology 257(1):125–134

Schröder W, Zimny M, Rudlowski C, Büll U, Rath W (1999) The role of 18F-fluoro-deoxyglucose positron emission tomography (18F-FDG PET) in diagnosis of ovarian cancer. Int J Gynecol Cancer 9(2):117–122

Schutter EM, Sohn C, Kristen P et al (1998) Estimation of probability of malignancy using a logistic model combining physical examination, ultrasound, serum CA 125, and serum CA 72-4 in postmenopausal women with a pelvic mass: an international multicenter study. Gynecol Oncol 69:56–63

Schwarz JK, Siegel BA, Dehdashti F, Grigsby PW (2007) Association of posttherapy positron emission tomography with tumor response and survival in cervical carcinoma. JAMA 298(19):2289–2295

Sebastian S, Lee SI, Horowitz NS et al (2008) PET-CT vs CT alone in ovarian cancer recurrence. Abdom Imaging 33:112–118

Sedlis A, Bundy BN, Rotman MZ et al (1999) A randomized trial of pelvic radiation therapy versus no further therapy in selected patients with stage IB carcinoma of the cervix after radical hysterectomy and pelvic lymphadenectomy: a gynecologic oncology group study. Gynecol Oncol 73:177–183

Shah CA, Goff BA, Lowe K, Peters WA 3rd, Li CI (2009) Factors affecting risk of mortality in women with vaginal cancer. Obstet Gynecol 113:1038–1045

Signorelli M, Guerra L, Buda A et al (2009) Role of the integrated FDG PET/CT in the surgical management of patients with high risk clinical early stage endometrial cancer: detection of pelvic nodal metastases. Gynecol Oncol 115:231–235

Simcock B, Neesham D, Quinn M (2006) The impact of PET/CT in the management of recurrent ovarian cancer. Gynecol Oncol 103:271–276

Sironi S, Buda A, Picchio M et al (2006) Lymph node metastasis in patients with clinical early-stage cervical cancer: detection with integrated FDG PET/CT. Radiology 238(1):272–279

Sironi S, Messa C, Mangili G et al (2004) Integrated FDG PET/CT in patients with persistent ovarian cancer: correlation with histological findings. Radiology 233:433–440

Son H, Kositwattanarerk A, Hayes MP et al (2010) PET/CT evaluation of cervical cancer: spectrum of disease. Radiographics 30(5):1251–1268

Sugiyama T, Nishida T, Ushijima K et al.(1995) Detection of lymph node metastasis in ovarian carcinoma and uterine corpus carcinoma by preoperative computerized tomography or magnetic resonance imaging. J Obstet Gynaecol (Tokyo 1995) 21:551–556

van der Burg ME, van Lent M, Buyse M et al (1995) The effect of debulking surgery after induction chemotherapy on the prognosis in advanced epithelial ovarian cancer. Gynecological Cancer Cooperative Group of the European Organization for Research and Treatment of Cancer. N Engl J Med 332:629–634

van der Veldt AA, Buist MR, van Baal MW, Comans EF, Hoekstra OS, Molthoff CF (2008) Clarifying the diagnosis of clinically suspected recurrence of cervical cancer: impact of 18F-FDG PET. J Nucl Med 49(12):1936–1943

Woelber L, Kock L, Gieseking F, Petersen C, Trillsch F, Choschzick M, Jaenicke F, Mahner S (2011) Clinical management of primary vulvar cancer. Eur J Cancer 47:2315–2321

Wu X, Matanoski G, Chen VW, Saraiya M, Coughlin SS, King JB, Tao XG (2008) Descriptive epidemiology of vaginal cancer incidence and survival by race, ethnicity, and age in the United States. Cancer 113(10):2873–2882

Yen TC, See LC, Lai CH et al (2004a) 18F-FDG uptake in squamous cell carcinoma of the cervix is correlated with glucose transporter 1 expression. J Nucl Med 45(1):22–29

Yen TC, See LC, Chang TC et al (2004b) Defining the priority of using 18F-FDG PET for recurrent cervical cancer. J Nucl Med 45(10):1632–1639

Yoshida Y, Kurokawa T, Kawahara K et al (2004) Incremental benefits of FDG positron emission tomography over CT alone for the preoperative staging of ovarian cancer. Am J Roentgenol 182(1):227–233

Musculoskeletal

Jeffrey J. Peterson

Contents

J. J. Peterson (✉)
Department of Radiology, Mayo Clinic,
4500 San Pablo Road, Jacksonville,
FL 32224-3899, USA
e-mail: Peterson.Jeffrey@mayo.edu

Abstract

PET imaging with Fluorine-18 2-Fluoro-2-Deoxyglucose or FDG PET can be quite useful for both primary bone tumors and soft tissue sarcomas. There are major indications for PET imaging for malignant processes including screening, diagnosis, staging, restaging, and monitoring response to therapy (Bestic et al. (Radiographics 29(5):1487–1500, 2009; Piperkova et al. Clin Nuclear Med 34 (3): 146–150, 2009). FDG PET has a limited role in the diagnosis of musculoskeletal tumors and has no role in screening for such lesions. PET has however proven quite efficacious for staging and restaging of musculoskeletal tumors (Bestic et al. Radiographics 29(5):1487–1500, 2009; Piperkova et al. Clin Nuclear Med 34(3):146–150, 2009). In addition PET can be useful for evaluating response to therapy of musculoskeletal tumors (Benz et al. Clin Cancer Res 15(8):2856–2863, 2009; Iagaru et al. Clin Nuclear Med 33(1):8–13, 2008). Most musculoskeletal lesions are sufficiently glucose-avid for FDG PET to reliably depict distant tumor involvement, local spread or recurrence (Charest et al. Euro J Null Med Mol Imaging 36:1944–1951, 2009). This chapter will examine the current utility and applications of FDG PET imaging for evaluation of musculoskeletal neoplasms.

1 Introduction

Positron emission tomography (PET) and PET combined with computed tomography (PET/CT) can be very helpful in the evaluation of musculoskeletal

P. Peller et al. (eds.), *PET-CT and PET-MRI in Oncology*, Medical Radiology. Diagnostic Imaging,
DOI: 10.1007/174_2011_529,

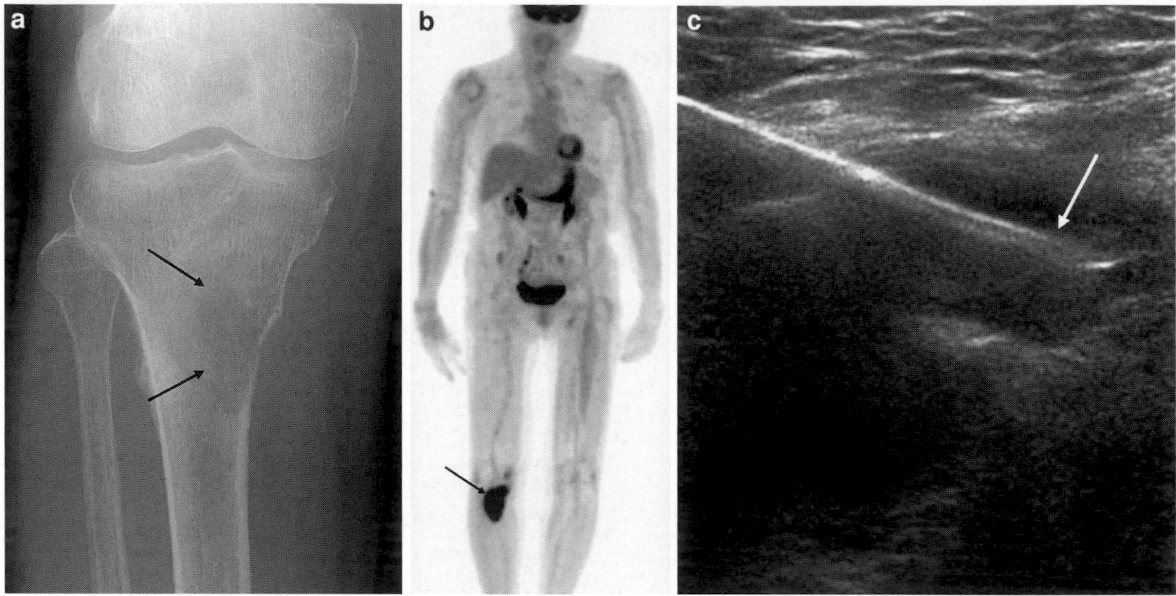

Fig. 1 **a** Anteroposterior radiograph of the knee depicts an ill-defined lesion (*arrows*) in the left proximal tibia with poorly defined non-sclerotic margins. Although nonspecific, the lesion presents features suggestive of a primary malignant bone tumor. **b** Whole-body FDG PET depicts increased metabolic activity within the lesion (*arrow*). No distant metastases were identified. PET proved useful for staging in this case but provided limited diagnostic information. Detecting activity within the lesion did not contribute to obtaining the exact diagnosis of this lesion and could not allow confident determination of malignancy. **c** The tissue diagnosis of malignant fibrous histiocytoma was obtained with an ultrasound-guided biopsy (*arrow*) of soft tissue extension of the osseous lesion

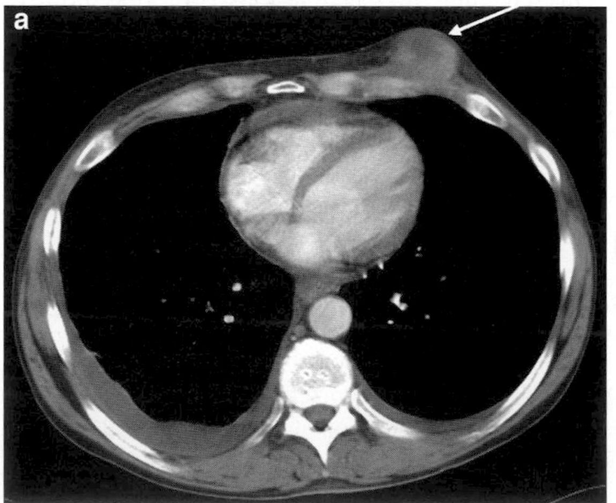

Fig. 2 **a** Axial CT depicts an enhancing soft tissue mass (*arrow*) in the left anterior chest corresponding to a palpable lesion. **b** PET imaging depicts increased FDG accumulation within the lesion (*arrow*) which, however, provided little diagnostic information. PET's lack of specificity made definite confirmation of malignancy impossible and percutaneous biopsy was necessary

neoplasms. (El-Zeftawy et al. 2001; Suzuki et al. 2004; Peterson 2007). PET imaging with Fluorine-18 2-Fluoro-2-Deoxyglucose or FDG PET can be useful for both primary bone tumors and soft tissue sarcomas (Charest et al. 2009). While FDG PET has a limited role in the diagnosis of such lesions, PET has proven efficacious for staging and restaging of musculoskeletal tumors (Volker et al. 2007; Piperkova et al. 2009)

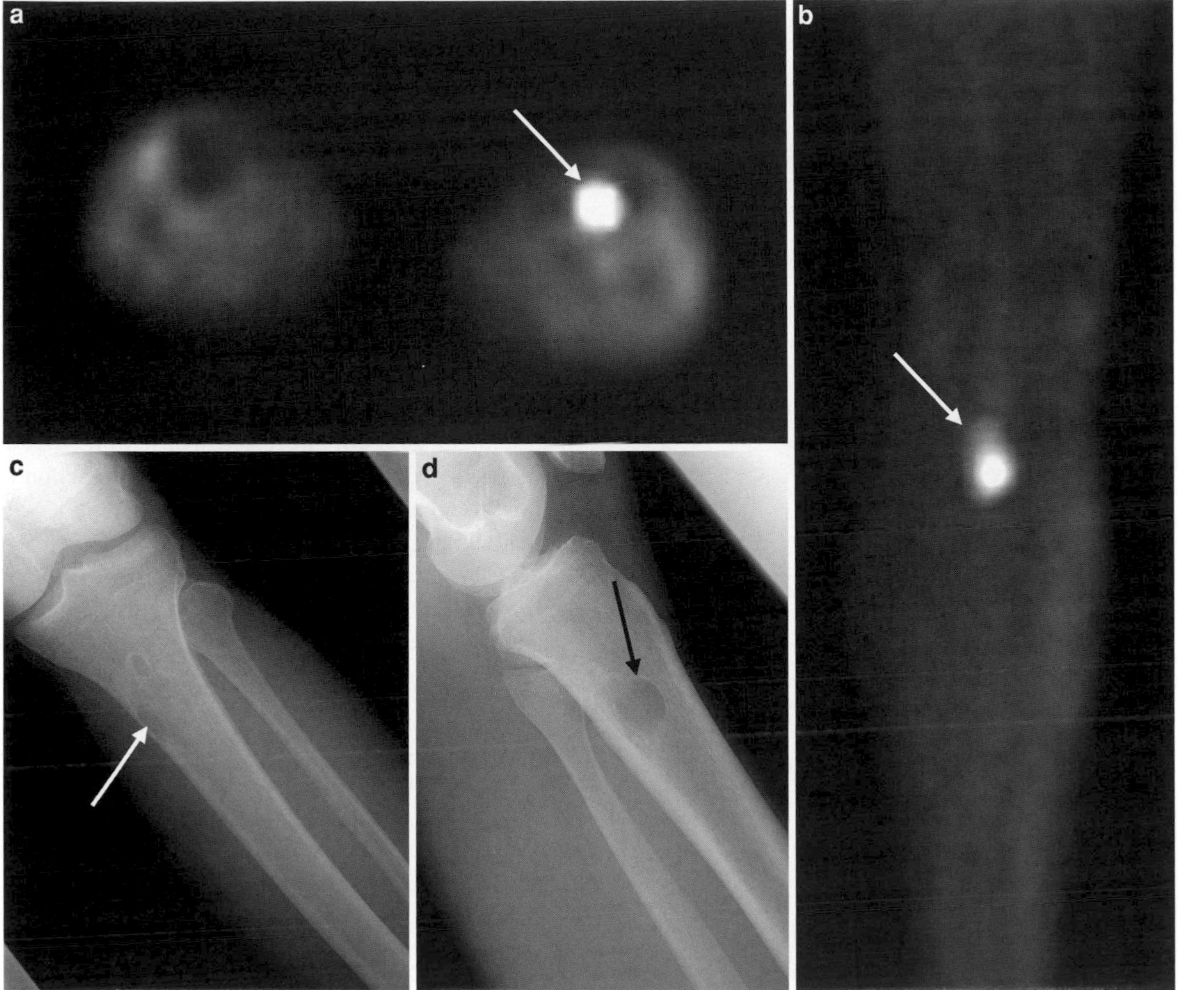

Fig. 3 Axial (**a**) and coronal (**b**) images from a PET scan shows increased metabolic activity within the left proximal tibia. Correlation with anteroposterior (**c**) and (**d**) lateral radiographs of the tibia confirms a benign fibro-osseous lesion (*arrows*) within the proximal tibia most compatible with a non-ossifying fibroma. Comparison with radiographs taken 2 years previously confirmed that the lesion was stable

including detection and depiction of osseous metastatic disease (Heusner et al. 2009; Peterson 2007; Peterson et al. 2003; Daldrup-Link et al. 2001). Most musculoskeletal lesions are sufficiently glucose-avid to allow FDG PET to reliably depict distant tumor involvement, local spread or recurrence (Bastiaannet et al. 2004; Charest et al. 2009). In addition PET can be useful to evaluate response to therapy of musculoskeletal tumors (Benz et al. 2009; Bredella et al. 2002; Iagaru et al. 2008; Hawkins et al. 2002a). Exact staging and restaging of these primary bone and soft tissue tumors are crucial to appropriate treatment planning (Volker et al. 2007; Piperkova et al. 2009). PET can also provide useful information for assessing ultimate patient prognosis (Costelloe et al. 2009; Lisle et al. 2009). This chapter will examine the current utility and applications of FDG PET imaging in the evaluation of musculoskeletal neoplasms.

There are major indications for PET imaging of malignant processes including screening, diagnosis, staging, restaging, and monitoring response to therapy. *Screening* refers to imaging asymptomatic patients for detection of disease that is not previously known or suspected. FDG PET is rarely indicated for screening purposes and is definitely not indicated for screening of musculoskeletal tumors (Peterson 2007). *Diagnosis*

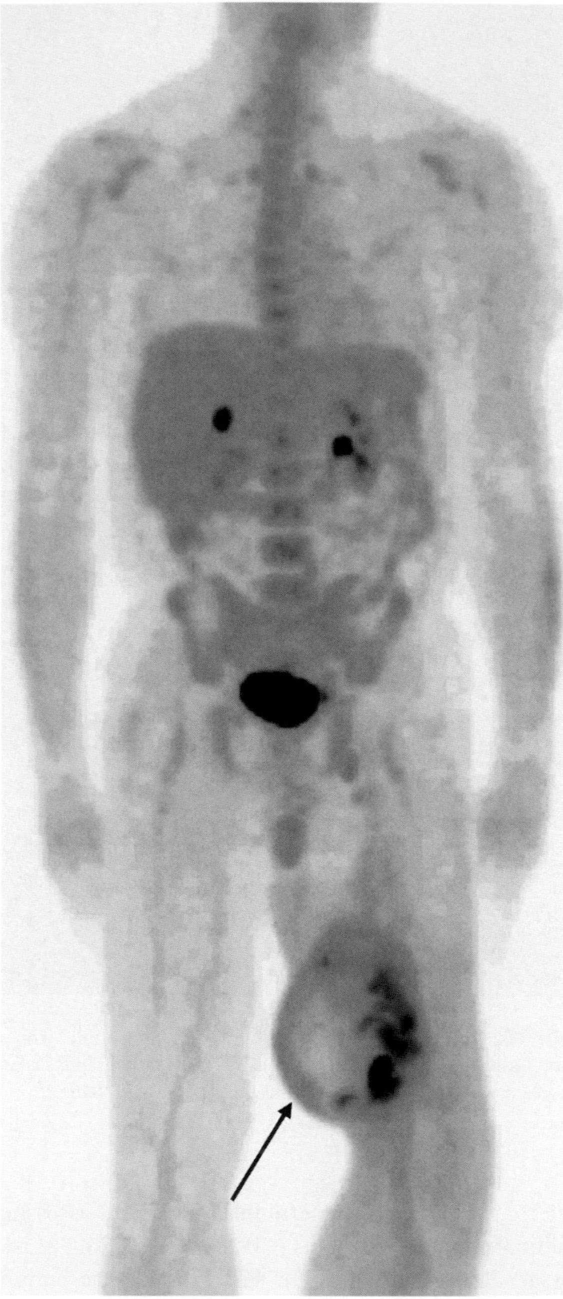

Fig. 4 FDG PET image of a large hemorrhagic soft tissue mass in the left thigh (*arrow*) reveals a large focus of diminished activity centrally, corresponding to central hemorrhage within the lesion as well as foci of increased metabolic activity in the periphery of the lesion, compatible with a viable tumor. Information from the PET image guided the percutaneous image-guided biopsy of the metabolically active tumor toward the periphery of the lesion

refers to the utilization of PET imaging to designate a lesion as malignant or benign prior to histologic evaluation or tissue confirmation. *Staging* with PET imaging involves imaging intended for detection of additional sites of involvement or metastatic disease before initial treatment but after tissue confirmation of the presence of a malignant lesion (Peterson 2007). *Restaging* entails imaging with PET following completion of therapy, to detect additional sites of involvement or to evaluate the extent of recurrent or residual disease. Restaging encompasses assessment of both primary and secondary lesions with evaluation of both the original tumor site/s and evaluation for metastatic disease. *Monitoring response to therapy* is defined as PET imaging before or after completion of therapy to appraise the efficacy of the therapy. Again this entails evaluation of both primary and secondary disease (Peterson 2007). There is obviously overlap in restaging and monitoring response to therapy. This chapter will further examine the utility and efficacy of FDG PET imaging for each of these indications.

2 Diagnosis

The imaging techniques most useful for the diagnosis of soft tissue and osseous lesions are typically anatomic imaging modalities including radiography, magnetic resonance imaging (MRI) and CT (Ho 2005; Peterson 2007). Imaging with these conventional methods reveals the morphological properties of the lesion such as tumor size and extent, tumor margins, and involvement of adjacent structures (Ho 2005; Peterson 2007). Anatomic imaging can also help to establish the diagnosis by evaluating the physical characteristics of the tumor according to its density and attenuation on radiographs and CT, and signal intensity on MRI. The most useful modality to assess osseous lesions initially and to establish the differential diagnosis is conventional radiography (Ho 2005; Peterson 2007). CT and MRI can be useful adjuncts to radiography to more precisely characterize the morphology and composition of both soft tissue and osseous lesions. Ultimately, histologic analysis of specimens obtained by image-guided biopsy or open surgical biopsy, is the definitive method of

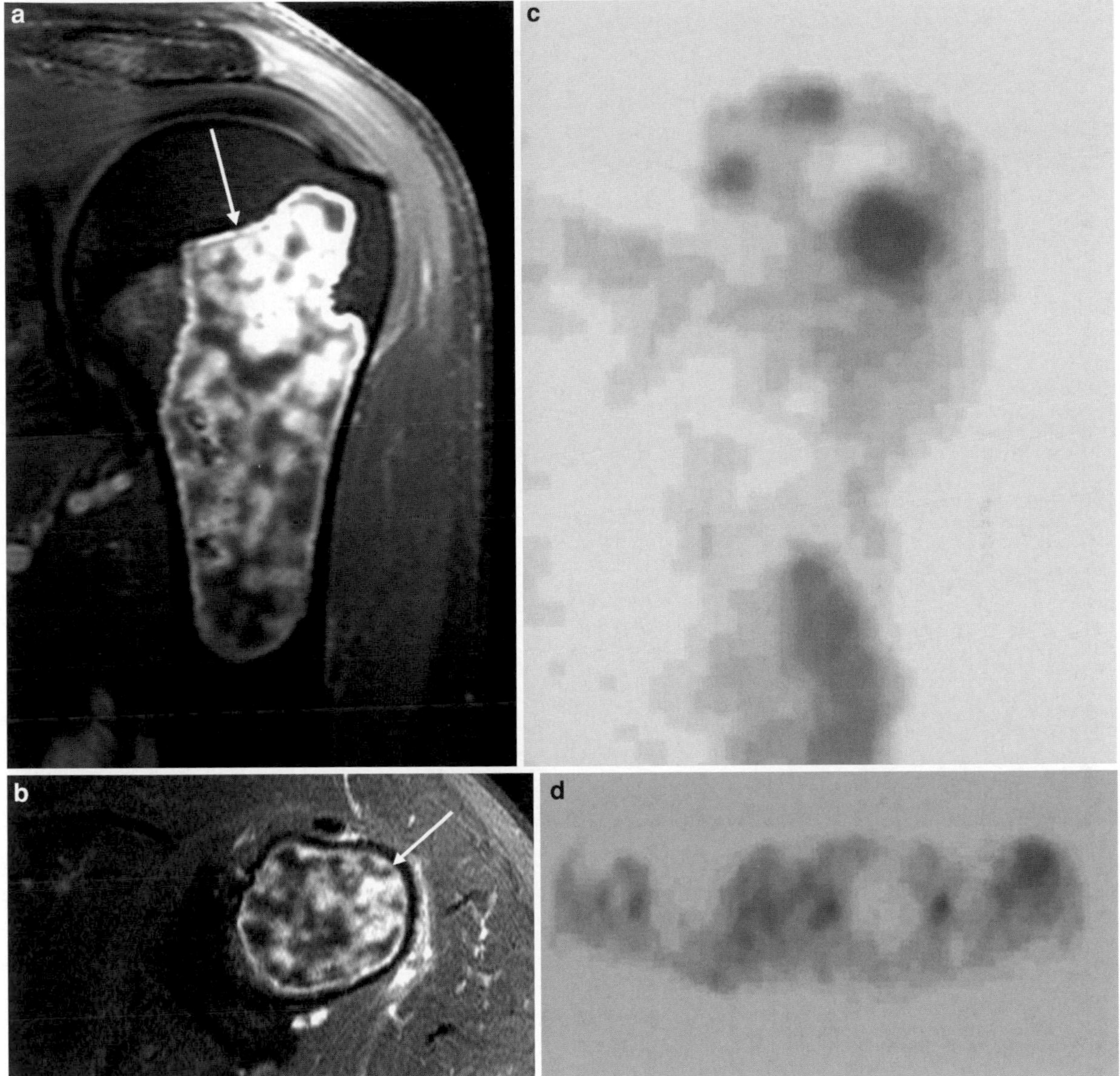

Fig. 5 Coronal (**a**) and axial (**b**) MRIs depict a cartilaginous lesion (*arrows*) in the left proximal humerus with associated endosteal scalloping. Subsequent coronal (**c**) and axial (**d**) FDG PET images demonstrate no significant abnormal metabolic activity corresponding to the lesion, suggesting benign enchondroma. The lesion remained stable in the appearance on follow-up radiographs and MRI examinations

establishing the diagnosis of musculoskeletal neoplasms (Fig. 1) (Ho 2005; Peterson 2007).

There are inherent limitations of the use of physiologic nuclear medicine techniques such as FDG PET imaging for the diagnosis of musculoskeletal tumors. While metabolic activity is accurately assessed with nuclear medicine techniques, morphology and tissue characterization, which are critical for diagnosis of lesions, are limited with nuclear medicine imaging (Fig. 2). In addition, specificity is a concern with PET for the diagnosis of musculoskeletal lesions. A wide variety of benign lesions including fibrous dysplasia, fibroxanthomas, and giant cell tumors may depict significant FDG accumulation (Fig. 3) (Aoki et al. 2001; Goodin et al. 2006). Currently, there is no well defined role for physiologic nuclear medicine imaging, such as FDG PET, in the initial diagnosis of primary osseous lesions.

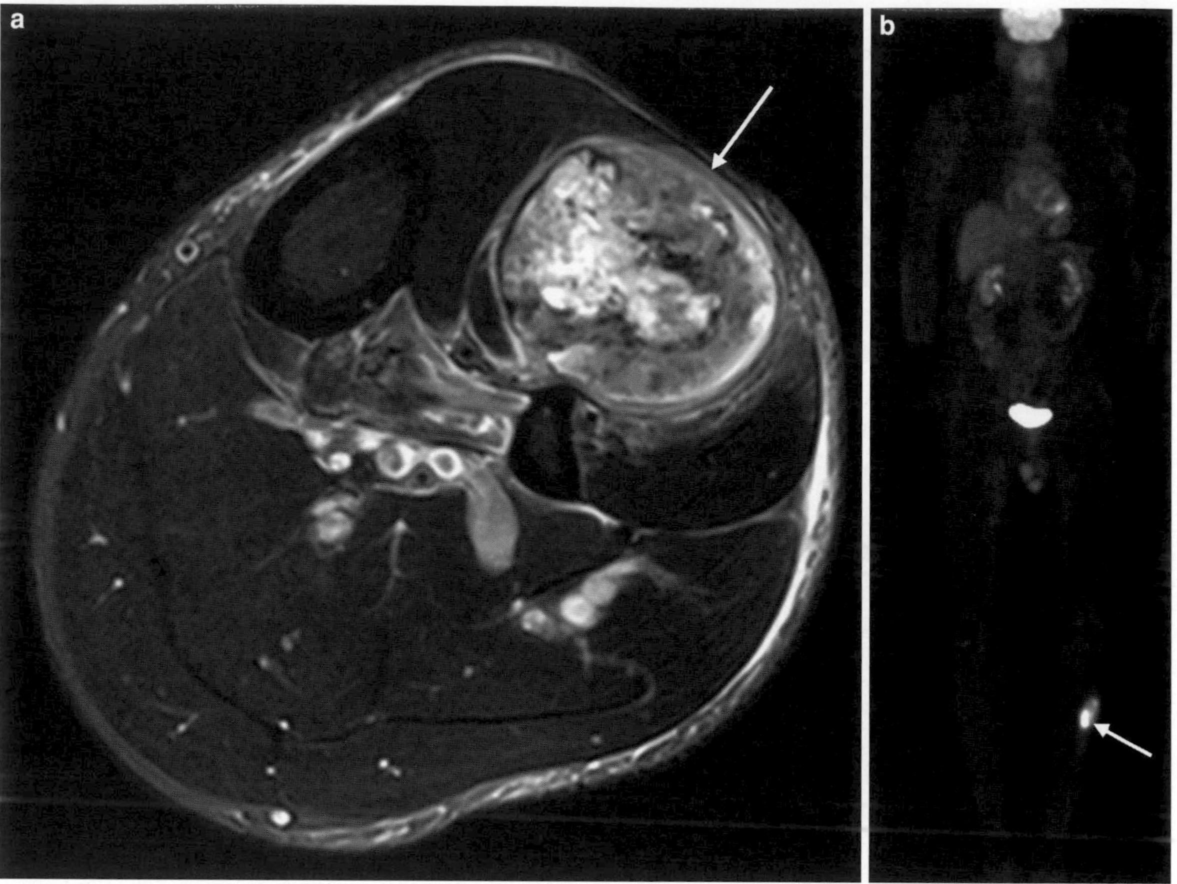

Fig. 6 **a** Axial MRI of the left calf depicts a mass (*arrow*) in the anterior compartment with imaging features suggesting a soft tissue sarcoma. **b** FDG PET obtained for staging depicts increased FDG accumulation within the primary lesion in the left calf (*arrow*) but no abnormal activity elsewhere to suggest local or distant metastases. Treatment planning thus focused on the local tumor with wide margin excision

The use of FDG PET imaging for the diagnosis of musculoskeletal tumors is being widely studied. In heterogeneous lesions with internal hemorrhage or necrosis PET imaging can be useful to guide the biopsy to sites of metabolically active tumor rather than areas of blood or necrosis (Klaeser et al. 2009; O'Sullivan et al. 2008) (Fig. 4). Feldman et al. have also reported the possibility of using FDG PET imaging to differentiate benign from malignant osteochondromas based on standard uptake values of the lesions (Fig. 5)(Feldman et al. 2005, 2006). Research is also underway to determine if FDG PET can provide diagnostic information by characterizing lesions as high or low grade based on metabolic activity. Examples include chondrosarcoma and liposarcoma in which subtypes of the lesion can be either high, intermediate, or low grade (Bastiaannet et al. 2004; Feldman et al. 2005; Brenner et al. 2004).

3 Staging

Staging of a lesion entails detection of additional sites of involvement or metastatic disease before initial treatment, but after tissue confirmation of a malignant lesion (Peterson 2007). Initial staging of musculoskeletal lesions is essential for establishing treatment planning (Volker et al. 2007; Piperkova et al. 2009). Prompt detection and localization of both local and distant spread of disease can allow timely initiation of appropriate treatment options and can improve the prognosis of patients with newly diagnosed primary bone tumors and soft tissue sarcomas (El-Zeftawy

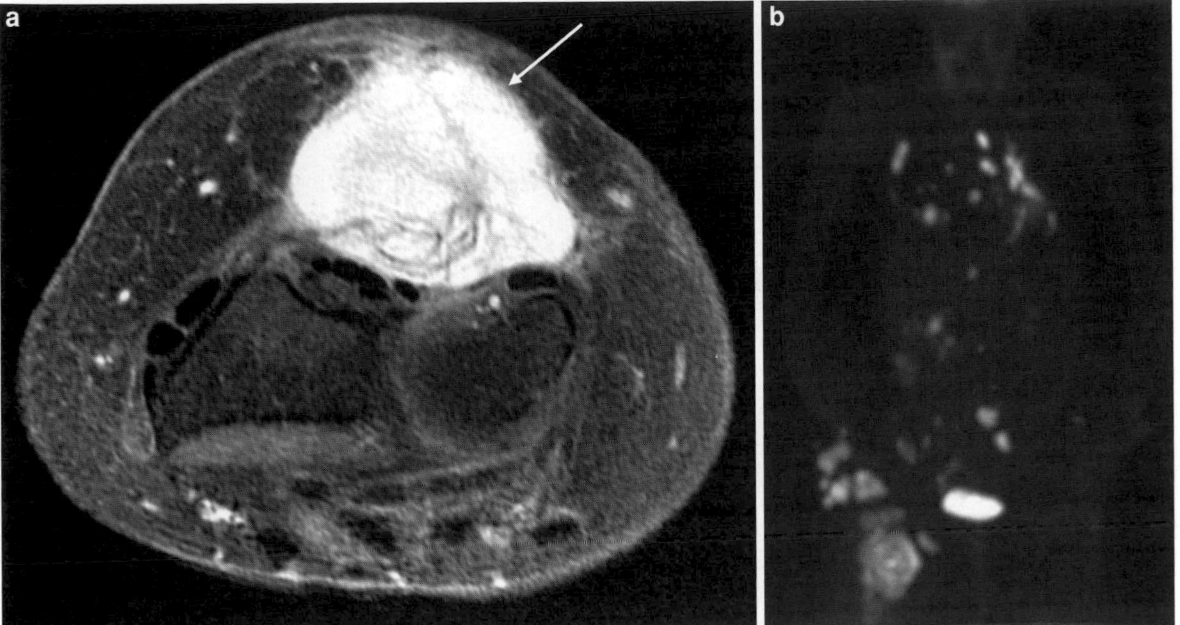

Fig. 7 **a** Post contrast MRI of the wrist in a patient with a palpable mass (*arrow*) along the dorsum depicts an enhancing mass corresponding to the palpable abnormality. **b** FDG PET obtained for staging unexpectedly depicts numerous foci of metabolic activity which are consistent with metastases scattered throughout the body. This significantly changed the treatment plan and prognosis for the patient

et al. 2001; Volker et al. 2007) (Fig. 6). Staging involves assessing both local tumor extent and the presence or absence of distant metastatic disease. This information is crucial for development of effective treatment plans for patients with primary bone tumors and soft tissue sarcomas (Volker et al. 2007; Ho 2005; Jadvar et al. 2004) (Fig. 7). Soft tissue sarcomas arise from the mesenchymal tissues and can invade the surrounding tissues or disseminate hematogenously, most frequently to the lungs (Ho 2005) (Fig. 8). Similarly osseous tumors can extend locally to involve adjacent structures or can spread hematogenously to the lungs, bones, or other organs. In addition to development of an appropriate plan for therapy, accurate detection and delineation of sites and locations of foci of distant metastatic disease may help clarify the overall prognosis for the patient (Volker et al. 2007) (Fig. 9).

Conventional anatomic imaging with radiography, CT, and MRI can demonstrate metastatic disease related to primary bone and soft tissue tumors, although physiologic imaging with nuclear medicine techniques such as bone scintigraphy or FDG PET imaging is often more sensitive (Heusner et al. 2009; McCarville et al. 2005). In the last decade FDG PET has been suggested to have significant advantages over bone scintigraphy for staging malignant tumors (Peterson et al. 2003). FDG PET can identify metastatic disease earlier and with more accuracy than bone scintigraphy. In addition to characterization of the primary tumor, FDG PET provides an excellent method for evaluating the entire body for the presence of metastatic disease involving both the osseous and soft tissue structures (Peterson et al. 2003). McCarville, in a series of 61 patients with childhood sarcoma (including Ewing sarcoma, osteosarcoma, chondrosarcoma, and others), found that FDG PET imaging could be very useful for staging musculoskeletal lesions, especially for identifying previously unsuspected metastases (McCarville et al. 2005). Volker et al. (2007) in a multicenter study of 46 pediatric patients with proven sarcoma showed PET to provide important additional information when compared to conventional imaging modalities with relevant impact on therapy planning.

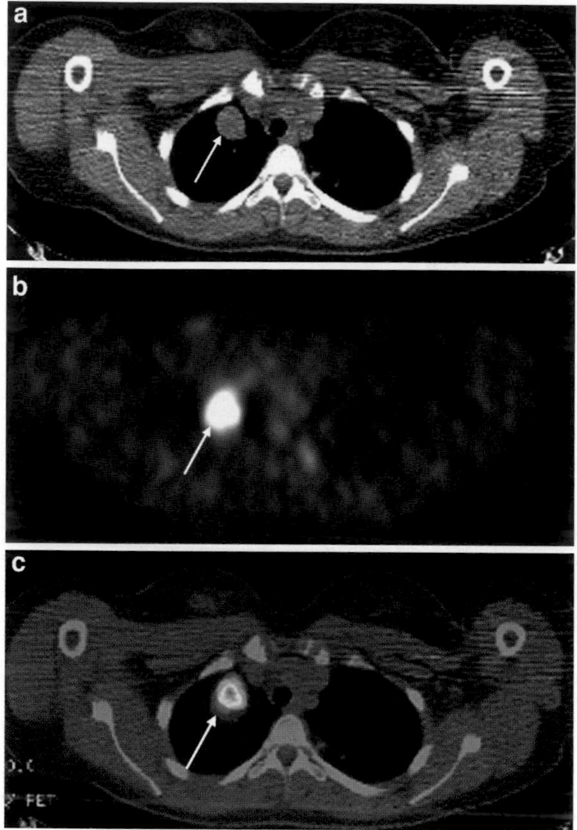

Fig. 8 **a** Axial non-enhanced CT, **b** FDG PET **c** PET/CT fusion images obtained for staging in a young patient with Ewing sarcoma delineate a large mass (*arrows*) in the upper lobe of the right lung with increased metabolic activity, most compatible with a pulmonary metastasis. Therapy was altered to account for the secondary lung lesion as well as the lower extremity primary tumor (*not shown*)

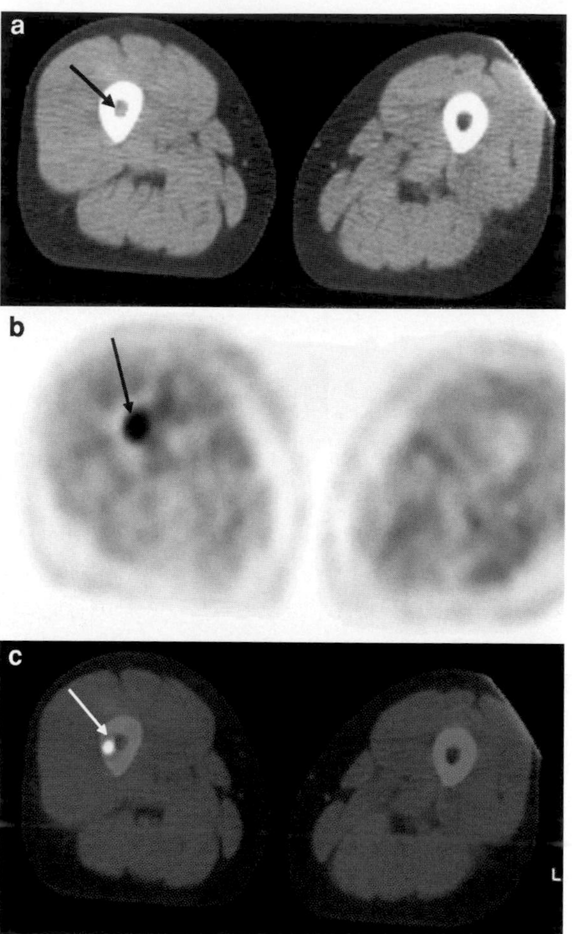

Fig. 9 **a** Axial non-enhanced CT, **b** FDG PET and **c** PET/CT fusion images of the lower extremities in a patient with a left lower extremity Ewing sarcoma depict a focus of increased FDG accumulation (*arrows*) along the lateral cortex of the right proximal femur. Anatomic imaging with CT (A) shows very subtle increased attenuation (*arrow*) of the medullary canal in this region. Subsequent image-guided biopsy confirmed this to be a focus of osseous metastatic disease. This previously unsuspected finding significantly changed the stage and treatment plan

FDG PET has also been shown to be of utility in predicting patient outcomes based on the avidity of FDG accumulation (Costelloe et al. 2009; Franzius et al. 2002a; Eary et al. 2002, Lisle et al. 2009). Franzius, in a study of 29 patients with primary osteosarcoma, concluded that high maximum standard uptake values with FDG PET imaging correlated with poor clinical outcome (Franzius et al. 2002a.) Eary et al. investigated 209 patients with sarcoma and suggested that FDG PET had utility in predicting disease-free survival in tumors; again, tumors with higher maximum standard uptake values had a significantly poorer SUV prognosis (Eary et al. 2002). Costelloe et al. in a study of 31 patients with osteosarcoma found PET imaging to provide useful information related to progression-free survival, overall survival, and tumor necrosis (Costelloe et al. 2009). It appears that FDG PET may be useful for predicting tumor behavior based on lesional characterization at the time of diagnosis (Costelloe et al. 2009; Franzius et al. 2002a; Eary et al. 2002).

Presence of metastatic disease has a considerable influence upon treatment planning and ultimate outcomes in patients with malignant processes (Peterson et al. 2003, Volker et al. 2007). Detection, localization, and characterization of metastases are essential

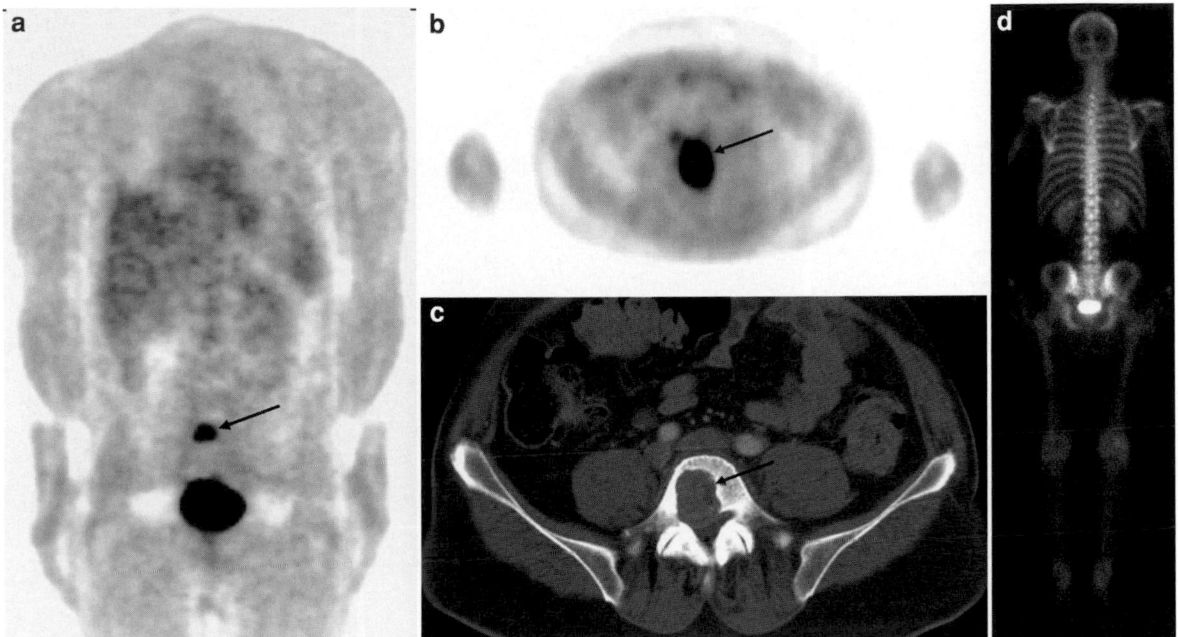

Fig. 10 Coronal (**a**) and axial (**b**) images from an FDG PET obtained for staging purposes in a patient with melanoma depict a hypermetabolic focus (*arrow*) in the L5 vertebra. **c** Axial CT depicts a corresponding lytic lesion (*arrow*) compatible with an osseous metastatic focus. **d** Bone scintigraphy obtained for staging in the same week as the PET scan depicts very little scintigraphic activity in the region of L5. It was postulated that this aggressive lytic lesion progressed faster than the underlying bone could mount a reparative response, limiting the activity seen on the bone scan

to accurate staging of patients with malignancy and in turn have great impact on therapeutic planning (Peterson et al. 2003). The modality best suited for detecting and evaluating metastatic disease varies with the tumor cell type (Peterson et al. 2003). The current standard of practice for the detection of osseous metastatic disease is whole-body scintigraphy. The typical radiopharmaceutical is technetium 99m methylene diphosphonate (Tc-99m MDP) (Peterson 2007). Tc99m MDP is incorporated into the matrix of the osseous structures with uptake based on local blood flow and osteoblastic activity (Peterson et al. 2003; Malhotra and Berman 2002). Bone scintigraphy is very sensitive for advanced osseous metastatic disease, although early involvement can be underdiagnosed as bone scintigraphy depicts the osseous reparative process associated with the lesion rather than delineating the actual tumor (Malhotra and Berman 2002; Peterson 2007). This gives FDG PET the ability to show foci of metastatic disease at an earlier stage than conventional bone scans (Fig. 10) (Peterson et al. 2003; Fogelman et al. 2005). FDG PET imaging has additional advantages over traditional bone scans, including a shorter examination time, with image acquisition and interpretation possible in as little as 2 h (Peterson 2007). PET also has inherently higher spatial resolution compared to conventional gamma cameras used for bone scintigraphy (Peterson et al. 2003). PET imaging also provides multiplanar capability and routinely obtains tomographic images providing excellent anatomic and morphologic detail. Single photon emission computed tomography (SPECT) images must be acquired in addition to standard whole-body planar images for bone scintigraphy to provide equal capability (Peterson et al. 2003).

Over the past decade FDG PET has proven to be an effective alternative to bone scintigraphy with Tc-99m MDP for the detection of metastatic disease in many types of malignancies (Suzuki et al. 2004; Yang et al. 2002; Cook et al. 1998) Staging and the search for metastatic disease has become one of the most widely used musculoskeletal applications of FDG PET imaging (Peterson 2007). PET has been proven to be superior to bone scintigraphy for the detection of osseous metastases for lymphoma,

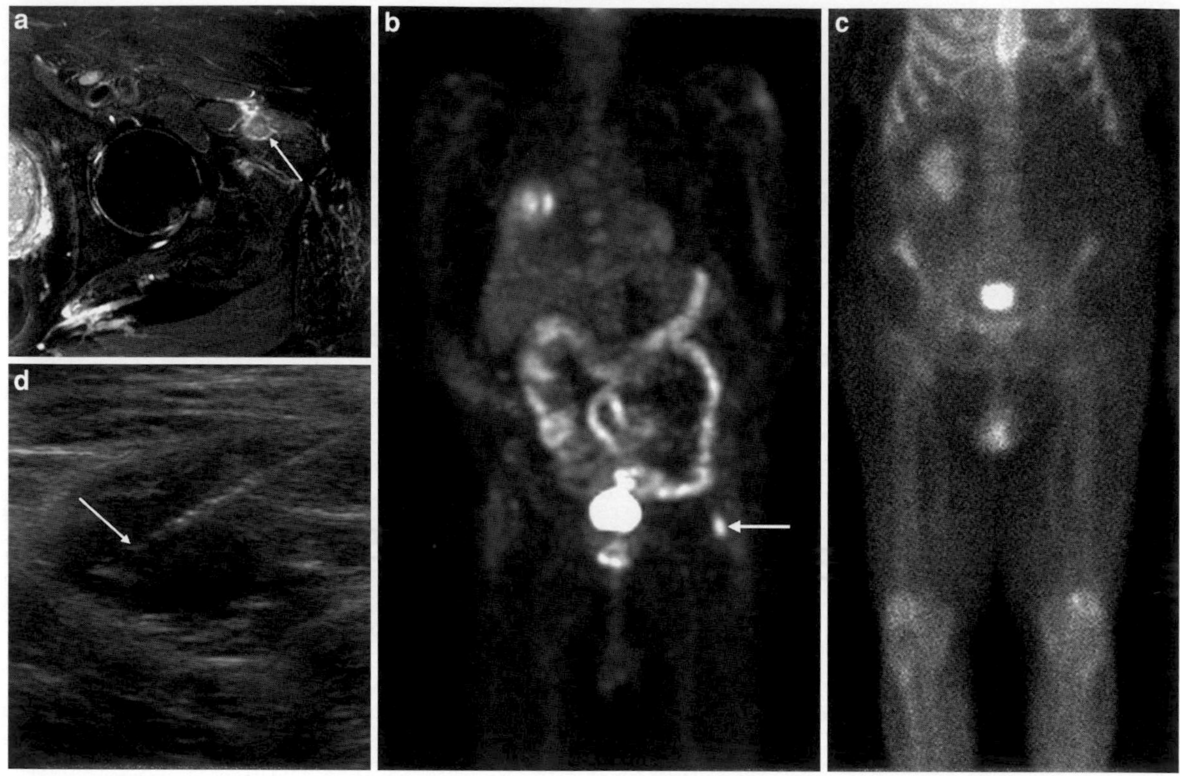

Fig. 11 **a** Axial T2-weighted MRI with fat saturation depicts a nonspecific soft tissue mass (*arrow*) in the soft tissue's anterior and lateral to the left hip. **b** PET scan obtained for staging depicts a hypermetabolic focus corresponding to the soft tissue nodule but no other lesions could be identified. **c** Bone scan also obtained for staging shows no abnormal scintigraphic activity. FDG PET has the advantage of detecting both soft tissue and osseous disease while bone scans can identify only osseous lesions reliably. **d** Subsequent ultrasound-guided biopsy (*arrow*) showed this to be an undifferentiated pleomorphic sarcoma

breast cancer, and non-small cell lung carcinoma (Peterson et al. 2003; Yang et al. 2002; Cook et al. 1998; Fogelman et al. 2005; Bury et al. 1998, Moog et al. 1999). Moog et al. (1999) studied 56 patients with lymphoma, and found that FDG PET was more sensitive and specific when compared to bone scintigraphy for detection of lymphomatous involvement of bone. FDG PET imaging is superior to bone scanning for evaluation of multifocal malignancies that produce purely lytic lesions, such as multiple myeloma and certain metastases (Schirrmeister et al. 2002). Cook et al. (1998) reported PET to be better than bone scanning for evaluation of osteolytic breast cancer metastases. In general, lytic metastases involving only the bone marrow are not as well depicted with bone scintigraphy, as these lesions may not induce an osteoblastic response or osseous reparative changes (Peterson et al. 2003; Hawkins et al. 2002a; Rybak and Rosenthal 2001; Heike et al. 2001). It has been suggested that aggressive osseous lesions can also outstrip their blood supply, inherently limiting the distribution of the radiotracer to the lesion and diminishing its conspicuity on bone scintigraphy (Peterson et al. 2003).

One of the most important advantages of FDG PET and PET/CT is that PET evaluates both the osseous and soft tissue structures. Bone scintigraphy only evaluates the osseous structures, and additional imaging (such as CT) is required to identify foci of pulmonary, nodal or soft tissue tumor involvement (Fig. 11) (Peterson et al. 2003). Imaging with a single test to evaluate both the bones and soft tissues is not only easier for the patient, it is cost effective, time efficient, and puts less strain on the health care system (Heusner et al. 2009).

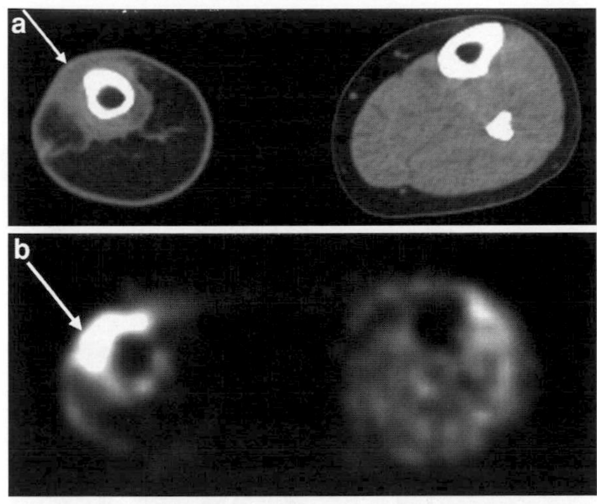

Fig. 12 **a** CT of the lower extremities in a patient with prior Ewing sarcoma with soft tissue fullness in the anterior right calf, in the area of prior surgery and radiation therapy, shows soft tissue thickening (*arrow*) worrisome for residual or recurrent disease. **b** FDG PET image depicts increased metabolic activity (*arrow*) corresponding to the soft tissue seen on CT, consistent with residual or recurrent Ewing sarcoma, which was confirmed by percutaneous biopsy. As exemplified in this case, FDG PET imaging can be very useful for restaging of primary bone tumors and soft tissue sarcomas

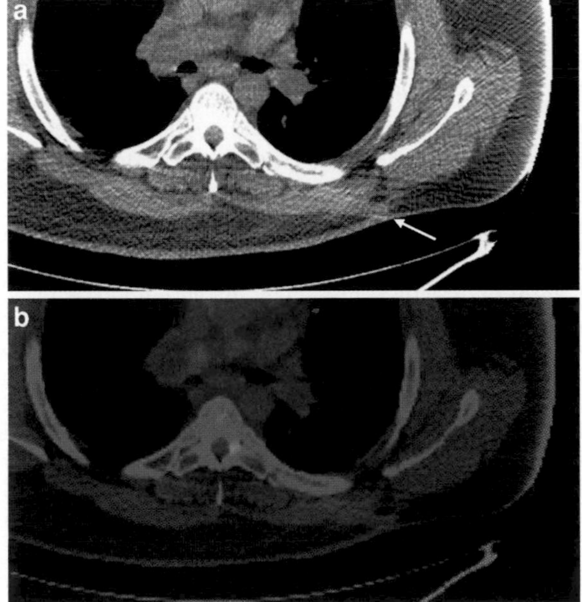

Fig. 13 FDG PET can be very helpful for evaluation of the surgical bed. **a** CT of the chest in a patient with Ewing sarcoma depicts architectural distortion and soft tissue fullness (*arrow*) in the operative bed. **b** FDG PET imaging confirms no abnormal metabolic activity in this region to suggest residual or recurrent disease

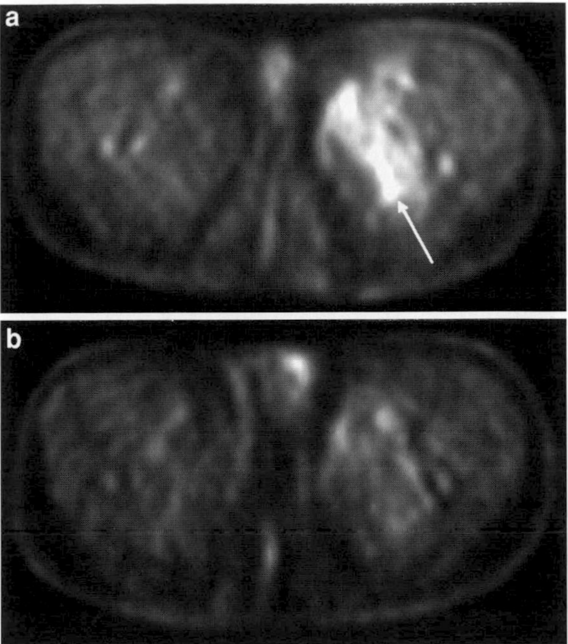

Fig. 14 **a** Postoperative restaging FDG PET scan 2 months following surgery depicts significant uptake (*arrow*) within the operative bed. At this time point PET imaging offers little useful information related to the surgical site. **b** Follow-up FDG PET examination for restaging 6 months following surgery depicts marked reduction in postoperative FDG accumulation in the operative bed with no abnormal focus of activity to suggest residual or recurrent tumor

The efficacy of FDG PET for the detection of osseous metastases can alleviate the need for an additional bone scan, resulting in a more cost effective workup of patients with musculoskeletal lesions (Heusner et al. 2009; Yang et al. 2002; Bury et al. 1998).

4 Restaging

PET is also quite useful for restaging primary osseous lesions and soft tissue sarcomas and for evaluating response to therapy (Benz et al. 2009; Iagaru et al. 2008; Peterson 2007). Restaging entails imaging with PET after completion of therapy to detect additional sites of involvement or to evaluate the extent of recurrent or residual disease (Peterson 2007). Restaging encompasses both primary and secondary lesions with evaluation of both the original tumor site/s and evaluation for local and distant metastatic disease (Piperkova et al. 2007). An estimated 40–60% of patients with soft tissue sarcomas

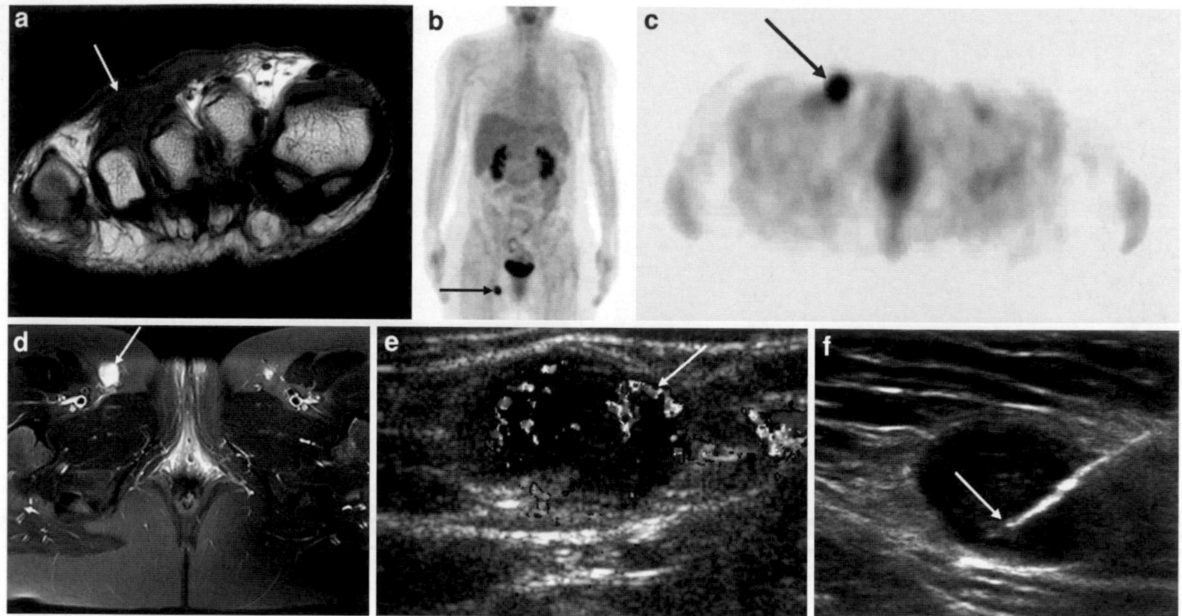

Fig. 15 **a** T1-weighted MRI of the right foot depicts an ill-defined lesion (*arrow*) extending along the dorsum of the foot overlying the 3rd and 4th metatarsals. Percutaneous biopsy proved this to be a synovial sarcoma and the foot was amputated. Nearly 2 years later, coronal (**b**) and axial (**c**) restaging PET images depicted a focus of abnormal activity (*arrow*) in the region of the right groin. **d** Post contrast MRI confirmed an enlarged enhancing node (*arrow*) in the right inguinal region corresponding to the focus of increased metabolic activity. **e** Ultrasound reveals a hypervascular hypoechoic lesion (*arrow*) in the right groin which was subsequently biopsied **f** and shown to be a focus of nodal metastatic disease

will develop local or distant recurrence of disease, and FDG PET imaging has the ability to identify these sites and to provide useful information for restaging (Fig. 12) (El-Zeftawy et al. 2001; Jadvar et al. 2004; Piperkova et al. 2009).

For local assessment FDG PET can be useful to differentiate recurrent tumor from post-surgical or post-therapeutic changes at the operative site. Detection of recurrence within the surgical bed can be quite challenging. Anatomic imaging is often hindered at sites of prior surgery by alterations in normal anatomy, distortion of tissue planes, artifacts from metal clips/hardware, and underlying radiation changes (Fig. 13) (El-Zeftawy et al. 2001, Peterson 2007, Bredella et al. 2002). Sensitivity for detection of sites of recurrence is high, but specificity is less certain and activity simply related to postoperative changes and healing can be seen for up to 6 months following surgery with significant uptake seen for 2–3 months. Because of this, restaging with PET imaging should be avoided for approximately 3 months following surgery to allow resolution of postoperative uptake in the operative bed (Bestic et al. 2009) (Fig. 14). FDG PET imaging, however, can be very useful for restaging of the surgical bed and is often very helpful in delineating focal areas of increased metabolic activity that suggests recurrence. PET can help focus imaging efforts and specifically target suspicious areas for follow-up anatomic imaging and can be helpful in directing subsequent image-guided biopsies to sites of maximum metabolic activity (Klaeser et al. 2009; O'Sullivan et al. 2008).

FDG PET can also be useful for whole-body evaluation for distant sites of metastatic disease that may not be clinically suspected. PET allows detection of sites of distant metastatic disease that may have developed since the prior treatment or follow-up (Fig. 15), which can have a dramatic effect on future treatment plans and therapy for the patient. In 2002b, Franzius et al., in a study of 27 patients with osteosarcoma and Ewing sarcoma, demonstrated PET to be sensitive, specific, and accurate in the detection of both local and distant recurrence of tumor. McCarville et al. (2005) also showed FDG PET to be very helpful for

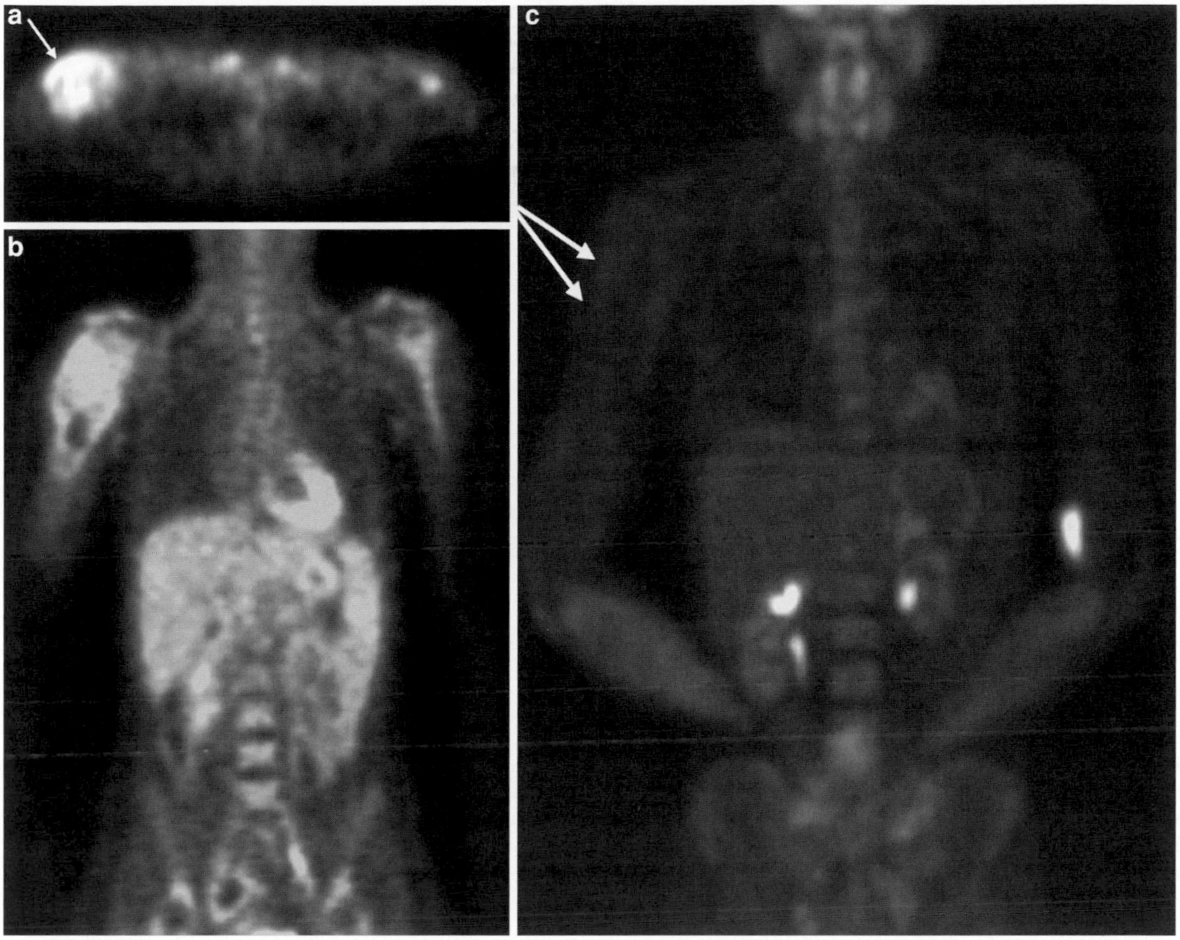

Fig. 16 Axial (**a**) and coronal (**b**) images from an FDG PET examination in a patient with Ewing sarcoma depict increased metabolic activity (*arrow*) about the right proximal humerus corresponding to the primary lesion. **c** Follow-up PET scan following radiation and chemotherapy depicts excellent response to treatment with marked decrease in abnormal metabolic activity in the right proximal humeral lesion (*arrow*). After wide margin resection and proximal humeral replacement, histologic analysis confirmed an excellent response to the neoadjuvant therapy

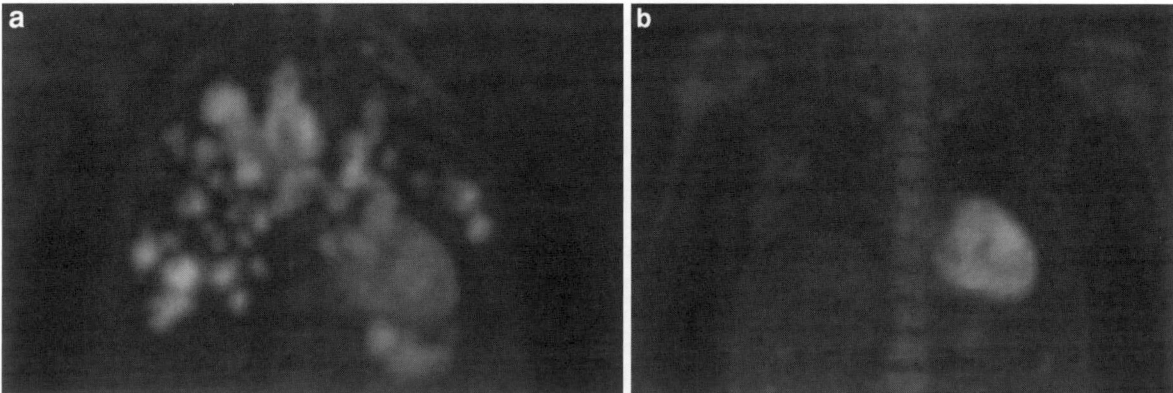

Fig. 17 **a** Coronal image of the chest from an FDG PET examination shows extensive pulmonary metastatic disease related to Ewing sarcoma. **b** Coronal PET image following therapy shows excellent response with near complete resolution of abnormal metabolic activity throughout both lungs

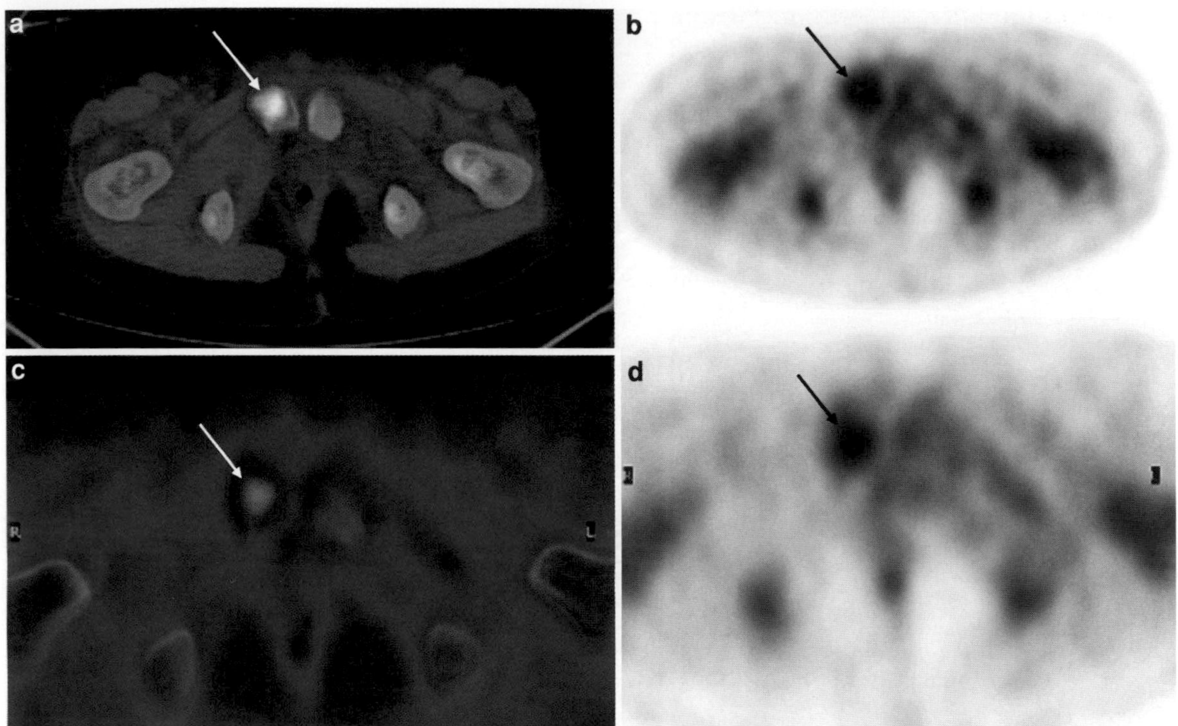

Fig. 18 Axial FDG PET (**a**) and PET/CT fusion (**b**) images in a patient with Ewing sarcoma involving the right pubic bone show a hypermetabolic focus (*arrows*) corresponding to the lesion. Axial FDG PET (**c**) PET/CT fusion (**d**) images following therapy show very poor response to therapy with significant residual activity associated with the lesion (*arrow*). Therapy was discontinued and the lesion was resected with histology confirming a large percentage of the tumor was still viable. In this case PET imaging was helpful both to assess the current therapy and guide future treatment

restaging and detecting tumor recurrence with musculoskeletal tumors, in addition to evaluating response to chemotherapy and radiation therapy. Further and larger trials of the efficacy of FDG PET for restaging primary bone and soft tissue sarcomas are needed.

5 Monitoring Response to Therapy

FDG PET imaging can be very useful for assessing treatment response in patients with primary bone tumors and soft tissue sarcomas (Benz et al. 2009; Iagaru et al. 2008; Hawkins et al. 2002b). In addition to surgical excision, neoadjuvant chemotherapy has proven beneficial for some types of primary osseous and soft tissue malignances. It can be challenging to differentiate viable from non-viable tumor on post treatment CT and MRI examination (Bredella et al. 2002). FDG PET imaging could prove to be the best non-invasive imaging examination for determining response to therapy in patients with primary bone lesions and soft tissue sarcoma (El-Zeftawy et al. 2001; Bredella et al. 2002; Hawkins et al. 2002b; Jadvar et al. 2004). Because PET reflects the internal metabolism of the lesion, it permits non-invasive differentiation of viable and non-viable tissue and thereby assesses the efficacy of treatment (Benz et al. 2009; Bredella et al. 2002) (Fig. 16). Histological response is typically determined by estimating the percentage of necrotic tumor cells remaining after neoadjuvant therapy. Benz et al. (2009) in a study of 50 patients with soft tissue sarcomas showed that a 35% reduction in FDG uptake was a sensitive predictor of histopathologic tumor response. Similarly, Hawkins and colleagues, in a study of 33 patients with both osteosarcoma and Ewing sarcoma, showed significant differences in response to treatment based upon the standard uptake value of the lesion. The authors suggest that FDG PET imaging could allow non-invasive prediction of response to treatment in patients with osteosarcoma and Ewing sarcoma (Fig. 17) (Hawkins et al. 2002b).

It appears that FDG PET imaging, by delineating areas of glucose utilization within musculoskeletal lesions, can provide a non-invasive method to evaluate therapy response, and can facilitate changes in treatment if the desired response is not achieved (Hawkins et al. 2002b). Response to treatment represents critical information in the treatment of musculoskeletal tumors. The response can determine whether effective chemotherapy is continued or ineffective chemotherapy is discontinued (Benz et al. 2009) (Fig. 18). It can also determine whether limb salvage procedures are possible or avoid unnecessary surgical intervention if metastatic disease is detected (Bredella et al. 2002; Jadvar et al. 2004).

References

Aoki J, Watanabe H, Shinozaki T, Takagishi K, Ishijima H, Oya N, Sato N, Inoue T, Endo K (2001) FDG PET of primary benign and malignant bone tumors: standardized uptake value in 52 lesions. Radiology 219:774–777

Bastiaannet E, Groen H, Jager PL, Cobben DC, van der Graff WT, Vaalburg W, Hoekstra HJ (2004) The value of FDG-PET in the detection, grading, and response to therapy of soft tissue and bone sarcomas; a systematic review and meta-analysis. Cancer Treat Rev 30:83–101

Benz MR, Czernin J, Allen-Aurbach MS, Tap WD, Dry SM, Elashoff D, Chow K, Evilevitch V, Eckardt JJ, Phelps ME (2009) FDG PET/CT imaging predicts histopathologic treatment responses after the initial cycle of neoadjuvant chemotherapy in high-grade soft-tissue sarcomas. Clin Cancer Res 15:2856–2863

Bestic JM, Peterson JJ, Bancroft LW (2009) Use of FDG PET in staging, restaging, and assessment of therapy response in Ewing sarcoma. Radiographics. Sep–Oct 29: 1487–1500

Bredella MA, Caputo GR, Steinbach LS (2002) Value of FDG positron emission tomography in conjunction with MR imaging for evaluating therapy response in patients with musculoskeletal sarcomas. AJR 179:1145–1150

Brenner W, Conrad EU, Eary JF (2004) FDG PET imaging for grading and prediction of outcome in chondrosarcoma patients. Eur J Nucl Med Mol Imaging 31:189–195

Bury T, Bareto A, Daenen F, Barthelemy N, Ghaye B, Rigo P (1998) Fluorine-18 deoxyglucose positron emission tomography for the detection of bone metastases in patients with non-small cell lung cancer. Eur J Nucl Med 25:1244–1247

Charest M, Hickeson M, Lisbona R, Novales-Diaz JA, Derbekyan V, Turcotte RE (2009) FDG PET/CT imaging in primary osseous and soft tissue sarcomas: a retrospective review of 212 cases. Euro J Null Med Mol Imaging 36:1944–1951

Cook GJ, Houston S, Rubens R, Maisey MN, Fogelman I (1998) Detection of bone metastases in breast cancer by (18)FDG PET: differing metabolic activity in osteoblastic and osteolytic lesions. J Clin Oncol 16:3375–3379

Costelloe CM, Macapinlac HA, Madewell JE, Fitzgold NE, Mawlawi OR, Rohren EM, Raymond AK, Lewis VO, Anderson PM, Bassett RL, Harrell RK, Marom EM (2009) 18F-FDG PET/CT as an indicator of progression-free and overall survival in osteosarcoma. J Nucl Med 50:340–347

Daldrup-Link HE, Franzius C, Link TM, Laukamp D, Sciuk J, Jurgens H, Schober O, Rummeny EJ (2001) Whole-body MR imaging for detection of bone metastases in children and young adults: comparison with skeletal scintigraphy and FDG PET. AJR 177:229–236

Eary JF, O'Sullivan F, Powitan Y, Chandhury KR, Vernon C, Bruckner JD, Conrad EU (2002) Sarcoma tumor FDG uptake measured by PET and patient outcome: a retrospective analysis. Eur J Nucl Med Mol Imaging 29:1149–1154

El-Zeftawy H, Heiba SI, Jana S, Rosen G, Salem S, Santiago JF, Abdel-Dayem HM (2001) Role of repeated F-18 fluorodeoxyglucose imaging in management of patients with bone and soft tissue sarcoma. Cancer Biother Radiopharm 16:37–46

Feldman F, Van Heertum R, Saxena C (2006) 18-Fluorodeoxyglucose positron emission tomography evaluation of benign versus malignant osteochondromas: preliminary observations. J Comput Assist Tomogr 30:858–864

Feldman F, Van Heertum R, Saxena C, Parisien M (2005) 18-FDG-PET applications for cartilage neoplasms. Skeletal Radiol 34:367–374

Franzius C, Bielack S, Flege S, Sciuk J, Jurgens H, Schober O (2002a) Prognostic significance of 18F-FDG and 99mTc-methylene diphosphonate uptake in primary osteosarcoma. J Nucl Med 43:1012–1017

Franzius C, Daldrup-Link HE, Wagner-Bohn A, Sciuk J, Heindel WL, Jurgens H, Schober O (2002b) FDG-PET for detection of recurrences from malignant primary bone tumors: comparison with conventional imaging. Ann Oncol 13:157–160

Fogelman I, Cook G, Israel O, Van der Wall H (2005) Positron emission tomography and bone metastases. Semin Nucl Med 35:135–142

Goodin GS, Shulkin BL, Kaufman RA, McCarville MB (2006) PET/CT characterization of fibroosseous defects in children:18F-FDG uptake can mimic metastatic disease. AJR 187:1124–1128

Hawkins DS, Rajendran JG, Conrad III EU, Bruckner JD, Eary JF (2002a) Evaluation of chemotherapy response in pediatric bone sarcomas by [F-18]-fluorodeoxy-D-glucose positron emission tomography. Am Cancer Soc 94:3277–3284

Hawkins DS, Rajendran JG, Conrad III EU, Bruckner JD, Eary JF (2002b) Evaluation of chemotherapy response in pediatric bone sarcoma by [f-18]-fluorodeoxy-D-glucose positron emission tomography. Cancer 94:3277–3284

Heike ED, Christiane F, Link TM, Laukamp D, Sciuk J, Jurgens H et al (2001) Whole-body MR imaging for detection of bone metastases in children and young adults: comparison with skeletal scintigraphy and FDG PET. Am J Roentgenol 177:229–236

Heusner T, Golitz P, Hamami M, Eberhardt W, Stefan E, Forsting M, Bockisch A, Antoch G (2009) "One-stop-shop" staging: should we prefer FDG PET/CT or MRI for the detection of bone metastases? Eur J Radiol. doi:10.1016/j.ejrad.2009.10.031

Ho YY (2005) Review of non-positron emission tomography functional imaging or primary musculoskeletal tumours: beyond the humble bone scan. Austral Radiol 49:445–459

Iagaru A, Masamed R, Chawla SP, Menendez LR, Fedenko A, Conti PS (2008) F-18 FDG PET and PET/CT Evaluation of response to chemotherapy in bone and soft tissue sarcomas. Clin Nuclear Med 33:8–13

Jadvar H, Gamie S, Romanna L, Conti PS (2004) Musculoskeletal system. Semin Nucl Med 34:254–261

Klaeser B, Mueller MD, Schmid RA, Guevara C, Krause T, Wiskerchen J (2009) PET-CT-guided interventions in the management of FDG-positive lesions in patients suffering from solid malignancies: initial experiences. Eur Radiol 19:1780–1785

Lisle JW, Eary JF, O'Sullivan J, Conrad EU (2009) Risk assessment based on FDG-PET imaging in patients with synovial sarcoma. Clin Orthop Relat Res 467:1605–1611

Malhotra P, Berman CG (2002) Evaluation of bone metastases in lung cancer. Imag Oncol 9:254–260

McCarville MB, Christe R, Daw NC, Spunt SL, Kaste SC (2005) PET/CT in the evaluation of childhood sarcomas. AJR 184:1293–1304

Moog F, Kotzerke J, Reske SN (1999) FDG PET can replace bone scintigraphy in primary staging of malignant lymphoma. J Nucl Med 40:1407–1413

O'Sullivan PJ, Rohren EM, Madewell JE (2008) Positron emission tomography-CT imaging in guiding musculoskeletal biopsy. Radiol Clin North Am 46:475–486

Peterson JJ (2007) F-18 FDG-PET for detection of osseous metastatic disease and staging, restaging, and monitoring response to therapy of musculoskeletal tumors. Semin Musculoskelet Radiol 11:246–260

Peterson JJ, Kransdorf MJ, O'Connor MI (2003) Diagnosis of occult bone metastases: positron emission tomography. Clin Orthop Relat Res 415S:S120–S128

Piperkova E, Mikhaeil M, Mouasavi A, Libes R, Viejo-Rullan LH, Rosen G, Abdel-Dayem H (2009) Impact of PET and CT in PET/CT studies for staging and evaluating treatment response in bone and soft tissue sarcomas. Clin Nuclear Med 34: 146–150

Rybak LD, Rosenthal DI (2001) Radiological imaging for the diagnosis of bone metastases. J Nucl Med 45:53–64

Schirrmeister H, Bommer M, Buck AK, Muller S, Messer P, Bunjes D, Mottaghy FM, Krause BJ, Neumaier B, Döhner H, Möller P, Reske SN (2002) Initial results in the assessment of multiple myeloma using 18F-FDG PET. Eur J Nucl Med 29:361–366

Suzuki H, Watanabe H, Shinozaki T, Yanagawa T, Suzuki R, Takagishi K (2004) Positron emission tomography imaging of musculoskeletal tumors in the shoulder girdle. J Shoulder Elbow Surg 13:635–647

Volker T, Denecke T, Steffen I, Misch D, Schonberger S, Plotkin M, Ruf J, Furth C, Stover B, Hautzel G, Henze G, Amthauer H (2007) Positron emission tomography for staging of pediatric sarcoma patients: results of a prospective multicenter trial. J Clin Oncol 25:5435–5441

Yang SN, Liang JA, Lin FJ, Kao CH, Lin CC, Lee CC (2002) Comparing whole body 18F-2-deoxyglucose positron emission tomography and technetium-99m methylene diphosphonate bone scan to detect bone metastases in patients with breast cancer. J Cancer Res Clin Oncol 128:325–328

Hematology

Rathan M. Subramaniam, Leonne Prompers, A. Agarwal, Ali Guermazi, and Felix M. Mottaghy

Contents

R. M. Subramaniam, L. Prompers, and F. M. Mottaghy are contributed equally.

A. Agarwal
Boston University School of Medicine, Boston, MA 02118, USA

L. Prompers · F. M. Mottaghy
Department of Nuclear Medicine, Maastricht University Medical Center, P. Debeylaan 25, 6229 HX, Maastricht, The Netherlands

A. Guermazi
Department of Radiology Director, Quantitative Imaging Center (QIC), Boston University School of Medicine Section Chief, Musculoskeletal Imaging Boston Medical Center, 820 Harrison Avenue, Boston, MA 02118, USA

F. M. Mottaghy (✉)
Clinic for Nuclear Medicine, University Hospital RWTH Aachen University, Pauwelsstr. 30, 52074 Aachen, Germany
e-mail: fmottaghy@ukaachen.de

R. M. Subramaniam
Russell H Morgan Departments of Radiology and Radiological Sciences Institutions, The Johns Hopkins Medical Institutions, 601 N. Caroline Street/ JHOC 3235, Baltimore , MD 21287, USA

Abstract

Malignant lymphoma is the most common hematologic malignancy and one of the most common malignant diseases in the general population. These lymphoproliferative disorders can be broadly divided into Hodgkin lymphoma (HL) and non-Hodgkin lymphoma (NHL). Patients with NHL have an especially poor prognosis with an average 5-year survival rate of 64%. NHL accounts for 2.6% of all cancer deaths. However, the 5-year survival has been gradually improving because of refinements in clinical management. Imaging has

P. Peller et al. (eds.), *PET-CT and PET-MRI in Oncology*, Medical Radiology. Diagnostic Imaging,
DOI: 10.1007/174_2012_594,

traditionally played a key role in the initial staging and surveillance of lymphoma. The first reports of PET for lymphoma imaging were published more than 20 years ago. Today 18F-FDG PET is the cornerstone of disease-staging in state-of-the-art management of HL and high grade NHL. In the past decades several studies investigated the value of PET/CT for the diagnosis and staging of lymphomas, and the great majority showed very high sensitivity and specificity in patients with HL and aggressive NHL. Greater variations have been reported in the sensitivity and specificity in patients with indolent lymphomas. PET is less commonly used for staging of these indolent lymphomas. Over the last few years, the efficacy of PET has been evaluated at all steps of lymphoma management including interim treatment monitoring, post-treatment response evaluation, and follow-up. Another important hematologic cancer is leukemia; however, even today, the role of functional (and morphologic) imaging in patients with leukemia is very limited. The role of PET/CT in multiple myeloma is evolving. PET/CT is superior to standard radiographic staging for multiple myeloma. It appears to be a prognostic marker for predicting outcome at baseline, after induction therapy and after transplantation for patients with multiple myeloma. Further studies may be necessary to validate these initial findings for incorporation of PET/CT in the guidelines for management of multiple myeloma.

1 Lymphoma

1.1 Classification of Lymphoma

Hodgkin's lymphoma (HL) is differentiated from other lymphomas by the microscopic detection of Reed-Sternberg cells within the tumor. In the current World Health Organization system, NHL is categorized into more than 20 subtypes on the basis of cell of origin (B or T cell precursor) and morphologic and immunophenotypic data (Harris et al. 2000). Fifty percent of the cases of NHL are patients with diffuse large B cell lymphoma or follicular lymphoma.

FDG PET is more sensitive and specific than CT in detecting extranodal spread of lymphoma (Moog et al. 1998). PET seems superior to CT alone for the initial staging of lymphoma (Hutchings et al. 2006; Delbeke et al. 2009), although PET alone cannot replace CT for pretreatment staging (Bangerter et al. 1998; Jerusalem et al. 2001). FDG PET is most often used in treatment assessment. An algorithm for the recommended timing of PET/CT and CT is shown in Fig. 1 [according to the study of Delbeke et al. (2009)], indicating that PET is superior to CT for assessing treatment response in patients with lymphoma (Hutchings et al. 2006; Jerusalem et al. 1999). However, two important reviews show only moderate positive predictive value (PPV) for FDG PET in post-therapy evaluation of HL (Terasawa et al. 2008; Zijlstra et al.2006). Zijlstra et al. reported a range of 60–100% of PPV in 5 studies and Terasawa a range of 13–100% in 10 studies with a weighted average of 62%. However, both studies show a very high negative-predictive value (NPV) for FDG PET in post-therapy evaluation of HL ranging from 84 to 100% in the Zijlstra report and ranging from 71 to 100% in the Terasawa report, with a weighted average of 94%. The rate of PET scans with positive findings after treatment ranges from 8 to 61% in the Terasawa review, with a weighted average of 30%. This means that the rate of PET scans with negative findings is about 70 (39–92%). Zijlstra reported similar findings. Combined, the 70% frequency of negative PET findings and the NPV of 94% indicate that patients are misclassified by disease status in only 4% of cases. This very low false negative rate, which does not seem significantly different from that in patients with negative CT findings (no residual mass), explains the high prognostic value and clinical utility of a negative post-therapy PET in patients with HL (Juweid 2008). Even in the case of patients with a residual mass, patients who have negative post-therapy PET do not need a biopsy and can safely be observed until there is clinical or radiologic evidence of relapse. Patients with aggressive NHL show similar findings. False positive PET findings affect only 3% of the patients, while false negative PET findings affect 14% of patients (PPV 90, NPV 80%). This false negative rate is the same as the false negative rate associated with patients with negative CT findings (Juweid et al. 2005). The prognostic value of a PET-negative finding is therefore maintained in patients with aggressive NHL. Although the PPV of PET in post-therapy residual mass assessment shows PET's efficacy to be somewhat limited, it is still superior to that of conventional imaging with CT or MRI, which cannot reliably differentiate between necrosis or fibrosis and viable tumor (Juweid

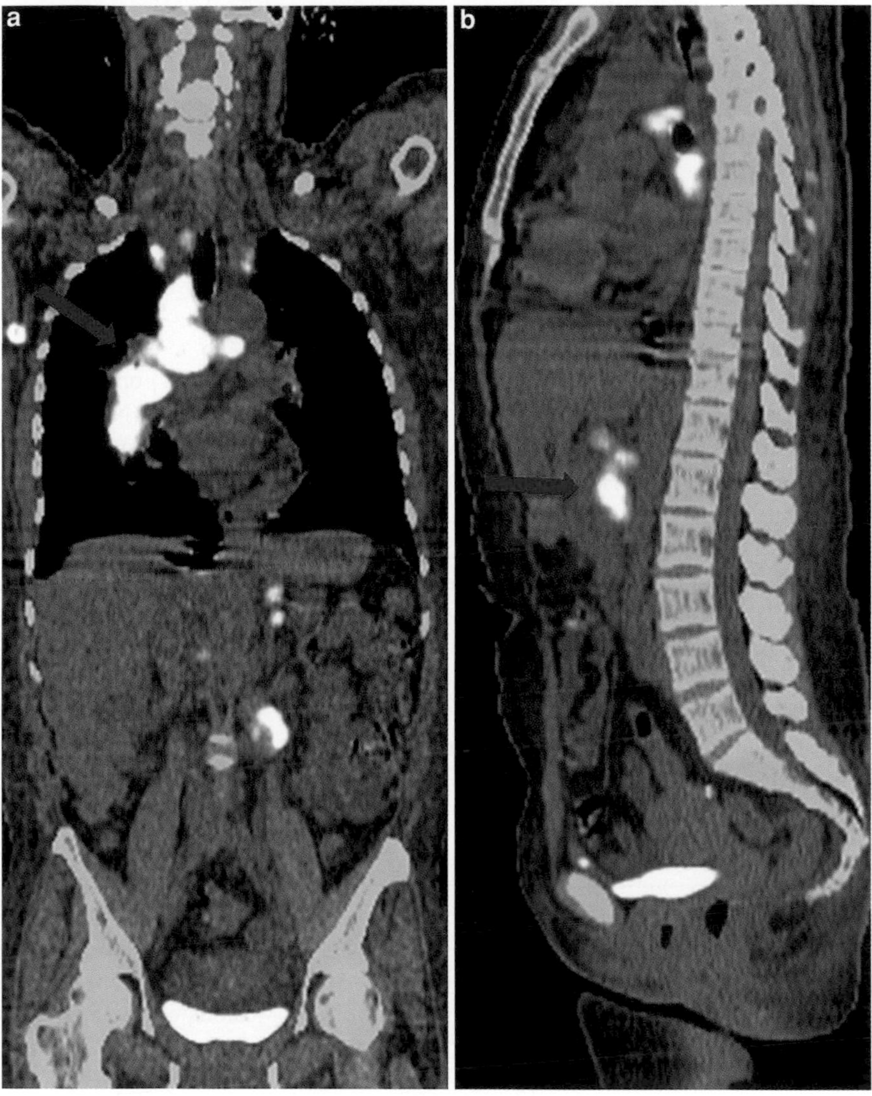

Fig. 1 Staging: Angioimmunoblastic T cell lymphoma. This 53-year-old woman presented with angioimmunoblastic T cell lymphoma. Coronal fused PET/CT (**a**) and sagittal fused PET/CT (**b**) demonstrate disease *above* and *below* the diaphragm

et al. 2005). Juweid showed in one of the few studies in which CT and PET were compared in the same patients with aggressive NHL that the PPV of CT was 43 versus 74% for PET (Juweid et al. 2005; Seam et al. 2007). The data available support PET even more in patients with HL (Juweid 2006). Integrated PET/CT is at the moment the most efficient diagnostic tool for initial staging and post-treatment assessment. The sensitivity and specificity of PET/CT are higher than those of contrast-enhanced CT alone (Delbeke et al. 2009; Juweid et al. 2007; Fueger et al. 2009; Yang et al. 2009; Le Dortz et al. 2010; Hutchings and Barrington 2009; Kwee et al. 2008; Blodgett et al. 2007; von Schulthess et al. 2006) In patients with aggressive NHL or HL, pretherapy FDG PET has significantly higher patient and site sensitivity than 67-Ga scintigraphy (100 vs. 80 and 100 vs. 71.5%) (Kostakoglu et al. 2002), the former standard in metabolic imaging of lymphoma (Wirth et al. 2002). Whole-body MRI using a diffusion-weighted sequence shows a higher spatial resolution for imaging of patients with lymphoma, although it has only limited ability in detecting mediastinal lesions (Kwee et al. 2008).

1.2 Tracers

In clinical practice the most frequently used tracer for diagnosing lymphoma is 18-FDG. Recently, 3'-deoxy-3'-[(18)F]fluorothymidine (FLT), a cell proliferation PET tracer, has been shown in numerous tumors to be more specific but less sensitive than 2-deoxy-2-[(18)F]fluoro-D:-glucose ([(18)F]FDG) (Graf et al. 2008; Buck et al. 2008). Since FLT is not generally used in clinical practice yet, this chapter will focus on 18F-FDG PET.

1.3 Standardized Uptake Value

Findings on PET/CT can be analyzed quantitatively with the help of the SUV (Huang 2000). This parameter is used to estimate the level of glucose metabolic activity in patients with lymphoma and to evaluate residual activity after therapy. The SUV in aggressive NHL and HL is generally significantly higher than in indolent lymphoma (Menda and Graham 2005). Visual assessment of treatment response is sufficient in clinical practice and is adequate for determining whether or not a PET/CT scan is positive for disease (Juweid et al. 2007). Quantitative evaluations of relative decrease in FDG uptake may be an important parameter used clinically for interim assessments in the future. Several prospective studies on this topic are currently underway.

2 Baseline Staging

The modified Ann Arbor staging classification system is widely used for lymphoma (Cabanillas and Fuller 1990). The system is based on location and number of lymph nodes involved and the presence or absence of extranodal disease. Accurate staging is critical for formulating management strategies. Patients with stage I or II lymphoma can be candidates for involved-field radiation rather than chemotherapy; patients with more advanced disease usually receive chemotherapy.

2.1 Prognostic Assessment

Accurate prognostic assessment is critical for formulating management strategies. The International Prognostic Index is usually used for NHL. It involves age, disease stage (Ann Arbor), performance status, serum lactate dehydrogenase (LDH), and the number of extranodal sites of disease. In HL, 7 clinical parameters are generally observed to predict outcome: age, sex, stage, hemoglobin concentration (Hb), albumin concentration, lymphocyte count, and white blood cell count. Determining the histological features of the tumor, prognostic indicators, and stage of disease are critical to creating an effective treatment plan (Hasenclever and Diehl 1998).

2.2 Staging of Aggressive NHL

The most common type of aggressive Non-Hodgkin's lymphoma (NHL) is large B cell lymphoma. Aggressive lymphomas are generally highly FDG avid. Tables 1 and 2 show the FDG avidity of the different subtypes of lymphoma. 18F-FDG PET is one of the cornerstones in treatment decision making and is strongly advised at baseline (Fig. 1) in the management of all patients with aggressive lymphomas. Use of PET generally leads to upstaging the tumor stage in comparison to CT alone (Naumann et al. 2004; Buchmann et al. 2001; Schoder et al. 2001).

2.3 Staging of Indolent NHL

Indolent lymphoma includes both B cell (for example, chronic lymphocytic leukemia, follicular lymphoma, marginal zone lymphoma, and small lymphocytic lymphoma) and T cell proliferative disorders. These lesions characteristically have low metabolic activity and low or no FDG uptake. Nevertheless, PET has a relatively high sensitivity for indolent lymphoma (Elstrom et al. 2003). The study of Fueger et al. 2009 reported that hybrid PET/CT added clinically important information that PET or CT alone did not offer. PET/CT performed significantly better in classifying lymph node groups as positive or negative for lymphoma and was better able to detect additional extranodal sites of disease. Progression of disease in indolent lymphoma is very slow and the disease is considered incurable in most cases. Treatment is primarily guided by manifestation of clinical symptoms. Since these clinical manifestations are more important for decision making than the stage of disease, PET is not routinely used for staging. Nevertheless, PET can still be clinically useful in patients with indolent lymphoma in several cases. Firstly, it can be useful in patients who present with a single

Table 1 FDG avidity in lymphoma according to Weiler-Sagie, Tsukamoto and Elstrom at all

Histology	Weiler Sagie *(62)*	Tsukamato *(57)*	Elstrom *(62)*
Hodgkin disease	100% (n=233)	97% (n=23)	98% (n=47)
Burkitt lymphoma	100% (n=18)	100% (n=5)	100% (n=1)
Mantle Cell lymphoma	100% (n=14)	100% (n=9)	100% (n=7)
Anaplastic large T-cell lymphoma	100% (n=14)	100% (n=5)	100% (n=2)
Marginal zone lymphoma, nodal	100% (n=8)		
Lymphoblastic lymphoma	100% (n=6)		
Angioimmunoblastic T-cell lymphoma	100% (n=4)	100% (n=5)	
Natural killer/T-cell lymphoma	100% (n=2)	100% (n=7)	100% (n=1)
Diffuse large B-cell lymphoma	97% (n=222)	97% (n=81)	100% (n=51)
Follicular lymphoma	95% (n=140)	91% (n=44)	98% (n=42)
Peripheral T-cell lymphoma	90% (n=10)	98% (n=9)	40% (n=5)
Small lymphotic lymphoma	83% (n=29)	50% (n=4)	100% (n=1)
Enteropathy-type T-cell lympoma	67% (n=3)		
Marignal zone lymphoma, unspecified			67% (n=12)
Marginal zone lymphoma, splenic	67% (n=3)	53% (n=10)	
MALT marginal zone lymphoma	54% (n=50)	82% (n=52)	
Lymphomatoid papulosis	50% (n=2)		
Primary cutaneous anaplastic large T-cell lymphoma	40% (n=5)		
Mycosis fungoides			100% (n=1)
Subcutaneous paniculitis-like T-Cell lymphoma		71% (n=1)	
Cutaneous B-cell lymphoma			0% (n=2)

Table 2 FDG Avidity of NHL according to clinical subtype

Clinical subtype	n	FDG-avid	% FDG -avidity
Aggressive	293	285	97
Indolent	240	200	83

lymph node region or 2 lymph node regions on the same side of the diaphragm (stage I or II). Patients with indolent and aggressive lymphoma in these early stages without bulky disease can be treated with curative intent with involved-field radiotherapy (Tsang et al. 2001; MacDermed et al. 2004). Secondly, indolent lymphoma can occasionally transform into aggressive lymphoma (most common is Richter transformation in large B cell lymphoma), which is associated with a very poor prognosis. Transformation of indolent into aggressive lymphoma is generally suspected in patients with very rapidly enlarging lymph nodes, increasing LDH level, or new onset of B cell symptoms (fever, night sweats and weight loss). PET is especially effective at detecting abnormally high FDG uptake at sites of transformation. Thirdly, staging by PET can be useful for baseline evaluation of patients undergoing new treatment regiments (e.g., tyrosine kinase inhibitors) in order to facilitate measurement of treatment response. This is also the case in patients undergoing radioimmuno-therapies with radiolabeled anti-CD20 monoclonal antibodies like 90Y-ibritumomab tiuxetan [Zevalin and 131I-tositumomab (Bexxar)]. The study of Jacene et al. (2009) showed that FDG PET/CT is a useful imaging technique for monitoring the response of NHL to radioimmunotherapy.

2.4 Staging of HL

Nodular sclerosing HL is the most common histologic type of HL. In almost all cases, HL displays significant FDG avidity and PET is more accurate in staging than CT alone. In clinical practice, PET is especially important for post-treatment response evaluation (Juweid et al. 2007).

2.5 Pitfalls

Some subtypes of lymphoma are difficult to detect by PET because they are difficult to differentiate from normal physiologic tissue uptake. These lymphomas include gastric lymphoma, lymphoma of the central nervous system (CNS), and testicular lymphoma. Gastric lymphoma characteristically has no or variable FDG uptake and is very difficult to differentiate from normal FDG uptake in the mucosa of the gastric wall. In testicular lymphoma, it is impossible to differentiate FDG uptake by the tumor from normal physiologic testicular uptake. In CNS lymphoma, it is also very difficult to differentiate uptake due to lymphoma from normal FDG uptake because of the very intense physiologic FDG uptake of normal cerebral tissue. FDG can therefore not be recommended as a primary staging tool. In these cases, beside MRI, FLT PET/CT might be of additional value (Buck et al. 2006).

Furthermore, it is known that frequent false positive findings on PET/CT are caused by diffuse FDG uptake secondary to reactive marrow hyperplasia. In addition, microscopic involvement of the bone marrow can be below the detection limit of PET, accounting for the relatively low sensitivity of PET in the detection of bone marrow lymphoma (43% for NHL) (Pakos et al. 2005). However, focal areas of intense FDG uptake in the bone marrow remain suspicious for lymphoma even when iliac crest biopsy is negative. If the clinical management of the patient could be influenced, further evaluation by targeted biopsy or MRI is recommended.

The clinical features of lymphoma observed by PET can be mimicked by sarcoidosis, and thus it is very difficult to differentiate between sarcoidosis and malignant lymphoma using only PET (Hunt et al. 2009). In addition, high FDG uptake can be observed in patients with high levels of brown adipose tissue. In the case of PET/CT, (low dose) CT can help to differentiate between a lymph node and brown adipose tissue (Karam et al. 2008; Sonet et al. 2007).

3 Assessment of Therapeutic Response

The use of PET/CT for assessment of therapeutic response in patients with lymphoma is strongly encouraged by the International Harmonization Project (Juweid et al. 2007). The initial recommendation by Cheson et al. (1999) was adapted to include PET and thereby streamline the classification of response (Fig. 2). This project recommends PET/CT to be performed at least 3 weeks after completion of therapy, preferably 6–8 weeks after chemotherapy and 8–12 weeks after radiation therapy alone or in combination with chemotherapy. In addition, early monitoring of lymphoma treatment is also recommended. As mentioned previously, well-established pretreatment prognostic factors have been shown to reliably predict survival in both HL and NHL. The disease stage and these prognostic factors determine the initial treatment regimen. A precise early prediction of the response to therapy might be able to divide patients who could be cured with less intensive and less toxic regimens from patients for whom an early switch to alternative, more aggressive treatment strategies could improve the likelihood and duration of remission. This model of risk-adapted therapy is being increasingly recognized as a method to achieve a higher cure rate with a lower or equal risk of treatment-related morbidity and mortality. Several studies have shown that early metabolic changes (after 1–3 cycles of chemotherapy) on PET/CT in patients with NHL and HL are highly predictive of the final treatment response (Hutchings and Barrington 2009; Spaepen and Mortelmans 2001). In treatment response assessment, mediastinal blood pool activity is recommended as reference background activity for defining PET positivity for a residual mass larger than 2 cm in its greatest transverse diameter (Juweid et al. 2007). Smaller masses should be considered positive for residual disease if their activity is higher than that of the surrounding background. Focal lesions in the spleen or in the liver with FDG uptake greater than that of the surrounding spleen or liver are considered positive for residual disease. Also diffuse FDG uptake in the spleen with greater intensity than that of the liver is considered positive for lymphoma. Focal, elevated FDG uptake in the bone marrow also is considered positive for viable lymphoma.

3.1 Assessment of Therapeutic Response in Aggressive NHL

A complete metabolic response after treatment in patients with potentially curable disease is a good

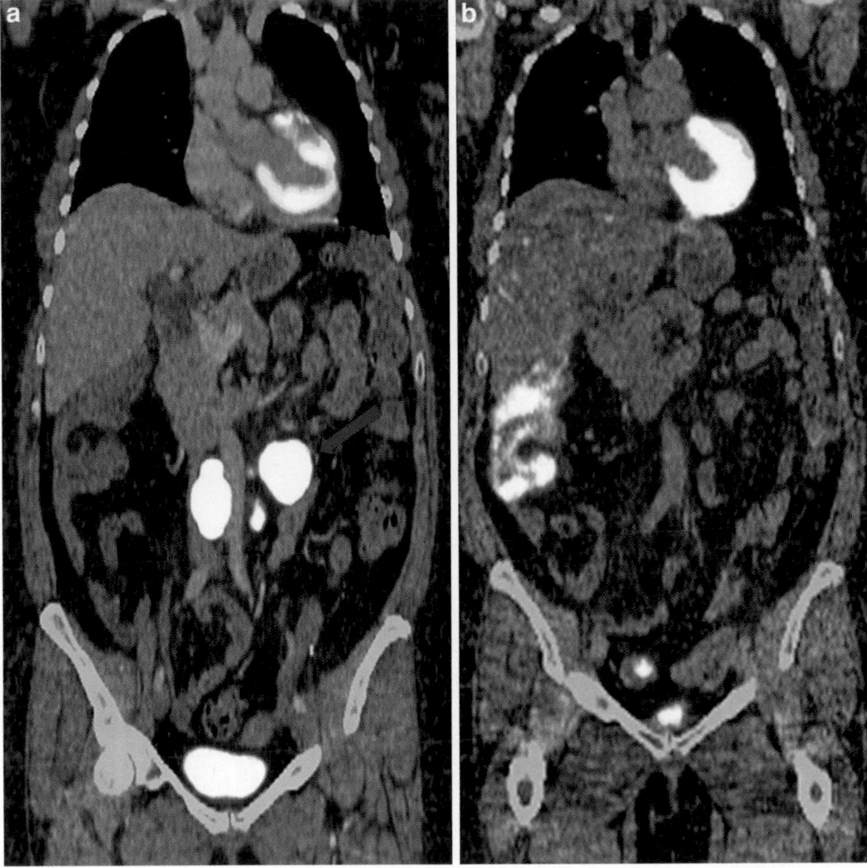

Fig. 2 End of therapy assessment. This 54-year-old woman originally presented with bulky mesenteric and retroperitoneal FDG-hypermetabolic (SUV_{max} 29.8) lymph nodes (**a**), with biopsy-proven diffuse large B cell lymphoma. Patient was treated with 6 cycles of R-CHOP and follow-up PET/CT study (**b**) demonstrated no FDG-hypermetabolic disease, consistent with complete metabolic response

prognostic indicator of long-term disease-free survival (Fig. 2). A complete metabolic response is defined as total absence of abnormal FDG uptake. FDG PET/CT is also useful in identifying residual or de-differentiated NHL (Fig. 3). In patients with residual disease, physicians should discuss the possible merits of continuing treatment, alterative treatments, and the possibility of stem cell transplantation with their patients. (Juweid et al. 2005; Juweid and Cheson 2005; Spaepen et al. 2003). For example, treatment with radiolabeled anti-CD20 monoclonal antibodies, 90Y-ibritumomab tiuxetan (Zevalin) and 131I-tositumomab (Bexxar), is available for treatment of refractory or relapsed NHL.

3.2 Assessment of Therapeutic Response in HL

Since in most cases HL is FDG avid, mid- or post-treatment PET/CT is useful in confirming or excluding complete remission (Fig. 4). PET/CT has a high ($\sim$90%) negative-predictive value (Jerusalem et al. 1999; Zijlstra 2006; Brepoels et al. 2007a, b). Persistent abnormal FDG uptake after therapy is an indication for a second-line chemotherapy agent and/or involved-field radiotherapy. In patients who have completed 6–8 cycles of chemotherapy, persistent abnormal FDG uptake is associated with a very poor long-term prognosis. Furthermore, interim evaluation of therapeutic response by PET/CT and CT was found to be a significant predictor of disease progression and may have an effect on therapeutic plans in patients with aggressive NHL (Yang et al. 2009).

3.3 Assessment of Therapeutic Response in Indolent NHL

Indolent lymphoma is usually incurable. Therapeutic response can be assessed by relief of clinical symptoms, progression- and event-free survival, and overall survival. If PET or PET/CT is implemented in therapeutic management, it is crucial to have a baseline PET in order to know the metabolic activity prior to treatment.

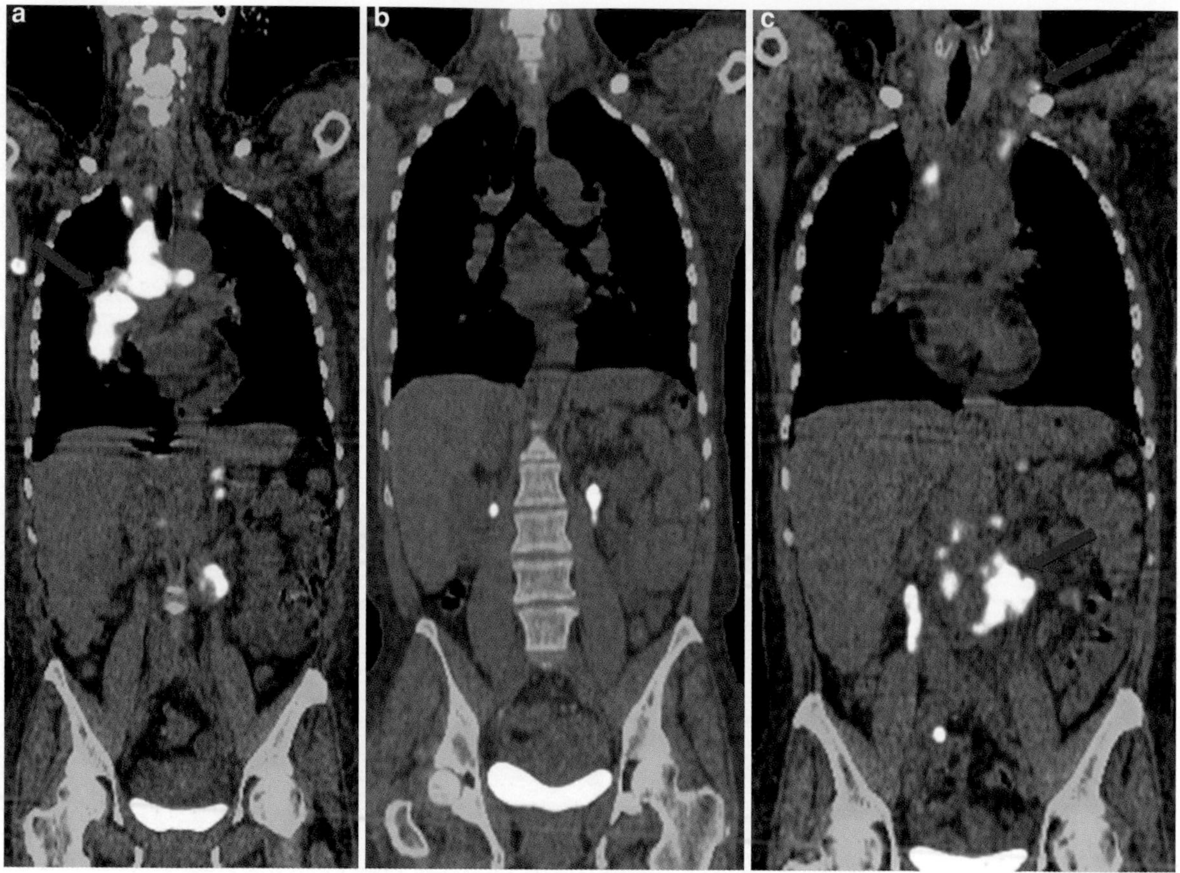

Fig. 3 De-differentiation into anaplastic large T cell lymphoma. This 53-year-old woman presented with angioimmunoblastic T cell lymphoma. Coronal fused PET/CT (**a**) demonstrated disease above and below the diaphragm that was treated successfully with CHOP showing no evidence of lymphoma (**b**), 8 months after (**c**), there was recurrence with de-differentiation into anaplastic large T cell lymphoma with increased FDG uptake in nodes throughout the neck, axillary, mediastinal, hilar, mesenteric, and retroperitoneal regions. The patient subsequently underwent treatment with 3 cycles of Brentuximab with good response

3.4 Pitfalls in Post-Treatment Assessment

One of the major issues in the interpretation of a post-treatment PET/CT scan is differentiating residual disease from FDG uptake due to post-treatment inflammation, normal physiologic activity, and coexisting infection (Prabhakar et al. 2007; Blake et al. 2006; Castellucci et al. 2005; Love et al. 2005; Cheson et al. 2007). Post-treatment inflammation can be present several weeks (usually 2–3) after finishing chemotherapy and until 3 months after chemoradiation. To differentiate coexisting infection from residual lymphoma, it is useful to have information about the presence or absence of neutropenia or a history of infection. Previous pneumonia can also be the cause of low to intermediate grade FDG uptake in draining lymph nodes in the mediastinum and hila. This can persist for several weeks after the acute infection. Correct interpretation of PET/CT images depends on knowing the clinical history of the patient, correlation with previous imaging studies, and awareness of any potential imaging artifacts. Another pitfall is due to diffusely increased FDG uptake throughout the marrow in post-therapy studies, which makes it difficult to assess success or failure of therapy in the bone marrow (Fig. 5).

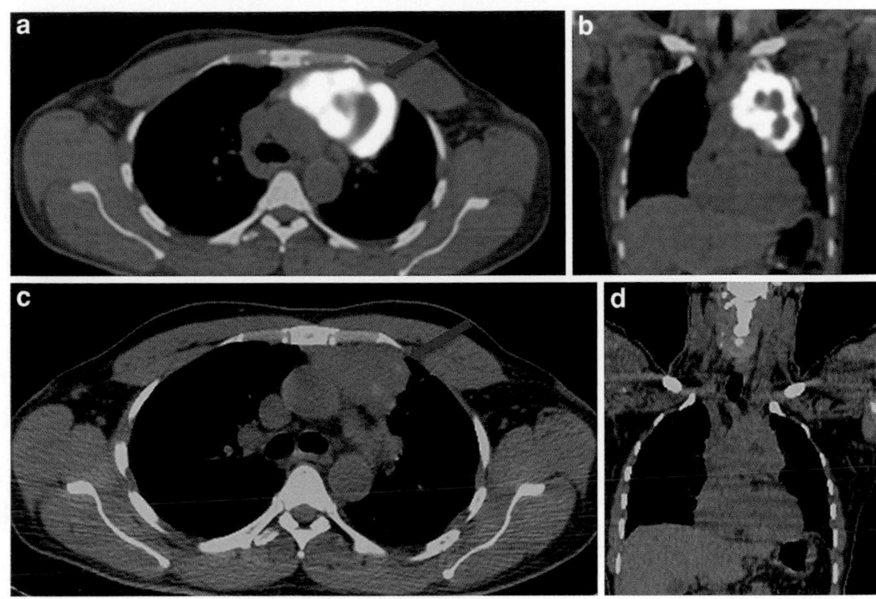

Fig. 4 Mid-therapy assessment. This 48-year-old man presented with stage IIA mixed cellularity HL in the anterior mediastinal mass with intense FDG hypermetabolism (SUVmax of 19.9) (**a**, **b**). No other focus of FDG-avid disease. The patient was treated with ABVD chemotherapy. Mid-therapy PET/CT images demonstrate (**c**, **d**) partial response to therapy with mild residual activity in the anterior mediastinal mass (SUV_{max} of 4.3)

4 Non-Hodgkin Lymphoma

4.1 Diffuse Large B cell Lymphoma

Diffuse large B cell lymphoma is the largest subtype of NHL and is curable in >50% of cases. It is often characterized by extranodal involvement at presentation. It occurs at all ages and in various locations (Fig. 6). The standard treatment is CHOP or R-CHOP. It is an aggressive type of lymphoma (often stage III or IV) and is FDG-avid in more than 90% of the cases (Juweid and Cheson 2005).

4.2 Mucosa-Associated Lymphoid Tissue

MALT lymphoma is related to chronic inflammation and autoimmune disease and is limited to organs. MALT lymphoma characteristically occurs in the orbital, lung, and stomach regions. Both orbital and gastric MALT lymphoma are difficult to detect by PET due to their relatively lower metabolic activity (Tsukamoto et al. 2007). In addition, normal physiologic FDG uptake in the stomach is common (high and variable background uptake), which makes it difficult to differentiate. Gastric MALT lymphoma has the ability to transform into high-grade diffuse large B cell lymphoma and is strongly related to Helicobacter pylori infection. In the case of MALT lymphoma in the lung, it is difficult to differentiate between lymphoma and pneumonia. Therefore the diagnosis is usually made by biopsy.

4.3 Follicular Lymphoma

FDG PET/CT has a high sensitivity (98%) and specificity (94%) for staging of follicular lymphoma. In clinical practice, PET/CT has the potential to upstage the tumor and thereby alter the management in 11% (study by Le Dortz et al. 2010)–46% (Wirth et al. 2008) of patients with apparent early-stage lymphoma (Le Dortz et al. 2010). A retrospective study of 45 patients diagnosed with follicular lymphoma PET/CT revealed 87 abnormal nodal areas not seen on CT (+51%) and 16 additional extra-nodal lesions (+89%) at initial staging of the patients. Furthermore PET/CT detected 13 cases of bone marrow involvement (11 not seen on CT) (Le Dortz et al. 2010). Patients with an early disease stage (I or II) are generally treated with radiation therapy, whereas patients with more advanced stage of follicular lymphoma are treated with rituximab. Therapeutic response was also assessed in the study by Le Dortz. Sensitivity and specificity for residual disease detection were, respectively, 100 and 97% with PET/CT versus 100 and 51% with CT.

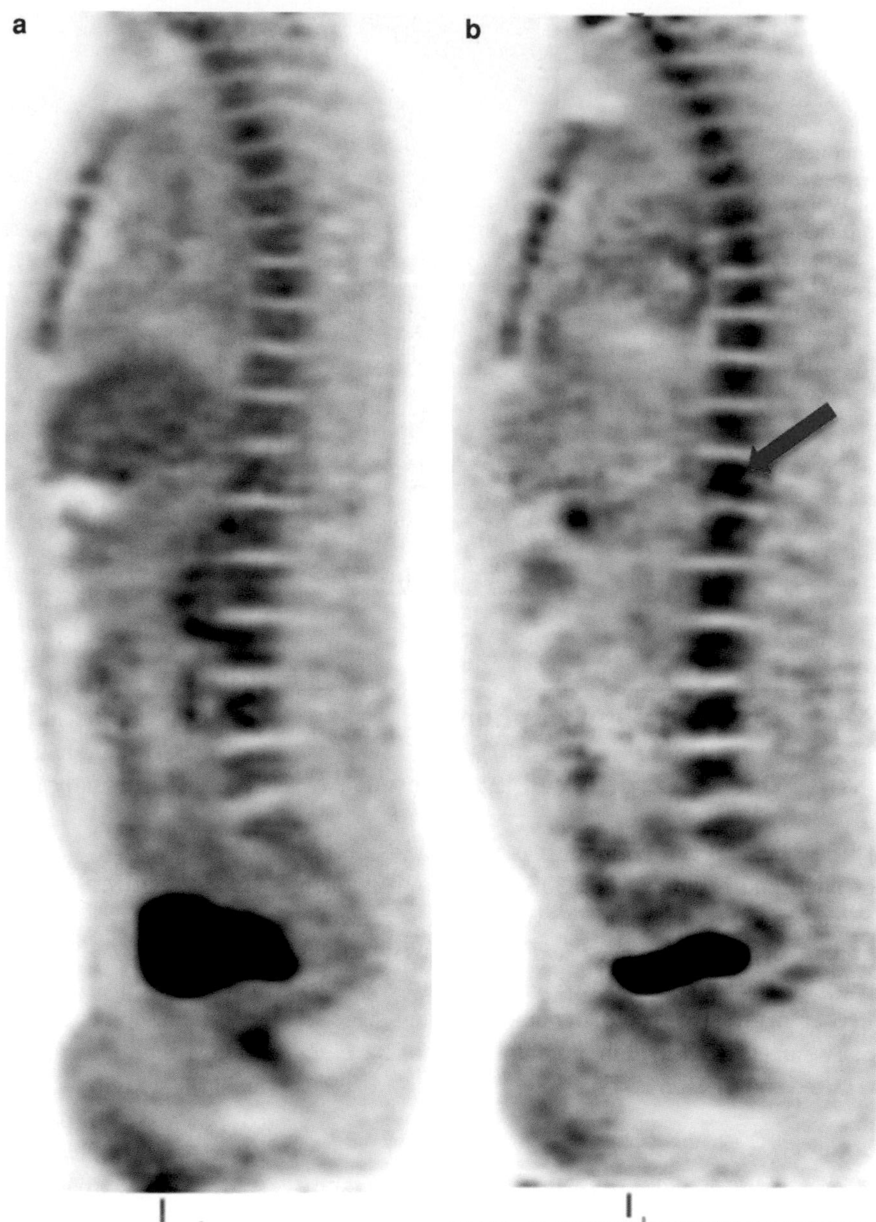

Fig. 5 Bone marrow activation in response to ABVD chemotherapy. This 43-year-old man presented with mixed cellularity HL. The pretreatment sagittal PET scan (**a**) showed physiological uptake in the bone marrow and a biopsy of the bone marrow taken at the time showed no lymphocytic involvement. Following treatment with ABVD chemotherapy, the patient showed a dramatic increase in uptake in the bone marrow (**b**)

4.4 Mantle Cell Lymphoma

Mantle cell lymphoma usually shows extra-nodal involvement and has a poor prognosis. It accounts for 4–8% of all NHLs. It shows clear uptake of FDG on PET (Brepoels et al. 2007a, b; Karam et al. 2006). Karam et al. showed that the overall survival and failure-free survival significantly decreased in patients with a mantle cell lymphoma and an SUV_{max} <5 on PET. The overall survival in patients with an SUV_{max} of >5 was 87.7% and in patients with an SUV_{max} of more than 5 was 34% (Karam et al. 2009).

4.5 Burkitt Lymphoma

Burkitt lymphoma is considered to be an aggressive type of lymphoma. It includes the endemic type

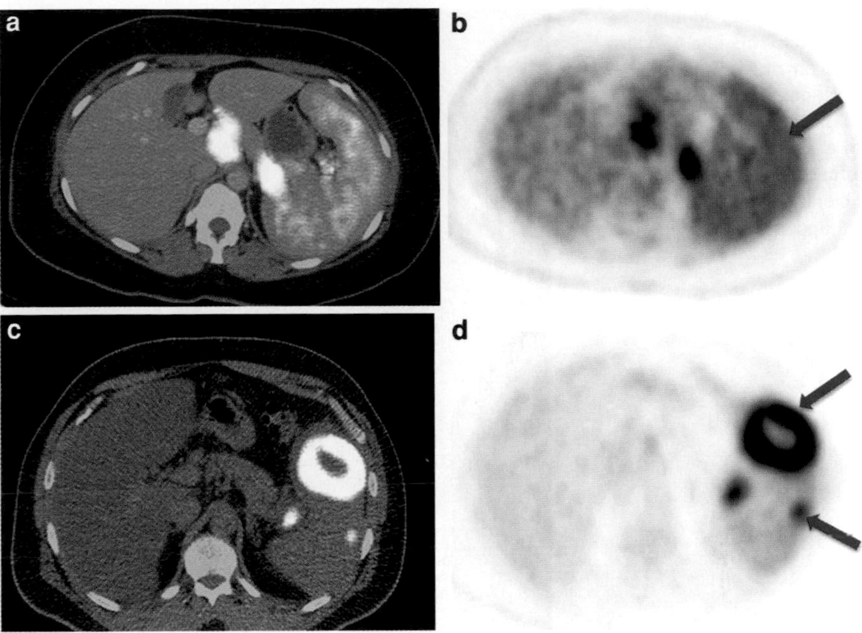

Fig. 6 Diffuse and focal splenic lymphoma. (**a**, **b**) Axial PET/CT and PET in a 45-year-old woman demonstrate hypermetabolic paraaortic lymphadenopathy and diffuse hypermetabolic (greater than liver, SUV_{max} 3.1) and enlarged spleen consistent with diffuse splenic lymphoma. (**c**, **d**) Axial PET/CT and PET in a 43-year-old male patient demonstrate intensely FDG-hypermetabolic focal splenic lesions (SUV_{max} up to 31.6) consistent with focal splenic lymphoma as well as mild splenic enlargement

(Africa), the sporadic type (Europe, Japan and the United States), and the immunodeficiency type. Non-African Burkitt lymphoma is extremely hypermetabolic and shows a high SUV_{max}. Treatment decreases the SUV in 85% of patients (Weiler-Sagie et al. 2010; Brepoels et al. 2007a, b).

5 Leukemia

Acute myeloid leukemia (AML) is a neoplasm of hematopoietic stem cells that do not retain the ability to differentiate but do retain proliferation capacity. Genetic factors are the most important predictors of outcome and response to therapy (Estey and Dohner 2006). Extramedullary disease seems to be more and more important in patients with relapse after allogenic stem cell transplantation (Kikushige et al. 2007). In contrast to malignant lymphoma, morphologic and functional imaging plays a minor role in the care of patients with leukemia. Increased FDG uptake in extramedullary leukemia has been shown earlier in a case report (Kuenzle et al. 2002). Buck et al. (2008) recently demonstrated uptake of 18-F FLT, a thymidine analog, in leukemia manifestations, indicating that molecular imaging of leukemia is feasible. Implications for clinical management and assessment of prognosis still need to be addressed.

6 Multiple Myeloma

6.1 Epidemiology and Disease Characteristics

Multiple myeloma is a cancerous malignancy of the blood that is characterized by clonal proliferation of the malignant plasma cells. It is the second most frequent malignancy of the blood after NHL and is the most common cause of primary malignancy in bones. Patients generally present with excess bone marrow plasma cells, osteolytic bone lesions, renal disease, and immunodeficiency (Hanrahan et al. 2010; Raab et al. 2009). In the United States, about 20,000 patients are diagnosed with and about 10,000 die from multiple myeloma every year (Laubach et al. 2009; Jemal et al. 2008). Despite advances in treatment such as the use of thalidomide, lenalidomide, the proteasome inhibitor bortezomib, stem cell transplantation, and monoclonal antibodies, the prognosis for patients with multiple myeloma remains poor. The disease has an average

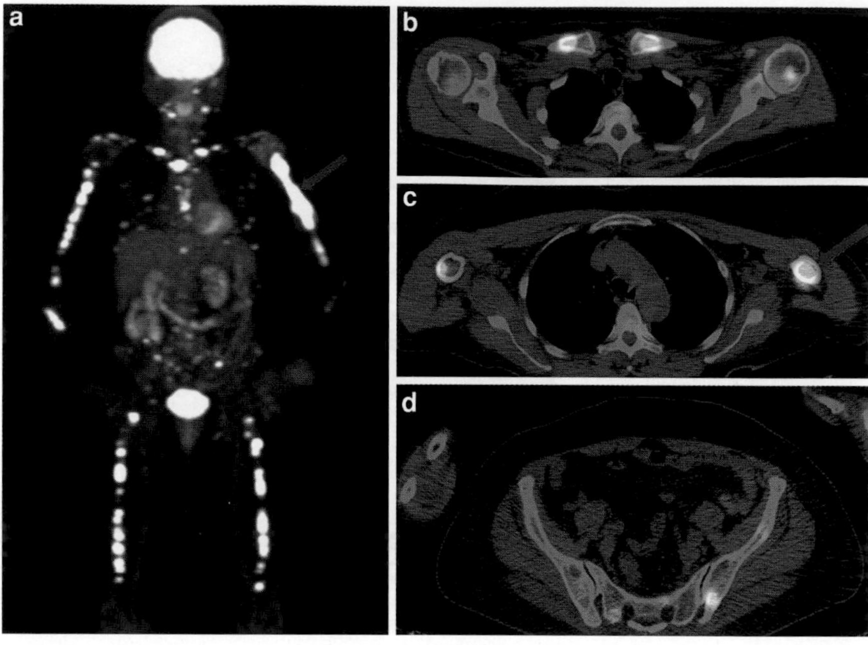

Fig. 7 Staging: Multiple myeloma. This is a 65-year-old woman with multiple myeloma. The MIP PET (**a**) and axial PET/CT (**b**, **c**, **d**) images demonstrate diffuse FDG-hypermetabolic skeletal lesions in the axial and appendicular skeleton

age of onset of 60 years and a 5-year survival of 45% (Lutje et al. 2009).

6.2 The Limitations of Conventional Imaging

The most widely used staging system for multiple myeloma, the Durie and Salmon myeloma staging system, determined that the detection of bone lesions by radiographic methods best correlated with measured myeloma cell mass (Durie and Salmon 1975). Most institutions assess the disease stage, disease progression, and treatment response using whole-body X-rays (Lutje et al. 2009). Indeed, in 2009, the International Myeloma Working Group (IMWG) established that conventional radiography remains the gold standard for staging patients with multiple myeloma and that PET/CT was not recommended for routine use in patients with multiple myeloma (Dimopoulos et al. 2009).

However, conventional imaging has many limitations compared to newer modalities such as MRI and FDG PET/CT that can lead to misdiagnosis. In a large prospective study involving 239 patients, Bartel et al. (2009) showed that the use of PET/CT to assess FDG suppression after induction therapy may offer a survival benefit by altering treatment in patients in whom FDG suppression cannot be achieved. Conventional imaging is unable to detect multiple myeloma early because lytic lesions are observable only when 30–50% of the bone mineral density is already lost (Lutje et al. 2009). In several studies comparing the sensitivity of radiography versus MRI for bone involvement in multiple myeloma, radiography had a false positive rate ranging from 30 to 70% (Ludwig et al. 1987; Fruehwald et al. 1988; Lecouvet et al. 1999). Furthermore, it is difficult to differentiate between osteopenia due to multiple myeloma from more common causes such as early signs of osteoporosis or excessive alcohol use (Dinter et al. 2009).

6.3 The Use of PET/CT

Newer imaging techniques such as PET/CT are integral to better diagnose and create more effective treatment regimens for patients with multiple myeloma. FDG PET is a superior modality for detecting bone marrow involvement in patients with multiple myeloma (Fig. 7). Bredella et al. (2005) showed that sensitivity of FDG PET in detecting myelomatous involvement was 85 and specificity was 92%. PET/CT is also able to distinguish between intramedullary and extramedullary lesions. In a study conducted by Nanni et al. (2006)

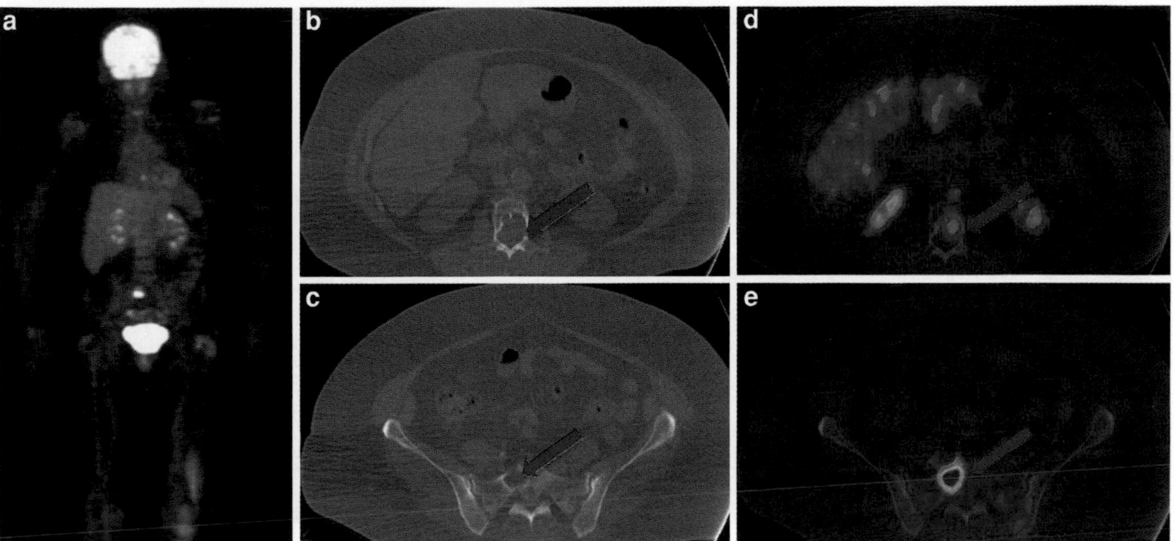

Fig. 8 Lesion biology: Multiple myeloma. This is a 68-year-old woman with lytic lesions (MIP PET, **a**) in the lumbar (**b**) and sacral (**c**) vertebral bodies. The lumbar vertebral body demonstrated mild FDG uptake (**d**) suggestive of less active disease, while the sacral vertebral body lesion demonstrated intense FDG hypermetabolism (**e**) suggestive of active disease

additional lesions in the skeleton were detected in 16 of 28 patients with newly diagnosed multiple myeloma when using FDG PET/CT compared to whole-body X-ray. Although MRI is also useful in cases of multiple myeloma, Fonti et al. (2008) showed that FDG PET/CT performed better than MRI in the detection of focal lesions in whole-body analysis.

6.4 Staging

Studies have shown that both FDG PET and FDG PET/CT can generally detect more lytic lesions and better stage multiple myeloma patients for treatment (Fig. 8). Zamangi et al. (2007) showed that in a prospective study of 46 newly diagnosed patients with multiple myeloma, FDG PET was superior in detecting lesions in 46% of patients, whereas whole-body radiography was superior in only 8% of patients. Van Lammeren-Venema et al. (2011) conducted a concordance assessment using 7 studies with a total of 242 patients between whole-body radiography and FDG PET. Of the 7 studies, 6 showed that FDG PET was able to detect more lesions at staging than whole-body radiography, with the exception of lytic lesions in the skull.

6.5 Therapy Assessment

FDG PET is especially useful during mid-therapy in ways that can significantly affect subsequent care (Fig. 9). Especially in cases of non-secretory multiple myeloma, residual glucose uptake shown by FDG PET mid-therapy can help to differentiate between high-risk and low-risk cases of multiple myeloma (Durie and Salmon 1975). In a study of 239 patients, Bartel et al. (2009) showed that the presence of 3 or more FDG-avid lesions in patients before autologous stem cell transplantation was associated with lower survival rates. However, the prognostic value of SUV mid-therapy is less clear. In a study of 19 patients, Dimitrakopoulou-Strauss demonstrated that although baseline SUV is a helpful tool to predict progression-free survival after chemotherapy, there was no correlation between the decrease in SUV after the first cycle of chemotherapy and progression-free survival (Dimitrakopoulou-Strauss et al. 2009). A recent prospective study involving 192 newly diagnosed multiple myeloma patients showed that the presence of at least 3 focal lesions, an SUV of more than 4.2, and extramedullary disease adversely affected progression-free survival (Zamagni et al. 2012). An SUV over 4.2 and the presence of extramedullary disease also correlated with

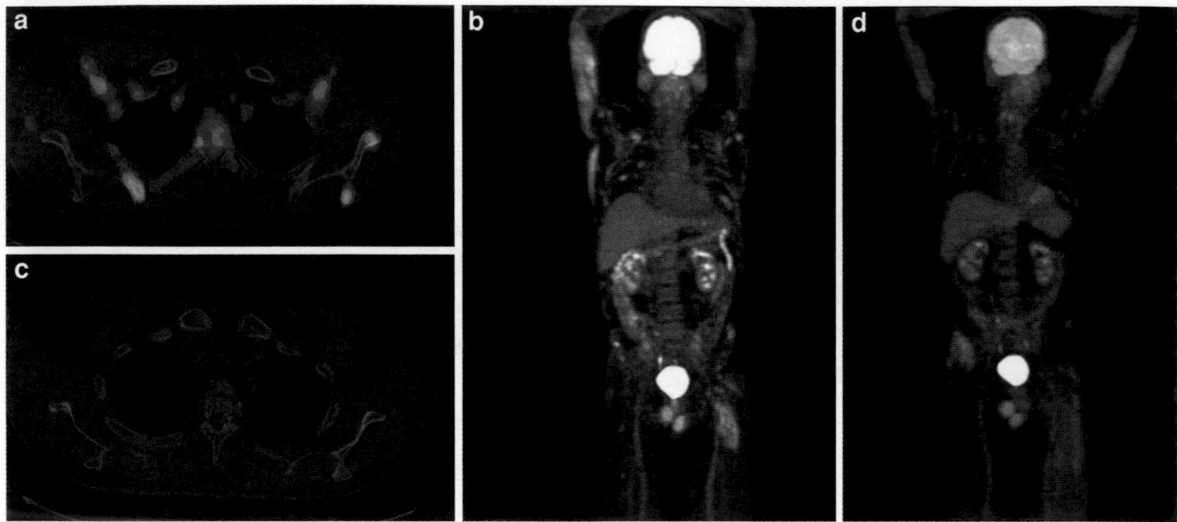

Fig. 9 Therapy response: Multiple myeloma. This is a 59-year-old man with multiple skeletal FDG-hypermetabolic lesions at baseline (**a** axial PET/CT and **b** MIP PET) and post-therapy (**c** axial PET/CT and **d** MIP PET). Images demonstrate complete metabolic resolution

shorter overall survival, with 4-year rates of 77 and 66%, respectively. Persistence of an SUV over 4.2 after thalidomide-dexamethasone induction therapy is also associated with shorter survival rates. Four-year overall survival of patients with a negative PET/CT 3 months after double auto transplantation was superior to those who had a positive PET/CT, with a progression-free survival rate of 66 and overall survival of 89%. Multivariate analysis showed that extramedullary disease, an SUV over 4.2 at baseline and a positive PET/CT 3 months after double transplantation were associated with shorter progression-free survival (Zamagni et al. 2012).

6.6 Pitfalls

Despite the many benefits of FDG PET/CT, there are still several pitfalls to the use of PET/CT in cases of multiple myeloma. Breyer et al. (2006) showed that PET/CT alone, can fail to detect diffuse spine involvement and lytic skeletal lesions smaller than 10 mm. In addition, treatment with corticosteroids concurrently during the time of PET/CT use can result in false positives (Hanrahan et al. 2010).

7 Conclusion

FDG PET/CT plays a key role in the diagnosis and evaluation of both HL and NHL and has become the first-line imaging modality for staging and end of therapy assessment. FDG PET/CT is more accurate than anatomic imaging alone. Imaging professionals should be aware of the different grades of lymphoma (indolent or aggressive) that generally correlate with management and FDG avidity. PET/CT is most efficiently employed if its uses and limitations in the context of treatment are understood. Furthermore, the level of metabolic activity indicated by PET/CT provides important prognostic information. FDG PET/CT improves primary diagnosis and assessment of treatment response in patients with lymphoma. Other radiotracers like FLT, hypoxia, or apoptosis imaging (De Saint-Hubert et al. 2008) as well as targeted molecular imaging of specific surface characteristics (Neumaier et al. 2008) are not yet ready for broad clinical use; however, they possess great potential to further improve molecular imaging of malignant lymphoma. Recently, molecular imaging of leukemia has also been shown to be feasible;

however, the clinical importance of this finding is yet to be adequately addressed. PET/CT is superior to standard radiographic staging for multiple myeloma. It appears to be a prognostic marker for predicting outcome at baseline, after induction therapy and after transplantation for patients with multiple myeloma. Further studies may be necessary for validation of these initial findings for incorporation of PET/CT in the guidelines for management for multiple myeloma.

References

Bangerter M, Moog F, Buchmann I et al (1998) Whole-body 2-[18F]-fluoro-2-deoxy-D-glucose positron emission tomography (FDG-PET) for accurate staging of Hodgkin's disease. Ann Oncol 9(10):1117–1122

Bartel TB, Haessler J, Brown TL et al (2009) F18-fluorodeoxyglucose positron emission tomography in the context of other imaging techniques and prognostic factors in multiple myeloma. Blood 114(10):2068–2076

Blake MA, Singh A, Setty BN et al (2006) Pearls and pitfalls in interpretation of abdominal and pelvic PET-CT. Radiographics 26(5):1335–1353

Blodgett TM, Meltzer CC, Townsend DW (2007) PET/CT: form and function. Radiology 242(2):360–385

Bredella MA, Steinbach L, Caputo G, Segall G, Hawkins R (2005) Value of FDG PET in the assessment of patients with multiple myeloma. Am J Roentgenol 184(4):1199–1204

Brepoels L, Stroobants S, De Wever W et al (2007a) Aggressive and indolent non-Hodgkin's lymphoma: response assessment by integrated international workshop criteria. Leuk Lymphoma 48(8):1522–1530

Brepoels L, Stroobants S, De Wever W et al (2007b) Hodgkin lymphoma: response assessment by revised international workshop criteria. Leuk Lymphoma 48(8):1539–1547

Breyer RJ 3rd, Mulligan ME, Smith SE, Line BR, Badros AZ (2006) Comparison of imaging with FDG PET/CT with other imaging modalities in myeloma. Skeletal Radiol 35(9):632–640

Buchmann I, Reinhardt M, Elsner K et al (2001) 2- (fluorine-18)fluoro-2-deoxy-D-glucose positron emission tomography in the detection and staging of malignant lymphoma a bicenter trial. Cancer 91(5):889–899

Buck AK, Bommer M, Stilgenbauer S et al (2006) Molecular imaging of proliferation in malignant lymphoma. Cancer Res 66(22):11055–11061

Buck AK, Herrmann K, Buschenfelde CM et al (2008) Imaging bone and soft tissue tumors with the proliferation marker [18F]fluorodeoxythymidine. Clin Cancer Res 14(10):2970–2977

Cabanillas F, Fuller LM (1990) The radiologic assessment of the lymphoma patient from the standpoint of the clinician. Radiol Clin North Am 28(4):683–695

Castellucci P, Nanni C, Farsad M et al (2005) Potential pitfalls of 18F-FDG PET in a large series of patients treated for malignant lymphoma: prevalence and scan interpretation. Nucl Med Commun 26(8):689–694

Cheson BD, Horning SJ, Coiffier B et al (1999) Report of an international workshop to standardize response criteria for non-Hodgkin's lymphomas. NCI sponsored international working group. J Clin Oncol 17(4):1244

Cheson BD, Pfistner B, Juweid ME et al (2007) Revised response criteria for malignant lymphoma. J Clin Oncol 25(5):579–586

De Saint-Hubert M, Wang H, Devos E et al (2008) Preclinical Imaging of Therapy Response Using Metabolic and Apoptosis Molecular Imaging. Mol Imaging Biol 18(7):1422–1430

Delbeke D, Stroobants S, de Kerviler E, Gisselbrecht C, Meignan M, Conti PS (2009) Expert opinions on positron emission tomography and computed tomography imaging in lymphoma. Oncologist 14(Suppl 2):30–40

Dimitrakopoulou-Strauss A, Hoffmann M, Bergner R, Uppenkamp M, Haberkorn U, Strauss LG (2009) Prediction of progression-free survival in patients with multiple myeloma following anthracycline-based chemotherapy based on dynamic FDG-PET. Clin Nucl Med 34(9):576–584

Dimopoulos M, Terpos E, Comenzo RL et al (2009) International myeloma working group consensus statement and guidelines regarding the current role of imaging techniques in the diagnosis and monitoring of multiple Myeloma. Leukemia 23(9):1545–1556

Dinter DJ, Neff WK, Klaus J et al (2009) Comparison of whole-body MR imaging and conventional X-ray examination in patients with multiple myeloma and implications for therapy. Ann Hematol 88(5):457–464

Durie BG, Salmon SE (1975) A clinical staging system for multiple myeloma. Correlation of measured myeloma cell mass with presenting clinical features, response to treatment, and survival. Cancer 36(3):842–854

Elstrom R, Guan L, Baker G et al (2003) Utility of FDG-PET scanning in lymphoma by WHO classification. Blood 101(10):3875–3876

Estey E, Dohner H (2006) Acute myeloid leukaemia. Lancet 368(9550):1894–1907

Fonti R, Salvatore B, Quarantelli M et al (2008) 18F-FDG PET/CT, 99mTc-MIBI, and MRI in evaluation of patients with multiple myeloma. J Nucl Med 49(2):195–200

Fruehwald FX, Tscholakoff D, Schwaighofer B et al (1988) Magnetic resonance imaging of the lower vertebral column in patients with multiple myeloma. Invest Radiol 23(3):193–199

Fueger BJ, Yeom K, Czernin J, Sayre JW, Phelps ME, Allen-Auerbach MS (2009) Comparison of CT, PET, and PET/CT for staging of patients with indolent non-Hodgkin's lymphoma. Mol Imaging Biol 11(4):269–274

Graf K, Dietrich T, Tachezy M et al (2008) Monitoring therapeutical intervention with ezetimibe using targeted near-infrared fluorescence imaging in experimental atherosclerosis. Mol Imaging 7(2):68–76

Hanrahan CJ, Christensen CR, Crim JR (2010) Current concepts in the evaluation of multiple myeloma with MR imaging and FDG PET/CT. Radiographics 30(1):127–142

Harris NL, Jaffe ES, Diebold J et al (2000) The World Health Organization classification of neoplastic diseases of the haematopoietic and lymphoid tissues: Report of the Clinical Advisory Committee Meeting, Airlie House, Virginia. Histopathology 36(1):69–86

Hasenclever D, Diehl V (1998) A prognostic score for advanced Hodgkin's disease. International prognostic factors project on advanced Hodgkin's disease. N Engl J Med 339(21):1506–1514

Huang SC (2000) Anatomy of SUV standardized uptake value. Nucl Med Biol 27(7):643–646

Hunt BM, Vallieres E, Buduhan G, Aye R, Louie B (2009) Sarcoidosis as a benign cause of lymphadenopathy in cancer patients. Am J Surg 197(5):629–632 (discussion 32)

Hutchings M, Barrington SF (2009) PET/CT for therapy response assessment in lymphoma. J Nucl Med 50(Suppl 1):21S–30S

Hutchings M, Loft A, Hansen M et al (2006) Position emission tomography with or without computed tomography in the primary staging of Hodgkin's lymphoma. Haematologica 91(4):482–489

Jacene HA, Filice R, Kasecamp W, Wahl RL (2009) 18F-FDG PET/CT for monitoring the response of lymphoma to radioimmunotherapy. J Nucl Med 50(1):8–17

Jemal A, Siegel R, Ward E et al (2008) Cancer statistics, 2008. CA Cancer J Clin 58(2):71–96

Jerusalem G, Beguin Y, Fassotte MF et al (1999) Whole-body positron emission tomography using 18F-fluorodeoxyglucose for posttreatment evaluation in Hodgkin's disease and non-Hodgkin's lymphoma has higher diagnostic and prognostic value than classical computed tomography scan imaging. Blood 94(2):429–433

Jerusalem G, Beguin Y, Fassotte MF et al (2001) Whole-body positron emission tomography using 18F-fluorodeoxyglucose compared to standard procedures for staging patients with Hodgkin's disease. Haematologica 86(3):266–273

Juweid ME (2006) Utility of positron emission tomography (PET) scanning in managing patients with Hodgkin lymphoma. Hematology/the Education Program of the American Society of Hematology American Society of Hematology 259(65):510–511

Juweid ME (2008) 18F-FDG PET as a routine test for posttherapy assessment of Hodgkin's disease and aggressive non-Hodgkin's lymphoma: where is the evidence? J Nucl Med 49(1):9–12

Juweid ME, Cheson BD (2005) Role of positron emission tomography in lymphoma. J Clin Oncol 23(21): 4577–4580

Juweid ME, Wiseman GA, Vose JM et al (2005) Response assessment of aggressive non-Hodgkin's lymphoma by integrated International Workshop Criteria and fluorine-18-fluorodeoxyglucose positron emission tomography. J Clin Oncol 23(21):4652–4661

Juweid ME, Stroobants S, Hoekstra OS et al (2007) Use of positron emission tomography for response assessment of lymphoma: consensus of the imaging subcommittee of international harmonization project in lymphoma. J Clin Oncol 25(5):571–578

Karam M, Novak L, Cyriac J, Ali A, Nazeer T, Nugent F (2006) Role of fluorine-18 fluoro-deoxyglucose positron emission tomography scan in the evaluation and follow-up of patients with low-grade lymphomas. Cancer 107(1):175–183

Karam M, Roberts-Klein S, Shet N, Chang J, Feustel P (2008) Bilateral hilar foci on 18F-FDG PET scan in patients without lung cancer: variables associated with benign and malignant etiology. J Nucl Med 49(9):1429–1436

Karam M, Ata A, Irish K et al (2009) FDG positron emission tomography/computed tomography scan may identify mantle cell lymphoma patients with unusually favorable outcome. Nucl Med Commun 30(10):770–778

Kikushige Y, Takase K, Sata K et al (2007) Repeated relapses of acute myelogenous leukemia in the isolated extramedullary sites following allogeneic bone marrow transplantations. Intern med (Tokyo, Japan) 46(13):1011–1014

Kostakoglu L, Leonard JP, Kuji I, Coleman M, Vallabhajosula S, Goldsmith SJ (2002) Comparison of fluorine-18 fluorodeoxyglucose positron emission tomography and Ga-67 scintigraphy in evaluation of lymphoma. Cancer 94(4):879–888

Kuenzle K, Taverna C, Steinert HC (2002) Detection of extramedullary infiltrates in acute myelogenous leukemia with whole-body positron emission tomography and 2-deoxy-2-[18F]-fluoro-D-glucose. Mol Imaging Biol 4(2):179–183

Kwee TC, Kwee RM, Nievelstein RA (2008) Imaging in staging of malignant lymphoma: a systematic review. Blood 111(2):504–516

Laubach JP, Mitsiades CS, Mahindra A et al (2009) Novel therapies in the treatment of multiple myeloma. J Natl Compr Canc Netw 7(9):947–960

Le Dortz L, De Guibert S, Bayat S et al (2010) Diagnostic and prognostic impact of (18)F-FDG PET/CT in follicular lymphoma. Eur J Nucl Med Mol Imaging 37:2307–2314

Lecouvet FE, Malghem J, Michaux L et al (1999) Skeletal survey in advanced multiple myeloma: radiographic versus MR imaging survey. Br J Haematol 106(1):35–39

Love C, Tomas M, Tronco G, Palestro C (2005) FDG PET of Infection and Inflammation. RadioGraphics 25:1357–1368

Ludwig H, Fruhwald F, Tscholakoff D, Rasoul S, Neuhold A, Fritz E (1987) Magnetic resonance imaging of the spine in multiple myeloma. Lancet 2(8555):364–366

Lutje S, de Rooy JW, Croockewit S, Koedam E, Oyen WJ, Raymakers RA (2009) Role of radiography, MRI and FDG-PET/CT in diagnosing, staging and therapeutical evaluation of patients with multiple myeloma. Ann Hematol 88(12): 1161–1168

MacDermed D, Thurber L, George TI, Hoppe RT, Le QT (2004) Extranodal nonorbital indolent lymphomas of the head and neck: relationship between tumor control and radiotherapy. Int J Radiat Oncol Biol Phys 59(3):788–795

Menda Y, Graham MM (2005) Update on 18F-Fluorodeoxyglucose/positron emission tomography and positron emission tomography/computed tomography imaging of squamous head and neck cancers. Semin Nucl Med 35(4):214–219

Moog F, Bangerter M, Diederichs CG et al (1998) Extranodal malignant lymphoma: detection with FDG PET versus CT. Radiology 206(2):475–481

Nanni C, Zamagni E, Farsad M et al (2006) Role of 18F-FDG PET/CT in the assessment of bone involvement in newly diagnosed multiple myeloma: preliminary results. Eur J Nucl Med Mol Imaging 33(5):525–531

Naumann R, Beuthien-Baumann B, Reiss A et al (2004) Substantial impact of FDG PET imaging on the therapy decision in patients with early-stage Hodgkin's lymphoma. Br J Cancer 90(3):620–625

Neumaier B, Mottaghy F, Buck A et al (2008) 18)F-immuno-PET: Determination of anti-CD66 biodistribution in a patient with high-risk leukemia. Cancer Biother Radiopharm (23): 819–824

Pakos EE, Fotopoulos AD, Ioannidis JP (2005) 18F-FDG PET for evaluation of bone marrow infiltration in staging of lymphoma: a meta-analysis. J Nucl Med 46(6):958–963

Prabhakar HB, Sahani DV, Fischman AJ, Mueller PR, Blake MA (2007) Bowel Hot Spots at PET-CT. Radiographics 27(1):145–159

Raab MS, Podar K, Breitkreutz I, Richardson PG, Anderson KC (2009) Multiple myeloma. Lancet 374(9686):324–339

Schoder H, Meta J, Yap C et al (2001) Effect of whole-body (18)F-FDG PET imaging on clinical staging and management of patients with malignant lymphoma. J Nucl Med 42(8):1139–1143

Seam P, Juweid ME, Cheson BD (2007) The role of FDG-PET scans in patients with lymphoma. Blood 110(10): 3507–3516

Sonet A, Graux C, Nollevaux MC, Krug B, Bosly A (2007) Vander Borght T. Unsuspected FDG-PET findings in the follow-up of patients with lymphoma. Ann Hematol 86(1):9–15

Spaepen K, Mortelmans L (2001) Evaluation of treatment response in patients with lymphoma using [18F]FDG-PET: differences between non-Hodgkin's lymphoma and Hodgkin's disease. Q J Nucl Med 45(3):269–273

Spaepen K, Stroobants S, Dupont P et al (2003) Prognostic value of pretransplantation positron emission tomography using fluorine 18-fluorodeoxyglucose in patients with aggressive lymphoma treated with high-dose chemotherapy and stem cell transplantation. Blood 102(1):53–59

Terasawa T, Nihashi T, Hotta T, Nagai H (2008) 18F-FDG PET for posttherapy assessment of Hodgkin's disease and aggressive Non-Hodgkin's lymphoma: a systematic review. J Nucl Med 49(1):13–21

Tsang RW, Gospodarowicz MK, Pintilie M et al (2001) Solitary plasmacytoma treated with radiotherapy: impact of tumor size on outcome. Int J Radiat Oncol Biol Phys 50(1):113–120

Tsukamoto N, Kojima M, Hasegawa M et al (2007) The usefulness of (18)F-fluorodeoxyglucose positron emission tomography ((18)F-FDG-PET) and a comparison of (18) F-FDG-pet with (67) gallium scintigraphy in the evaluation of lymphoma: relation to histologic subtypes based on the World Health Organization classification. Cancer 110(3):652–659

van Lammeren-Venema D, Regelink JC, Riphagen, II, Zweegman S, Hoekstra OS, Zijlstra JM (2011) (18) F-fluoro-deoxyglucose positron emission tomography in assessment of myeloma-related bone disease: A systematic review. Cancer. doi:10.1002/cncr.26467 [1 Sep 2011]

von Schulthess GK, Steinert HC, Hany TF (2006) Integrated PET/CT: current applications and future directions. Radiology 238(2):405–422

Weiler-Sagie M, Bushelev O, Epelbaum R et al (2010) (18) F-FDG avidity in lymphoma readdressed: a study of 766 patients. J Nucl Med 51 (1):25–30

Wirth A, Seymour JF, Hicks RJ et al (2002) Fluorine-18 fluorodeoxyglucose positron emission tomography, gallium-67 scintigraphy, and conventional staging for Hodgkin's disease and non-Hodgkin's lymphoma. Am J Med 112(4):262–268

Wirth A, Foo M, Seymour JF, Macmanus MP, Hicks RJ (2008) Impact of [18f] fluorodeoxyglucose positron emission tomography on staging and management of early-stage follicular non-hodgkin lymphoma. Int J Radiat Oncol Biol Phys 71(1):213–219

Yang DH, Min JJ, Jeong YY et al (2009) The combined evaluation of interim contrast-enhanced computerized tomography (CT) and FDG-PET/CT predicts the clinical outcomes and may impact on the therapeutic plans in patients with aggressive non-Hodgkin's lymphoma. Ann Hematol 88(5):425–432

Zamagni E, Nanni C, Patriarca F et al (2007) A prospective comparison of 18F-fluorodeoxyglucose positron emission tomography-computed tomography, magnetic resonance imaging and whole-body planar radiographs in the assessment of bone disease in newly diagnosed multiple myeloma. Haematologica 92(1):50–55

Zamagni E, Petrucci A, Tosi P et al (2012) Long-term results of thalidomide and dexamethasone (thal-dex) as therapy of first relapse in multiple myeloma. Ann Hematol 91(3):419–426

Zijlstra JM (2006) Lindauer-van der Werf G, Hoekstra OS, Hooft L, Riphagen, II, Huijgens PC. 18F-fluoro-deoxyglucose positron emission tomography for post-treatment evaluation of malignant lymphoma: a systematic review. Haematologica 91(4):522–529

Dermatological

David Brandon and Bruce Barron

Contents

D. Brandon (✉) · B. Barron
Department of Radiology,
Emory University School of Medicine,
Atlanta, GA, USA
e-mail: david.brandon@emoryheathcare.org

Abstract

FDG PET/CT is a valuable tool to evaluate many dermatologic malignancies, especially in more advanced disease states. The literature supporting the use of FDG PET/CT in staging, restaging, or treatment assessment is greatest in melanoma. When compared to conventional imaging, FDG PET/CT is superior due to better lesion sensitivity and the extended imaging coverage. Changes in management due to PET/CT results are frequently reported in more than 30% of patients with skin cancers.

1 Overview of the Skin

The skin provides the primary surface for interaction with the world and thus has an array of functions including providing a physical barrier to pathogens, trauma, toxins, solar radiation, and water. Furthermore, it acts as an immunologic organ, thermoregulator, and sensory perception system. The skin is composed of three layers: the epidermis, dermis, and subcutaneous tissue. The epidermis directly provides many of the barrier functions through the layers of keratinocytes which continually replenish themselves and melanin produced by melanocytes. Langerhans cells also reside in the epidermis, collecting and presenting foreign antigens to the lymphocytes. The epidermis relies on the dermis for nutrition and waste elimination through the dermo-epidermal junction as it has no blood or lymphatic vessels. The dermis contains a network of fibrous tissue which imparts strength and flexibility to the skin as well as fibroblasts to maintain the fibrous tissue. The subcutaneous tissue cushions the skin with a layer of adipose tissue.

P. Peller et al. (eds.), *PET-CT and PET-MRI in Oncology*, Medical Radiology. Diagnostic Imging,
DOI: 10.1007/174_2011_498,

FDG PET has been used to evaluate differences in a variety of skin properties among different races, sexes, and ages. Overall, black patients have a slightly higher skin maximum standard uptake value (SUV) and skin thickness than white patients (Wehrli et al. 2007). However, there is no statistically significant difference in the maximum SUV of the skin of men and women despite well-documented differences in skin thickness. As age increases, there is a statistically significant increase in the skin maximum SUV of white patients and an upward trend in the black patients that does not reach significance. As skin ages due to chronologic and photoaging, orderly differentiation of keratinocytes begins to fail as do other processes that contribute to a robust barrier system leading to increased inflammation and keratinocyte turnover. These factors may account for the increase in skin maximum SUV in white patients with age and the anti-oxidative properties of melanin could help explain the lack of statistically significant change in black patients.

2 Melanoma

2.1 Background and Epidemiology

Melanoma is an aggressive skin malignancy arising from melanocytes residing on the basement membrane of the epidermis. Melanocytes produce the photoprotective pigment melanin and deliver melanin packaged in melanosomes to adjacent keratinocytes, imparting color to the skin, eyes, and hair. Originating from neural crest tissue, melanoblasts migrate during development and differentiate into melanocytes upon reaching the target organ. Melanocytes can be found in the cutaneous epidermis, eye, hair follicles, leptomeninges, inner ear, and heart (Bosserhoff 2011). In contrast to the short-lived keratinocyte, the melanocyte has a robust anti-apoptotic system and lives for decades, affording a long time horizon in which to acquire genetic mutations (Plettenberg et al. 1995; Quevado et al. 1969).

Over the past 30 years, the incidence of melanoma has increased in the United States, with an estimated 70,230 new cases of melanoma in 2011 and 8790 melanoma-related deaths (Society 2011a, b). The lifetime risk of melanoma is highest in fair-skinned individuals (approximately 1 in 50) and much lower in dark-skinned individuals (1 in 1,000). Melanoma is common over a wide age range and the incidence increases with age with the highest rates in the ninth decade of life. Based on Surveillance, Epidemiology and End Results (SEER) data, two incidence peaks are observed at 54 and 74 years with truncal melanoma peaking near the former and ear and face melanoma peaking near the latter (Lachiewicz et al. 2008). Men 65 and older have more than double the rate of melanoma than women 65 and older but the incidence is similar for men and women less than 65 (Society 2011a, b).

Additional risk factors for developing melanoma include UV exposure (both solar and artificial), nevi density, presence and size of congenital nevi, personal history of melanoma, familial history of melanoma, immune suppression, and xeroderma pigmentosum, where DNA repair mechanisms are defective. A personal history of melanoma confers a 5–10% risk of a second melanoma developing. Approximately, 10% of melanoma patients have a first degree relative who has had melanoma and gene mutations have been found in 10–40% of families with high incidences of melanoma (Society 2011a, b). Chemical environmental risk factors such as pesticides and arsenic are undergoing further study (Bosserhoff 2011).

2.2 Histopathology

The majority of melanomas are grouped into five clinicopathological categories: superficial spreading, lentigo maligna, acral lentiginous, desmoplastic, and nodular. Superficial spreading melanoma accounts for approximately 70% of melanomas followed by nodular melanoma (15–20%), lentigo maligna (4–15%), acral lentiginous (2–8% in whites, 30–75% in blacks, Hispanics, and Asians), and desmoplastic (<1%) (Habif 2010). Initially most melanoma categories have a radial growth phase lasting for months to years, where atypical melanocytes proliferate within the epidermis with the exception of nodular melanoma which has no significant radial growth phase and shows rapid growth over weeks to months. When the atypical melanocytes extend through the basement membrane to invade the reticular dermis, the melanoma has entered the vertical growth phase and has metastatic potential.

The thickness of the primary melanoma as measured from the top of the granular layer to the deepest level of invasion (Breslow thickness) is the strongest prognostic factor with a thickness of 0.75 mm or less having an excellent prognosis. Ulceration of the primary lesion is the second most important histologic finding for prognosis, indicating a higher risk of metastatic disease and upstaging the lesion. Other significant prognostic histologic findings include mitotic rate, histologic regression, and tumor infiltrating lymphocytes. For melanomas <1 mm thick, the anatomic measure of tumor invasion (Clark level) is more predictive of survival than ulceration (Balch et al. 2001).

Melanoma can spread unpredictably by both lymphatic and hematogenous routes and metastases can be found virtually anywhere in the body. Hematogenous metastases in the absence of lymph node involvement are well known and associated with primary tumors with aggressive features. The most common first sites of distant metastases for stage III patients are the skin (38%), lung (36%), liver (20%), and brain (20%), alone or in combination (Balch 1983). Stage I melanoma has better than a 90% five-year survival rate, but survival drops off quickly for metastatic disease with a five-year survival of 69.5% for stage IIIA and 6.7% for stage IV with lung metastases (M1b).

2.3 Molecular Genetics

While multiple steps are needed for cutaneous melanoma to develop, as with other malignancies, recent discoveries have pointed to two initiation routes for melanoma formation and provided targets for personalized molecular-based therapies.

The mitogen-activated protein kinase (MAPK) pathway is a signaling cascade that helps regulate proliferation, differentiation, senescence, and apoptosis with mutations removing checks on growth (Da Forno and Saldanha 2011). Mutations of the MAPK pathway in melanoma were initially described in NRAS that lead to continuous activation of the entire pathway without external growth signals. Oncogene NRAS mutations are seen in about 20% of cutaneous melanomas. More recently, mutations in the downstream ras effector BRAF have been described that lead to deregulation of proliferation pathways. BRAF mutations are reported in 50–70% of cutaneous melanomas and are more common in younger individuals with multiple nevi and melanomas of intermittently UV-exposed areas (e.g truncal). However, UV radiation is not a significant causative factor of BRAF mutations, and BRAF mutation frequency is low in melanomas in long-term UV exposure areas and is unrelated to UV exposure (acral and mucosal) (Bosserhoff 2011). Furthermore, BRAF mutations are not common in other types of skin cancers in high UV exposure areas. The etiologies of BRAF mutations remain unclear and are a major focus of research. Of note, germline BRAF mutations have not been identified.

NRAS and BRAF mutations are nearly mutually exclusive in melanoma, which is to be expected as they lie in the same pathway, and collectively are seen in 75% of melanomas (Hocker and Tsao 2007) presenting an attractive target for therapies that will be discussed later.

A second important initiation route for melanoma involves mutations in CDKN2A which encodes for both $p16^{INK4a}$ and $p14^{ARF}$ and for which both somatic and germline mutations have been described. $p16^{INK4a}$ acts a tumor suppressor by halting the G1 to S phase transition; function tends to remain preserved in early melanoma but is absent in advanced primary and metastatic melanomas (Da Forno and Saldanha 2011). $p14^{ARF}$ also acts as a tumor suppressor by inhibiting MDM2 which promotes p53 degradation. p53 plays an important role in cell cycle arrest and apoptosis and the loss of control over these cellular functions is crucial in the formation of melanoma.

The PI3K pathway, in which NRAS also plays a key initiating role, helps promotes cell proliferation and survival. In contrast to other cancers in which PI3K pathway mutations are oncogenic, melanomas tend to have mutations in PTEN which normally functions as a tumor suppressor on the PI3K pathway. PTEN deletions are very uncommon in primary melanoma but are common in metastatic melanoma with a 30–50% incidence. Simultaneous BRAF and PTEN mutations in melanoma are well described in the literature.

2.4 Staging

Cutaneous melanoma TNM staging was most recently updated in 2009 with the seventh edition of the American Joint Committee on Cancer (AJCC) Cancer Staging manual (see Table 1) Edge et al. (2009). Stage I and II (localized melanoma) are defined by the primary tumor characteristics (T) and absence of nodal or metastatic disease (see Table 1). Stage III melanoma has spread to regional lymph nodes with distant metastases and is stratified by the pattern of nodal

Table 1 Melanoma of the skin staging, 2009

Primary tumor (T)			
TX	Primary tumor cannot be assessed (for example, curettaged or severely regressed melanoma)		
T0	No evidence of primary tumor		
Tis	Melanoma in situ		
T1	Melanomas 1.0 mm or less in thickness		
T2	Melanomas 1.01–2.0 mm		
T3	Melanomas 2.01–4.0 mm		
T4	Melanomas more than 4.0 mm		
T classification			
	Thickness (mm)		Ulceration status/mitoses
T1	≤1.0		a: w/o ulceration and mitosis <1/mm^2
			b: with ulceration or mitoses ≥1/mm^2
T2	1.01–2.0		a: w/o ulceration
			b: with ulceration
T3	2.01–4.0		a: w/o ulceration
			b: with ulceration
T4	>4.0		a: w/o ulceration
			b: with ulceration
Clinical staging			
Stage 0	Tis	N0	M0
Stage IA	T1a	N0	M0
Stage IB	T1b	N0	M0
	T2a	N0	M0
Stage IIA	T2b	N0	M0
	T3a	N0	M0
Stage IIB	T3b	N0	M0
	T4a	N0	M0
Stage IIC	T4b	N0	M0
Stage III	Any T	≥N1	M0

Source. Adapted from AJCC 7th edition
Note: a and b subcategories of T are assigned based on ulceration and number of mitoses per mm^2

metastases (N). Stage IV melanoma is characterized by the presence of distant metastases and stratified by metastasis location. Additionally, elevated serum LDH at initial presentation upstages the patient to M1c regardless of the site of metastasis.

For melanomas >1 mm in depth or when ulceration is present, sentinel lymph node biopsy (SNLB) has a very high sensitivity (≥95%) and has had a significant impact on clinical care by upstaging patients who were deemed clinically node-negative (Yu et al. 1999). SLNB is not indicated when lymph node metastases have been confirmed prior to surgery. AJCC 7 also added immunohistochemical detection of lymph node metastases which significantly lowers the threshold for detecting micrometastases and accounts in part for the shift from a micrometastases-only rate of 50% to over 80% in stage III patients (Leong et al. 2011).

3 FDG PET in Melanoma Staging

In the early 1990s, radiolabeled glucose analogs were shown to localize well, first in mouse models with both murine melanomas and human melanoma

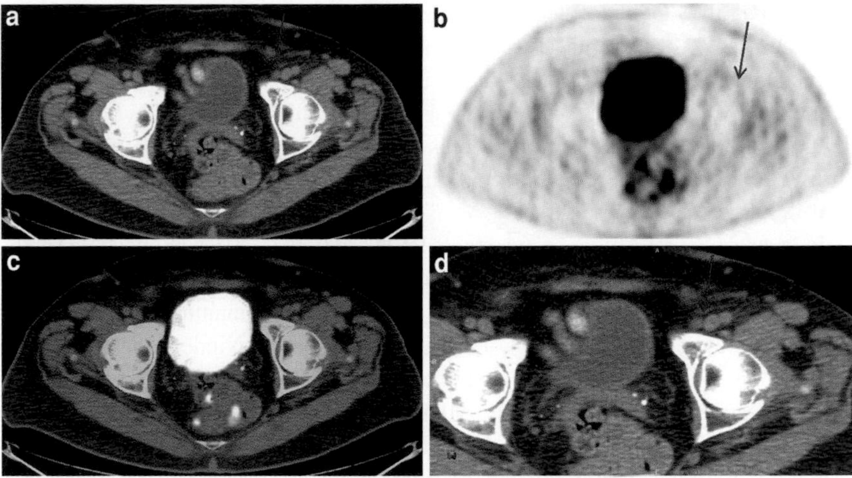

Fig. 1 False negative: CT, PET, fused, and zoomed CT images (**a**–**d**). False-negative lymph node (*red arrow*) in a patient with a left heel melanoma. On pathology, the maximum length of the metastasis was 1.2 mm resulting in a tumor volume of <78 mm^3 which correlates with very poor FDG sensitivity for melanoma lymph node metastases

xenografts and then in patients with melanoma (Gritters et al. 1993; Kern 1991; Wahl et al. 1991). Subsequently, the role of FDG PET and FDG PET/CT in staging, prognosis, restaging, and therapy monitoring has been investigated.

Due to the visibility of cutaneous lesions and PET technical limitations, FDG PET does not have a role in the diagnosis of melanoma, although primary lesions can occasionally be seen. The sensitivity of FDG PET for lesions less than 78 mm^3 is very poor (14%) which has implications for both primary lesions and nodes with micrometastases (Fig. 1) (Wagner et al. 2001). Therefore, FDG PET is not recommended for patients with pathologic stage I through IIIA when regional nodes are negative or have a low metastatic burden due to poor sensitivity, as demonstrated in two large recent meta-analyses (2096 PET only patients, 809 PET/CT patients in Krug et al.) (Jimenez-Requena et al. 2010; Krug et al. 2008). The overall sensitivity of 60% for early stage disease in the meta-analysis by Krug was much lower than the sensitivity of SLNB (Krug et al. 2008). Of note, both meta-analyses focused primarily on FDG PET alone as the FDG PET/CT literature was limited and their data covered a long period when PET technology was rapidly improving and AJCC melanoma staging categories were changed.

In patients with a greater regional node tumor burden or distant metastases (stages IIIB-IV), FDG PET performs much better with an overall sensitivity of 86% and specificity of 87% (Krug et al. 2008). By comparison, ultrasound, chest and abdomen CT, brain MRI, and bone scintigraphy have sensitivities ranging from 57 to 81% and specificities from 45 to 87% (Uren et al. 2011). Compared to conventional imaging, FDG PET has better sensitivity for deep soft-tissue, lymph node, and visceral metastases, which are the most frequently missed metastases noted on autopsy. The metastases which PET most frequently misses are reported to be sub-centimeter lung metastases, brain, liver, predominantly necrotic metastases, and subcutaneous metastases. False-positive lesions on PET due to infection and inflammation are another source of error.

When CT is acquired in the same session, PET/CT showed improved sensitivity and specificity over FDG PET in both a meta-analysis and a more recent prospective trial including improved sensitivity for the lesions that PET-only imaging misses (Krug et al. 2008; Strobel et al. 2007). The prospective trial also compared PET/CT to PET/CT with a dedicated CT read in 124 patients; the dedicated CT read improved sensitivity from 85 to 98%. The sensitivity for brain metastases on FDG PET remains low, and is often specifically excluded from analysis in many papers, necessitating a brain MRI if there is clinical concern. In patients with palpable lymph nodes, PET/CT prior to surgery had a sensitivity of 87% and specificity of 98% for detection of other metastases, changing the surgical plan in 37% of patients (Aukema et al. 2010). In this study, brain MRI was also employed, finding brain metastases in 7% of patients. In 49 patients with surgery planned for metastases based on CT chest, abdomen, and pelvis and MRI brain findings, FDG PET found additional metastases in 55% of patients leading to treatment changes in 24 patients (49%) and surgical cancelation in 12 patients (24%) (Gulec et al.

2003). Overall, FDG PET leads to a change in management in 33% of patients (8 studies, range 15–64%) with advanced disease primarily due to upstaging and delineation of metastatic burden, though in 1 study FDG PET did downstage 4% of patients thought to be unresectable based on conventional imaging (Krug et al. 2008; Valk et al. 1996).

In a prospective study of 64 stage III/IV patient comparing FDG PET/CT with whole-body MRI, the overall accuracy of PET/CT was 87% compared to 79% (Pfannenberg et al. 2007). PET/CT was more accurate in N-staging and skin, subcutaneous, and lung metastases with whole-body MRI being more accurate for liver bone and brain metastases. While it is clear that PET/CT staging can be augmented by organ-specific MRI, especially for the brain and liver, the role of whole-body MRI, including PET/MR, remains under investigation.

Recently, elevation of the serum tumor marker LDH was added to the AJCC M staging criteria due to an associated worse prognosis. Elevation in other tumor markers has been shown to predict relapse of disease prior to detection on conventional imaging (S100B) or to signal the progression from local to metastatic disease (melanoma inhibitory activity—MIA) but the role of non-LDH serum marker in the management of melanoma remains unclear. In a retrospective study of 125 consecutive high risk melanoma patients, the prognostic value for cancer-related mortality of FDG PET/CT was greater than both serum S100B and MIA with sensitivities of 96.8, 45.2, and 36.1%, respectively (Essler et al. 2011). In 31% of patients with metastatic disease on PET, the two tumor markers were never elevated.

In summary, for stage IIIB, IIIC, and IV cutaneous melanoma, FDG PET/CT is the most accurate modality for staging, has a significant effect on patient management, and can be augmented by dedicated anatomic imaging when clinically indicated, especially brain MRI.

4 FDG PET Imaging Protocol

Standard preparations for FDG PET/CT (fasting, exogenous insulin avoidance, etc.) have been discussed in prior chapters and should be followed by the patient. The imaging field typically extends from the vertex of the skull to at least mid-thigh, though some institutions acquire the entirety of the lower extremities on all cutaneous melanoma patients. Patients with primaries in the lower extremities should have their entire body imaged. Two studies found the addition of the lower extremities to be of no clinical value in 295 total patients with no isolated metastases found and several false positives due to benign lesions (Querellou et al. 2010; Niederkohr et al. 2007). One of these studies also found that the addition of vertex to skull base found no unanticipated lesions in 297 scans on 173 patients (Niederkohr et al. 2007). This raises the possibility of reducing both scan time and CT dose to the patient by more narrowly tailoring the examination.

The role of intravenous contrast with PET/CT remains investigational. In a study of 50 patients with metastatic melanoma, contrast- enhanced PET/CT had minimal improvement in sensitivity over low-dose PET/CT (100% vs 97%) and no difference in specificity (93%) (Pfluger et al. 2011).

In a group of 34 patients with a variety of cancers (four with melanoma) and hepatic metastases, dual time point imaging of the liver at 69 and 100 min had 90% sensitivity for liver metastases compared to 59% for the first scan (Dirisamer et al. 2008). The effect of delaying the initial scan time to 100 min or greater on detection of metastases throughout the body has not been adequately studied.

5 Treatment of Melanoma

Surgery is the mainstay for early stage melanomas. For small tumors (less than 1 mm thick and without ulceration), excision with a 1–2 cm margin alone is sufficient. For thicker tumors (T2 and higher) or a T1b, SLNB is performed in addition to excision and provides valuable staging data. If the sentinel node is positive, then a lymphadenectomy of the nodal basin is performed. For patients with positive regional nodes or a melanoma greater than 4 mm in the absence of positive nodes, systemic therapy or enrollment in a clinical trial should strongly be considered. In retrospective studies, radiotherapy in patients with multiple tumor-positive lymph nodes or lymph nodes with extracapsular extension has been shown to improve local control (Abeloff et al. 2008). In selected patients, localized treatments such as isolated limb perfusion or infusion can help with local control but do not affect survival.

For patients with advanced disease, accurate assessment of the metastatic burden by appropriate imaging is paramount for proper treatment planning. In carefully selected patients with an isolated distant metastasis, surgery can provide palliation and possibly increase survival. Unfortunately, multiple chemotherapy regimens studied in metastatic melanoma have low response rates and do not provide a survival benefit. Immunotherapy with high-dose IL-2 demonstrates durable responses in a small fraction of patients (less than 5%) but requires hospitalization during administration due to possible severe renal, cardiac, and neurologic toxicity effects. Immunotherapy with low-dose IL-2 and interferon-alfa have similar response rates to chemotherapy and no overall survival benefit.

As a result of the limited efficacy of adjuvant therapies, new therapies are being investigated that take advantage of the robust immunogenic properties of melanoma and our understanding of the molecular genetics of aggressive melanomas (Abeloff et al. 2008). Melanoma vaccines have shown promise in phase I/II trials as solitary agents but phase III trials consistently show no efficacy (Yang 2011). The solitary phase III trial showed benefit compared to high-dose IL-2 and a peptide vaccine demonstrating increased overall and completed response. Unfortunately, the peptide vaccine formulation primarily used is no longer produced and newer formulations of the vaccine have conflicting efficacy data.

Recent promising phase III trials have also been published on ipilimumab, a fully human monoclonal immunoglobulin that blocks CTLA-4 on T lymphocytes leading to increased anti-tumor activity by T cells. Improved overall survival was seen with ipilimumab alone and in combination with dacarbazine (Hodi et al. 2010; Robert et al. 2011). Blockage of CTLA-4 also leads to T lymphocytes targeting normal tissues resulting in significant immune-related adverse events involving the skin, GI tract, adrenals, and pituitary gland.

Its key role in the formation of melanoma makes the MAPK pathway an attractive target for molecular therapies. Initial attempts to target BRAF with the multikinase inhibitor sorafenib were unsuccessful both as a solitary and combined agent (Abeloff et al. 2008). More recently, phase I and II multicenter clinical trial of the BRAF kinase inhibitor vemurafenib showed better overall and progression-free survival when compared to dacarbazine (DTIC) in unresectable, previously treated stage IIIC and IV patients. Therapies targeting NRAS are still in the early research stages (Hamid et al. 2011).

6 Post-Treatment FDG PET

While PET/CT has no role early in stage I and II melanoma, recurrences are not uncommon but are frequently local. More than 70% of melanoma recurrences are detected by patients themselves and by clinical examination (Abeloff et al. 2008). However, 15% of patients with melanomas less than 1 mm thick will develop metastases (Kalady et al. 2003). In one series, 11 patients with local recurrence had no regional or distant metastases detected except for two with false-positive FDG findings (Etchebehere et al. 2010). FDG PET/CT has not been extensively studied in this patient population and the decision to use FDG PET should be based on clinical concern for metastases.

Restaging of stage III and IV patients with FDG PET and PET/CT has been shown to be valuable and sensitive in several studies (Fig. 2) (Strobel et al. 2007; Etchebehere et al. 2010; Reinhardt et al. 2006; Akcali et al. 2007). In 78 patients with restaging PET/CT, 22% of 23 patients were upstaged from locoregional recurrence to distant recurrence and management was changed in 27% of all patients (Etchebehere et al. 2010). Also in this study, while PET could not upstage stage IV patients, it did change management in 30% of patients by altering radiotherapy, surgical, and chemotherapy planning. The timing and frequency of restaging PET/CT has not been adequately studied.

The use of FDG as biomarker for therapy response also has a relatively small body of literature although it is frequently incorporated in clinical drug trials. Hoffman et al. found FDG PET useful in evaluating the effect of palliative chemotherapy after two or three cycles with differing survivals for complete and partial metabolic responders as well as for patients with disease progression (Hofman et al. 2007). In 25 stage IV melanoma patients, PET/CT and CT had similar response assessment to chemotherapy while serum S100B was inferior to both (Strobel et al. 2008). FDG PET also showed a trend toward longer overall survival and significantly longer progression-free survival in responders compared with nonresponders which was information not provided by CT.

FDG PET after isolated limb perfusion therapy demonstrated early response to therapy, although all patients progressed by 11 months after therapy (Mercier et al. 2001). Increased uptake throughout the treated limb due to inflammation was also seen in patients scanned 1 month after therapy.

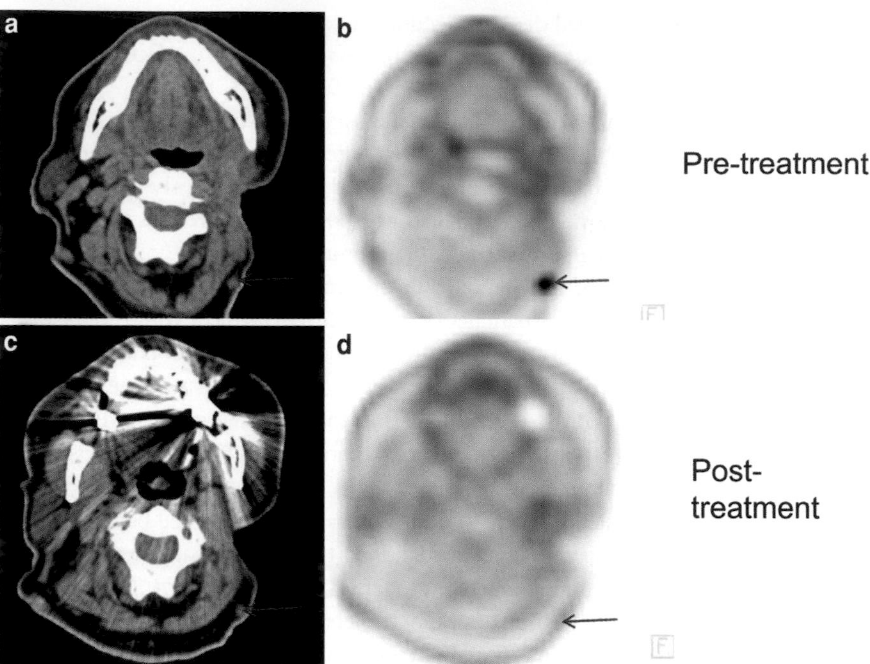

Fig. 2 Therapy response: **a** CT and **b** FDG PET images show one of many subcutaneous metastases (*red arrow*) in a patient with stage IV melanoma. *Bottom row*: After chemotherapy, **c** CT shows minimal decrease in size of the metastases but **d** FDG PET demonstrates resolution of abnormal activity suggestive of treatment response

Melanoma vaccine therapy activates the immune system and inflammation-related false-positive PET findings have been posited. A false-positive PET scan due to inflammation at the vaccine injection site has been reported but no false positives in lymph nodes and other sites have been described (Friedman and Wahl 2004). False-positive mediastinal and hilar lymphadenopathy on PET/CT have been reported in a patient receiving low-dose interferon-alpha-2b after high-dose interferon therapy due to reactive lymph nodes (Kalkanis et al. 2011).

Because of the high risk for metastases in advanced stage melanoma, surveillance FDG PET/CT imaging is frequently clinically employed although significant data on the sensitivity, timing, management changes, and cost-effectiveness are not available.

7 Other PET Radiopharmaceuticals

A wide variety of molecular PET probes have been studied in melanoma focusing on angiogenesis, hypoxia, apoptosis, generic tumor biomarkers, and melanoma-specific target such as melanin, MCR1, and high molecular weight-associated antigen (Ren et al. 2010). The majority of these tracers remain in the preclinical phase or have unsatisfactory imaging characteristics in humans.

In the early 1990s, C-11 methionine PET demonstrated good sensitivity for lesions greater than 1.5 cm though the high physiologic liver uptake would likely make liver metastasis detection difficult (Lindholm et al. 1995). F-18 6-fluoro-L dopa (FDOPA) and analogs have shown lower sensitivity than FDG (64% compared to 86%) (Dimitrakopoulou-Strauss et al. 2001; Mishima et al. 1997). However, FDOPA did have high accumulation in lesions missed by FDG including within the liver and the sensitivity of the two studies together was 95% (Dimitrakopoulou-Strauss et al. 2001).

More recently, cell proliferation after administration of the CTLA4 blocking agent tremelimumab was studied with 3′-deoxy-3′ F-18 fluorothymidine (FLT) and compared to FDG as in vitro tests have difficulty in demonstrating a response (Ribas et al. 2010). Increased splenic activity was detected on FLT but not on FDG after tremelimumab administration providing a non-invasive method of assessing immune activation. Further study is needed to determine whether FLT in this setting will have clinical relevance, with a likely goal of identifying the subset of patients who will benefit from CTLA4 blockade.

In preclinical studies, the melanin-specific 18F-6-fluoro-N-[2-(diethylamino)ethyl] pyridine-3-carboxamide (MEL050) showed rapid tumor accumulation in primary lesions and lymph node metastases with high tumor retention and low background by 3 h (Denoyer et al. 2010, 2011). MEL050, in initial human studies with five patients with stage III melanoma visualized melanotic primary tumors with good target to background characteristics, had a predominantly renal clearance pathway, and was without adverse events after seven days of monitoring (Ware et al. 2011). MEL050 has the potential for a better sensitivity and specificity than FDG PET in melanotic melanoma, especially for smaller volume tumor and liver metastases, but further human trials are needed.

8 Non-Cutaneous Melanoma

Ocular melanoma is uncommon with an incidence of 6 per million. It arises in the uveal tissues (Laver et al. 2010) and metastasizes hematogenously with the first site primarily being the liver. Approximately 50% of patients with intraocular melanomas will have metastatic disease and, similar to stage IV cutaneous melanoma, prognosis is poor with an average life expectancy of seven months (Laver et al. 2010). FDG PET has a very poor sensitivity for the primary ocular tumor akin to cutaneous melanoma primary sensitivity (Spraul et al. 2001). When FDG PET/CT was used in the initial staging of 333 patients with ocular melanoma, seven patients were found to have metastases (Freton et al. 2011). These patients had either T3 or T4 tumors with metastases mostly found in the liver (7 of 7 patients) and bone (2 of 7). Of note, 20% of patients with T4 tumors were found to have metastases by PET. In contrast, Strobel et al. found FDG PET/CT to have low sensitivity for liver metastases from ocular melanoma in six patients with 59% being FDG negative (Strobel et al. 2009). In patients with FDG-avid liver metastases, extra-hepatic metastases were also FDG avid, but no FDG-avid extra-hepatic metastases were seen in patients with FDG-negative liver metastases.

Primary mucosal melanomas are rare accounting for 1.3–1.4% of melanomas (Seetharamu et al. 2010). The head and neck is the most common primary site accounting for 25–50% of cases with other primary sites including the esophagus, gastrointestinal tract, anorectal region, female genitalia, and conjunctiva. Unlike cutaneous melanoma, most mucosal melanomas are lentiginous followed by superficial spreading and nodular types. Metastatic disease is common at presentation as the primary lesions are often not visible and are asymptomatic until very advanced. In sinonasal malignant melanoma, FDG PET/CT was useful in the initial staging including assessment of the primary tumor and follow-up after resection with good visualization of all metastases except a brain metastasis found only by MRI (Haerle et al. 2011; Lamarre et al. 2011). False-positive results were described at the primary site after therapy due to residual inflammation resulting in a very high negative predictive value but a lower positive predictive value. In both initial staging and restaging groups totaling 14 patients with conjunctival melanoma, FDG PET demonstrated systemic metastases in one patient and none in the other 13 patients, who were also negative on conventional imaging (Kurli et al. 2008).

9 Merkel Cell Carcinoma

Merkel cell carcinoma (MCC) is a rare cutaneous neuroendocrine cancer with an aggressive course that appears to be rising in incidence with an estimated 1500 cases per year in the United States (Abeloff et al. 2008; Wong and Wang 2010). Merkel cells are found in the basal epidermal layer of the skin functioning as mechanoreceptors and have a neuroectodermal origin. The pathogenesis is still under investigation but Merkel cell polyomavirus (MCV) DNA is found in 80% of cases and mounting evidence suggests MCV is a causal factor for many patients. MCC has a peak at around 69 years and affects primarily white patients. Fifty percent of MCC arises in the head and neck, especially in sun exposed areas, with the extremities and trunk the next most likely sites of origin (Fig. 3) (Abeloff et al. 2008). MCC does occur in non-sun exposed areas such as the genitalia and the bladder.

At present, 30% of patients have regional lymph node metastases and over the course of the disease 50–75% of patients will have lymph node relapse after treatment and up to 49% will have distant metastases (Abeloff et al. 2008; Peloschek et al. 2010). Early stage disease requires wide local excision followed by radiotherapy to the primary site and regional lymph node bed, as MCC is considered radiosensitive. The use of SLNB versus regional lymphadenectomy in small tumors has not been settled. Regional lymphadenectomy is advocated for primary tumors that are large, in the head and neck, have lymphovascular invasion, or are the small cell subtype (Abeloff et al. 2008). In unresectable lesions, radiotherapy is the primary treatment or can be utilized in a

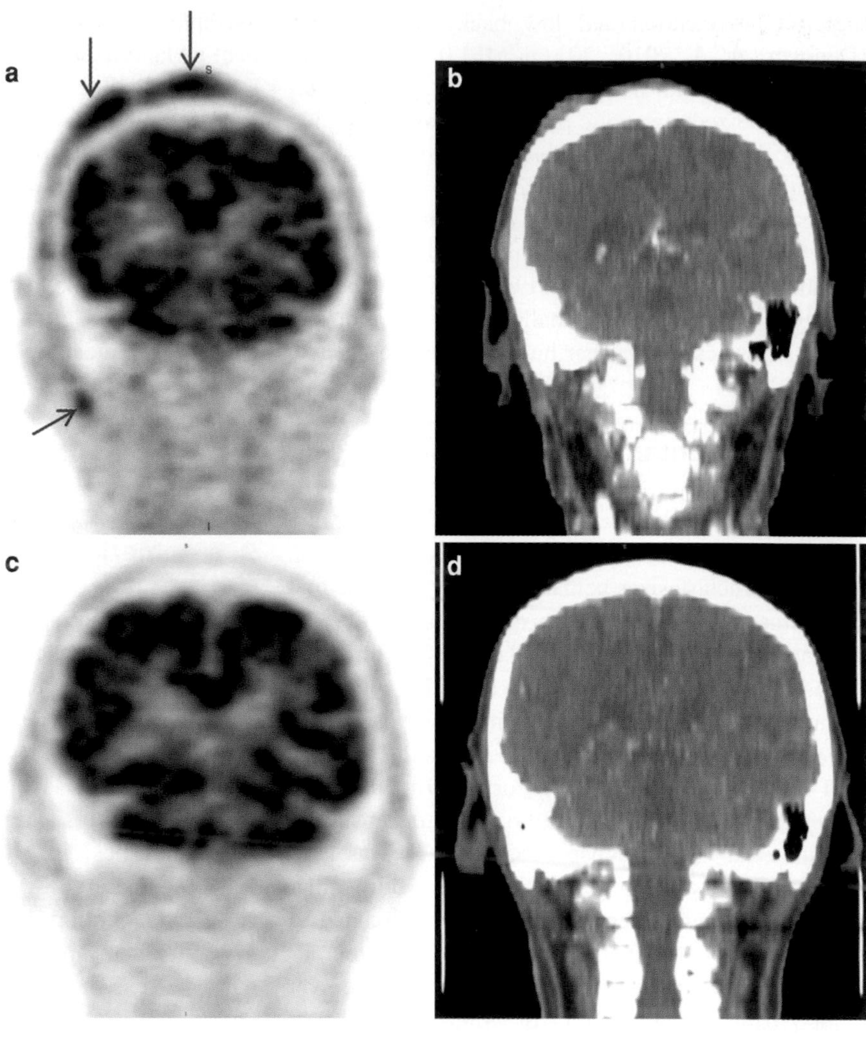

Fig. 3 Therapy response: Initial staging (**a**) PET and (**b**) CT in a patient with stage IIIB Merkel cell carcinoma of the scalp and ipsilateral cervical lymph node metastases. **c** PET and (**d**) CT after two cycles of chemotherapy with carboplatin and Taxol show a very good response to therapy

palliative role. Adjuvant chemotherapy has not demonstrated a definite clinical benefit to date. In patients with systemic disease, salvage chemotherapy is the principal therapy and may increase overall survival somewhat. Unfortunately, nearly all patients with metastatic MCC will die of the disease and the overall mortality at three years is 33% (Wong and Wang 2010).

Given the rarity of MCC, the imaging literature consists of only small case series and those using FDG are primary FDG PET only. Peloschek compared 24 FDG PET studies in 16 patients to regional ultrasound, CT, and MRI with a region-based sensitivity of 85.7% and specificity of 96.2% for FDG PET as opposed to 95.5 and 89.1% for conventional imaging. FDG PET upstaged one patient compared to conventional imaging with patient-based staging being otherwise very similar between the two modalities. Similar results when comparing FDG PET/CT and CT were described by Maury in 15 patients with a sensitivity of 89% for both (Maury et al. 2011). PET found additional metastatic lesions outside of the CT field of view in one patient, but this did not change management as other known metastatic disease was present. Concannon used FDG PET/CT in the initial staging of 12 patients and restaging of 9 patients (Concannon et al. 2010). PET/CT changed the management in 43% of cases (9 patients) including the downstaging of a patient who was then treated with curative intent. Of note, all proven sites of MCC larger than 5 mm were visualized on PET/CT with a sensitivity of 94% for pathologically proven disease. In six patients, Iagaru found FDG PET/CT useful in staging and restaging with one false negative in a 6 mm tumor. Of note, occult second primaries found on PET are frequently reported in the MCC case series despite the small number of patients and could represent a selection bias as immune suppression is a risk factor for MCC development (Concannon et al. 2010; Iagaru et al. 2006). FDG PET before and after isolated limb perfusion therapy demonstrated a complete metabolic resolution in one patient suggesting FDG may have a role in this setting (Lampreave et al. 1998).

As MCC is a neuroendocrine tumor, gamma camera and PET radiopharmaceuticals that target the neuroendocrine system have been used with varying success. FDG PET has been shown to be superior to indium-111 pentetreotide (Wong et al. 2000). FDOPA has shown mixed results in the literature with a higher false negative rate than FDG and a lower tumor to background ratio (Peloschek et al. 2010; Talbot et al. 2005).

In summary, while the literature is limited, FDG PET/CT appears to have an important role in the initial staging of high risk patients as well as in restaging as MCC shows good FDG avidity and PET/CT offers total body imaging. The role of FDG PET in therapy monitoring will need further study.

10 Basal and Squamous Cell Carcinoma of the Skin

Approximately 2.2 million patients are diagnosed with basal and squamous cell carcinomas of the skin, with basal cell representing 80% of the cases (Society 2011a, b; Habif 2010). As in melanoma, patients with light skin tone are most at risk and sun exposure is a driving factor, especially for squamous cell. Both are also increasing in incidence at an estimated rate of 2–3% per year (Abeloff et al. 2008).

Basal cell carcinomas (BCC) develop from basal keratinocytes in the epidermis and skin adnexa. The majority of BCCs are found on the head and neck (85%) with 25–30% arising on the nose (Habif 2010). BCC also occurs in sun protected areas such as the breast and genitalia. BCC primarily grows by direct extension with an unpredictable course and relies on adjacent stroma for growth support, which may be the reason for very low rates of hematogenous and lymphatic metastases. Five major histologic subtypes have been described: nodular, superficial, micronodular, infiltrative, and morpheaform. The two most common subtypes, nodular and superficial, have well defined borders, are the least aggressive, and most amenable to treatment. The other three have poorly defined borders leading to a higher rate of positive margins after resection and a higher recurrence rate (Habif 2010).

Surgical management is the principal treatment but radiation therapy, photodynamic, immunotherapy, and topical chemotherapy have been used with varying success (Abeloff et al. 2008). Primary BCCs over 1 cm in six patients were evaluated by FDG PET and three were FDG avid, all of the nodular subtype (Fosko et al. 2003). In a patient with multiple BCCs with an enlarging chest BCC and palpable left axillary lymphadenopathy, FDG PET visualized the primary and pathologically proven left axillary lymph node metastases. Thus, FDG PET may play a role in patients with known or suspected metastatic BCC but is not indicated for evaluation of primary lesions or for recurrence.

Cutaneous squamous cell carcinoma (SCC) arises from keratinocytes in skin or mucosal surfaces (Fig. 4). While light skin tone is a significant risk factor, SCC occurs in blacks and Asians more often than BCC (Abeloff et al. 2008). SCCs are found most frequently in the head and neck in white patients and are associated with sun exposure but there is no site predilection in black patients. SCC spreads locally by invading the soft tissue, shelving along harder tissues such as bone and muscle, and tracking along nerves. SCC more frequently metastasizes than BCC, initially to superficial and then deep lymph nodes (Fig. 5). In SCC with $\geq$4 mm depth of invasion, the rate of metastasis is 45.7% (Habif 2010). SCC arising in prior areas of trauma such as a chronic thermal burn or scars tends to follow a more aggressive course with metastases in nearly 40% of cases. Distant metastases are the result of hematogenous spread and occur most frequently in the lung, liver, brain, skin, and bone (Habif 2010). As with BCC, surgical management is the mainstay, though radiotherapy can be used alone or after surgical excision to reduce local recurrence rates in SCCs greater than 2 cm in size. Chemotherapy can be used in SCCs with high risk features or in patients who are not good surgical candidates.

In a case series by Cho, FDG PET was used to stage 11 patients and restage one patient with SCC (Cho et al. 2005). Overall, the primary lesions in 9 staging patients were FDG avid with all high risk lesions seen but only 1 of 3 low risk lesions visualized. An SCC was classified as high risk in the study if one of the following conditions were present: ear or lip location, scar origin, immunosuppression of the

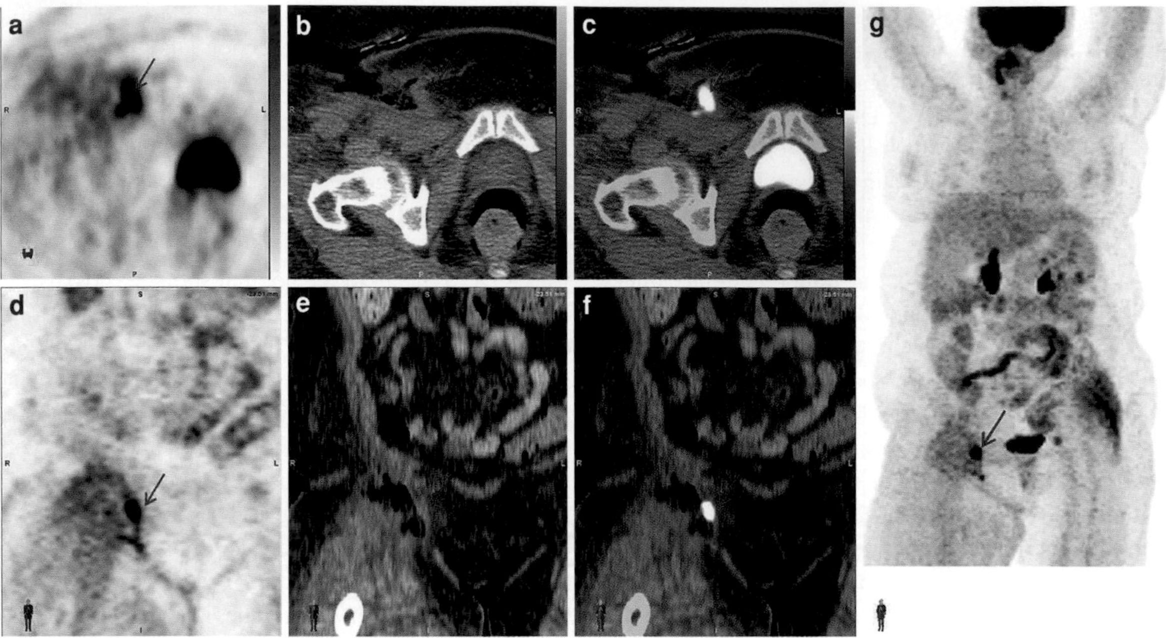

Fig. 4 Recurrence early diagnosis: **a–f** PET, CT, Fused PET/CT, and MIP images. Vulvar squamous cell carcinoma that recurred in a nonhealing wound after excision of metastatic inguinal lymph nodes. The pathologically proven recurrence at this site (*red arrowhead*) was not clinically evident until two months later

patient, poorly differentiated histology, depth great than 4 mm, or diameter greater than 2 cm. Lymph node involvement was seen in three patients and distant metastases were present only in the restaged patient. All metastatic lesions were pathologically proven to be SCC. In a patient being re-irradiated for SCC, FDG PET performed before therapy and after 44 Gy showed no change suggesting the cancer was not responding to radiotherapy (Nieder and Grosu 2005). The course of 64 Gy was completed but the tumor grew rapidly within eight weeks of therapy completion. In the limited current literature, high risk primary lesions and metastatic SCC appears to have adequate tumor to background visualization but the sensitivity for these processes is unknown.

Solid organ transplant recipients have up to a 65-fold greater risk of SCC than the general population and are also at greater risk for BCC, melanoma, and Kaposi sarcoma due to immune suppression (Fig. 6) (Zwald and Brown 2011). The SCCs in the organ transplant population tend to follow an aggressive course and are frequently multiple. There is no published literature on the sensitivity or specificity of FDG PET for primary or metastatic SCC or BCC in this patient population.

11 Primary Cutaneous Lymphoma

Primary cutaneous lymphomas are a heterogeneous group of non-Hodgkin lymphomas that are primarily T cell (CTCL) in origin with B cell cutaneous lymphomas accounting only for 10–20% of cases (Habif 2010; A-beloff et al. 2008). The two most common CTCLs are mycosis fungoides (50%) and Sézary syndrome (roughly 30%) which have a combined incidence of 1 in 100,000 and an average age of diagnosis in the sixth decade. Unlike other cutaneous malignancies, CTCL are more likely to develop in the black population.

The cutaneous findings in CTCLs vary widely from non-specific dermatitis-like lesions to exfoliative erythema of the entire dermis (Fig. 7). Thus, the average time to diagnosis from the initial appearance of skin lesions is 6 years (Abeloff et al. 2008). Mycosis fungoides typically follows an indolent course with erythematous patches that can progress to plaques and, eventually, a tumor phase. At presentation, 40% of patients will have very limited disease with 25% demonstrating a tumor phase or an erythrodermic phase (Abeloff et al. 2008). In addition to blood and peripheral lymph nodes, extracutaneous disease in CTCLs is

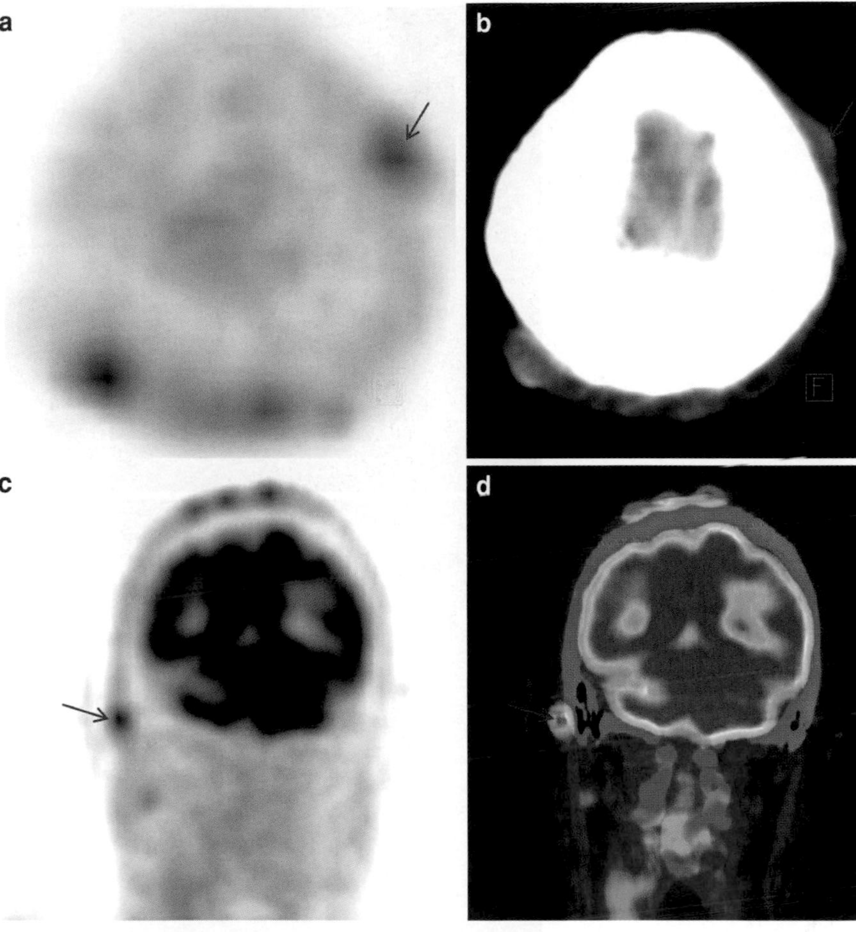

Fig. 5 Dermal metastasis: **a**, **b** axial FDG PET and CT demonstrating multiple dermal metastases from a scalp SCC. **c**, **d** coronal PET and fused images also show a post-auricular lymph node metastasis

present at autopsy in 54–100% of cases with common sites including abdominopelvic lymph nodes, bone marrow (27–47%), and nodular lymphoid infiltration of the portal tracts in the liver (8–16%) (Abeloff et al. 2008). Sézary syndrome presents with exfoliative erythroderma of the entire skin surface, thickening of the palms and soles, and intense pruritus and requires the presence of Sézary cells in the peripheral blood to make the diagnosis. There are multiple subtypes of Sézary syndrome with different hematopathologic findings and variable aggressiveness.

The prognosis of CTCL also varies greatly but parallels the level of skin involvement. In mycosis fungoides, patients with less than 10% skin involvement in the patch or plaque stage have a 90% survival at 15 years but patients with lymph node metastases have only a 40% 5-year survival. Sézary syndrome has a 2–4 year medial survival. Death is often due to infection including viral and fungal diseases that accompany advanced disease. CTCLs patients are at increased risk for second primaries including non-small-cell and small-cell lung cancer, Hodgkin lymphoma, and non-Hodgkin lymphoma which are also frequent causes of death in this patient population (Abeloff et al. 2008).

Primary cutaneous B cell lymphomas (CBCL) tend to be less aggressive than CTCLs, though the primary cutaneous large B-cell lymphoma, in the leg, has 37% overall 5-year survival. Extracutaneous metastases are less common than with CTCL although intravascular large B cell lymphoma frequently has lung and central nervous system involvement in addition to skin lesions.

Early case series studies using FDG PET only to evaluate CTCLs found low sensitivities but this was partially due to the inclusion of many stage Ia patients who were falsely negative (Elstrom et al. 2003; Valencak et al. 2004). Advanced disease was uniformly positive on FDG PET in the early study which reported staging (Valencak et al. 2004). In a mixed group of 15 CTCL patients and 4 CBCL patients with 11 initial staging studies and 20 restaging studies,

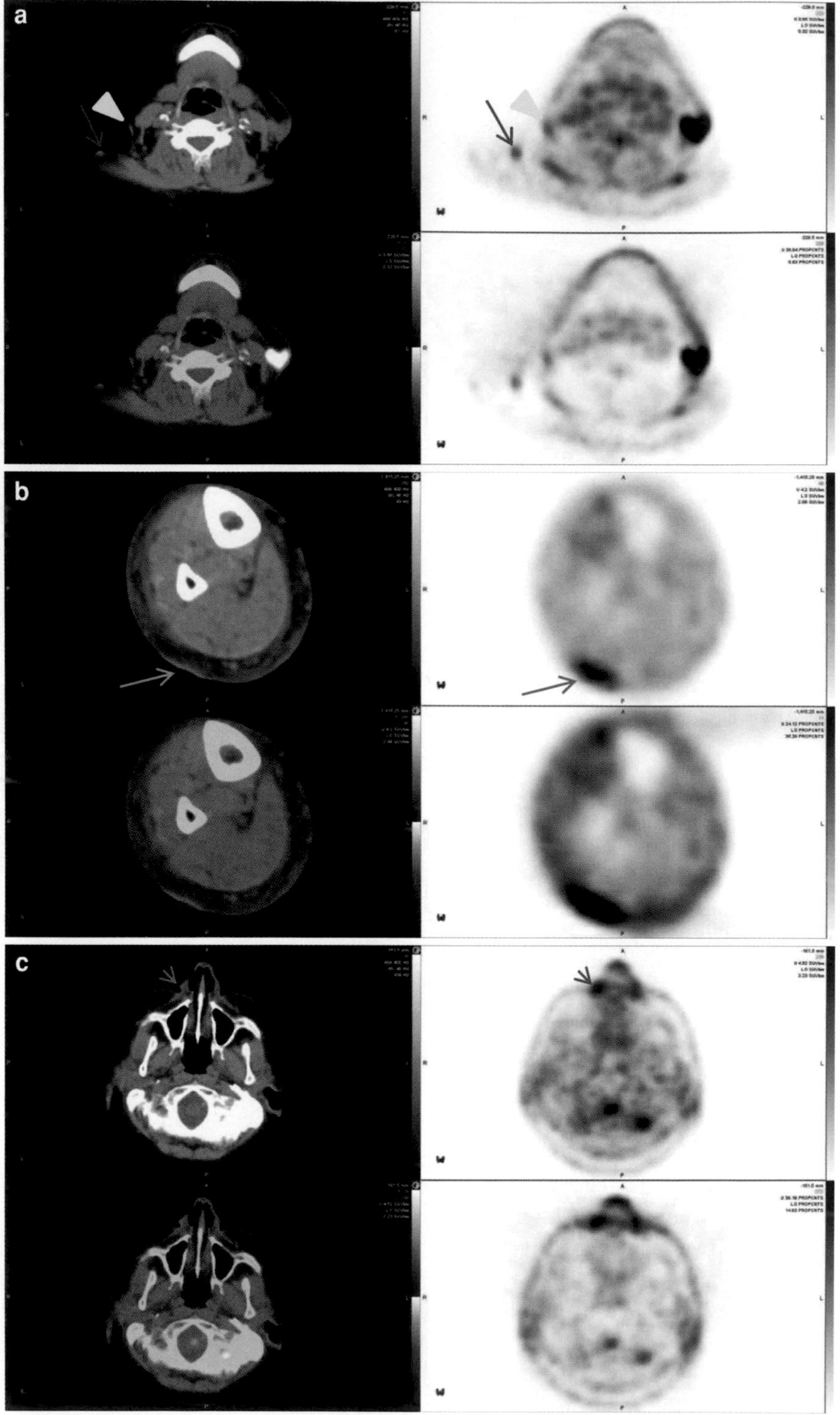

Fig. 6 CT, FDG PET attenuation correction, fused images, and FDG PET non-attenuation correction in a immuno-suppressed renal transplant patient with an SCC of the shoulder (**a**, *red arrow*), *right neck* (**a**, *yellow arrowhead*), *left neck* SCC metastasis (**a**, *unmarked*), and *right calf* (**b**, *blue arrow*) as well as a BCC on the lateral right nasal ala (**c**, *orange arrow*)

FDG PET was more sensitive than CT for local disease at both staging and restaging and similar to CT for distant disease with an overall accuracy of 97% for PET and 82% for CT (Kumar et al. 2006).

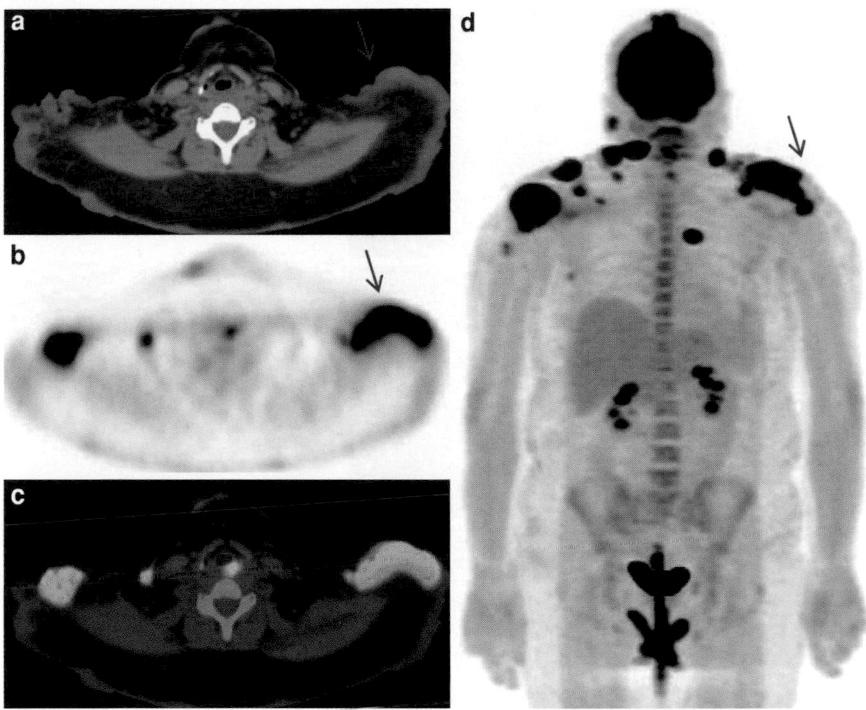

Fig. 7 T cell lymphoma: **a–d** CT, FDG PET, fused PET/CT, and MIP images. Cutaneous T cell lymphoma affecting the head, neck, and upper chest with intense FDG activity

More recently, FDG PET/CT has been found useful in a variety of CTCLs although none of these studies were designed to assess sensitivity or specificity (Feeney et al. 2010; Kuo et al. 2008; Tsai et al. 2006). Feeney retrospectively analyzed FDG PET/CTs ordered for initial staging or relapse prior to further therapies of 135 T cell lymphoma patients, 55 of whom had cutaneous involvement. All histologic subtypes had patients with FDG-avid lesions. The highest mean maximum SUV was seen in mycosis fungoides, supporting the findings of another study (Feeney et al. 2010; Tsai et al. 2006). In that study, 71% of patients had extranodal disease that in 48% of cases fell outside the normal range for a CT of the chest, abdomen, and pelvis. In a group of 13 patients with mycosis fungoides or Sézary syndrome, Tsai found lymph node metastases in all patients on PET/CT but in only five patients on CT (Tsai et al. 2006). Additionally, Kuo describes a case of cutaneous panniculitic CTCL in which physical examination significantly underestimated the disease burden seen on PET/CT, though the effect on staging was not described (Kuo et al. 2008a). Several case reports or small series have found FDG PET useful in the assessment of response to therapy of CTCL and CBCL but the role for PET/CT in this setting remains investigational (Kumar et al. 2006; Kim et al. 2010; Kuo et al. 2008b; Shapiro et al. 2002).

Due to partial volume effects, skin patches and plaques are frequently missed on FDG PET and PET/CT, especially in early stage disease. Feeney did report that FDG PET found more cutaneous patches in patients with mycosis fungoides than CT but was, of course, inferior to clinical examination (Feeney et al. 2010). Due to the frequent ulceration of cutaneous lesions in CTCLs and the underlying inflammation of erythrodermic processes such as Sézary syndrome, reactive lymph nodes leading to a false positive on FDG PET have been frequently described in the literature but the frequency or impact on staging has not been elucidated (Fig. 8) (Kumar et al. 2006; Feeney et al. 2010; Kuo et al. 2008a). Biopsy of FDG-avid lymph nodes that would result in a change in stage is recommended. As with other lymphomas, the sensitivity for bone marrow involvement is low (20% in Kako et al.) and a negative FDG PET does not obviate the need for a bone marrow biopsy if otherwise indicated (Kako et al. 2007).

Based on the limited literature, FDG PET/CT can play a valuable role in the staging and restaging of aggressive cutaneous T and B cell lymphomas by more accurately delineating tumor burden compared to FDG PET only or diagnostic CT. The role of PET/CT in treatment response needs further study. Careful examination of the cutaneous and subcutaneous tissues on PET and CT is needed to find subtle lesions.

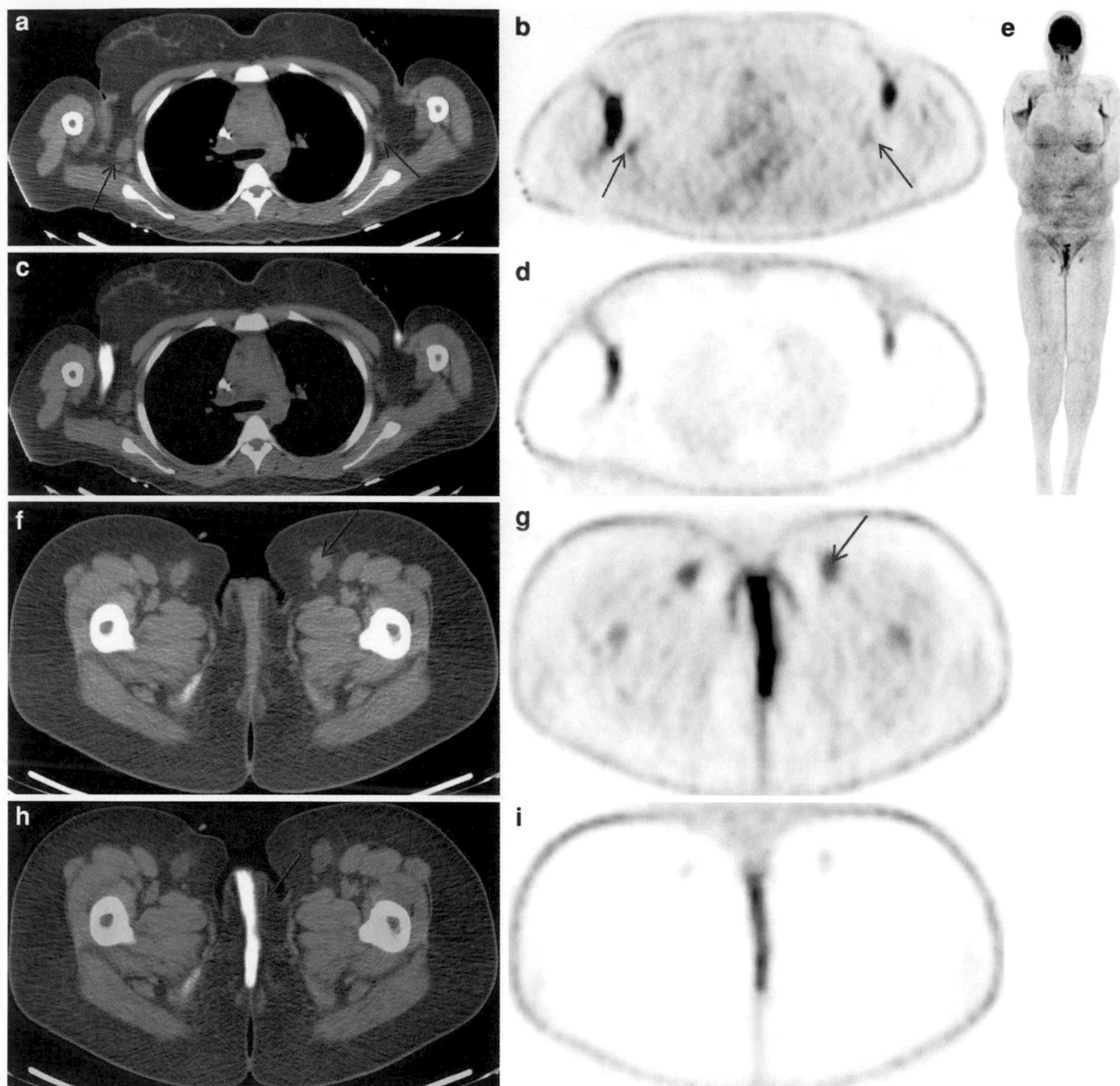

Fig. 8 A Mycosis fungoides: **a–d** CT, FDG PET attenuation correction (AC), FDG PET non-attenuation correction (non-AC), and fused images of a patient with erythrodermic phase mycosis fungoides (MF) showing intense uptake in thickened skin in both axilla. Careful inspection reveals uptake in the remaining AC PET is visually similar to non-AC PET consistent with widespread dermal involvement. Also note the mild FDG uptake in bilateral axillary lymph nodes (*red arrows*), which could be reactive as opposed to neoplastic due to the inflammation accompanying the erythroderma. **e** Attenuation corrected maximal intensity projection (MIP) with the appearance of a non-AC MIP due to widespread dermal involvement by MF. **f–i** Extensive vulvar involvement (*arrow*) with MF and bilateral FDG-avid inguinal lymph nodes (*arrow*) that have higher SUVs than the axillary lymph nodes and are concerning for metastases. Note again the increased uptake diffusely throughout the skin due to MF

12 Cutaneous Metastases

Cutaneous metastases occur in 2–10% of cancer patients and manifest in three basic patterns (Habif 2010). Flesh-colored nodules that rapidly appear and grow to around 2 cm before stabilizing are most common and are hematogenous in origin. Incorrect initial clinical diagnosis of these lesions as a benign process such as a cyst is common. The lesions may also have the appearance of a vascular tumor such as Kaposi sarcoma. The next most common presentation is

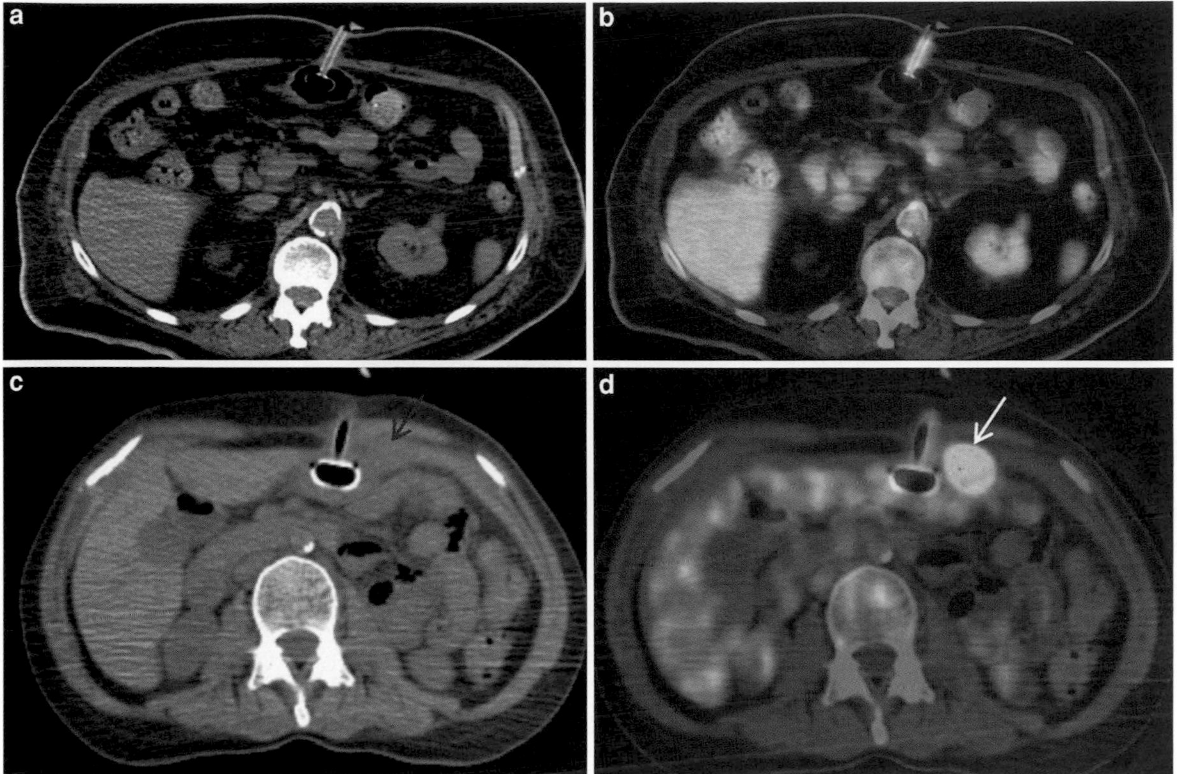

Fig. 9 Inflammatory uptake versus metastasis: **a**, **b** CT, FDG PET, fused images demonstrate increased FDG accumulation in the subcutaneous tissue which the percutaneous epigastric (PEG) tube transits due to inflammation, which is a common benign finding. **c**, **d** CT and fused images show an intensely FDG-avid soft-tissue nodule (*red arrow*) in the subcutaneous tissue lateral to the PEG tube consistent with a metastasis. The patient had a large laryngeal squamous cell carcinoma and the PEG tube was placed using a pull through method which include passing the tube through the pharynx. Unfortunately, the abdominal wall subcutaneous tissue was seeded with tumor and the occult metastases were found on a restaging PET/CT after surgery and adjuvant radiotherapy successfully treated the primary site. This metastasis was surgically removed and was identical to the primary on pathology

similar to a cutaneous infectious or inflammatory process with redness, swelling, tenderness, and warmth caused by tumor infiltration and obstruction of subepidermal lymphatics. This inflammatory pattern is most often seen in breast cancer and frequently treated as a bacterial infection. Least common, cicatricial plaques similar in appearance to discoid lupus erythematosus can cause alopecia and frequently affects the scalp, originating from breast cancer in women and renal and lung cancer in men. This pattern can also rarely appear as a hard fibrotic plaque on the chest or upper extremities due to breast cancer and is termed carcinoma en cuirasse, after a type of chest armor originally made of leather. Overall, the cancers most likely to have cutaneous metastases are the colon, lung, breast, ovarian, renal, oral cavity squamous cell, and melanoma.

13 Benign Cutaneous Uptake

Increased FDG accumulation in benign cutaneous and subcutaneous processes has been well described in the literature with both PET and PET/CT (Blumer et al. 2009; Metser and Even-Sapir 2007; Metser et al. 2007). Many of the foci of increased FDG uptake are due to immune response with activated white blood cells in sterile inflammation or infection from a wide range of etiologies accounting for 73% of foci of benign uptake in 1 study of 289 patients (Metser et al. 2007). Activated white blood cells upregulate glucose transporters, especially GLUT3, and are driven by cytokines and growth factors to increase their metabolic rate (Metser et al. 2007). Trauma, frequently iatrogenic, is a main factor leading to increased uptake in surgical wounds, post-surgical changes such as hematomas or seromas, ostomies (Fig. 9), injections of medications such as insulin or anticoagulants (Fig. 10), therapeutic injections such as bacillus Calmett-Guérin, and post-radiotherapy changes. Non-iatrogenic trauma such as lacerations, insect bites (Fig. 11), or thermal injuries (Fig. 12) can also be FDG avid. Regional lymph nodes can be reactive to infection or sterile inflammation, resulting in false-positive FDG findings in reactive lymph nodes, though the SUVs tend to be low.

A wide variety of benign dermatologic diseases can show increased FDG avidity such as acne, seborrheic dermatitis, rhinophyma, and skin vasculitis attributable to the accompanying inflammation. As many cancer patients have weakened immune systems, cutaneous infectious processes can have florid or unusual presentations that can be difficult to distinguish from malignancy (Figs. 13 and 14). Systemic granulomatous diseases such as sarcoidosis may present with both skin findings and subcutaneous lymphadenopathy with variable FDG accumulation. Systemic lymph node disorders such as Castleman or Rosai-Dorfman disease are also reported to be FDG avid (Metser and Even-Sapir 2007).

Physiologic uptake in muscles or brown fat is also frequently seen. Brown fat, also known as metabolically active fat, has significant sympathetic innervation and, upon stimulation by a cold environment, uncouples the mitochondrial energy storage processes in favor of heat production for non-shivering thermogenesis. Prior to PET/CT, false interpretation of brown fat as malignancy was reported in 2.3–4% of patients (Wehrli et al. 2007). The proportion of brown fat is highest in newborns and decreases quickly with age. The typical distribution is relatively symmetric in the neck, supraclavicular regions, and/or axilla but it can be seen along the sternum or spine in the paravertebral area and in the mediastinum and renal fossa (Metser and Even-Sapir 2007). Hibernomas, a benign proliferation of brown fat, have intense FDG uptake and cannot be distinguished from liposarcomas by PET (Metser and Even-Sapir 2007).

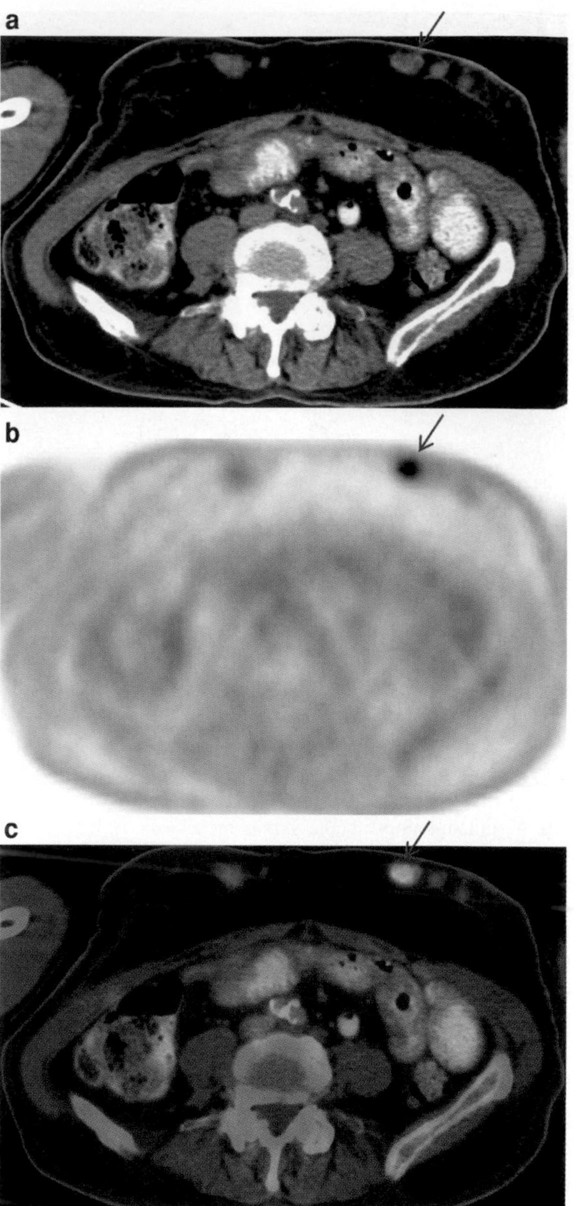

Fig. 10 Injection granulomas: (**a** = **c**) CT, FDG PET, and fused images demonstrating multiple enoxaparin injection sites in the subcutaneous tissue with rounded, irregular shapes and varying FDG activity. Feeny noted that this appearance could mimic subacute panniculitis-like T cell lymphoma(78)

FDG dose infiltration into the tissue or skin contamination with tracer presents several problems. Both represent highly concentrated FDG and can obscure adjacent PET findings. Depending on the size of infiltration, an insufficient amount of FDG may have been introduced intravenously and the images may be nondiagnostic. As the entire dose was not administered and the actual dose distributed through the body is not easily calculable, the calculated SUVs will be falsely low. Increased FDG uptake in normal axillary lymph nodes accompanying dose infiltration are common and may reduce the sensitivity for malignancy in the ipsilateral axilla, though many will have a benign appearance on CT (Blumer et al. 2009).

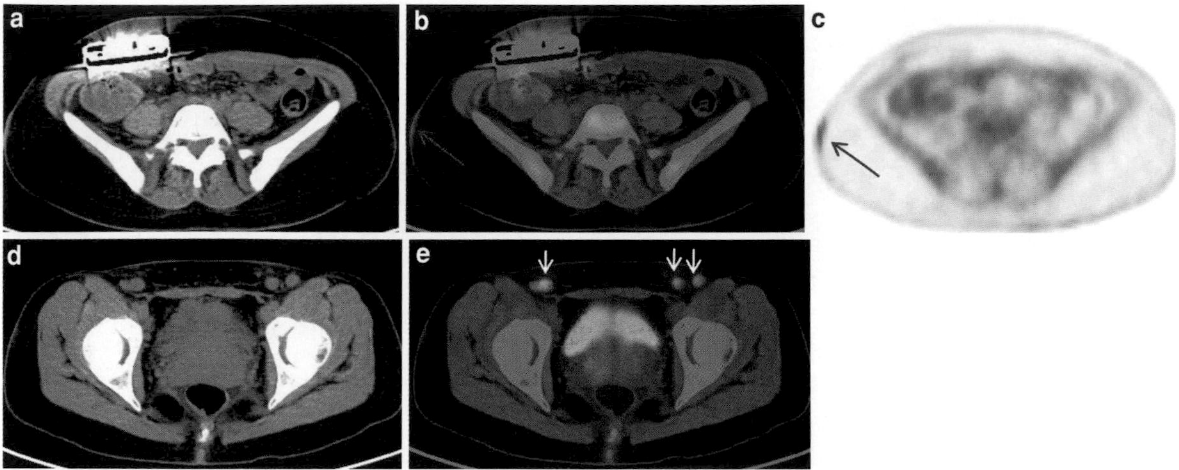

Fig. 11 Insect bites: **a–c** CT and fused PET/CT images demonstrate FDG-avid skin thickening of the lateral abdomen (*arrow*) in a patient with treated lymphoma undergoing surveillance imaging. **d**, **e** CT and fused PET/CT images show bilateral FDG-avid inguinal lymph nodes (*arrow*). The patient had been camping the prior weekend and received multiple insect bites over her entire body that were visible on PET and CT. The findings resolved on future imaging without interval therapy

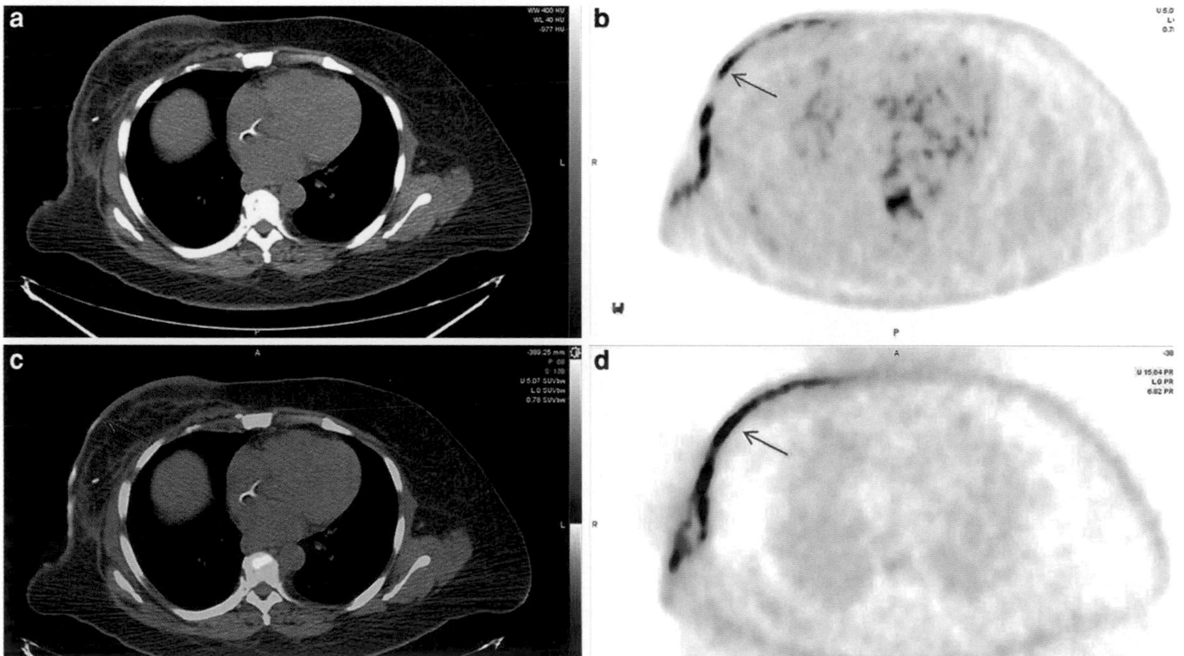

Fig. 12 Thermal injury: **a–d** CT, AC FDG PET, fused, and non-AC PET images in a patient with right breast cancer treated with mastectomy. The patient fell asleep with a heating pad on her reconstructed right breast a few days before her PET-CT resulting in a thermal burn that is indistinguishable on imaging from dermal metastases (carcinoma in cuirasse). A vertebral metastasis is also visible on the AC PET image and the PET/CT was ordered to evaluate the treatment responses of her widespread osseous disease and not to evaluate local recurrence

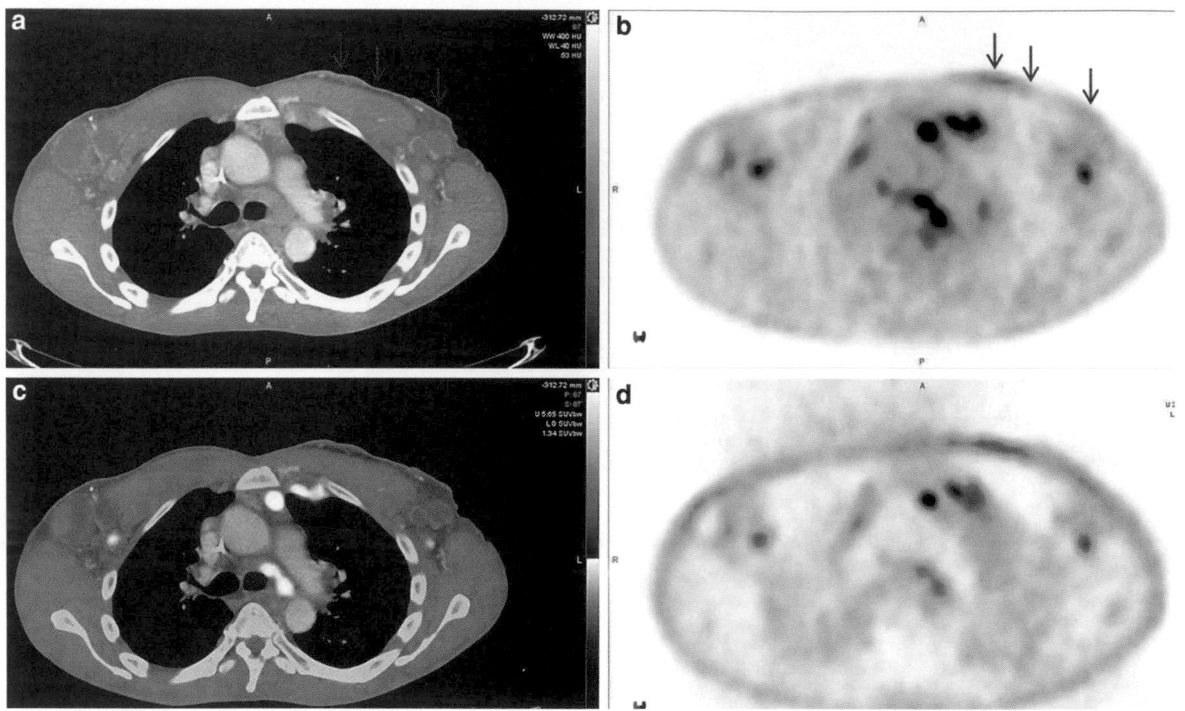

Fig. 13 Infection: **a–d** CT, AC FDG PET, fused, and non-AC PET images in a patient with refractory B cell lymphoma who had a shingles outbreak in the left upper chest at the time of his PET/CT (*red arrows*). Note the asymmetric skin thickening

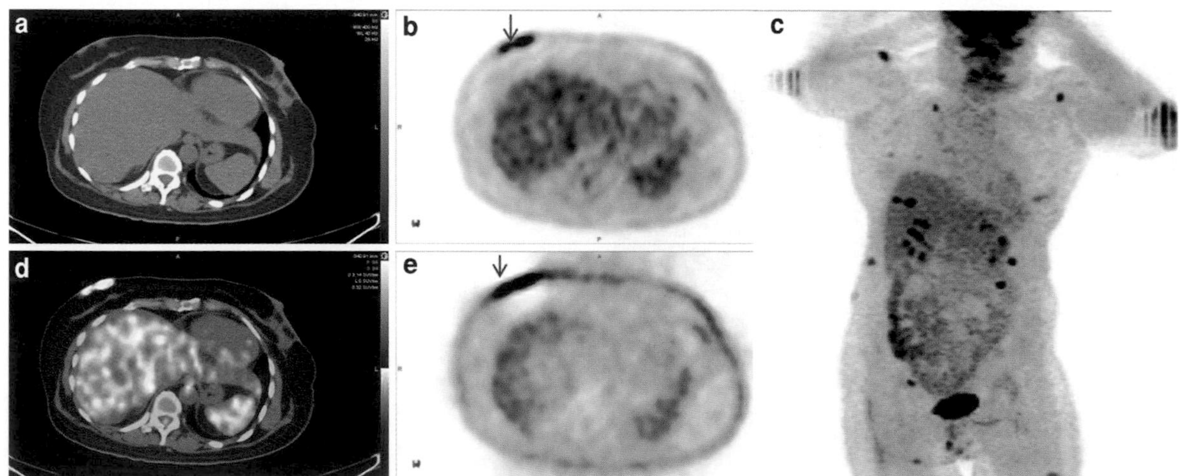

Fig. 14 Infection: **a–e** CT, AC FDG PET, MIP, fused, and non-AC PET images in a patient with stage IV infiltrating ductal carcinoma of the left breast. The MIP show multiple foci of increased tracer activity scattered throughout the body. Axial images show two adjacent lesions involving the dermis and subcutaneous tissue of the right breast and are representative of the other lesions seen on the MIP. On pathology, these lesions were multifocal Staphylococcus aureus abscesses but many were indistinguishable from cutaneous metastases on imaging

14 Conclusion

FDG PET/CT provides a valuable functional tool for evaluating many malignancies that arise in or affect the skin, especially in more advanced disease states. As many of these conditions are uncommon, the literature supporting the use of FDG PET/CT in staging, restaging, or treatment monitoring is limited but changes in patient management are frequently reported in more than 30% of patients. When compared to conventional imaging, FDG PET/CT, but not necessarily FDG PET, is superior due to better lesion sensitivity and the extended imaging range. FDG PET does have limitations: lower sensitivity for brain metastases than MRI, the inability to image micrometastases, and increased uptake in a variety of benign processes. Appropriate ordering of complementary imaging, a close review of accompanying CT images, and a thorough clinical history can overcome many of these limitations, and biopsy of indeterminate lesions can be held in reserve. Non-FDG radiopharmaceuticals remain investigational but hold the promise of molecularly targeting cancer cells or processes with a goal of patient-specific therapy.

Acknowledgments The authors would like to thank Khalil Salman, MD, and Robert Lucaj, MD, for their help in preparing some of the cases.

References

Abeloff MD et al (eds) (2008) Abeloff's clinical oncology. 4th edn. Churchill Livingstone Elsevier, Philadelphia, p 2592

Akcali C et al (2007) Detection of metastases in patients with cutaneous melanoma using FDG-PET/CT. J Int Med Res 35(4):547–553

Aukema T et al (2010) Utility of preoperative 18F-FDG PET/CT and brain MRI in melanoma patients with palpable lymph node metastases. Ann Surg Oncol 17(10):2773–2778

Balch CM et al (1983) A multifactorial analysis of melanoma. IV. Prognostic factors in 200 melanoma patients with distant metastases (stage III). J Clin Oncol Off J Amer Soc Clin Oncol 1(2):126–134

Balch CM et al (2001) Prognostic factors analysis of 17, 600 melanoma patients: validation of the American Joint Committee on Cancer melanoma staging. J Clin Oncol 19(16):3622–3634

Blumer SL et al (2009) Cutaneous and subcutaneous imaging on FDG-PET: benign and malignant findings. Clin Nucl Med 34(10):675–683

Bosserhoff A (ed) (2011) Melanoma development: molecular biology. Springer-Verlag, New York, p 390

Cho SB et al (2005) Fluorodeoxyglucose positron emission tomography in cutaneous squamous cell carcinoma: retrospective analysis of 12 patients. Dermatol Surg 31(4):442–446 (Discussion 446–447)

Concannon R, Larcos GS, Veness M (2010) The impact of ^{18}F-FDG PET-CT scanning for staging and management of Merkel cell carcinoma: results from Westmead Hospital, Sydney, Australia. J Am Acad Dermatol 62(1):76–84

Da Forno PD, Saldanha GS (2011) Molecular aspects of melanoma. Clin Lab Med 31(2):331–343

Denoyer D et al (2010) High-contrast PET of melanoma using (18)F-MEL050, a selective probe for melanin with predominantly renal clearance. J Nucl Med 51(3):441–447

Denoyer D et al (2011) Improved detection of regional melanoma metastasis using 18F–6-fluoro-N-[2-(diethylamino)ethyl] pyridine-3-carboxamide, a melanin-specific PET probe, by perilesional administration. J Nucl Med 52(1):115–122

Dimitrakopoulou-Strauss A, Strauss LG, Burger C (2001) Quantitative PET studies in pretreated melanoma patients: a comparison of 6-[18F]fluoro-L-dopa with 18F-FDG and (15)O-water using compartment and noncompartment analysis. J Nucl Med 42(2):248–256

Dirisamer A et al (2008) Dual-time-point FDG-PET/CT for the detection of hepatic metastases. Mol Imag Biology 10(6):335–340

Edge S et al (eds) (2009) AJCC cancer staging manual, 7th edn. Springer, New York

Elstrom R et al (2003) FDG-PET scanning in lymphoma by WHO classification. Blood 101(10):3875–3876

Essler M et al (2011) Prognostic value of [18F]-fluoro-deoxy-glucose PET/CT, S100 or MIA for assessment of cancer-associated mortality in patients with high risk melanoma. PLoS ONE 6(9):e24632

Etchebehere EC et al (2010) Impact of [F-18] FDG-PET/CT in the restaging and management of patients with malignant melanoma. Nucl Med Commun 31(11):925–930

Feeney J et al (2010) Characterization of T-cell lymphomas on FDG PET/CT. Am J Roentgenol 195(2):333–340

Fosko SW et al (2003) Positron emission tomography for basal cell carcinoma of the head and neck. Arch Dermatol 139(9):1141–1146

Freton A et al (2011) Initial PET/CT staging for choroidal melanoma: AJCC correlation and second nonocular primaries in 333 patients. Eur J Ophthalmol 22(2):236–243

Friedman KP, Wahl RL (2004) Clinical use of positron emission tomography in the management of cutaneous melanoma. Semin Nucl Med 34(4):242–253

Gritters L et al (1993) Initial assessment of positron emission using 2-fluorine-18-fluoro-2-deoxy-D-glucose in the imaging of malignant melanoma. J Nucl Med 34:1420–1427

Gulec SA et al (2003) The role of fluorine-18 deoxyglucose positron emission tomography in the management of patients with metastatic melanoma: impact on surgical decision making. Clin Nucl Med 28(12):961–965

Habif TP (2010) Clinical dermatology. 5th edn. Elsevier, Mosby

Haerle SK et al (2011) The value of (18)F-FDG-PET/CT imaging for sinonasal malignant melanoma. Eur Arch Otorhinolaryngol 269(1):127–33

Hamid O et al (2011) Systemic treatments of metastatic melanoma: new approaches. J Surg Onc 104:425–429

Hocker T, Tsao H (2007) Ultraviolet radiation and melanoma: a systematic review and analysis or reported sequence variants. Hum Mutat 28(6):578–588

Hodi F et al (2010) Improved survival with ipilimumab in patients with metastatic melanoma. N Engl J Med 363:711–723

Hofman MS et al (2007) Assessing response to chemotherapy in metastatic melanoma with FDG PET: early experience. Nucl Med Commun 28(12):902–906

Iagaru A et al (2006) Merkel cell carcinoma: Is there a role for 2-deoxy-2-[f-18]fluoro-D-glucose-positron emission tomography/computed tomography? Mol Imag Biology : MIB : Off Publ Acad Mol Imag 8(4):212–217

Jimenez-Requena F et al (2010) Meta-analysis of the performance of ^{18}F-FDG PET in cutaneous melanoma. Eur J Nucl Med Mol Imag 37:284–300

Kako S et al (2007) FDG-PET in T-cell and NK-cell neoplasms. Ann Oncol 18:1685–1690

Kalady MF et al (2003) Thin melanomas: predictive lethal characteristics from a 30-year clinical experience. Ann Surg 238(4):528–535 Discussion 535–537

Kalkanis D et al (2011) F-18 FDG PET positive hilar and mediastinal lymphadenopathy mimicking metastatic disease in a melanoma patient treated with interferon-alpha-2b. Clin Nucl Med 36(2):154–155

Kern K (1991) [14C]deoxyglucose uptake and imaging in malignant melanoma. J Surg Res 50:643–647

Kim J-S et al (2010) Before and after treatment ^{18}F-FDG PET/CT images in a patient with cutaneous T-cell lymphoma. Eur J Nucl Med Mol Imag 37:1995

Krug B et al (2008) Role of PET in the initial staging of cutaneous malignant melanoma: systematic review. Radiology 249(3):836–844

Kumar R et al (2006) 18F-fluorodeoxyglucose-positron emission tomography in evaluation of primary cutaneous lymphoma. Br J Dermatol 155:357–363

Kuo PH et al (2008a) FDG-PET/CT in the evaluation of cutaneous T-cell lymphoma. Mol Imag Biol 10:74–81

Kuo PH et al (2008b) FDG-PET/CT for the evaluation of response to therapy of cutaneous T-cell lymphoma to vorinostat (suberoylanilide hydroxamic acid, SAHA) in a phase II trial. Mol Imag Biol 10:306–314

Kurli M, Chin K, Finger PT (2008) Whole-body 18 FDG PET/CT imaging for lymph node and metastatic staging of conjunctival melanoma. Br J Ophthalmol 92(4):479–482

Lachiewicz AM et al (2008) Epidemiologic support for melanoma heterogeneity using the surveillance, epidemiology, and end results program. J Invest Dermatol 128(5):1340–1342

Lamarre ED et al (2011) Role of positron emission tomography in management of sinonasal neoplasms-a single institution's experience. Amer J Otolaryngol. PMID 21925763 [Epub ahead of print]

Lampreave JL et al (1998) PET evaluation of therapeutic limb perfusion in Merkel's cell carcinoma. J Nucl Med 39(12):2087–2090

Laver NV, McLaughlin ME, Duker JS (2010) Ocular melanoma. Arch Pathol Lab Med 134(12):1778–1784

Leong SP et al (2011) Cutaneous melanoma: a model to study cancer metastasis. J Surg Onc 103:538–549

Lindholm P et al (1995) Carbon-11-methionine PET imaging of malignant melanoma. J Nucl Med 36(10):1806–1810

Maury F et al (2011) Interest of (18)F-FDG PET-CT scanning for staging and management of merkel cell carcinoma: a retrospective study of 15 patients. J Eur Acad Dermatol Venereol doi: 10.1111/j.1468-3083.2011.03994.x

Mercier GA, Alavi A, Fraker DL (2001) FDG positron emission tomography in isolated limb perfusion therapy in patients with locally advanced melanoma: preliminary results. Clin Nucl Med 26(10):832–836

Metser U, Even-Sapir E (2007) Increased (18)F-fluorodeoxyglucose uptake in benign, nonphysiologic lesions found on whole-body positron emission tomography/computed tomography (PET/CT): accumulated data from four years of experience with PET/CT. Semin Nucl Med 37(3):206–222

Metser U et al (2007) Benign nonphysiologic lesions with increased 18F-FDG uptake on PET/CT: characterization and incidence. Am J Roentgenol 189(5):1203–1210

Mishima Y et al (1997) In vivo diagnosis of human malignant melanoma with positron emission tomography using specific melanoma-seeking 18F-DOPA analogue. J Neurooncol 33(1–2):163–169

Nieder C, Grosu AL (2005) Response monitoring by positron emission tomography during radiotherapy of a squamous cell skin carcinoma. Onkologie 28(10):505–507

Niederkohr RD et al (2007) Clinical value of including the head and lower extremities in 18F-FDG PET/CT imaging for patients with malignant melanoma. Nucl Med Commun 28(9):688–695

Peloschek P et al (2010) Diagnostic imaging in Merkel cell carcinoma: lessons to learn from 16 cases with correlation of sonography, CT, MRI and PET. Eur J Radiol 73(2):317–323

Pfannenberg C et al (2007) Prospective comparison of 18F-fluorodeoxyglucose positron emission tomography/computed tomography and whole-body magnetic resonance imaging in staging of advanced malignant melanoma. Eur J Cancer 43(3):557–564

Pfluger T et al (2011) PET/CT in malignant melanoma: contrast-enhanced CT versus plain low-dose CT. Eur J Nucl Med Mol Imag 38(5):822–831

Plettenberg A et al (1995) Human melanocytes and melanoma cells constitutively express the Bcl-2 proto-oncogene in situ and in cell culture. Am J Pathol 146(3):651–659

Querellou S et al (2010) Clinical and therapeutic impact of 18F-FDG PET/CT whole-body acquisition including lower limbs in patients with malignant melanoma. Nucl Med Commun 31(9):766–772

Quevado W, Szabo GJ (1969) Influence of age and UV on the populations of dopa-positive melanocytes in human skin. J Invest Dermatol 52(3):287–290

Reinhardt MJ et al (2006) Diagnostic performance of whole body dual modality 18F-FDG PET/CT imaging for N- and M-staging of malignant melanoma: experience with 250 consecutive patients. J Clin Oncol 24(7):1178–1187

Ren G, Pan Y, Cheng Z (2010) Molecular probes for malignant melanoma imaging. Curr Pharm Biotechnol 11(6):590–602

Ribas A et al (2010) Imaging of CTLA4 blockade-induced cell replication with (18)F-FLT PET in patients with advanced melanoma treated with tremelimumab. J Nucl Med 51(3):340–346

Robert C et al (2011) Ipilimumab plus dacarbazine for previously treated metastatic melanoma. N Engl J Med 364:2517–2526

Seetharamu N, Ott PA, Pavlick AC (2010) Mucosal melanomas: a case-based review of the literature. The Oncologist 15(7):772–781

Shapiro M et al (2002) Assessment of tumor burden and treatment response by 18F-fluorodeoxyglucose injection and positron emission tomography in patients with cutaneous T- and B-cell lymphomas. J Am Acad Dermatol 47(4):623–628

Society AC (2011a) Cancer Facts & Figures 2011. American Cancer Society, Atlanta

Society AC (2011b) Melanoma skin cancer. In: American Cancer Society, A.C. Society, Editor 2011, American Cancer Society, Atlanta

Spraul CW, Lang GE, Lang GK (2001) Value of positron emission tomography in the diagnosis of malignant ocular tumors. Ophthalmologica. J Int d'ophtalmologie. Int J Ophthalmol. Zeitschrift fur Augenheilkunde 215(3):163–168

Strobel K et al (2007) High risk melanoma: accuracy of FDG PET/CT with added CT morphologic information for detection of metastases. Radiology 244(2):566–574

Strobel K et al (2008) Chemotherapy response assessment in stage IV melanoma patients-comparison of 18F-FDG-PET/CT, CT, brain MRI, and tumormarker S-100B. Eur J Nucl Med Mol Imag 35(10):1786–1795

Strobel K et al (2009) Limited value of 18F-FDG PET/CT and S-100B tumour marker in the detection of liver metastases from uveal melanoma compared to liver metastases from cutaneous melanoma. Eur J Nucl Med Mol Imag 36(11):1774–1782

Talbot J-N et al (2005) 6-[F-18]Fluoro-L-DOPA positron emission tomography in the imaging of merkel cell carcinoma: preliminary report of three cases with 2-Deoxy-2-[F-18]Fluoro-D-glucose positron emission tomography or pentetreotide-(111In) SPECT data. Mol Imaging Biol 7:257–261

Tsai EY et al (2006) Staging accuracy in mycosis fungoides and Sezary syndrome using positron emission tomography and computed tomography. Arch Dermatol 142:577–584

Uren RF et al (2011) Guidelines for lymphoscintigraphy and F18 FDG PET scans in melanoma. J Surg Onc 104: 405–419

Valencak J et al (2004) Positron emission tomography with [^{18}F] 2-fluoro-D-2-deoxyglucose in primary cutaneous T-cell lymphomas. Haematologica 89(1):115–116

Valk P et al (1996) Cost-effectiveness of PET imaging in clinical oncology. Nucl Med Biol 23(6):737–743

Wagner J et al (2001) FDG-PET sensitivity for melanoma lymph node metastases is dependent on tumor volume. J Surg Onc 77(4):237–242

Wahl R et al (1991) 18F–2-deoxyglucose-2-fluoro-D-glucose uptake into human tumor xenografts. Feasibility studies for cancer imaging with positron-emission tomography. Cancer 67:1544–1550

Ware R et al (2011) First human study of N-(2-(diethylamino)ethyl)-6-[F-18]fluoropyridine-3-carboxamide (MEL050). J Nucl Med 52(Suppl 1):415

Wehrli NE et al (2007) Determination of age-related changes in structure and function of skin, adipose tissue, and skeletal muscle with computed tomography, magnetic resonance imaging, and positron emission tomography. Semin Nucl Med 37(3):195–205

Wong HH, Wang J (2010) Merkel cell carcinoma. Arch Pathol Lab Med 134(11):1711–1716

Wong CO, Pham AN, Dworkin HJ (2000) F-18 FDG accumulation in an octreotide negative Merkel cell tumor. Clin Positron Imag 3(2):71–73

Yang J (2011) Melanoma vaccines. Cancer J 17(5):277–282

Yu L et al (1999) Detection of microscopic melanoma metastases in sentinel lymph nodes. Cancer 86:617–627

Zwald FOR, Brown M (2011) Skin cancer in solid organ transplant recipients: advances in therapy and management. part I. Epidemiology of skin cancer in solid organ transplant recipients. J Am Acad Dermatol 65(2):253–261

Pediatric

Hossein Jadvar, Frederic H. Fahey, and Barry L. Shulkin

Contents

H. Jadvar (✉)
Division of Nuclear Medicine, Keck School of Medicine, University of Southern California, 2250 Alcazar Street, Los Angeles, CA 90033, USA
e-mail: jadvar@usc.edu

H. Jadvar
Division of Nuclear Medicine, Department of Radiology, Keck School of Medicine, University of Southern California, Los Angeles, CA, USA

F. H. Fahey
Division of Nuclear Medicine, Harvard Medical School, Children's Hospital Boston, Boston, MA, USA

B. L. Shulkin
Division of Diagnostic Imaging, St. Jude's Children's Research Hospital, Memphis, TN, USA

Abstract

Positron emission tomography (PET) has emerged as an important diagnostic tool in the imaging evaluation of children with cancer. The recent advent of hybrid positron emission tomography/computed tomography (PET/CT) imaging systems has provided additional diagnostic capability by providing precise anatomic localization of metabolic information and metabolic characterization of normal and abnormal structures. The use of CT transmission scanning for attenuation correction has shortened the total acquisition time, which is a desirable attribute in pediatric imaging. Moreover, accumulating clinical experience, expansion of the regional distribution of the most common PET radiotracer, fluorine-18 fluorodeoxyglucose (FDG), and the introduction of mobile PET units have improved access to this powerful diagnostic imaging technology. In this chapter, we review the clinical applications of PET and PET/CT in pediatric oncology. General considerations in patient preparation and radiation dosimetry will be discussed.

1 Introduction

Positron emission tomography (PET) has emerged as an important diagnostic tool in the imaging evaluation of children with cancer. The recent advent of hybrid positron emission tomography/computed tomography (PET/CT) imaging systems has provided additional diagnostic capability by providing precise anatomic localization of metabolic information and metabolic

P. Peller et al. (eds.), *PET-CT and PET-MRI in Oncology*, Medical Radiology. Diagnostic Imaging,
DOI: 10.1007/174_2012_576,

characterization of normal and abnormal structures. The use of CT transmission scanning for attenuation correction has shortened the total acquisition time, which is a desirable attribute in pediatric imaging. Moreover, accumulating clinical experience, expansion of the regional distribution of the most common PET radiotracer, fluorine-18 fluorodeoxyglucose (FDG), and the introduction of mobile PET units have improved access to this powerful diagnostic imaging technology. In this chapter, we review the clinical applications of PET and PET/CT in pediatric oncology. General considerations in patient preparation and radiation dosimetry will be discussed.

2 Patient Preparation

Preparation of children and parents for nuclear medicine imaging has been thoroughly reviewed elsewhere (Gordon 1998; Treves 1995). Sheets wrapped around the body, sandbags, and/or special holding devices are often sufficient for immobilization. Parents may accompany the child during the course of the imaging study to provide emotional support. Establishing reliable intravenous access is critical in pediatric imaging as patients and parents do not tolerate multiple access attempts. In this regard, utilization of experienced personnel skilled in pediatric anesthesiology is helpful. Bladder catheterization may also be needed to avoid the possibility of spontaneous voiding during image acquisition with resultant radioactive urine contamination and obscuring of pelvic lesions due to reconstruction artifacts. Moreover, a full bladder may also cause discomfort and lead to patient motion and image degradation (Shulkin 2004). Sedation is indicated when it is anticipated that simple methods will be inadequate to assure acceptable image quality. Guidelines, such as those advanced by the Society of Nuclear Medicine, the American Academy of Pediatrics, and the American Society of Anesthesiology are useful in developing an institutional pediatric sedation program (Mandell et al. 1997; American Academy of Pediatrics, Committee on Drugs 1992; American Society of Anesthesiologists, Task Force on Sedation and Analgesia by Non-Anesthesiologists 2002). Although many sedatives may affect cerebral metabolism, they are not known to cause significant changes in tumor metabolism and can be administered at any time relative to FDG administration for studies of tumors outside the central nervous system (CNS) (Shulkin 1997).

With combined PET/CT devices, imaging protocols are kept simple and reasonable to facilitate patient tolerance of the imaging procedure (McQuattie 2008; Shore 2008; Townsend and Beyer 2002; Kaste 2004; Borgwardt et al. 2003; Beyer et al. 2004; Cohade and Wahl 2003). Oral contrast may be given to outline the bowel without significant untoward effects on image quality, although semi-quantitative measures such as the standardized uptake value (SUV) may be slightly altered (Visvikis et al. 2003; Nehmeh et al. 2003; Dizendorf et al. 2002). The optimum SUV calculation in pediatric patients may be different from that used in adult patients due to the body changes that occur during childhood. Specifically, in pediatric patients it appears that SUVs based on body surface area are a more uniform parameter than SUVs based on body weight (Yeung et al. 2002). Currently, intravenous contrast is not administered routinely in PET/CT imaging studies due to the need for different contrast protocols for optimal CT imaging of various anatomic regions and the induction of potential attenuation correction-related artifacts. However, with appropriate imaging protocols, which may include alternative contrast application schemes or variations to the attenuation correction procedure, PET/CT diagnostic capacity may be improved with little or no compromise on image quality. Kaste has reviewed the experience with implementing PET/CT at a tertiary pediatric hospital (Kaste 2004). Issues such as the physical location of the PET/CT unit, the roles of CT and nuclear medicine technologists, and the methodology for study interpretation are discussed. Additional important considerations are the use of intravenous and sugar-free oral contrasts for the CT portion of the PET/CT examinations and the management of hyperglycemia. Procedure guidelines for tumor imaging with PET and PET/CT have been published (Schelbert et al. 1998; Delbeke et al. 2006).

3 Radiation Dosimetry

3.1 Pediatric Patient Dosimetry

Several factors affect the dosimetry of positron emitters relative to single photon imaging agents. On the one hand, the energy per photon is higher

Table 1 Radiation Dosimetry for FDG

	1 y	5 y	10 y	15 y	Adult
Mass (kg)	9.8	19.0	32.0	55.0	70.0
Administered activity (MBq)	54.5	105.6	177.8	305.6	389.0
Bladder	32.1	33.8	49.8	64.2	62.2
Brain	2.6	3.6	5.3	8.6	10.9
Heart	19.1	21.1	21.3	24.8	24.1
Kidneys	5.2	5.7	6.4	7.6	8.2
Red marrow	3.3	3.4	3.9	4.3	4.3
Effective dose (mSv)	5.2	5.3	6.4	7.6	7.4

The doses are reported in mSv [ICRP Report 80]. Patient masses represent the 50% percentile for that age [ICRP Report 56, Age-dependent doses to members of the public from intake of radionuclides: Part 1, International Commission on Radiation Protection, 1989, p 4]

Table 2 Effective dose in pediatrics for a variety of radiopharmaceuticals

Radiopharmaceutical	Maximum administered activity (MBq)	1 y	5 y	10 y	15 y	Adult
FDG	389	5.2	5.3	6.4	7.6	7.4
Ga-67 Citrate	222	19.9	19.9	20.3	22.7	22.2
99mTc HMPAO	740	5.1	5.4	5.8	6.4	6.9
99mTc MDP	740	2.8	2.8	3.7	4.1	4.2
99mTc MIBI	740	4.7	4.6	5.4	5.8	5.8

The doses are reported in mSv. The Maximum Administered Activity is that which would be administered to a 70-kg adult. The pediatric dose is scaled by the patient's weight as in Table 1 [ICRP Report 80, Radiation dose to patients from radiopharmaceuticals, International Commission on Radiation Protection, 1998, pp 49–110; ICRP Report 56, Age-dependent doses to members of the public from intake of radionuclides: Part 1, International Commission on Radiation Protection, 1989, p 4]

(511 keV as compared to 140 keV for ^{99m}Tc), and there are two photons emitted per annihilation event. This leads to higher energy fluence per unit activity than with most single photon agents. However, the higher photon energy also leads to a smaller fraction of the photons being absorbed within the patient. Table 1 summarizes the dosimetry of FDG for selected organs as well as the effective dose in the pediatric population based upon the administered activity of 5.55 kBq/kg (0.15 μCi/kg).

Since the administered activities are scaled by body weight, the doses are similar across the age range and slightly higher in adults. The effective dose is 5.1 and 7.4 mSv for the 1-year old and the adult, respectively. The critical organ is the bladder wall with the dose being 6–8 times higher than the effective dose (based on a 2-h voiding; however patients routinely void before image acquisition starts about 1 h post-injection). Table 2 compares the effective dose from FDG to a number of commonly used, single photon imaging agents. From this table, it can be seen that the radiation absorbed dose to the patient from an FDG PET scan is similar to the dose received from other nuclear medicine imaging procedures (Jones et al. 1982; Ruotsalainen et al. 1996; Gelfand 2009).

3.2 Parent Dosimetry

In many cases in pediatric imaging, the parents prefer to remain with the patient during the procedure. The exposure rate constants for ^{18}F and ^{99m}Tc are 0.0154 and 0.00195 mR/h per MBq at 1 m, respectively. The difference is primarily due to the higher photon energy for ^{18}F as compared to ^{99m}Tc and the fact that two photons are emitted per disintegration. It is therefore prudent to consider the radiation exposure to the parent during these procedures. As shown in

Table 3 Total exposure to the parent from a patient receiving 260 MBq of 18F for an FDG PET study

Distance from patient during uptake period (m)	Distance from patient during imaging period (m)	Total exposure to parent (mR)
1	1	5.5
1	2	4.0
2	2	1.4
2	3	1.1

It is assumed that the parent stayed with the patient during a 60-min uptake period and a 60-min imaging period

Table 4 Dose from CT

kVp	Newborn	1 y	5 y	10 y	Med adult
80	7.0	5.7	4.5	3.8	1.5
100	13.5	11.3	9.0	7.9	3.5
120	21.4	18.2	14.9	12.9	6.0
140	30.1	25.8	21.8	18.9	9.0

All doses are reported in mGy. All data were obtained at 130 mAs and a pitch of helical 1.5:1

Table 1, pediatric patients receive a range of administered activities depending on patient size. Consider the following assumptions: the patient receives 260 MBq and is considered to be a point source with no self-absorption. The patient sits in a preparatory room for 60 min during uptake and then is imaged for 60 min. These assumptions are quite conservative leading to an overestimation of the radiation dose to the parent. Table 3 estimates the total exposure to the parent during both the uptake and imaging periods, provided the parent maintains the distance from the patient specified.

Even if the parent stayed within 1 m of the patient during the entire uptake and imaging periods, the exposure to the parent would be no more than 5.5 mR. Therefore, the parents can be allowed to stay with the patient during the procedure but are instructed to stay as far from the patient as they feel comfortable. However, we do not allow siblings of patients to remain with the patient during the uptake or imaging periods.

3.3 Pediatric PET/CT Dosimetry

Hybrid PET/CT scanners use the CT portion of the examination for attenuation correction, anatomical correlation, and possibly diagnosis. The dose to the patient from CT can vary greatly depending on the tube voltage, tube current, rotation speed, pitch, slice thickness, patient size, and volume of the patient that is imaged (Gelfand and Lemen 2007; Fahey 2009). Table 4 summarizes the dose to patients of various agents (based on a phantom study using phantoms of various sizes) as a function of tube voltage. Smaller patients receive a substantially higher dose from the same CT acquisition parameters. For example, a 10-year-old will receive approximately twice the radiation dose of a medium-sized adult for the same CT acquisition parameters.

Comparing the values in Tables 1 and 4, the dose to the patient from the CT portion of the scan can be equal to, if not higher, than the dose received from the radiopharmaceutical. Thus, the acquisition parameters for the CT portion of the scan should be tailored to the patient's size. For diagnostic CT, reduction of exposure by 30–50% relative to adult has been suggested (Brenner et al. 2001). Reducing the mAs proportionately decreases the absorbed radiation dose without significant loss in the information provided. In addition, there is the potential to further reduce the tube voltage and current without adversely affecting the quality of the attenuation correction in those cases where precise anatomical correlation is less important. In an anthropomorphic phantom investigation, it was noted that for pediatric patients, adequate attenuation correction of PET images could be obtained with very low-dose CT (80 kVp, 5 mAs, 1.5:1 pitch) while reducing the dose 100-fold relative to diagnostic CT. It was noted that for adults, when keeping

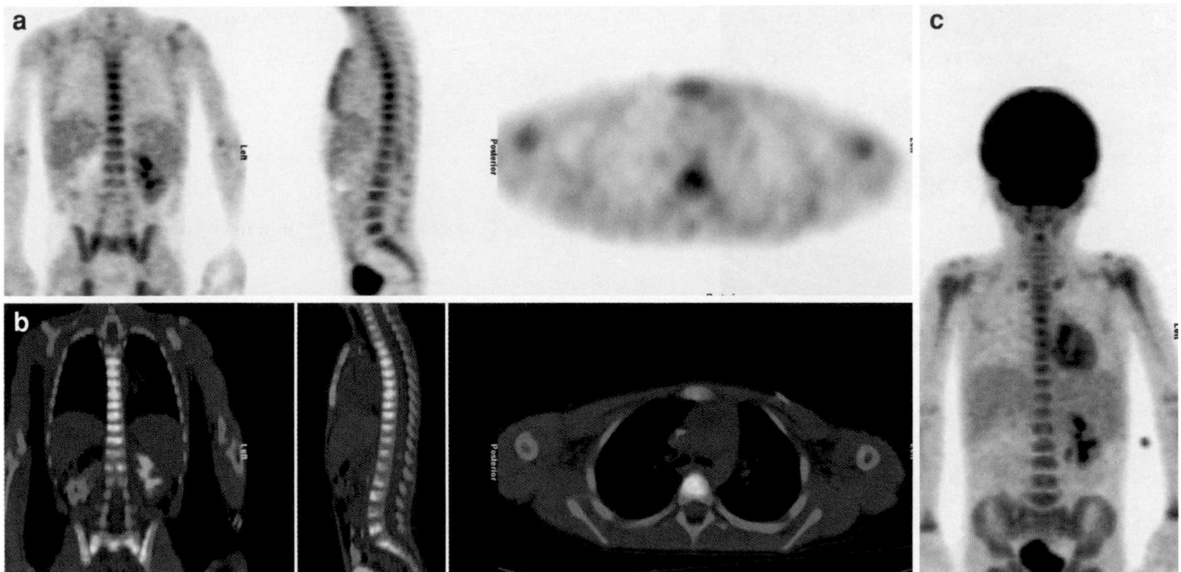

Fig. 1 FDG PET/CT images of a 3-year-old boy treated for Wilms tumor showing marked GCSF activation of the bone marrow. **a** FDG PET images of the torso show markedly increased uptake in the bone marrow (*left* coronal, *middle* sagittal, *right* transverse). **b** Fusion images of same planes. **c** Anterior view of the maximal intensity projection images

the same tube current and pitch, the tube voltage needs to be increased to 120 kVp to avert undercorrection (Fahey et al. 2007).

A retrospective study examining the radiation dose delivered in 248 clinical PET/CT studies performed in 78 pediatric patients (average 3.2 scans per child) demonstrated an average individual whole-body effective dose of 20.3 mSv (range 2.7–54.2 mSv) for the CT, average of 4.6 mSv (range 0.4–7.7 mSv) for PET, and average of 24.8 mSv (range 6.2–60.7 mSv) for PET/CT. The average cumulative radiation dose per patient from CT studies was 64.4 mSv (range 2.7–326 mSv), from PET studies 14.5 mSv (range 2.8–73 mSv), and from PET/CT studies 78.9 mSv (range 6.2–399 mSv). The authors concluded that the radiation exposure from serial PET/CT studies in children with cancer is considerable and that ALARA principles must be employed in pediatric PET/CT studies (Chawla et al. 2010). Similar concerns have been raised by others (Robbins 2008). In this regard, a weight-based injected activity and CT tube current used for anatomical calibration has been suggested (Alessio et al. 2009). Using this technique, the radiation dose was found to be 20–50% of the dose from PET/CT protocols that use a fixed technique of 120 mAs and 120 kVp. Additionally, it has been demonstrated that pediatric PET of constant image quality (in terms of noise-equivalent count rate density) can be performed with time or dose savings of up to 50% for the lightest patients (10–20 kg) (Accorsi et al. 2010).

4 Pediatric Variants and Pitfalls

Before reviewing the applications of PET in pediatric oncology, it is important to consider potential causes of misinterpretation of FDG PET that relate to physiologic FDG distribution in children. Important physiological variations in FDG distribution encountered in children include a more extensive distribution of hematopoietic marrow than in the adult and the occurrence of high FDG uptake in the thymus (Weinblatt et al. 1997; Patel et al. 1996), in the adenoids and the tonsils and in the skeletal growth centers, particularly those of the long bone physes. Other potential pitfalls, similar to imaging adults, include variable FDG uptake in working skeletal muscles, brown fat, myocardium, thyroid gland, and gastrointestinal tract, as well as accumulation of excreted FDG in the renal pelves, ureters, and bladder, and possible tracer accumulation in draining

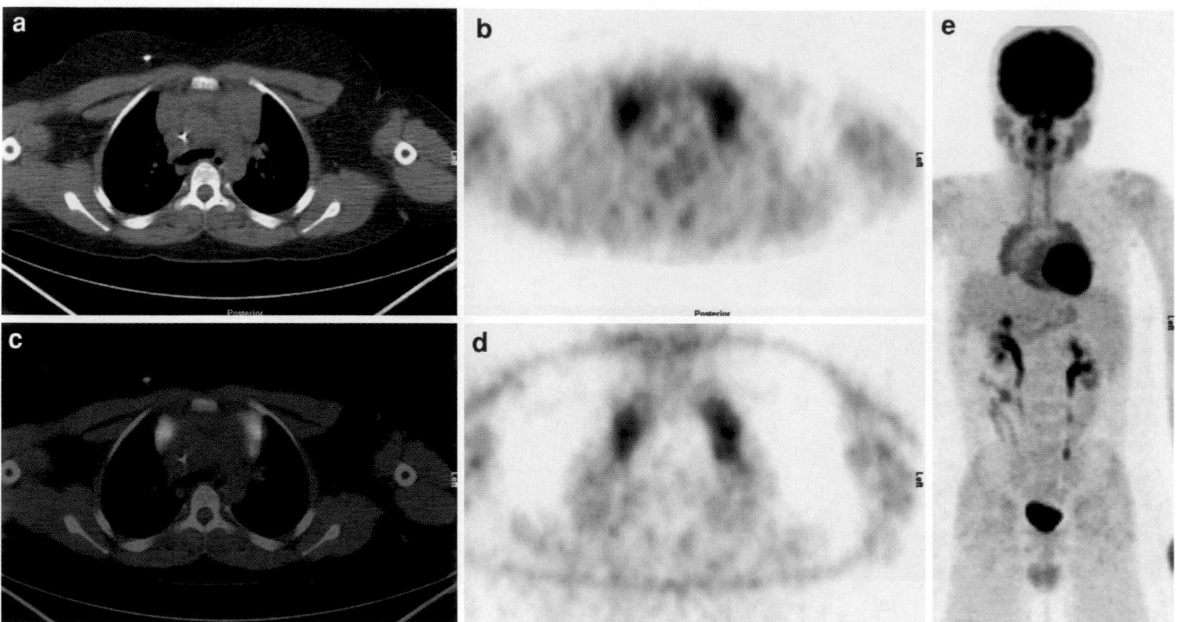

Fig. 2 FDG PET/CT images of a 12-year-old boy treated for embryonal sarcoma of the liver. Images of the upper chest show markedly increased uptake in the thymus, which appears prominent. **a** transaxial CT, **b** transaxial attenuation corrected PET, **c** fusion images, **d** PET non-attenuation corrected images and **e** anterior view of the maximal intensity projection image

lymph nodes from extravasated tracer at the time of intravenous tracer administration (Delbeke 1999; Yeung et al. 2003; Minotti et al. 2004; Hany et al. 2002; Cohade et al. 2003; Shammas et al. 2009). Diffuse high bone marrow and splenic FDG uptake following administration of hematopoietic stimulating factors may also resemble disseminated metastatic disease (Sugawara et al. 1998; Hollinger et al. 1998). Elevated bone marrow FDG uptake has been observed in patients as many as 4 weeks following completion of treatment with granulocyte colony-stimulating factor (Sugawara et al. 1998) (Fig. 1). Thymic activity may also be elevated in a minority of young adults after chemotherapy because of reactive thymus hyperplasia (Brink et al. 2001; Philip et al. 2005; Andre et al. 2008) (Fig. 2). Physiologic thymic hypermetabolism may also be seen in younger children prior to chemotherapy. With the introduction of PET/CT imaging systems, it has been recognized that elevated FDG uptake in the normal brown adipose tissue may also be a source of false-positive finding (Yeung et al. 2003; Cohade et al. 2003; Truong et al. 2004). The common anatomic areas involved include the neck and shoulder region, axillae, mediastinum, and the paravertebral and perinephric regions. Neck brown fat hypermetabolism is seen significantly more in the pediatric population than in the adult population (15 vs. 2%, $p < 0.01$) and appears to be stimulated by cold temperatures (Yeung et al. 2003; Cohade et al. 2003). Recent data have shown that brown fat metabolic activity may be suppressed pharmacologically (e.g. propranolol, fentanyl) (Tatsumi et al. 2004; Gelfand et al. 2005) or by the simple measure of controlling environmental temperature in the hours before injection and during the uptake phase (Garcia et al. 2006). High FDG uptake may also occasionally be seen in some normal organs (e.g. testis) and benign lesions (Goethals et al. 2009). Among these, fibroosseous defects (Goodin et al. 2006), which are very common in the growing skeleton, nonosifying fibromas that can mimic residual lymphoma (Von Falck et al. 2007a), and osteochondromas (Feldman et al. 2006), which can develop secondary to radiation therapy, are particularly important to note (Fig. 3).

Some artifacts are unique to the hybrid PET/CT imaging systems. These artifacts may be due to metallic objects, respiration, and the use of oral and intravenous contrast agents. Overcorrection of dense metallic objects may result in hot spot artifacts in the

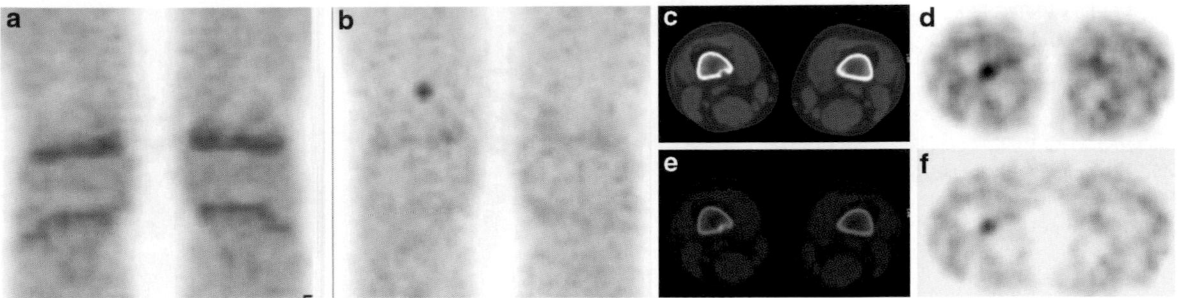

Fig. 3 FDG PET/CT images of a 6-year-old girl treated for melanoma. **a** Anterior MIP images of the knees acquired at diagnosis and **b** 6 months later show a new focus of uptake in the right distal femur. FDG PET/CT images of the lower thighs and femur at 6 months show markedly increased uptake in the right femur, **c** transaxial CT, **d** transaxial attenuation corrected PET, **e** fusion images and **f** PET non-attenuation corrected images

attenuation-corrected PET images (Bujenovic et al. 2003). Transient hot spot artifacts may also be seen on PET as a result of the bolus passage of undiluted intravenous contrast material. This is uncommon with proper contrast infusion protocols. The overestimation bias is modest (less than 15%) on the PET emission images of organs except the kidneys which may display higher bias (Nakamoto et al. 2003). Examination of the nonattenuation corrected images can be helpful in distinguishing this technical artifact from physiologic/pathologic hypermetabolism. It is also important to note that attenuation correction of PET emission data using an artifactual CT map can yield false semi-quantitative indices in the regions adjacent to metallic artifacts and probably in the presence of oral and intravenous contrasts (Visvikis et al. 2003).

5 Clinical Oncology Applications

Cancer is second only to trauma as a cause of death in children (Gurney et al. 1995). The approximately 10% of deaths during childhood that are attributable to cancer make it the leading cause of childhood disease-related death (Robison 1997). Of all the adult cancers to which FDG PET has been most widely applied, only lymphomas and brain tumors occur with an appreciable incidence in children (Shulkin 2004). However, the diagnostic utility of FDG PET and its impact on patient management have been reported for many pediatric cancers (Franzius and Schober 2003; Wegner et al. 2005; Pacak et al. 2004; Figarola et al. 2005; Kinoshita et al. 2005; Philip et al. 2005; Franzius et al. 2005; Sasi et al. 2005; Buchler et al. 2005; Mackie et al. 2006; Mody et al. 2006; McCarville 2009; Murphy et al. 2008; Kleis et al. 2009; Andre et al. 2008; Tatsumi et al. 2007). In decreasing order of frequency, PET led to important changes in clinical management of lymphoma (32%), brain tumors (15%), and sarcomas (13%) (Wegner et al. 2005). PET/CT has also been shown to improve upon PET alone by precise CT localization of metabolic abnormalities on PET and by metabolic characterization of abnormal and normal findings on CT, thereby increasing diagnostic confidence and reducing equivocal image interpretations (Bar-Sever et al. 2007; Nanni et al. 2006; Yeung et al. 2005; Moon and McHugh 2005). Moreover, with the advent of hybrid PET/MRI systems, the unique diagnostic information contents of both PET and MRI may be combined as merging the findings of separate evaluations with these imaging modalities is advantageous over conventional imaging (e.g. for detection of osseous metastases) (Kumar et al. 2008).

5.1 Central Nervous System Tumors

Tumors of the CNS account for about 20% of all pediatric cancers, second only to that of hematologic malignancies. The majority of pediatric brain tumors arise from neuroepithelial tissue. CNS tumors are subclassified histopathologically by cell type and graded for degree of malignancy using criteria that include mitotic activity, infiltration, and anaplasia (Kleihues et al. 1993; Robertson et al. 1997).

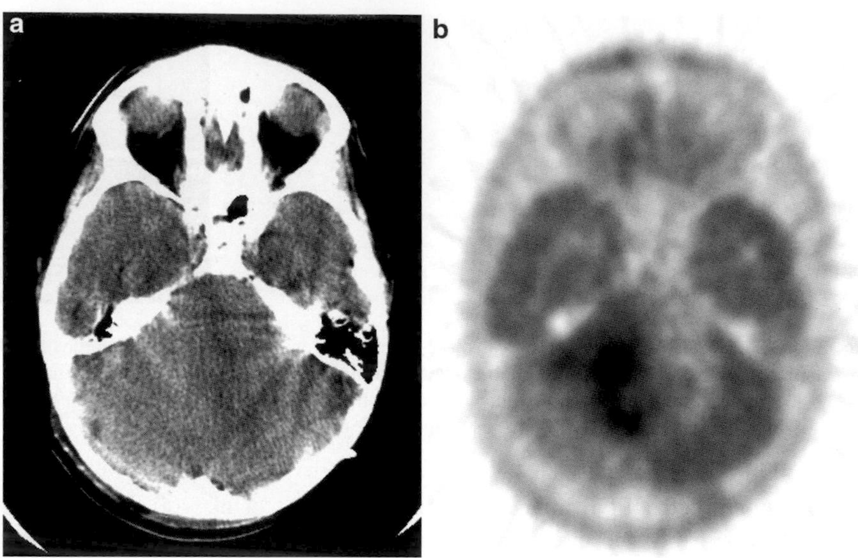

Fig. 4 FDG PET/CT images of an 8-year-old boy with a cerebellar glioblastoma. **a** transaxial CT and **b** transaxial attenuation corrected FDG PET. Markedly increased uptake of FDG is present in the right cerebellar tumor

The distribution of the most common CNS tumors may be categorized according to the major anatomic compartment involved. In the posterior fossa, medulloblastoma, cerebellar astrocytoma, ependymoma, and brain stem gliomas are most common. Tumors about the third ventricle include tumors that arise from suprasellar, pineal, and ventricular tissue. The most common neoplasms about the third ventricle are optic and hypothalamic gliomas, craniopharyngiomas, and germ cell tumors. Supratentorial tumors are most often astrocytomas, many of which are low-grade (Robertson et al. 1997).

MRI and CT are the principle imaging modalities used in staging and following children with CNS tumors. Their main limitation is distinguishing viable recurrent or residual tumor from post-therapy alterations. SPECT with thallium-201 (^{201}Tl) and ^{99m}Tc methoxyisobutylisonitrile (MIBI) have proven valuable for this determination in a number of pediatric brain tumors, generally demonstrating tracer uptake in the tumor and not in the scar tissue (Maria et al. 1997; O'Tuama et al. 1991, 1993; Rollins et al. 1995).

Use of FDG PET in brain tumors has been widely reported in adult patients for whom FDG PET has helped distinguish viable tumor from post-therapeutic changes (Valk et al. 1988; Di Chiro et al. 1988; Glantz et al. 1991). High FDG uptake relative to adjacent brain indicates residual or recurrent tumor whereas low or absent FDG uptake is observed in areas of necrosis (Fig. 4). This distinction is most readily made with high-grade tumors that show high uptake of FDG at diagnosis. FDG PET does not, however, exclude microscopic tumor foci. FDG PET results also may not correlate accurately with tumor progression after intensive radiation therapy (Janus et al. 1993). Moreover, elevated FDG uptake may persist in the immediate post-therapy period (Rozental et al. 1991).

The combined anatomic (MRI) and metabolic (PET) image information has been shown to improve the diagnostic yield of stereotactic brain biopsy in children with infiltrative, ill-defined brain lesions while reducing tissue sampling in high-risk functional areas (Pirotte et al. 2003, 2007). Combined imaging also facilitates tumor resection planning (Pirotte et al. 2006). In this regard, the recent development of hybrid PET/MRI imaging systems can facilitate the diagnostic evaluation (Kim et al. 2010). FDG PET has been applied to tumor grading and prognostication. Higher grade aggressive tumors typically have higher FDG uptake than do lower grade tumors, which may appear iso- or hypometabolic to the normal brain (Schifter et al. 1993; Borgwardt et al. 2005). The development of hypermetabolism as evidenced by increased FDG uptake in a low-grade tumor that appears hypometabolic at diagnosis indicates transformation to a higher grade (Francavilla et al. 1989). The degree of FDG uptake appears to correlate with the biological behavior of the tumor. Shorter survival times have been reported for patients whose tumors

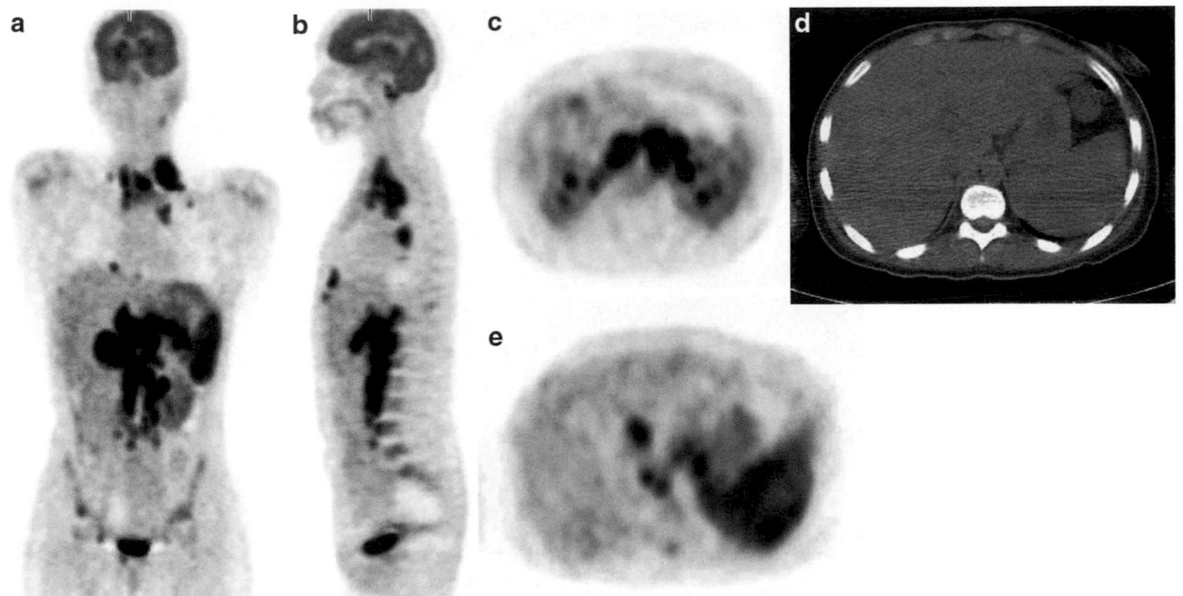

Fig. 5 FDG PET/CT images of a 17-year-old girl with widespread nodular sclerosing Hodgkin lymphoma at presentation, **a** anterior view of the maximal intensity projection image, **b** sagittal and **c** transaxial shows many nodal areas of abnormal uptake in the neck, chest, and abdomen. Transverse **d** CT and **e** attenuation corrected PET images of the upper abdomen show markedly increased FDG uptake in the spleen and central abdominal lymph nodes

show the highest degree of FDG uptake (Patronas et al. 1985). Limited available data suggest that FDG PET findings, including quantitative methods, also correlate well with histopathology and clinical outcome in children (Bruggers et al. 1993; Molloy et al. 1999a, b; Holthof et al. 1993; Hoffman et al. 1992; Gururangan et al. 2004; Wang et al. 2006). This has potential pediatric use as an excellent correlation between FDG PET findings and clinical outcome has been reported in children affected by neurofibromatosis who have low-grade astrocytomas (Williams et al. 2008). In that series, high tumor glucose metabolism shown by FDG PET was a more accurate predictor of tumor behavior than histological analysis.

Another positron emitting radiotracer that has been used to study pediatric brain tumors is the radiolabeled amino acid carbon-11 methionine (^{11}C-Met), which localizes to only a minimal degree in normal brains. Uptake of this radiotracer reflects transmethylation pathways that are present in some tumors. However, similar to FDG, some low-grade gliomas may escape detection without clear limits of tumor-to-normal brain ratios that can accurately assess malignancy grade (O'Tuama et al. 1990; Mosskin et al. 1987; Utriainen et al. 2002; Torii et al. 2005). ^{11}C-Met PET has been reported to be useful in differentiating viable tumor from therapy-induced changes (O'Tuama et al. 1990; Lilja et al. 1989; Pirotte et al. 2005; Ceyssens et al. 2006). However, it is worth noting that similar to FDG, ^{11}C-Met is not tumor-specific as it has been shown to accumulate in some benign CNS diseases, likely as a result of blood–brain barrier disruption (Mineura et al. 1997). Both FDG-PET and ^{11}C-Met PET have been shown to be independent predictors of event-free survival (Utriainen et al. 2002; Van Laere et al. 2005). ^{11}C-Met, because of the relatively short 20-min half-life of the ^{11}C label, must be produced locally for administration and is currently not commercially available. Potential uses of [^{18}F]3′-deoxy-3′-fluorothymidine, [^{11}C]methyl-L-tryptophan and [^{18}F]fluoroethyl-L-tyrosine in assessing brain tumors have recently been described (Choi et al. 2005; Juhasz et al. 2006; Floeth et al. 2005; Pauleit et al. 2005; Weckesser et al. 2005).

5.2 Lymphoma

Non-Hodgkin and Hodgkin lymphomas account for between 10 and 15% of pediatric malignancies

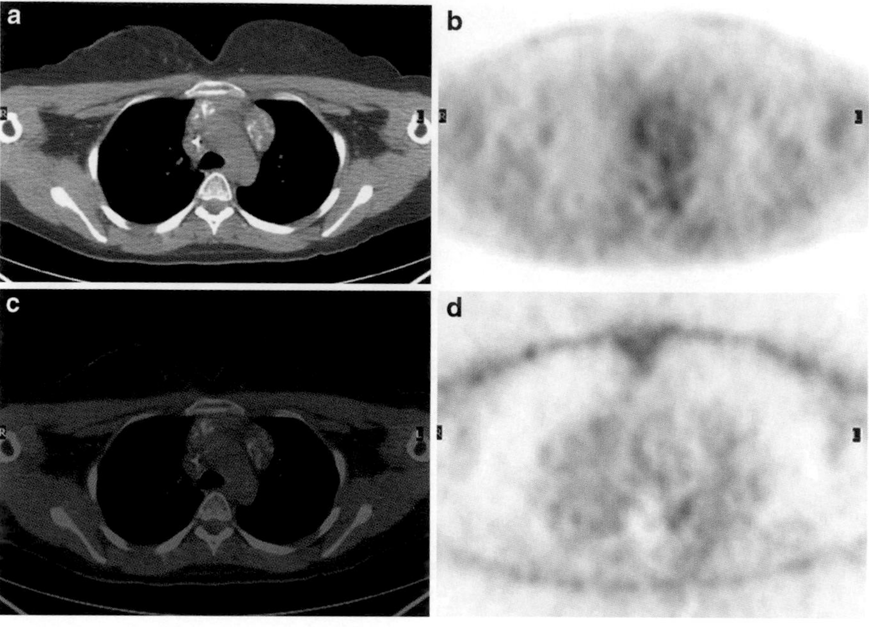

Fig. 6 FDG PET/CT images of a 20-year-old woman 1 year after treatment for Hodgkin lymphoma, **a** transaxial CT, **b** transaxial attenuation corrected PET, **c** fusion images and **d** PET non-attenuation corrected images. The CT shows calcified mediastinal masses without FDG uptake, consistent with scar tissue rather than active lymphoma

(Fig. 5). Non-Hodgkin lymphoma occurs throughout childhood. Lymphoblastic and small-cell tumors, including Burkitt lymphoma, are the most common histological types. The disease is usually widespread at diagnosis. Mediastinal and hilar involvement are common with lymphoblastic lymphoma. Burkitt lymphoma most often occurs in the abdomen. Hodgkin disease has a peak incidence during adolescence and accounts for about 6% of all childhood cancers (Kaste et al. 2005). Nodular sclerosing and mixed cellularity are the most common histologic types. The disease is rarely widespread at diagnosis and the majority of cases have intrathoracic nodal involvement (Gurney et al. 1995; Cohen 1992).

Gallium-67 citrate scintigraphy has proven useful in staging and monitoring therapeutic response in patients with non-Hodgkin and Hodgkin lymphomas (Nadel and Rossleigh 1995; Rossleigh et al. 1990; Howman-Giles et al. 1982; Yang et al. 1979; Sty et al. 1985). In numerous studies that predominantly included adult patients, FDG has been shown to accumulate in non-Hodgkin and Hodgkin lymphomas (Delbeke 1999; Barrington and Carr 1995; Bangerter et al. 1998; Jerusalem et al. 1999; Leskinen-Kallio et al. 1991; Moog et al. 1997, 1998a, b; Okada et al. 1991, 1992; Rodriguez et al. 1995; Paul 1987; Newman et al. 1994; de Wit et al. 1997; Cremerius et al. 1998; Hoh et al. 1997; Romer et al. 1998; Stumpe et al. 1998; Lapela et al. 1995; Carr et al. 1998; Segall 2001; Moody et al. 2001; Kostakoglu et al. 2000; Tatsumi et al. 2001; Hudson et al. 2004). Similar to gallium-67 citrate, FDG uptake is generally greater in higher grade lymphomas than in lower grade lymphomas (Okada et al. 1991; Rodriguez et al. 1995). FDG PET has been reported to reveal disease sites that are not detected by conventional staging methods, including those missed by gallium-67 citrate scan, resulting in upstaging of disease with potential therapeutic ramifications (Moog et al. 1998a, b; Paul 1987; Newman et al. 1994; de Wit et al. 1997). FDG PET when performed at the time of initial evaluation has also been shown to change disease stage and treatment in 10–23% of children with lymphoma (Montravers et al. 2002; Depas et al. 2005; Amthauer et al. 2005; Hernandez-Pampaloni et al. 2006; Kabickova et al. 2006). Identification of areas of intense FDG uptake within the bone marrow can be particularly useful in directing the site of biopsy or even eliminating the need for biopsy at staging (Moog et al. 1998b; Carr et al. 1998). FDG PET is also useful for assessing residual soft tissue masses shown by CT after therapy. Absence of FDG uptake in a residual mass is predictive of remission while high uptake indicates residual or recurrent tumor (de Wit et al. 1997; Moody et al. 2001; Keresztes et al. 2004) (Fig. 6). A negative FDG PET scan after completion of chemotherapy, however, does not exclude the presence of residual microscopic disease (Lavely et al. 2003). FDG PET can predict clinical outcome with a higher accuracy than conventional imaging (91 vs. 66%, respectively, $p < 0.05$) in patients previously treated for Hodgkin disease (Filmont et al. 2004).

In one recent study from Egypt that included 152 patients with lymphoma (117 Hodgkin disease and 35 non-Hodgkin lymphoma), FDG PET/CT was evaluated for initial staging of disease (Group 1, $n = 41$), early treatment response assessment after 2–3 cycles of chemotherapy (Group II, $n = 51$), treatment response assessment 4–8 weeks after completion of therapy (Group III, $n = 42$), and for long-term follow-up (Group IV, $n = 18$). In Group I, PET/CT upstaged the disease in 12.2% and downstaged the disease in 14.6% of patients. The sensitivity and specificity of PET/CT versus conventional imaging were 100 and 97.7% versus 83 and 66.6% for Group II, 100 and 90.9% versus 55.5 and 57.5% for Group III, and 100 and 100% versus 100 and 38.4% for Group IV (Riad et al. 2010).

Levine et al. (2006) reported on the frequency of false-positive studies with PET-only systems after completion of therapy. Scans were considered positive if the interpretation was most consistent with malignancy. Diagnostic validation was by pathologic evaluation, resolution on follow-up scan, or absence of disease progression over at least 1 year without intervention. A false-positive rate of 16% was observed with etiologies such as fibrosis, progressive transformation of germinal centers, abdominal wall hernia, appendicitis, thymus, and HIV associated lymphadenopathy. The authors contended that positive PET scans after treatment should be interpreted cautiously and therapeutic decisions should not be made without histologic confirmation. A similar sentiment has been adopted by others (Meany et al. 2007; Beker et al. 2008). Still, the hybrid systems which incorporate both structural and metabolic information will provide a more accurate assessment by precise localization of imaging findings, significantly reducing the potential for misinterpretation of such entities as abdominal wall hernia, etc. (Tatsumi et al. 2005). In fact a recent German study demonstrated that a correlative imaging strategy that includes FDG PET provides the most accurate imaging evaluation, improves diagnostic confidence, and impacts therapeutic management (Furth et al. 2006). Another study from Israel that utilized PET/CT in 24 Hodgkin and 7 non-Hodgkin lymphoma patients showed that PET/CT resulted in a stage change in 32% of patients (22% upstage and 10% downstage) (Miller et al. 2006). In general it is suggested that a negative PET/CT during routine follow-up for lymphoma in children strongly suggests absence of recurrence (high negative predictive value) but a positive finding should be interpreted with caution (low positive predictive value) (Rhodes et al. 2006). The potential role of FDG PET in radiation treatment planning for pediatric oncology including lymphoma has also been recently described (Swift 2002; Korholz et al. 2003; Krasin et al. 2004). Additionally, FDG PET/CT may be useful for detecting and monitoring treatment in pediatric solid organ transplant patients suffering from lymphoproliferative disease (Von Falck et al. 2007).

There has been an interest in determining whether FDG PET/CT performed early after treatment can stratify risk in patients with lymphoma. A recent report from Germany compared FDG PET/CT studies before chemotherapy, after two cycles of chemotherapy and after completion of chemotherapy in 40 pediatric patients with Hodgkin lymphoma (Furth et al. 2009). The mean follow-up was 46 months (range 26–72 months). The sensitivity and NPV of PET were 100% for both early and late post-therapy PET assessments. Moreover, the early PET identified two patients who relapsed during the follow-up period. The authors concluded that as previously noted in adults, PET assessment early after the initiation of chemotherapy can accurately stratify risk in pediatric patients.

FDG PET has been compared to ^{11}C Met PET in a relatively small series of 14 patients with non-Hodgkin lymphoma. ^{11}C Met PET provided superior tumor to background contrast while FDG PET was superior in distinguishing between high- and low-grade lymphomas (Leskinen-Kallio et al. 1991). In summary, the existing relatively large body of evidence indicates that PET will play an increasingly important role in staging, evaluating tumor response, planning radiation treatment fields, and monitoring after completion of therapy in pediatric lymphoma (Franzius and Schober 2003; Krasin et al. 2004).

5.3 Neuroblastoma

Neuroblastoma is the most common extracranial solid malignant tumor in children. The mean age of patients

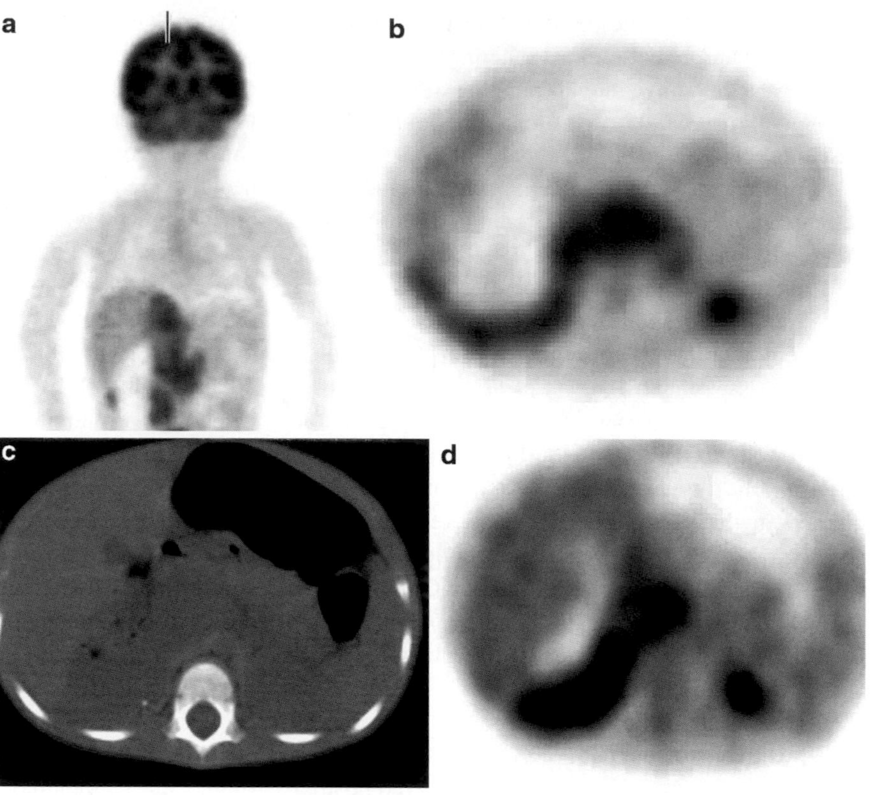

Fig. 7 FDG PET/CT images of a 2-year-old boy with recurrent neuroblastoma. Attenuation corrected FDG PET images show markedly increased uptake in abdominal masses representing tumor, **a** coronal and **b** transaxial. Transverse **c** CT and **d** attenuation corrected PET images show increased uptake in a large right retroperitoneal focus extending across the midline. Renal excretion of FDG is present on the left side

at presentation is 20–30 months and it is rare after the age of 5 years (Cohen 1992). The adrenal glands are the most common site of neuroblastoma. Other sites of origin include the paravertebral and presacral sympathetic chain, the organ of Zuckerkandl, posterior mediastinal sympathetic ganglia, and cervical sympathetic plexuses. Gross or microscopic calcification is often present in the tumor. Disseminated disease is present in up to 70% of neuroblastoma cases at diagnosis and most commonly involves cortical bone and bone marrow. Less frequently, there is involvement of liver, skin, and lung. A primary tumor is not detected in up to 10% of children with disseminated neuroblastoma or in those who present with paraneoplastic syndromes (Bousvaros et al. 1986).

Surgical excision is the preferred treatment of localized neuroblastoma. When local disease is extensive, intensive preoperative chemotherapy may be utilized. When distant metastases are present, prognosis is poor but high dose chemotherapy, total-body irradiation, and bone marrow reinfusion is beneficial for some children with this presentation.

Delineation of local disease is achieved with MRI, CT, and scintigraphy. These tests are also utilized in localizing the primary site in children who present with disseminated disease or with paraneoplastic syndrome. Metaiodobenzylguanidine (MIBG, an analog of guanethidine and norepinephrine) and indium 111 (^{111}In pentetreotide, a somatostatin type 2 receptor agonist) scintigraphy have been employed in these settings with a sensitivity of greater than 85% for detecting neuroblastoma. Uptake of MIBG into the neuroblastoma is by a neuronal sodium and energy-dependent transport mechanism. The localization of ^{111}In-pentetreotide in the neuroblastoma reflects the presence of somatostatin receptors on some neuroblastoma cells (Briganti et al. 1997).

Bone scintigraphy has been most widely used for detection of skeletal involvement for staging but cannot distinguish active disease from bony repair on the basis of tracer uptake. Patients with residual unresected primary tumors are periodically evaluated with MRI or CT. These studies, however, cannot distinguish viable tumor from treatment-related scar (Goo 2010). Specificity in establishing residual viable tumor can be improved with MIBG or ^{111}In pentetreotide imaging when the primary tumor had been shown to accumulate one of these agents. These agents are also useful in assessing residual skeletal disease in patients with MIBG or ^{111}In pentetreotide avid skeletal metastases. Neuroblastomas are metabolically active tumors (Fig. 7). Neuroblastomas and/or their metastases avidly concentrated FDG prior to chemotherapy or radiation therapy in 16 of 17 patients studied with FDG PET and MIBG imaging (Shulkin et al. 1996). Uptake after therapy varied but tended to be lower. FDG and MIBG results were concordant in most instances, although there were a few discordant cases when one tracer accumulated at a site of disease and the other did not. MIBG imaging was overall considered superior to FDG PET particularly in delineation of residual disease (Taggart et al. 2009). One advantage of FDG PET is that the FDG is administered only 30–60 min before imaging, while MIBG has to be given one or more days before imaging. A recent report indicated that FDG might be superior in depicting stage I and II disease and at major decision points during therapy (e.g. before stem cell transplantation or before surgery) (Sharp et al. 2009). In this same comparative study, I-123-MIBG scintigraphy was found to be superior to FDG PET for stage IV neuroblastoma, primarily due to better depiction of marrow involvement, as outlined below.

FDG PET may be limited for the evaluation of the bone marrow involvement of neuroblastoma due to mild FDG accumulation by the normal bone marrow (Shulkin et al. 1996). Pitfalls resulting from physiologic FDG uptake in the bowel and the thymus are additional factors that may limit the role for FDG PET in neuroblastoma. The current primary role of FDG PET in neuroblastoma is the evaluation of known or suspected neuroblastomas that do not demonstrate MIBG uptake. Some investigators have advocated inclusion of the brain in the imaging field of all advanced neuroblastoma cases due to the possibility of meningeal involvement (Chawla et al. 2010).

Carbon-11-hydroxyephedrine (^{11}C-HED), an analog of norepinephrine, and ^{11}C epinephrine PET have also been used in evaluating neuroblastoma. In a study with 7 neuroblastomas, all of them showed uptake of ^{11}C-HED (Shulkin et al. 1996) and 4 of 5 showed uptake of ^{11}C epinephrine (Shulkin et al. 1999). A recent study reported a higher sensitivity for [^{11}C]HED PET/CT than for [^{123}I]MIBG SPECT/CT (99 vs. 93%) (Franzius et al. 2006). Uptake of these tracers is demonstrated within minutes after tracer administration, which is an advantage over MIBG imaging. However, practical current limitations regarding cost and the need for on-site synthesis of short-lived ^{11}C for ^{99m}Tc (half-life of 20 min) hinder their clinical utility. Compounds labeled with F-18, such as fluoronorepinephrine, fluorometaraminol, and fluorodopamine may also be useful tracers (Brink et al. 2006). PET using 4-[fluorine-18] fluoro-3-iodobenzylguanidine (Vaidyanathan et al. 1995) and I 124 labeled MIBG (Ott et al. 1992) has also been described.

5.4 Wilms Tumor

Wilms tumor is the most common renal malignancy of childhood. Wilms tumor is predominantly seen in younger children and uncommonly encountered after the age of 5 years (Gurney et al. 1995). Bilateral renal involvement occurs in about 5% of all cases and can be synchronous or metachronous (Cohen 1992; Barnewolt et al. 1997). An asymptomatic abdominal mass is the typical mode of presentation. Nephrectomy with adjuvant chemotherapy is the treatment of choice. Radiation therapy is used in selected cases when resection is incomplete.

Radiography, ultrasonography, CT, and MRI are commonly employed in anatomic staging and detection of metastases, which predominantly involve lung, occasionally liver, and only rarely other sites. Anatomic imaging, however, is limited in the assessment for residual or recurrent tumor (Barnewolt et al. 1997). Uptake of FDG by Wilms tumor has been described (Shulkin et al. 1997) but a role for FDG PET in Wilms tumor has not been established. Normal excretion of FDG through the kidney is also a limiting factor. However, careful correlation with anatomic cross-sectional imaging usually allows distinction of tumor uptake from normal renal FDG excretion. We have found FDG PET most useful for identifying active tumor in residual masses that persist following radiation and/or chemotherapy, and for evaluating the effects of treatment on metastatic disease (Fig. 8). In a recent report from Germany, FDG PET was compared to conventional imaging in 12 patients with either primary ($n = 9$) or relapsed ($n = 3$) Wilms tumor (Misch et al. 2008). FDG PET did not provide additional diagnostic information to

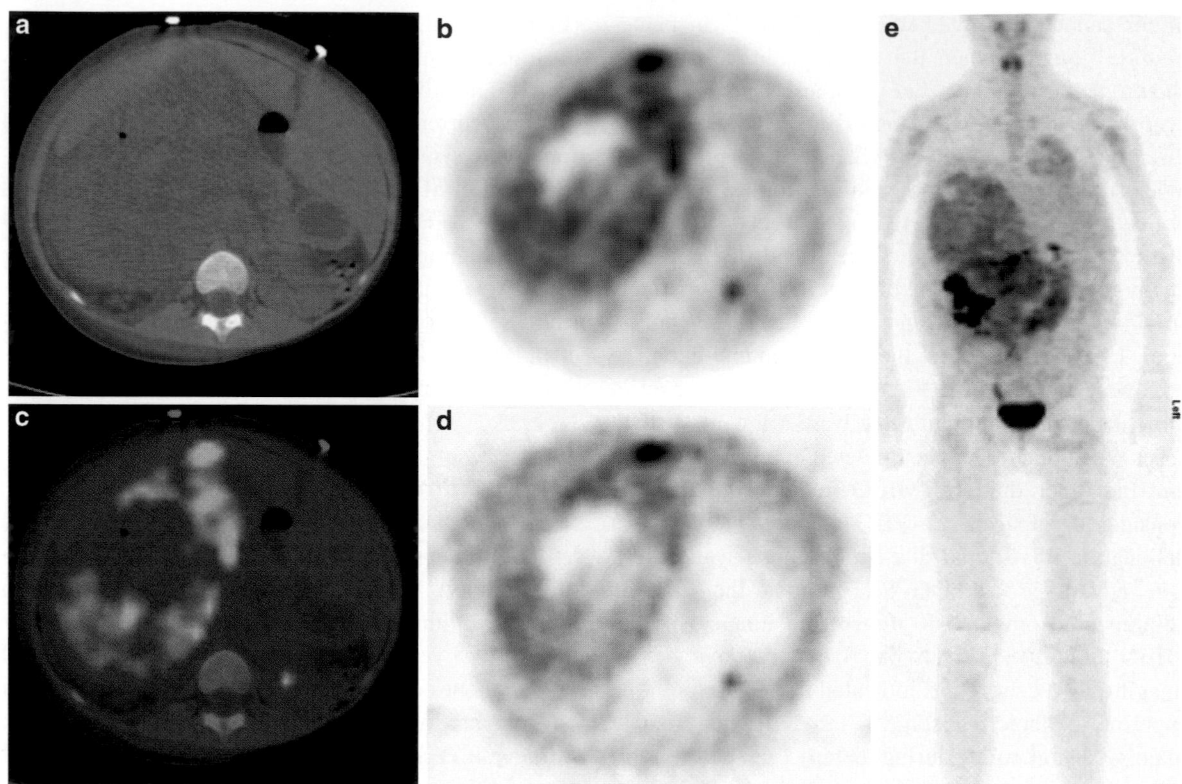

Fig. 8 FDG PET/CT images of a 4-year-old girl with Wilms tumor at presentation. Images of the abdomen show markedly increased uptake in the tumor, surrounding an area devoid of uptake, consistent with central necrosis, **a** transaxial CT, **b** transaxial attenuation corrected PET, **c** fusion images, **d** PET non-attenuation corrected images, and **e** anterior view of the maximal intensity projection image. The right kidney is displaced inferolaterally

the standard imaging work-up for staging, preoperative response assessment, or in predicting clinical outcome. However, PET was advantageous over conventional imaging for assessing residual disease after therapy and restaging before treatment.

5.5 Bone Tumors

Osteosarcoma and Ewing sarcoma are the two primary bone malignancies of childhood. Osteosarcoma is more common and predominantly affects adolescents and young adults with a second peak in older adults, principally in individuals with a history of radiation to bone or Paget disease. This tumor rarely affects children younger than 7 years of age. Osteosarcoma is typically a lesion of the long bones. The treatment of choice for osteosarcoma of an extremity is wide resection and limb-sparing surgery, which involves resection of tumor with a cuff of surrounding normal tissue at all margins and skeletal reconstruction. Limb sparing procedures can be appropriately performed in 80% of patients with the current chemotherapeutic regimens pre- and post-operatively and with imaging to define tumor extent and viability (McDonald 1994).

Almost all cases of Ewing sarcoma occur between the ages of 5 and 30 years with the highest incidence in the second decade of life. In patients younger than 20 years, Ewing sarcoma most often affects the appendicular skeleton. In patients over 20, pelvic, rib, and vertebral locations predominate. The tumor is believed to be of neuroectodermal origin and, along with the primitive neuroectodermal tumor, to be part of a spectrum of a single biologic entity (Triche 1993). Therapy for Ewing sarcoma involves irradiation and/or surgery for control of the primary lesion and multiagent chemotherapy for eradication of metastatic disease (O'Connor and Pritchard 1991).

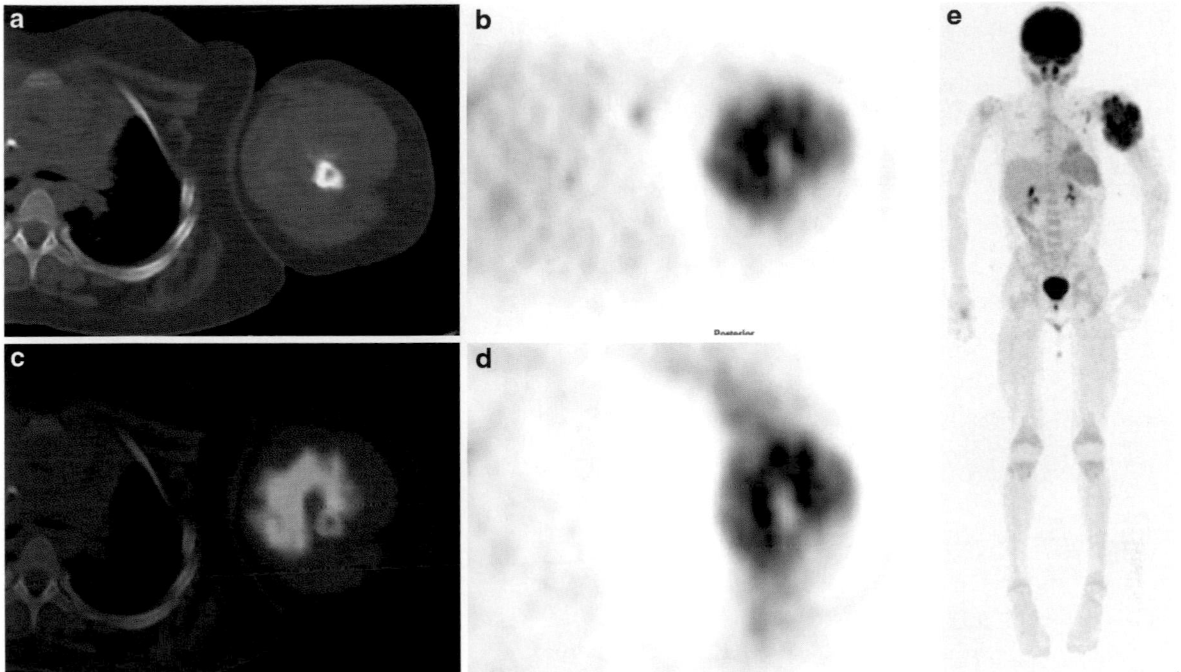

Fig. 9 FDG PET/CT images of an 8-year-old girl with osteosarcoma of the left humerus. *Top panel* Images of the left arm show markedly increased uptake in the bone and soft tissue mass, **a** transaxial CT, **b** transaxial attenuation corrected PET, **c** fusion images, **d** PET non-attenuation corrected images and **e** anterior view of the maximal intensity projection image

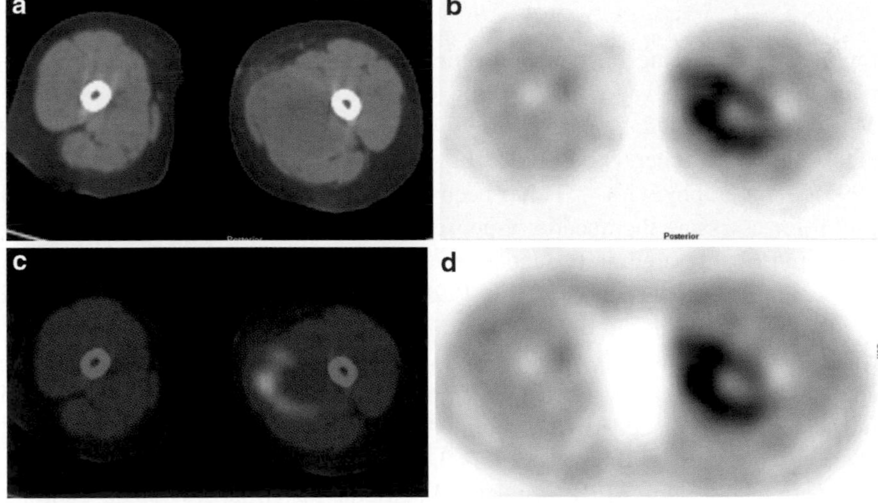

Fig. 10 FDG PET/CT images of a 2-year-old boy with rhabdomyosarcoma of the left thigh. Images of the thighs show markedly increased uptake in left sided soft tissue mass. The areas of decreased uptake within the tumor represent necrotic tissue, **a** transaxial CT, **b** transaxial attenuation corrected PET, **c** fusion images and **d** PET non-attenuation corrected images

MRI is used to define the local extent of osteosarcoma and Ewing sarcoma in bone and soft tissue. However, signal abnormalities caused by peritumoral edema can result in an overestimation of tumor extension (Jaramillo et al. 1996). Scintigraphy has been used primarily to detect osseous metastases of these tumors at diagnosis and during follow-up. With osteosarcoma, skeletal scintigraphy occasionally demonstrates extraosseous metastases, most often pulmonary, due to osteoid production by the metastatic deposits. Due to the nonspecific appearance of viable tumor on MRI, variable results have been

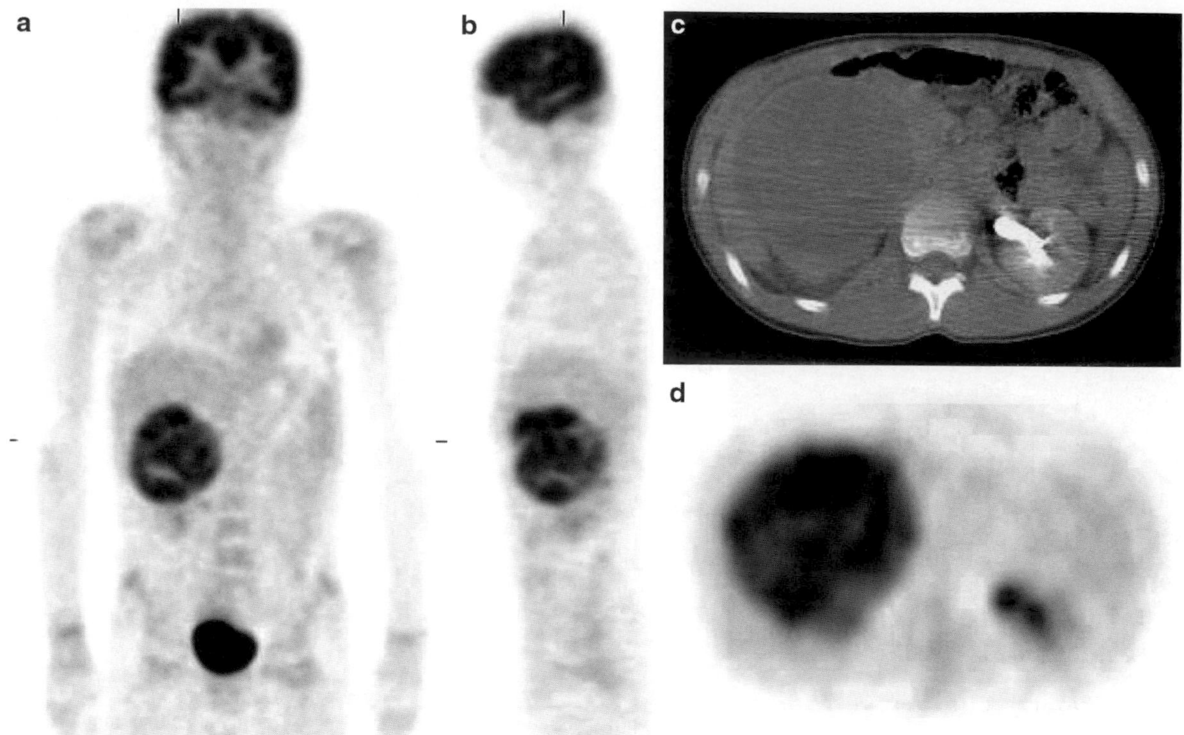

Fig. 11 FDG PET/CT images of an 8-year-old boy with adrenocortical carcinoma. **a** Anterior view of the maximal intensity projection image, **b** sagittal, transaxial **c** CT and **d** attenuation corrected PET images show markedly increased uptake in the right sided abdominal mass. Activity in the left kidney represents FDG excreted into the collecting system

reported for assessing chemotherapeutic response in planning for limb salvage surgery (Frouge et al. 1988; MacVicar et al. 1992; Lemmi et al. 1990; Erlemann et al. 1990; Holscher et al. 1992; Lawrence et al. 1993). Scintigraphy with ^{201}Tl has been shown to be useful for assessing therapeutic response in osteosarcoma and Ewing sarcoma (Connolly et al. 1996; Lin and Leung 1995; Menendez et al. 1993; Ramanna et al. 1990; Rosen et al. 1993; Ohtomo et al. 1996). Marked decrease in ^{201}Tl uptake by the tumor indicates a favorable response to chemotherapy. A change in therapy may be needed when tumor ^{201}Tl uptake does not decrease within weeks of chemotherapy. Technetium Tc 99m MIBI may also be useful in osteosarcoma but seemingly not with Ewing sarcoma (Bar-Sever et al. 1997; Caner et al. 1992).

The exact role of FDG PET in osteosarcoma and Ewing sarcoma is unclear. However, current experience suggests that in patients with bone sarcomas, FDG PET may play an important role in assessing the extent of disease, in monitoring response to therapy, and in predicting long-term outcome after therapy (Lenzo et al. 2000; Abdel-Dayem 1997; Shulkin et al. 1995; Franzius et al. 2000; Hawkins et al. 2002, 2005; Brisse et al. 2004; Jadvar et al. 2005; Gyorke et al. 2006; Bestic et al. 2009; Benz et al. 2009) (Fig. 9). The post-therapy level of FDG uptake may underestimate the extent of tumor necrosis when compared to histological assessment probably due to some increase in the metabolic activity in response to therapy-induced inflammation and healing (Huang et al. 2006). Compared to bone scintigraphy, FDG PET may be superior for detecting osseous metastases from Ewing sarcoma, but may be less sensitive for those from osteosarcoma (Franzius et al. 2000). A second potential role is in assessing patients with suspected or known pulmonary metastasis, which is particularly common with osteosarcoma. In a recent retrospective study of 55 patients with bone tumors, PET detected metastases in 22% of patients with 67% of these harboring disease outside the lung; 7% of patients were upstaged to Stage IV with the most important alteration in treatment decisions

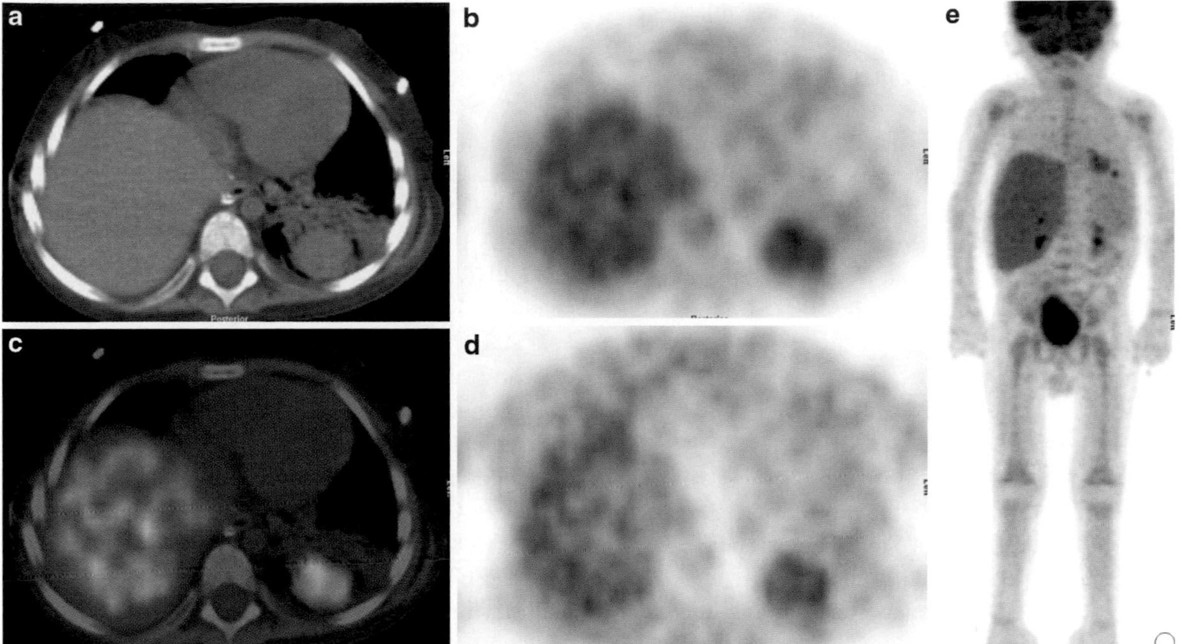

Fig. 12 FDG PET/CT images of a 4-year-old boy with metastatic hepatoblastoma. Images of the chest show markedly increased uptake in the metastatic deposit in the left lower lung, **a** transaxial CT, **b** transaxial attenuation corrected PET, **c** fusion images, **d** PET non-attenuation corrected images, and **e** anterior view of the maximal intensity projection image. The liver is massively enlarged

being the substitution of irradiation in lieu of surgery for local control (Kneisl et al. 2006). In another related recent prospective multi-center study comparing FDG PET with conventional imaging (including CT) in 46 pediatric patients with sarcoma (23 with Ewing, 11 with osteosarcoma, 12 with rhabdomyosarcoma), PET was found to be equally effective as conventional imaging for detection of the primary tumors, and superior to conventional imaging for detection of lymph node metastases, but inferior to CT for depicting lung metastases (Volker et al. 2007). As noted by others, the latter shortcoming of PET may be due to subcentimeter lesions with sizes below the spatial resolution of PET scintigraphy (Tateishi et al. 2007; Arush et al. 2007).

Recently, there has been a re-emergence of interest in ^{18}F sodium fluoride bone PET for evaluation of the skeleton (Lim et al. 2007; Ovadia et al. 2007). When compared to the traditional ^{99m}Tc MDP bone scintigraphy, ^{18}F sodium fluoride bone PET is associated with shorter time between injection and scanning (30 min vs. 3 h), similar radiation dosimetry (3.5 mGy for PET vs. 2.8 mGy for MDP), higher resolution, and higher cost of radiotracer. However, the higher cost may be offset by increased patient throughput given the shorter tracer uptake period with PET (Lim et al. 2007). Further studies will be needed to assess the exact clinical utility and cost-benefit ratio of ^{18}F sodium fluoride in comparison to the standard single photon bone scintigraphy.

5.6 Soft Tissue Tumors

Rhabdomyosarcoma is the most common soft-tissue malignancy of childhood. The peak incidence occurs between 3 and 6 years of age. Rhabdomyosarcomas can develop in any organ or tissue, but contrary to what the name implies, do not usually arise in muscle. The most common anatomic locations are the head, particularly the orbit and paranasal sinuses, the neck, and the genitourinary tract. CT or MRI is important for establishing the extent of local disease. Radiography and CT are used for detecting pulmonary metastases and skeletal scintigraphy is employed for identifying osseous metastases. Radiation therapy and surgery are utilized for local disease control and chemotherapy is employed for treatment of metastatic disease. Rhabdomyosarcomas show variable degrees of FDG accumulation. Although there are reports of diagnostic utility of FDG PET, its exact clinical role in rhabdomyosarcoma is currently not established (Shulkin 1997; Lenzo et al. 2000; Ben Arush et al. 2001, 2006; Peng et al. 2006) (Fig. 10). A recent study has shown that in patients with soft tissue sarcomas, the pretreatment tumor SUV_{max} and change in SUV_{max} after neoadjuvant chemotherapy independently identified patients at high risk of tumor recurrence (Schuetze et al. 2005).

5.7 Rare Tumors in Children

The utility of FDG PET in rare tumors is reported primarily in the form of single case reports (Jadvar and Fischman 1999; Chen et al. 2007; Lee et al. 2007; Kaste et al. 2007). Adrenocortical tumors in children are usually endocrinologically active and very aggressive clinically (Rodriguez-Galindo et al. 2005). A germline mutation is a major predisposing factor. Most patients with an adrenocortical tumor present with virilization. Two-thirds of patients have resectable tumors for which surgery currently holds the only realistic hope for cure. Preliminary experience indicates that these tumors are quite active metabolically, and FDG has been used to monitor them (Mackie et al. 2006; Binkovitz et al. 2008) (Fig. 11).

Hepatoblastoma is quite rare, accounting for less than 1% of childhood tumors (Rodriguez-Galindo et al. 2005; Roebuck and Perilongo 2006). With chemotherapy and surgery as primary treatment modalities, the prognosis has improved considerably over the past 20 years. Five-year survival has increased from 30 to 70%. These tumors are also metabolically active. In contrast to FDG uptake in hepatocellular carcinomas, hepatoblastomas accumulate and retain FDG much more reliably (Fig. 12). FDG PET has been found useful in monitoring hepatoblastomas during and after therapy (Mody et al. 2006).

PET has also been used for treatment planning of cancer in children. In one recent case report as proof of concept, I-124 PET was used for patient-specific three-dimensional radiobiologic dosimetry calculation of the optimal I-131 dose for treatment of a pediatric patient with differentiated papillary thyroid cancer (Hobbs et al. 2009). Another related study found that standard I-124 PET/CT dosimetry protocol was safe and informative in children with differentiated thyroid carcinoma (Freudenberg et al. 2007).

6 Conclusion

FDG PET is being increasingly applied to pediatric conditions, particularly in oncology (Federman and Feig 2007). PET and PET/CT scanning in children is not currently supported by Center for Medicare and Medicaid Services unless the disease condition coincides with a reimbursed adult condition. The recent merger of the Children's Cancer Group (CCG) and the Pediatric Oncology Group (POG) to form Children's Oncology Group (COG) brings the opportunity to examine the use of FDG PET in the management of childhood tumors in multi-institutional, co-operative efforts. Future data will, no doubt, show not only that FDG PET and FDG PET/CT can provide useful diagnostic information but that they will also play a pivotal role in the clinical management and care of children with cancer.

References

Abdel-Dayem HM (1997) The role of nuclear medicine in primary bone and soft tissue tumors. Semin Nucl Med 27:355–363

Accorsi R, Karp JS, Surti S (2010) Improved dose regimen in pediatric PET. J Nucl Med 51:293–300

Alessio AM, Kinahan PE, Manchanda V et al (2009) Weight-based, low-dose pediatric whole-body PET/CT protocols. J Nucl Med 50(10):1570–1577

American Academy of Pediatrics (1992) Committee on drugs. Guidelines for monitoring and management of pediatric patients during and after sedation for diagnostic and therapeutic procedures. Pediatrics 89:1110–1115

American Society of Anesthesiologists, Task Force on Sedation and Analgesia by Non-Anesthesiologists (2002) Practice guidelines for sedation and analgesia by non-anesthesiologists. Anesthesiology 96:1004–1017

Amthauer H, Furth C, Denecke T et al (2005) FDG-PET in 10 children with non-Hodgkin's lymphoma: initial experience in staging and follow-up. Klin Pediatr 217:327–333

Andre N, Fabre A, Colavolpe C et al (2008) FDG PET and evaluation of posttherapeutic residual tumors in pediatric oncology: preliminary experience. J Pediatr Hematol Oncol 30(5):343–346

Arush MW, Israel O, Postovsky S et al (2007) Positron emission tomography/computed tomography with 18fluoro-deoxyglucose in the detection of local recurrence and distant metastases of pediatric sarcoma. Pediatr Blood Cancer 49:901–905

Bangerter M, Moog F, Buchmann I et al (1998) Whole-body 2-[18F]-fluoro-2-deoxy-D-glucose positron emission tomography (FDG-PET) for accurate staging of Hodgkin's disease. Ann Oncol 9:1117–1122

Barnewolt CE, Paltiel HJ, Lebowitz RL, Kirks DR (1997) Genitourinary system. In: Kirks DR (ed) Practical pediatric imaging: diagnostic radiology of infants and children, 3rd edn. Lippincott-Raven, Philadelphia, pp 1009–1170

Barrington SF, Carr R (1995) Staging of Burkitt's lymphoma and response to treatment monitored by PET scanning. Clin Oncol 7:334–335

Bar-Sever Z, Connolly LP, Treves ST et al (1997) Technetium-99m MIBI in the evaluation of children with Ewing's sarcoma. J Nucl Med 38:13P

Bar-Sever Z, Keidar Z, Ben-Barak A et al (2007) The incremental value of 18F-FDG PET-CT in pediatric malignancies. Eur J Nucl Med Mol Imaging 34(5):630–637

Beker DB, Berrak SG, Canpolat C et al (2008) False positivity of FDG-PET/CT in a child with Hodgkin disease. Pediatr Blood Canecr 50(4):881–883

Ben Arush MW, Israel O, Kedar Z et al (2001) Detection of isolated distant metastasis in soft tissue sarcoma by fluorodeoxyglucose positron emission tomography: case report. Pediatr Hematol Oncol 18(4):295–298

Ben Arush MW, Bar Shalom R, Potovsky S et al (2006) Assessing the use of FDG-PET in the detection of regional and metastatic nodes in alveolar rhabdomyosarcoma of extremities. J Pediatr Hematol Oncol 28:440–445

Benz MR, Tchekmedyian N, Eilber FC et al (2009) Utilization of positron emission tomography in the management of patients with sarcoma. Curr Opin Oncol 21:345–351

Bestic JM, Peterson JJ, Bancroft LW (2009) Use of FDG PET in staging, restaging, and assessment of therapy response in Ewing sarcoma. Radiographics 29(5):1487–1500

Beyer T, Antoch G, Muller S et al (2004) Acquisition protocol considerations for combined PET/CT imaging. J Nucl Med 45(Suppl 1):25S–35S

Binkovitz I, Henwood M, Caniano D et al (2008) Early detection of recurrent pediatric adrenal cortical carcinoma using FDG PET. Clin Nucl Med 33(3):186–188

Borgwardt L, Larsen HJ, Pedersen K, Hojgaard L (2003) Practical use and implementation of PET in children in a hospital PET center. Eur J Nucl Med Mol Imaging 30(10): 1389–1397

Borgwardt L, Hojgaard L, Carstensen H et al (2005) Increased fluorine-18 2-fluoro-2-deoxy D-glucose (FDG) uptake in childhood CNS tumors is correlated with malignancy grade: a study with FDG positron emission tomography/magnetic resonance imaging coregistration and image fusion. J Clin Oncol 23:3030–3037

Bousvaros A, Kirks DR, Grossman H (1986) Imaging of neuroblastoma: an overview. Pediatr Radiol 16:89–106

Brenner D, Elliston C, Hall E, Berdon W (2001) Estimated risks of radiation-induced fatal cancer from pediatric CT. Am J Roentgenol 176:289–296

Briganti V, Sestini R, Orlando C et al (1997) Imaging of somatostatin receptors by indium-111-pentetreotide correlates with quantitative determination of somatostatin receptor type 2 gene expression in neuroblastoma tumor. Clin Cancer Res 3:2385–2391

Brink I, Reinhardt MJ, Hoegerle S et al (2001) Increased metabolic activity in the thymus gland studied with 18F-FDG PET: age dependency and frequency after chemotherapy. J Nucl Med 42:591–595

Brink I, Schaefer O, Walz M et al (2006) Fluorine-18 DOPA PET imaging of paraganglioma syndrome. Clin Nucl Med 31:39–41

Brisse H, Ollivier L, Edeline V et al (2004) Imaging of malignant tumors of the long bones in children: monitoring response to neoadjuvant chemotherapy and preoperative assessment. Pediatr Radiol 34:595–605

Bruggers CS, Friedman HS, Fuller GN et al (1993) Comparison of serial PET and MRI scans in a pediatric patient with a brainstem glioma. Med Pediatr Oncol 21(4):301–306

Buchler T, Cervinek L, Belohlavek O et al (2005) Langerhans cell histiocytosis with central nervous system involvement: follow up by FDG PET during treatment with cladribine. Pediatr Blood Cancer 44:286–288

Bujenovic S, Mannting F, Chakrabarti R et al (2003) Artifactual 2-deoxy-2-[(18)F]fluoro-D-deoxyglucose localization surrounding metallic objects in a PET/CT scanner using CT-based attenuation correction. Mol Imaging Biol 5:20–22

Caner B, Kitapel M, Unlu M et al (1992) Technetium-99m-MIBI uptake in benign and malignant bone lesions: a comparative study with technetium-99m-MDP. J Nucl Med 33:319–324

Carr R, Barrington SF, Madan B et al (1998) Detection of lymphoma in bone marrow by whole-body positron emission tomography. Blood 91:3340–3346

Ceyssens S, Van Laere K, de Groot T et al (2006) [11C]methionine PET, histopathology, and survival in primary brain tumors and recurrence. AJNR Am J Neurolradiol 27: 1432–1437

Chawla M, Reddy R, Kumar R et al (2009) PET-CT in detection of meningeal metastasis in neuroblastoma. Pediatr Surg Int 25:211–215

Chawla SC, Federman N, Zhange D et al (2010) Estimated cumulative radiation dose from PET/CT in children with malignancies: a 5-year retrospective review. Pediatr Radiol 40(5):681–686

Chen YW, Huang MY, Chang CC et al (2007) FDG PET/CT findings of epitheloid sarcoma in pediatric patient. Clin Nucl Med 32(11):898–901

Choi SJ, Kim JS, Kim JH et al (2005) [18F]3′-deoxy-3′-fluorothymidine PET for the diagnosis and grading of brain tumors. Eur J Nucl Med Mol Imaging 32:653–659

Cohade C, Wahl RL (2003) Applications of positron emission tomography/computed tomography image fusion in clinical positron emission tomography—clinical use, interpretation methods, diagnostic improvements. Semin Nucl Med 33(3): 228–237

Cohade C, Osman M, Pannu HK et al (2003) Uptake in supraclavicular area fat ("USA-Fat"): description on 18F-FDG PET/CT. J Nucl Med 44:170–176

Cohen MD (1992) Imaging of children with cancer. Mosby Yearbook, St. Louis

Connolly LP, Laor T, Jaramillo D et al (1996) Prediction of chemotherapeutic response of osteosarcoma with quantitative thallium-201 scintigraphy and magnetic resonance imaging. Radiology 201(P):349

Cremerius U, Fabry U, Neuerburg J et al (1998) Positron emission tomography with 18-F-FDG to detect residual disease after therapy for malignant lymphoma. Nucl Med Commun 19:1055–1063

de Wit M, Bumann D, Beyer W et al (1997) Whole-body positron emission tomography (PET) for diagnosis of residual mass in patients with lymphoma. Ann Oncol 8(Suppl 1):57–60

Delbeke D (1999) Oncological applications of FDG PET Imaging: colorectal cancer, lymphoma, and melanoma. J Nucl Med 40:591–603

Delbeke D, Coleman RE, Guiberteau MJ et al (2006) Procedure guideline for tumor imaging with 18F-FDG PET-CT 1.0. J Nucl Med 47:885–895

Depas G, De Barsy C, Jerusalem G et al (2005) 18F-FDG PET in children with lymphomas. Eur J Nucl Med Mol Imaging 32:31–38

Di Chiro G, Oldfield E, Wright DC et al (1988) Cerebral necrosis after radiotherapy and/or intraarterial chemotherapy for brain tumors: PET and neuropathologic studies. AJR Am J Roentgenol 150:189–197

Dizendorf EV, Treyer V, von Schulthess GK, Hany TF (2002) Application of oral contrast media in coregistered positron emission tomography-CT. AJR Am J Roentgenol 179(12): 477–481

Erlemann R, Sciuk J, Bosse A et al (1990) Response of osteosarcoma and Ewing sarcoma to preoperative chemotherapy: assessment with dynamic and static MR imaging and skeletal scintigraphy. Radiology 175:791–796

Fahey FH (2009) Dosimetry of pediatric PET/CT. J Nucl Med 50(9):1483–1491

Fahey FH, Palmer MR, Strauss KJ et al (2007) Dosimetry and adequacy of CT-based attenuation correction for pediatric PET: phantom study. Radiology 243:96–104

Federman N, Feig SA (2007) PET/CT in evaluating pediatric malignancies: a clinician's perspective. J Nucl Med 48(12): 1920–1922

Feldman F, Vanheertum R, Saxena C (2006) 18Fluorodeoxyglucose positron emission tomography evaluation of benign versus malignant osteochondromas: preliminary observations. J Comput Assist Tomogr 30:858–864

Figarola MS, McQuiston SA, Wilson F et al (2005) Recurrent hepatoblastoma with localization by PET-CT. Pediatr Radiol 35:1254–1258

Filmont JE, Yap CS, Ko F et al (2004) Conventional imaging and 2-deoxy-2-[18F]fluoro-D-glucose positron emission tomography for predicting the clinical outcome of patients with previously treated Hodgkin's disease. Mol Imaging Biol 6:47–54

Floeth FW, Pauleit D, Wittsack HJ et al (2005) Multimodal metabolic imaging of cerebral gliomas: positron emission tomography with [18F]fluoroethyl-L-tyrosine and magnetic resonance spectroscopy. J Neurosurg 102:318–327

Francavilla TL, Miletich RS, Di Chiro G et al (1989) Positron emission tomography in the detection of malignant degeneration of low-grade gliomas. Neurosurgery 24:1–5

Franzius C, Schober O (2003) Assessment of therapy response by FDG PET in pediatric patients. Q J Nucl Med 47:41–45

Franzius C, Sciuk J, Brinkschmidt C et al (2000a) Evaluation of chemotherapy response in primary bone tumors with F-18 FDG positron emission tomography compared with histologically assessed tumor necrosis. Clin Nucl Med 25:874–881

Franzius C, Sciuk J, Daldrup-Link HE et al (2000b) FDG-PET for detection of osseous metastases from malignant primary bone tumors: comparison with bone scintigraphy. Eur J Nucl Med 27:1305–1311

Franzius C, Juergens KU, Vomoor J (2005) PET-CT with diagnostic CT in the evaluation of childhood sarcoma. AJR Am J Roentgenol 184:1293–1304

Franzius C, Hermann K, Weckesser M et al (2006) Whole-body PET-CT with 11C-meta-hydroxyephedrine in tumors of the sympathetic system: feasibility study and comparison with 123I-MIBG SPECT-CT. J Nucl Med 47:1635–1642

Freudenberg LS, Jentzen W, Marlowe RJ et al (2007) 124-Iodine positron emission tomography/computed tomography dosimetry in pediatric patients with differentiated thyroid cancer. Exp Clin Endocrinol Diabetes 115(10):690–693

Frouge C, Vanel D, Coffre C et al (1988) The role of magnetic resonance imaging in the evaluation of Ewing sarcoma—a report of 27 cases. Skeletal Radiol 17:387–392

Furth C, Denecke T, Steffen I et al (2006) Correlative imaging strategies implementing CT, MR, and PET for staging of childhood Hodgkin disease. J Pediatr Hematol Oncol 28: 501–512

Furth C, Steffen IG, Amthauer H et al (2009) Early and late therapy response assessment with [18F]fluorodeoxyglucose positron emission tomography in pediatric Hodgkin's lymphoma: analysis of a prospective multicenter trial. J Clin Oncol 27(26):4365–4391

Garcia CA, Van Nostrand D, Atkins F et al (2006) Reduction of brown fat 2-deoxy-2-[F-18]fluoro-D-glucose uptake by controlling environmental temperature prior to positron emission tomography scan. Mol Imaging Biol 8:24–29

Gelfand MJ (2009) Dosimetry of FDG PET/CT and other molecular imaging applications in pediatric patients. Pediatr Radiol 39(Suppl 1):S46–S56

Gelfand MJ, Lemen LC (2007) PET/Ct and SPECT/CT dosimetry in children: the challenge to the pediatric imager. Semin Nucl Med 37(5):391–398

Gelfand MJ, O'Hara SM, Curtwright LA et al (2005) Premedication to block [(18)F]FDG uptake in the brown adipose tissue of pediatric and adolescent patients. Pediatr Radiol 35:984–990

Glantz MJ, Hoffman JM, Coleman RE et al (1991) Identification of early recurrence of primary central nervous system tumors by [18F]fluorodeoxyglucose positron emission tomograph. Ann Neurol 29:347–355

Goethals I, De Vriendt C, Hoste P et al (2009) Normal uptake of F-18 FDG in the testis as assessed by PET/CT in a pediatric study population. Ann Nucl Med 23(9): 817–820

Goo HW (2010) Whole body MRI of neuroblastoma. Eur J Radiol 75(3):306–314

Goodin GS, Shulkin BL, Kaufman RA et al (2006) PET-CT characterization of fibroosseous defects in children: 18F-FDG uptake can mimic metastatic disease. AJR Am J Roentgenol 187:1146

Gordon I (1998) Issues surrounding preparation, information, and handling the child and parent in nuclear medicine. J Nucl Med 39:490–494

Gurney JG, Severson RK, Davis S, Robison LL (1995) Incidence of cancer in children in the United States. Cancer 75:2186–2195

Gururangan S, Hwang E, Herndon JE 2nd et al (2004) [18F]fluorodeoxyglucose positron emission tomography in patients with medulloblastoma. Neurosurgery 55:1280–1288

Gyorke T, Zajic T, Lange A et al (2006) Impact of FDG PET for staging of Ewing sarcomas and primitive neuroectodermal tumors. Nucl Med Commun 27:17–24

Hany TF, Gharehpapagh E, Kamel EM et al (2002) Brown adipose tissue: a factor to consider in symmetrical tracer uptake in the neck and upper chest region. Eur J Nucl Med Mol Imaging 29:1393–1398

Hawkins DS, Rajendran JG, Conrad EU 3rd et al (2002) Evaluation of chemotherapy response in pediatric bone sarcomas by [F-18]-fluorodeoxy-D-glucose positron emission tomography. Cancer 94(12):3277–3284

Hawkins DS, Schuetze SM, Butrynski JE et al (2005) [18F]fluorodeoxyglucose positron emission tomography predicts outcome for Ewing sarcoma family of tumors. J Clin Oncol 23:8828–8834

Hernandez-Pampaloni M, Takalkar A, Yu JQ et al (2006) F-18 FDG-PET imaging and correlation with CT in staging and follow-up of pediatric lymphomas. Pediatr Radiol 36:524–531

Hobbs RF, Wahl RL, Javadi MS et al (2009) 124I PET-based 3D-RD dosimetry for a pediatric thyroid cancer patient: real-time treatment planning and methodologic comparison. J Nucl Med 50(11):1844–1847

Hoffman JM, Hanson MW, Friedman HS et al (1992) FDG-PET in pediatric posterior fossa brain tumors. J Comput Assist Tomogr 16:62–68

Hoh CK, Glaspy J, Rosen P et al (1997) Whole body FDG PET imaging for staging of Hodgkin's disease and lymphoma. J Nucl Med 38:343–348

Hollinger EF, Alibazoglu H, Ali A et al (1998) Hematopoietic cytokine-mediated FDG uptake simulates the appearance of diffuse metastatic disease on whole-body PET imaging. Clin Nucl Med 23:93–98

Holscher HC, Bloem JL, Vanel D et al (1992) Osteosarcoma: chemotherapy-induced changes at MR imaging. Radiology 182:839–844

Holthof VA, Herholz K, Berthold F et al (1993) In vivo metabolism of childhood posterior fossa tumors and primitive neuroectodermal tumors before and after treatment. Cancer 72(4):1394–1403

Howman-Giles R, Stevens M, Bergin M (1982) Role of gallium-67 in management of pediatric solid tumors. Aust Pediatric J 18:120–125

Huang TL, Liu RS, Chen TH et al (2006) Comparison between F-18-FDG positron emission tomography and histology for the assessment of tumor necrosis rates in primary osteosarcoma. J Chin Med Assoc 69:372–376

Hudson MM, Krasin MJ, Kaste SC (2004) PET imaging in pediatric Hodgkin's lymphoma. Pediatr Radiol 34(3): 190–198

Jadvar H, Fischman AJ (1999) Evaluation of rare tumors with [F-18]fluorodeoxyglucose positron emission tomography. Clin Positron Imaging 2:153–158

Jadvar H, Alavi A, Mavi A, Shulkin BL (2005) PET in pediatric diseases. Radiol Clin N Am 43:135–152

Janus T, Kim E, Tilbury R et al (1993) Use of [18F] fluorodeoxyglucose positron emission tomography in patients with primary malignant brain tumors. Ann Neurol 33:540–548

Jaramillo D, Laor T, Gebhardt M (1996) Pediatric musculoskeletal neoplasms. Evaluation with MR imaging. MRI Clin N Am 4:1–22

Jerusalem G, Warland V, Najjar F et al (1999) Whole-body 18F-FDG PET for the evaluation of patients with Hodgkin's disease and non-Hodgkin's lymphoma. Nucl Med Commun 20:13–20

Jones SC, Alavi A, Christman D et al (1982) The radiation dosimetry of 2-[18F]fluoro-2-deoxy-D-glucose in man. J Nucl Med 23:613–617

Juhasz C, Chugani DC, Muzik O et al (2006) In vivo uptake and metabolism of alpha-[11C]methyl-L-tryptophan in human brain tumors. J Cereb Blood Flow Metab 26: 345–357

Kabickova E, Sumerauer D, Cumlivska E et al (2006) Comparison of (18)F-FDG-PET and standard procedures for the pretreatment staging of children and adolescents with Hodgkin's disease. Eur J Nucl Med Mol Imaging 33:1025–1031

Kaste SC (2004) Issues specific to implementing PET-CT for pediatric oncology: what we have learned along the way. Pediatr Radiol 34(3):205–213

Kaste SC, Howard SC, McCarville EB et al (2005) 18F-FDG-avid sites mimicking active disease in pediatric Hodgkin's. Pediatr Radiol 35:141–154

Kaste SC, Rodriguez-Galindo C, McCarville ME et al (2007) PET-CT in pediatric Langehans cell histiocytosis. Pediatr Radiol 37(7):615–622

Keresztes K, Lengyel Z, Devenyi K et al (2004) Mediastinal bulky tumor in Hodgkin's disease and prognostic value of positron emission tomograhy in the evaluation of post treatment residual masses. Acta Haematol 112:194–199

Kim S, Salamon N, Jackson HA et al (2010) PET imaging in pediatric neuroradiology: current and future applications. Pediatr Radiol 40(1):82–96

Kinoshita H, Shimotake T, Furukawa T et al (2005) Mucoepidermal carcinoma of the lung detected by positron emission tomography in a 5-year-old girl. J Pediatr Surg 40:E1–E3

Kleihues P, Burger P, Scheithauer B (1993) The new WHO classification of brain tumors. Brain Pathol 3:255–268

Kleis M, Daldrup-Link H, Matthay K et al (2009) Diagnostic value of PET/CT for the staging and restaging of pediatric tumors. Eur J Nucl Med Mol Imaging 36(1):23–36

Kneisl JS, Patt JC, Johnson JC et al (2006) Is PET useful in detecting occult nonpulmonary metastases in pediatric bone sarcomas? Clin Orthop Relat Res 450:101–104

Korholz D, Kluge R, Wickmann L et al (2003) Importance of F18-fluorodeoxy-D-2-glucose positron emission tomography (FDG-PET) for staging and therapy control of Hodgkin's lymphoma in childhood and adolescence—consequences for the GPOH-HD 2003 protocol. Onkologie 26:489–493

Kostakoglu L, Leonard JP, Coleman M et al (2000) Comparison of FDG-PET and Ga-67 SPECT in the staging of lymphoma. J Nucl Med 41(Suppl 5):118P

Krasin MJ, Hudson MM, Kaste SC (2004) Positron emission tomography in pediatric radiation oncology: integration in the treatment-planning process. Pediatr Radiol 34:214–221

Kumar J, Seith A, Kumar A et al (2008) Whole-body MR imaging with the use of parallel imaging for detection of skeletal metastases in pediatric patients with small cell neoplasms: comparison with skeletal scintigraphy and FDG PET/CT. Pediatr Radiol 38(9):953–962

Lapela M, Leskinen S, Minn HR et al (1995) Increased glucose metabolism in untreated non-Hodgkin's lymphoma: a study with positron emission tomography and fluorine-18-fluorodeoxyglucose. Blood 86:3522–3527

Lavely WC, Delbeke D, Greer JP et al (2003) FDG PET in the follow-up of management of patients with newly diagnosed Hodgkin and non-Hodgkin lymphoma after first-line chemotherapy. Int J Radiat Oncol Biol Phys 57:307–315

Lawrence JA, Babyn PS, Chan HS et al (1993) Extremity osteosarcoma in childhood: prognostic value of radiologic imaging. Radiology 189:43–47

Lee EY, Vargus SO, Sawicki GS et al (2007) Mucoepidermoid carcinoma of bronchus in a pediatric patient: (18)F-FDG PET findings. Pediatr Radiol 37(12):1278–1282

Lemmi MA, Fletcher BD, Marina NM et al (1990) Use of MR imaging to assess results of chemotherapy for Ewing sarcoma. AJR Am J Roentgenol 155:343–346

Lenzo NP, Shulkin B, Castle VP, Hutchinson RJ (2000) FDG PET in childhood soft tissue sarcoma. J Nucl Med 41(Suppl 5):96P

Leskinen-Kallio S, Ruotsalainen U, Nagren K et al (1991) Uptake of carbon-11-methionine and fluorodeoxyglucose in non-Hodgkin's lymphoma: a PET study. J Nucl Med 32: 1211–1218

Levine JM, Weiner M, Kelly KM (2006) Routine use of PET scans after completion of therapy in pediatric Hodgkin disease results in a high false positive rate. J Pediatr Hematol Oncol 28:711–714

Lilja A, Lundqvist H, Olsson Y et al (1989) Positron emission tomography and computed tomography in differential diagnosis between recurrent or residual glioma and treatment-induced brain lesion. Acta Radiol 38:121–128

Lim R, Fahey FH, Drubach LA et al (2007) Early experience with fluorine-18 sodium fluoride bone PET in young patients with back pain. J Pediatr Orthop 27(3):277–282

Lin J, Leung WT (1995) Quantitative evaluation of thallium-201 uptake in predicting chemotherapeutic response of osteosarcoma. Eur J Nucl Med 22:553–555

Mackie GC, Shulkin BL, Ribeiro RC et al (2006) Use of [18F]fluorodeoxyglucose positron emission tomography in evaluating locally recurrent and metastatic adrenocortical carcinoma. J Clin Endocrinol Metab 91:2665–2671

MacVicar AD, Olliff JFC, Pringle J et al (1992) Ewing sarcoma: MR imaging of chemotherapy-induced changes with histologic correlation. Radiology 184:859–864

Mandell GA, Cooper JA, Majd M et al (1997) Procedure guidelines for pediatric sedation in nuclear medicine. J Nucl Med 38:1640–1643

Maria B, Drane WB, Quisling RJ, Hoang KB (1997) Correlation between gadolinium-diethylenetriaminepentaacetic acid contrast enhancement and thallium-201 chloride uptake in pediatric brainstem glioma. J Child Neurol 12: 341–348

McCarville MB (2009) PET-CT imaging in pediatric oncology. Cancer Imaging 9:35–43

McDonald DJ (1994) Limb salvage surgery for sarcomas of the extremities. AJR 163:509–513

McQuattie S (2008) Pediatric PET/CT imaging: tips and techniques. J Nucl Med Technol 36(4):171–180

Meany HJ, Gidvani VK, Minniti CP (2007) Utility of PET scans to predict disease relapse in pediatric patients with Hodgkin lymphoma. Pediatr Blood Cancer 48(4):399–402

Menendez LR, Fideler BM, Mirra J (1993) Thallium-201 scanning for the evaluation of osteosarcoma and soft tissue sarcoma. J Bone Joint Surg 75:526–531

Miller E, Metser U, Avrahami G et al (2006) Role of 18F-FDG PET/CT in staging and follow-up of lymphoma in pediatric and young adult patients. J Comput Assist Tomogr 30:689–694

Mineura K, Sasajima T, Kowada M et al (1997) Indications for differential diagnosis of nontumor central nervous system diseases from tumors. A positron emission tomography study. J Neuroimaging 7:8–15

Minotti AJ, Shah L, Keller K (2004) Positron emission tomography/computed tomography fusion imaging in brown adipose tissue. Clin Nucl Med 29(1):5–11

Misch D, Steffen IG, Schonberger S et al (2008) Use of positron emission tomography for staging, preoperative response assessment and posttherapeutic evaluation in children with Wilms tumor. Eur J Nucl Med Mol Imaging 35:1642–1650

Mody RJ, Pohlen JA, Malde S et al (2006) FDG PET for the study of primary hepatic malignancies in children. Pediatr Blood Cancer 47:51–55

Molloy PT, Belasco J, Ngo K, Alavi A (1999a) The role of FDG PET imaging in the clinical management of pediatric brain tumors. J Nucl Med 40:129P

Molloy PT, Defeo R, Hunter J et al (1999b) Excellent correlation of FDG PET imaging with clinical outcome in patients with neurofibromatosis type I and low grade astrocytomas. J Nucl Med 40:129P

Montravers F, McNamara D, Landman-Parker J et al (2002) [(18)F]FDG in childhood lymphoma: clinical utility and impact on management. Eur J Nucl Med Mol Imaging 29: 1155–1165

Moody R, Shulkin B, Yanik G et al (2001) PET FDG Imaging in Pediatric Lymphomas. J Nucl Med 42(Suppl 5):39P

Moog F, Bangerter M, Diederichs CG et al (1997) Lymphoma: role of whole-body 2-deoxy-2-[F-18]fluoro-D-glucose (FDG) PET in nodal staging. Radiology 203:795–800

Moog F, Bangerter M, Kotzerke J et al (1998a) 18-F-fluorodeoxyglucose positron emission tomography as a new approach to detect lymphomatous bone marrow. J Clin Oncol 16: 603–609

Moog F, Bangerter M, Diederichs CG et al (1998b) Extranodal malignant lymphoma: detection with FDG PET versus CT. Radiology 206:475–481

Moon L, McHugh K (2005) Advances in pediatric tumor imaging. Arch Dis Child 90:608–611

Mosskin M, von Holst H, Bergstrom M et al (1987) Positron emission tomography with 11C-methionine and computed tomography of intracranial tumors compared with histopathologic examination of multiple biopsies. Acta Radiol 28:673–681

Murphy JJ, Tawfeeq M, Chang N et al (2008) Early experience with PET/CT scan in the evaluation of pediatric abdominal neoplasms. J Pediatr Surg 43(2):2186–2192

Nadel HR, Rossleigh MA (1995) Tumor imaging. In: Treves ST (ed) Pediatric nuclear medicine, 2nd edn. Springer, New York, pp 496–527

Nakamoto Y, Chin RB, Kraitchman DL et al (2003) Effects of nonionic intravenous contrast agents at PET/CT imaging: phantom and canine studies. Radiology 227:817–824

Nanni C, Rubello D, Castelluci P et al (2006) 18F-FDG PET-CT fusion imaging in pediatric solid extracranial tumors. Biomed Pharmacother 60:593–606

Nehmeh SA, Erdi YE, Kalaigian H et al (2003) Correction for oral contrast artifacts in CT attenuation-corrected PET images obtained by combined PET/CT. J Nucl Med 44(12): 1940–1944

Newman JS, Francis IR, Kaminski MS, Wahl RL (1994) Imaging of lymphoma with PET with 2-[F-18]-fluoro-2-deoxy-D-glucose: correlation with CT. Radiology 190: 111–116

O'Connor MI, Pritchard DJ (1991) Ewing's sarcoma. Prognostic factors, disease control, and the reemerging role of surgical treatment. Clin Orthop 262:78–87

Ohtomo K, Terui S, Yokoyama R et al (1996) Thallium-201 scintigraphy to assess effect of chemotherapy to osteosarcoma. J Nucl Med 37:1444–1448

Okada J, Yoshikawa K, Imazeki K et al (1991) The use of FDG-PET in the detection and management of malignant lymphoma: correlation of uptake with prognosis. J Nucl Med 32:686–691

Okada J, Yoshikawa K, Itami M et al (1992) Positron emission tomography using fluorine-18-fluorodeoxyglucose in malignant lymphoma: a comparison with proliferative activity. J Nucl Med 33:325–329

Ott RJ, Tait D, Flower MA et al (1992) Treatment planning for 131I-mIBG radiotherapy of neural crest tumors using 124I-mIBG positron emission tomography. Br J Radiol 65:787–791

O'Tuama LA, Phillips PC, Strauss LC et al (1990) Two-phase [11C]L-methionine PET in childhood brain tumors. Pediatr Neurology 6:163–170

O'Tuama L, Janicek M, Barnes P et al (1991) Tl-201/Tc-99m HMPAO SPECT imaging of treated childhood brain tumors. Pediatr Neurol 7:249–257

O'Tuama L, Treves ST, Larar G et al (1993) Tl-201 versus Tc-99m MIBI SPECT in evaluation of childhood brain tumors. J Nucl Med 34:1045–1051

Ovadia D, Metser U, Lievshitz G et al (2007) Back pain in adolescents: assessments with integrated 18F-fluoride positron emission tomography-computed tomography. J Pediatr Orthop 27:90–93

Pacak K, Ilias I, Chen CC et al (2004) The role of 18F-fluorodeoxyglucose positron emission tomography and In-111-diethylenetriaminepentaacetate-D-Phe-pentetreotide scintigraphy in the localization of ectopic adrenocorticotropin-secreting tumors causing Cushing's syndrome. J Clin Endocrinol Metab 89:2214–2221

Patel PM, Alibazoglu H, Ali A et al (1996) Normal thymic uptake of FDG on PET imaging. Clin Nucl Med 21:772–775

Patronas NJ, Di Chiro G, Kufta C et al (1985) Prediction of survival in glioma patients by means of positron emission tomography. J Neurosurg 62:816–822

Paul R (1987) Comparison of fluorine-18-2-fluorodeoxyglucose and gallium-67 citrate imaging for detection of lymphoma. J Nucl Med 28:288–292

Pauleit D, Floeth F, Hamacher K et al (2005) O-(2-[18F]fluoroethyl)-L-tyrosine PET combined with MRI improves the diagnostic assessment of cerebral gliomas. Brain 128(Pt 3): 678–687

Peng F, Rabkin G, Muzik O (2006) Use of 2-deoxy-[F-18]-fluoro-D-glucose positron emission tomography to monitor therapeutic response by rhabdomyosarcoma in children: report of a retrospective case. Clin Nucl Med 31:394–397

Philip I, Shun A, McCowage G et al (2005) Positron emission tomography in recurrent hepatoblastoma. Pediatr Surg Int 21:341–345

Pirotte B, Goldman S, Salzberg S et al (2003) Combined positron emission tomography and magnetic resonance imaging for the planning of stereotactic brain biopsies in children: experience in 9 cases. Pediatr Neurosurg 38(3): 146–155

Pirotte B, Levivier M, Morelli D et al (2005) Positron emission tomography for the early postsurgical evaluation of pediatric brain tumors. Childs Nerv Syst 21:294–300

Pirotte B, Goldman S, Dewitte O et al (2006) Integrated positron emission tomography and magnetic resonance imaging-guided resection of brain tumors: a report of 103 consecutive procedures. J Neurosurg 104:238–253

Pirotte B, Acerbi F, Lubeansu A et al (2007) PET imaging in surgical management of pediatric brain tumors. Childs Nerv Syst 23(7):739–751

Ramanna L, Waxman A, Binney G et al (1990) Thallium-201 scintigraphy in bone sarcoma: comparison with gallium-67 and technetium-99m MDP in the evaluation of chemotherapeutic response. J Nucl Med 31:567–572

Rhodes MM, Delbeke D, Whitlock JA et al (2006) Utility of FDG PET-CT in follow-up of children treated for Hodgkin and non-Hodgkin lymphoma. J Pediatr Hematol Oncol 28:300–306

Riad R, Omar W, Kotb M et al (2010) Role of PET/CT in malignant pediatric lymphoma. Eur J Nucl Med Mol Imaging 37(2):319–329

Robbins E (2008) Radiation risks from imaging studies in children with cancer. Pediatr Blood Cancer 51(4):453–457

Robertson R, Ball WJ, Barnes P (1997) Skull and brain. In: Kirks D (ed) Practical pediatric imaging. Diagnostic radiology of Infants and children. Lippincott-Raven, Philadelphia, pp 65–200

Robison L (1997) General principles of the epidemiology of childhood cancer. In: Pizzo P, Poplack D (eds) Principles and practice of pediatric oncology. Lippincott-Raven, Philadelphia, pp 1–10

Rodriguez M, Rehn S, Ahlstrom H et al (1995) Predicting malignancy grade with PET in non-Hodgkin's lymphoma. J Nucl Med 36:1790–1796

Rodriguez-Galindo C, Figueiredo BC, Zambetti GP et al (2005) Biology, clinical characteristics, and management of adrenocortical tumors in children. Pediatr Blood Cancer 45(3):265–273

Roebuck DJ, Perilongo G (2006) Hepatoblastoma: an oncological review. Pediatr Radiol 36(3):183–186

Rollins N, Lowry P, Shapiro K (1995) Comparison of gadolinium-enhanced MR and thallium-201 single photon emission computed tomography in pediatric brain tumors. Pediatr Neurosurg 22:8–14

Romer W, Hanauske AR, Ziegler S et al (1998) Positron emission tomography in non-Hodgkin's lymphoma: assessment of chemotherapy with fluorodeoxyglucose. Blood 91:4464–4471

Rosen G, Loren GJ, Brien EW et al (1993) Serial thallium-201 scintigraphy in osteosarcoma. Correlation with tumor necrosis after preoperative chemotherapy. Clin Orthop 293: 302–306

Rossleigh MA, Murray IPC, Mackey DWJ (1990) Pediatric solid tumors: evaluation by gallium-67 SPECT studies. J Nucl Med 31:161–172

Rozental JM, Levine RL, Nickles RJ (1991) Changes in glucose uptake by malignant gliomas: preliminary study of prognostic significance. J Neuro-Oncol 10:75–83

Ruotsalainen U, Suhonen-Povli H, Eronen E et al (1996) Estimated radiation dose to the newborn in FDG-PET studies. J Nucl Med 37:387–393

Sasi OA, Sathiapalan R, Rifai A et al (2005) Colonic neuroendocrine carcinoma in a child. Pediatr Radiol 35: 339–343

Schelbert H, Hoh CK, Royal HD et al (1998) Procedure guideline for tumor imaging using Fluorine-18-FDG. J Nucl Med 39:1302–1305

Schifter T, Hoffman JM, Hanson MW et al (1993) Serial FDG-PET studies in the prediction of survival in patients with primary brain tumors. J Comput Assist Tomogr 17:509–561

Schuetze SM, Rubin BP, Vernon C et al (2005) Use of positron emission tomography in localized extremity soft tissue sarcoma treated with neoadjuvant chemotherapy. Cancer 103:339–348

Segall GM (2001) FDG PET imaging in patients with lymphoma: a clinical perspective. J Nucl Med 42(4): 609–610

Shammas A, Lim R, Charron M (2009) Pediatric FDG PET/CT: physiologic uptake, normal variants, and benign conditions. Radiographics 29(5):1467–1486

Sharp SE, Shulkin BL, Gelfand MJ et al (2009) 123I-MIBG scintigraphy and 18F-FDG PET in neuroblastoma. J Nucl Med 50(8):1237–1243

Shore RM (2008) Positron emission tomography/computed tomography (PET/CT) in children. Pediatr Ann 37:404–412

Shulkin BL (1997) PET applications in Pediatrics. Q J Nucl Med 41:281–291

Shulkin BL (2004) PET imaging in pediatric oncology. Pediatr Radiol 34:199–204

Shulkin BL, Mitchell DS, Ungar DR et al (1995) Neoplasms in a pediatric population: 2-[F-18]-fluoro-2-deoxy-D-glucose PET studies. Radiology 194:495–500

Shulkin BL, Hutchinson RJ, Castle VP et al (1996a) Neuroblastoma: positron emission tomography with 2-[fluorine-18]-fluoro-2-deoxy-D-glucose compared with metaiodobenzylguanidine scintigraphy. Radiology 199:743–750

Shulkin BL, Wieland DM, Baro ME et al (1996b) PET hydroxyephedrine imaging of neuroblastoma. J Nucl Med 37:16–21

Shulkin BL, Chang E, Strouse PJ et al (1997) PET FDG studies of Wilms tumors. J Pediatr Hem/Onc 19:334–338

Shulkin BL, Wieland DM, Castle VP et al (1999) Carbon-11 epinephrine PET imaging of neuroblastoma. J Nucl Med 40:129P

Stumpe KD, Urbinelli M, Steinert HC et al (1998) Whole-body positron emission tomography using fluorodeoxyglucose for staging of lymphoma: effectiveness and comparison with computed tomography. Eur J Nucl Med 25:721–728

Sty JR, Kun LE, Starshak RJ (1985) Pediatric applications in nuclear oncology. Semin Nucl Med 15:171–200

Sugawara Y, Fisher SJ, Zasadny KR, Kison PV, Baker LH, Wahl RL (1998) Preclinical and clinical studies of bone marrow uptake of fluorine-1-fluorodeoxyglucose with or without granulocyte colony-stimulating factor during chemotherapy. J Clin Oncol 16:173–180

Swift P (2002) Novel techniques in the delivery of radiation in pediatric oncology. Pediatr Clin N Am 49:1107–1129

Taggart DR, Han MM, Quach A et al (2009) Comparison of iodine-123 metaiodobenzylguainidine (MIBG) scan and [18F]fluorodeoxyglucose positron emission tomography to evaluate response after iodine-131 MIBG therapy for relapsed neuroblastoma. J Clin Oncol 27(32):5343–5349

Tateishi U, Hosono A, Makimoto A et al (2007) Accuracy of 18F fluorodeoxyglucose positron emission tomography/computed tomography in staging pediatric sarcomas. J Pediatr Hematol Oncol 29(9):608–612

Tatsumi M, Kitayama H, Sugahara H et al (2001) Whole-body hybrid PET with 18F-FDG in the staging of non-Hodgkin's lymphoma. J Nucl Med 42(4):601–608

Tatsumi M, Engles JM, Ishimori T et al (2004) Intense (18)F-FDG uptake in brown fat can be reduced pharmacologically. J Nucl Med 45:1189–1193

Tatsumi M, Cohade C, Nakamoto Y et al (2005) Direct comparison of FDG PET and CT findings in patients with lymphoma: initial experience. Radiology 237:1038–1045

Tatsumi M, Miller JH, Wahl RL (2007) 18F-FDG PET in evaluating non-CNS pediatric malignancies. J Nucl Med 48(12):1923–1931

Torii K, Tsuyuguchi N, Kawabe J et al (2005) Correlation of amino-acid uptake using methionine PET and histological classification in various gliomas. Ann Nucl Med 19: 677–683

Townsend DW, Beyer T (2002) A combined PET-CT scanner: the path to true image fusion. Br J Radiol 75(Suppl): S24–S30

Treves ST (1995) Introduction. In: Treves ST (ed) Pediatric nuclear medicine, 2nd edn. Springer, New York, pp 1–11

Triche TJ (1993) Pathology of pediatric malignancies. In: Pizzo PA, Poplack DG (eds) Principles and practice of pediatric oncology, 2nd edn. JB Lippincott, Philadelphia, pp 115–152

Truong MT, Erasmus JJ, Munden RF et al (2004) Focal FDG uptake in mediastinal brown fat mimicking malignancy: a potential pitfall resolved on PET-CT. AJR Am J Roentgenol 183:1127–1132

Utriainen M, Metsahonkala L, Salmi TT et al (2002) Metabolic characterization of childhood brain tumors: comparison of 18F-fluordeoxyglucose and 11C-methionine positron emission tomography. Cancer 95(6):1376–1386

Vaidyanathan G, Affleck DJ, Zalutsky MR (1995) Validation of 4-[fluorine-18]fluoro-3-iodobenzylguanidine as a positron-emitting analog of MIBG. J Nucl Med 36:644–650

Valk PE, Budinger TF, Levin VA et al (1988) PET of malignant cerebral tumors after interstitial brachytherapy. Demonstration of metabolic activity and correlation with clinical outcome. J Neurosurg 69:830–838

Van Laere K, Ceyssens S, Van Calenbergh F et al (2005) Direct comparison of 18F-FDG and 11C-methionine PET in suspected recurrence of glioma: sensitivity, inter-observer variability and prognostic value. Eur J Nucl Med Mol Imaging 32:39–51

Visvikis D, Costa DC, Croasdale I et al (2003) CT-based attenuation correction in the calculation of semi-quantitative indices of [18F]FDG uptake in PET. Eur J Nucl Med Mol Imaging 30(3):344–353

Volker T, Denecke T, Steffen I et al (2007) Positron emission tomography for staging of pediatric sarcoma patients: results of a prospective multicenter trial. J Clin Oncol 25(34):5435–5441

Von Falck C, Rosenthal H, Gratz KF et al (2007a) Nonossifying fibroma can mimic residual lymphoma in FDG PET: additional value of combined PET/CT. Clin Nucl Med 32:640–642

Von Falck C, Maecker B, Schirg E et al (2007b) Post transplant lymphoproliferative disease in pediatric solid organ transplant patients: a possible role for [18F]-FDG PET(/CT) in initial staging and therapy monitoring. Eur J Radiol 63:427–435

Wang SX, Boethus J, Ericson K (2006) FDG-PET on irradiated brain tumor: ten years summary. Acta Radiol 47:85–90

Weckesser M, Langen KJ, Rickert CH et al (2005) O-(2-[18F]fluorethyl)-L-tyrosine PET in the clinical evaluation of primary brain tumors. Eur J Nucl Med Mol Imaging 32:422–429

Wegner EA, Barrington SF, Kingston JE et al (2005) The impact of PET scanning on management of pediatric oncology patients. Eur J Nucl Med Mol Imaging 32:23–30

Weinblatt ME, Zanzi I, Belakhlef A et al (1997) False-positive FDG-PET imaging of the thymus of a child with Hodgkin's disease. J Nucl Med 38:888–890

Williams G, Fahey FH, Treves ST, Kocak M et al (2008) Exploratory evaluation of two-dimensional and three-dimensional methods of FDG PET quantification in pediatric anaplastic astrocytoma: a report from the pediatric brain tumor consortium (PBTC). Eur J Nucl Med Mol Imaging 35(9):1651–1658

Yang SL, Alderson PO, Kaizer HA, Wagner HA (1979) Serial Ga-67 citrate imaging in children with neoplastic disease: concise communication. J Nucl Med 20:210–214

Yeung HW, Sanches A, Squire OD et al (2002) Standardized uptake value (SUV) in pediatric patients: an investigation to determine the optimum measurement parameter. Eur J Nucl Med Mol Imaging 29(1):61–66

Yeung HW, Grewal RK, Gonen M et al (2003) Patterns of (18)F-FDG uptake in adipose tissue and muscle: a potential source of false-positives for PET. J Nucl Med 44(11): 1789–1796

Yeung HW, Schoder H, Smith A et al (2005) Clinical value of combined positron emission tomography/computed tomography imaging in the interpretation of 2-deoxy-2-[F-18]fluoro-D-glucose positron emission tomography studies in cancer patients. Mol Imaging Biol 7:229–235

Assessment of Response to Therapy

Ali Gholamrezanezhad, Alin Chirindel, and Rathan Subramaniam

Contents

Abstract

In modern clinical oncology, there is a growing need to identify response to treatment to detect improvement or worsening of the disease as early as possible. Anatomical imaging modalities that rely on morphologic or structural data, though precise in the delineation of lesions, do not provide functional information about response and have limited reproducibility. The accuracy of anatomical parameters is limited partly due to the delay between the treatment and the appearance of tumor shrinkage. As the changes in tumor metabolism precede the changes in tumor size, functional imaging modalities are more clinically useful and allow visualization of tumor response at earlier stages. PET provides information regarding the metabolic behavior of the disease, independent of morphological and anatomical criteria. This chapter reviews the current evidence on the potential contribution of PET to evaluation of response to therapy and the challenges ahead, especially the standardization of performing clinical PET/CT across centers, to be meaningful in patient care.

A. Gholamrezanezhad · A. Chirindel ·
R. Subramaniam (✉)
Russell H Morgan Department of Radiology and Radiological Science, Johns Hopkins Medical Institutions, Baltimore, MD, USA
e-mail: rsubram4@jhmi.edu

P. Peller et al. (eds.), *PET-CT and PET-MRI in Oncology*, Medical Radiology. Diagnostic Imaging,
DOI: 10.1007/174_2012_707,

1 Introduction

In modern clinical oncology, there is a growing demand to identify response to treatment in patients treated for cancers and to detect improvement or worsening of the disease as early as possible. It is clear that evaluation of tumor response to treatment remains difficult because of the unknown course of tumor reaction to therapy for most malignancies. In fact, the presence of numerous determinants and underlying factors for response to treatment (such as type of tumor, type of treatment procedures (e.g. choice of chemotherapeutic regimens and radiotherapy plans), patient's age, stage of the disease, etc) make it clinically difficult to reliably assess tumor response to treatment, which emphasizes the need for effective imaging methods in these settings.

Currently, conventional anatomical imaging methods are the mainstay of evaluation of response to treatment in most clinical settings and cancer therapies. They define response to treatment solely as reduction of tumor size, without considering molecular or functional phenomena that appear earlier than the structural or anatomic alterations. These modalities that rely on morphologic or structural data, although very precise in the delineation of lesions, frequently present a limited diagnostic efficacy in the evaluation of response to treatments. Anatomic parameters suffer from limited reproducibility and frequently are unable to distinguish between fibrotic scar and viable tumor tissue. The accuracy of anatomical parameters is limited partly due to the delay between the treatment and the appearance of tumor shrinkage. Usually, several cycles of chemotherapy are necessary to significantly affect the tumor size. The available anatomical imaging modalities are unable to predict response to treatment in an appropriate and timely manner. Therefore, anatomical imaging methods such as CT cannot differentiate between necrotic tumor or scar tissue and residual tumor early after treatment (Delgado-Bolton and Delgado 2009; Buyse et al. 2000).

As the change in tumor metabolism precedes the changes in tumor size, functional imaging modalities (the most important of which is PET) seem to be more clinically useful and allow visualization of tumor response at earlier stages (Pons et al. 2009). PET has the potential to contribute significantly to treatment planning and to evaluation of response to therapy in patients with solid tumors. It provides information regarding the metabolic behavior of the disease, independent of morphological and anatomical criteria (Spaepen and Mortelmans 2001). In fact, PET imaging provides information noninvasively to predict the response to treatment at the earliest possible time, and response assessment provided by serial metabolic imaging strongly correlates to survival and prognosis (Baum and Przetak 2001). Available reports confirm how metabolic imaging may change the outcome of some cancer types. However, the role of PET in the context of patient management and the cost-effectiveness of this approach with several cancers types warrants further investigation. Also, therapy monitoring by PET could help to optimize neoadjuvant therapy protocols and to avoid ineffective preoperative treatments in nonresponders, although proof is needed for this idea. Furthermore, which patients benefit most from metabolic imaging and how much the regional tracer uptake varies are still unknown.

2 Functional Versus Anatomical Imaging Modalities: Advantages and Disadvantages

The traditional approach to treatment monitoring through imaging modalities relies on assessing anatomical changes in tumor size, before and after treatment. The original World Health Organization (WHO) criteria consist of bi-dimensional measurements of the tumor and the response is defined as a decrease in the product of two perpendicular diameters of the tumor by at least 50 %. The more recent response evaluation criteria in solid tumors (RECIST) introduced by the National Cancer Institute (NCI) and the European association for research and treatment of cancer (EO-RTC) defines response to treatment as a 30 % decrease in the sum of the diameters of target lesions (Allen-Auerbach and Weber 2009; Eisenhauer et al. 2009) (Table 1). Given these somewhat arbitrary response criteria, it is not surprising that high spatial resolution inherent to anatomical imaging modalities such as CT and MRI is a great advantage. However, a consistent correlation between tumor response (as determined by WHO or the RECIST criteria) and patient survival has not been proven yet (Allen-Auerbach and Weber 2009). A reduction in tumor diameter does not always significantly correlate with a histopathologic response.

Table 1 A review of different criteria for assessing response to treatment (Cheson 2007a; Wahl et al. 2009)

	IWG[a]	WHO[b]	RECIST[c]	PERCIST[d]	EORTC[e]
Complete remission	A. FDG-avid or PET positive before therapy: mass of any size permitted if PET negative; b. Variably FDG-avid or PET negative: regression to normal size on CT	Measurable disease: disappearance of all known disease, confirmed at ≥ 4 weeks; Nonmeasurable disease: disappearance of all known disease, confirmed at ≥ 4 weeks	Target lesions: disappearance of all target lesions, confirmed at ≥ 4 weeks; Nontarget lesions: disappearance of all nontarget lesions and normalization of tumor markers, confirmed at ≥ 4 weeks	Complete resolution of 18F-FDG uptake within measurable target lesion so that it is less than mean liver activity and indistinguishable from surrounding background blood-pool levels. Disappearance of all other lesions to background blood pool levels. No new 18F-FDG–avid lesions in pattern typical of cancer. If progression by RECIST, must verify with follow-up	Complete resolution of 18F-FDG uptake within tumor volume so that it is indistinguishable from surrounding normal tissue
Partial remission	≥50 % decrease in SPD of up to 6 largest dominant masses. No increase in size of other nodes; a. FDG-avid or PET positive before therapy: 1 or more PET positive at previously involved site; b. Variably FDG-avid or PET negative: regression on CT	Measurable disease: ≥ 50 % decrease from baseline, confirmed at ≥ 4 week; Nonmeasurable disease: estimated decrease of ≥ 50 %, confirmed at 4 wk	Target lesions: ≥ 30 % decrease from baseline, confirmed at 4 weeks; Nontarget lesions: No definite criteria for PR (persistence of one or more nontarget lesions or tumor markers above normal limits is described as nonPD)	Reduction of minimum of 30 % in target measurable tumor 18F-FDG SUL peak. Absolute drop in SUL must be at least 0.8 SUL units, as well. Measurement is commonly in same lesion as baseline but can be another lesion if that lesion was previously present and is the most active lesion after treatment. No increase, > 30 % in SUL or size of target or nontarget lesions (i.e., no PD by RECIST or IWC) (if PD anatomically, must verify with follow-up). Reduction in extent of tumor 18F-FDG uptake is not requirement for PMR. No new lesions	Reduction of minimum of 15 % ± 25 % in tumor 18F-FDG SUV after 1 cycle of chemotherapy, and > 25 % after more than 1 treatment cycle; reduction in extent of tumor 18F-FDG uptake is not a requirement for PMR

(continued)

Table 1 (continued)

	IWG[a]	WHO[b]	RECIST[c]	PERCIST[d]	EORTC[e]
Stable disease	A. FDG-avid or PET positive before therapy: PET positive at prior sites of diseases and no new sites on CT or PET; b. Variably FDG-avid or PET negative: no change in size of previous lesions on CT	Measurable disease: neither PR nor PD criteria met; Nonmeasurable disease: neither PR nor PD criteria met	Target lesions: neither PR nor PD criteria met; Nontarget lesions: No definite criteria for SD (persistence of one or more nontarget lesions or tumor markers above normal limits is described as nonPD)	Not CMR, PMR, or PMD	Increase in tumor 18F-FDG SUV < 25 % or decrease of < 15 % and no visible increase in extent of 18F-FDG tumor uptake (20 % in longest dimension)
Progressive disease	Appearance of a new lesion > 1.5 cm in any axis; - ≥ 50 % in the longest diameter of a previously identified node > 1 cm in short axis or in the SPD of more than one node; - Lesions PET positive if FDG-avid lymphoma or PET positive before therapy	Measurable disease: ≥ 25 % increase of one or more lesions or appearance of new lesions; Nonmeasurable disease: estimated increase of ≥ 25 % in existent lesions or new lesions	Target lesions: ≥ 20 % increase over smallest sum observed or appearance of new lesions; Nontarget lesions: unequivocal progression of nontarget lesions or appearance of new lesions	>30 % increase in 18F-FDG SUL peak, with > 0.8 SUL unit increase in tumor SUV peak from baseline scan in pattern typical of tumor and not of infection/treatment effect. OR: Visible increase in extent of 18F-FDG tumor uptake (75 % in TLG volume with no decline in SUL. OR: New 18F-FDG–avid lesions that are typical of cancer and not related to treatment effect or infection. PMD other than new visceral lesions should be confirmed on follow-up study within 1 mo unless PMD also is clearly associated with progressive disease by RECIST 1.1	Increase in 18F-FDG tumor SUV of > 25 % within tumor region defined on baseline scan; visible increase in extent of 18F-FDG tumor uptake (20 % in longest dimension) or appearance of new 18F-FDG uptake in metastatic lesions

[a] Revised international working group (IWG): the international harmonization project for response criteria in lymphoma clinical trials

[b] Measurable disease: change in sum of products of the longest diameter and greatest perpendicular diameters, no maximal number of lesions specified

[c] Target lesions: change in sum of LD, maximum of 5 per organ up to 10 total (more than 1 organ)

[d] PERCIST Positron emission tomography response criteria in solid tumors

[e] EORTC European organization for research and treatment of cancer

On the other hand, PET reveals functional information about cell metabolic activity including glucose or other nutrient metabolism, proliferation, angiogenesis, hypoxia, apoptosis, and other important aspects of biology of malignant cells. This allows localization of the most active lesion the potentially radiation or chemotherapy-resistant or susceptible parts of a tumor, as well as cancerous metabolic activities outside the CT-drawn tumor boundaries, which seems to be the most clinically important advantage inherent to the technique. One of the main strengths of PET is that it permits whole-body imaging and in contrast to histopathologic approaches is not limited to the characterization of one or a few (sometimes very heterogeneous) target lesions. In fact, PET enables physicians to evaluate multiple tumor sites at the same time (de Geus-Oei et al. 2009). Moreover, serial scanning makes it possible to follow functional changes over time during treatment, particularly on a quantitative scale. However, the disadvantages of PET relative to techniques such as MRI, including limited resolution and radiation burden, should not be ignored. Therefore, these modalities should be considered complementary, rather than competitive, as they visualize and measure different aspects of tumor behavior (de Geus-Oei et al. 2009).

As mentioned before, PET suffers from lower anatomical resolution than MRI. Present data show that a combination of PET and conventional imaging (i.e. PET/CT or PET/MRI) mostly outperforms conventional imaging on its own, in its ability to predict histopathological reference findings. In fact PET combined with CT or MRI is superior to both anatomical and physiological techniques alone, and PET/CT has largely replaced stand-alone PET in clinical use (Allen-Auerbach and Weber 2009; Lonsdale and Beyer 2010; Townsend et al. 2004). PET/CT allows for precise anatomic localization of abnormalities noted on PET, thereby reducing the number of false-positive studies and improving the diagnostic accuracy significantly over PET or CT alone (Czernin et al. 2007). The shorter scan times result in greater patient throughput and have increased overall patients' access to PET/CT imaging (Allen-Auerbach and Weber 2009). Moreover, from a clinical point of view, the anatomic information gained from a PET/CT study allows for more confident interpretations and easier communication between the treating physicians and the nuclear clinicians reading the scans (Allen-Auerbach and Weber 2009).

It has been thought that radiotherapy-induced inflammatory changes may cause increased radiotracer activity both in the region of the tumor and in the other radiosensitive tissues in the field of radiotherapy, limiting the diagnostic accuracy of PET imaging (Pons et al. 2009). Although there is no doubt that radiation-induced inflammation intensifies 18F-FDG activity, the intensity of 18F-FDG uptake may still be lower than in highly metabolically active untreated primary tumors, such as non-small cell lung cancer or esophageal cancer. Moreover, the configuration of increased 18F-FDG uptake in radiation-induced inflammation is often markedly different from a malignant tumor (Weber 2005). It is therefore frequently possible to differentiate between radiation-induced inflammatory responses and residual tumor lesion, particularly when comparing a pre-treatment with a post-treatment PET scan (Weber 2005).

3 Technical Issues of PET in the Assessment of Response to Treatment

3.1 Visual Interpretation Versus Quantitative Measurement of Tumor 18F-FDG Uptake

To assess tumor response after completion of therapy, visual assessment of tumor 18F-FDG uptake has been considered sufficient and the technical requirements for PET/CT imaging do not differ significantly from those of a routine whole-body PET/CT scan applied for tumor staging. However, if PET scans are performed during treatment to evaluate subsequent tumor response to ongoing regimen, quantitative analysis of tumor metabolism becomes necessary, as at this point there is still considerable residual 18F-FDG uptake, even in patients responding to treatment (Allen-Auerbach and Weber 2009). Those studies that looked at the time course of tumor uptake during treatment indicate that, besides a baseline scan performed prior to treatment initiation, quantitative analysis of changes in 18F-FDG uptake is needed to evaluate early response (Ott et al. 2003). For example, evaluation of changes in 18F-FDG uptake in patients with locally advanced esophageal cancer treated with chemoradiotherapy and followed by surgical resection shows that it is only after the completion of neoadjuvant therapy that the 18F-FDG uptake of responding lesions decreases almost to background levels. Although 18F-FDG uptake of responding tumors had decreased significantly compared with nonresponding tumors, most of the responding tumors still showed significant 18F-FDG uptake at PET/CT scans performed 2 weeks after the start of therapy, a fact which emphasizes the importance of quantitative analysis to detect small, visually undetectable changes (Wieder et al. 2004).

3.2 Anatomic and Functional Imaging Together

Combining the metabolic and volumetric quantitative changes observed with PET/CT could improve accuracy for gauging tumor response (Allen-Auerbach and Weber 2009). Larson et al. suggested combining anatomic and functional information and monitoring changes derived from multiplying the tumor volume on CT with the 18F-FDG uptake on PET, resulting in a highly accurate technique for assessing the response of tumors to treatment (Larson et al. 1999).

3.3 Acquisition Reproducibility

Biologic and technologic factors such as scanner and reconstruction parameters can significantly affect standardized uptake value (SUV) measurements, which are the most commonly applied measure of quantitative analysis of PET imaging. Spatial resolution and other factors vary significantly from one PET scanner to another. Even different models of scanners from the same manufacturer may measure substantially different SUVs. Each scanner has a specific calibration factor to convert measured counts to radioactivity. How this calibration is performed significantly affects the underlying quantitative accuracy of output results. Therefore, when using serial SUV measurements to assess response to treatment, imaging should be performed on the same scanner using the same image acquisition and reconstruction protocols. In addition, attention to details is mandatory for accurate measurement of the radiopharmaceutical dose. Calibration of the clocks on a PET scanner and dose calibrator is important to reduce error in SUV measurement based on the injected radioactivity (Adams et al. 2010).

Differences in body size and weight can significantly change SUV output data; hence, this factor should be controlled by using the same body size measurement between baseline and follow-up studies (Adams et al. 2010). Such an important consideration should not be ignored, as patients' weight can change significantly during the course of cancer treatments. The Women's Healthy Eating and Living study examining more than 3,000 women undergoing treatment for breast cancer showed that approximately 45 % of patients had significant weight gain (defined as more than 5 % positive change) after treatment. At 4 years after treatment, fewer than 5 % of patients with significant weight gain had returned to baseline weight (Saquib et al. 2007). The more extreme weight changes within these populations have the potential to affect the validity of SUV change measurements (Adams et al. 2010).

As it is clearly described by Hicks, the maximum SUV (SUV_{max}) of a lesion is the most reproducible index and is widely accepted for monitoring the response to treatment. However, the major concern regarding the use of the SUV_{max} for this purpose is that it ignores alterations in the distribution of a tracer within a lesion. "Accordingly, a rapidly growing tumor undergoing central necrosis may show no change in the SUV_{max} or may even show a reduction as the thin rim of viable tumor becomes subject to partial-volume effects. Therefore, alternative metabolic parameters that integrate both tumor volume and the intensity of uptake have been suggested" (Hicks 2009).

4 Metabolic Markers in PET Imaging

4.1 Imaging of Glycolysis with 18F-FDG

In human tumors, 18F-FDG PET uptake correlates well with the rate of glycolysis, which is known to be markedly greater in cancer tissues than in the normal counterparts from which malignancy arises (Larson and Schwartz 2006). Although there are different PET radiotracers that supply information on different aspects of tumor biology, such as amino acid uptake, enzymatic expression, receptor density, cell proliferation, presence and activity of neurotransmitters, blood flow, hypoxia, and angiogenesis, the most frequently used PET tracer for monitoring therapy and the assessment of treatment response is 18F-fluorodeoxyglucose (18F-FDG), which supplies information on glucose metabolism (Delgado-Bolton and Delgado 2009). Accumulating evidence indicates that 18F-FDG PET is very useful for monitoring during treatment and assessing response after therapy ends. (Larson and Schwartz 2006).

Numerous studies in lung cancer, lymphoma, breast cancer, and some other tumors have demonstrated that 18F-FDG PET can detect an early response to treatment, which correlates well with clinical evolution. It has been confirmed that 18F-FDG PET can supply prognostic information and improve management decisions in oncologic settings, allowing for early identification of the response to treatment. To assess early response to treatment, 18F-FDG PET can be performed as soon as 7 days after starting the chemotherapy (Delgado-Bolton and Delgado 2009). As mentioned earlier, PET images can be analyzed visually and semiquantitatively, and the latter provides more precise evaluation of changes related to treatment response (Delgado-Bolton and Delgado 2009).

Thresholds ranging from 20 to 70 % reduction of SUV are used for 18F-FDG tumor uptake as the reference value for response evaluation and the appropriate percentage SUV reduction threshold depends, among other things, on technical and clinical factors that differ among studies and institutions (Weber 2006; Kim et al. 2004). There is no standardized protocol with a SUV cutoff value that is generally accepted to indicate a response to treatment. However, for early-effect evaluation on chemotherapy, after one cycle for example, smaller SUV threshold values are used than for late assessment (Boellaard et al. 2008). Unfortunately, a clear consensus of what constitutes a significant change has yet to be reached. Based on reproducibility studies of 18F-FDG uptake in untreated tumors, relative changes of more than 20 % are unlikely to be caused by measurement errors or variations in tumor metabolic activity. However, this only applies if significant baseline metabolic activity is present (Allen-Auerbach and Weber 2009).

Due to biological changes in tumors during chemotherapy, there are some general limitations in the evaluation of response to treatment using 18F-FDG PET. Tumor response to treatment is in general associated with a drop in the intensity of FDG uptake (Larson and Schwartz 2006; Barrington and Carr 1995; Heron et al. 2008). However, a small number of patients seem to display anomalous behavior; their tumors have reduced in size on anatomical imaging, they do not relapse during prolonged clinical follow-ups, their histopathologic assessments are negative for viable tumor cells, and there is no remarkable change, or even a rise, in 18F-FDG uptake at the site of the original disease. In almost all these cases, PET scanning was undertaken within 1 week of completing a full course of radiotherapy or chemotherapy. Hence, it has been suggested that this early persistence of 18F-FDG uptake is due to inflammatory changes within the lesion as a result of the therapy itself and that this limits the usefulness of PET in immediate evaluation of tumor response. Remarkably high 18F-FDG uptake has been observed in macrophages and granulation tissue surrounding necrotic tumor, which adds weight to this hypothesis (Barrington and Carr 1995). In fact, the newly formed granulation tissue around the tumor and macrophages, which can massively infiltrate the marginal areas surrounding necrotic areas of the tumors, shows a higher uptake of 18F-FDG than the viable tumor cells. A maximum of 29 % of the glucose utilization in some models has been attributed to these nontumor tissues (Kubota et al. 1992). Especially after anti-neoplastic treatment, high accumulation of 18F-FDG in the tumor is considered to represent high metabolic activity of the viable tumor cells, but it is possible that the nonneoplastic cellular elements are also a source of metabolic activity (Kubota et al. 1992). However, in clinical practice it has been shown that generally, when rapid lysis of malignant cells occurs, abnormal 18F-FDG uptake can be eliminated simultaneously, even when there has been extensive visceral inflammation and infiltration. In these settings, improvement can be seen on PET, associated with rapid clinical response, return of biochemical indices to normal levels, and complete clearance of tumoral cells (Barrington and Carr 1995).

4.1.1 Timing of Imaging with 18F-FDG PET

It has been shown that 18F-FDG metabolic activity of some tumor types decreases rapidly in the early stages of chemotherapy and reaches a plateau in the later stages, sometimes irrespective of pathological response status (Wieder et al. 2004; McDermott et al. 2007; Krak et al. 2005; Avril et al. 2005). This limits the optimal time for monitoring chemotherapy response using 18F-FDG PET to the time between the end of the first cycle and the midpoint of chemotherapy in some situations (McDermott et al. 2007). The underlying causes for minimal changes in tumor 18F-FDG uptake between the midpoint and endpoint of chemotherapy are not fully understood, but it could be due to a reduction in vascular delivery caused by the therapy. Based on the MRI evidence, the cellular transport rate between plasma and the extracellular compartment falls during chemotherapy and by a greater extent in

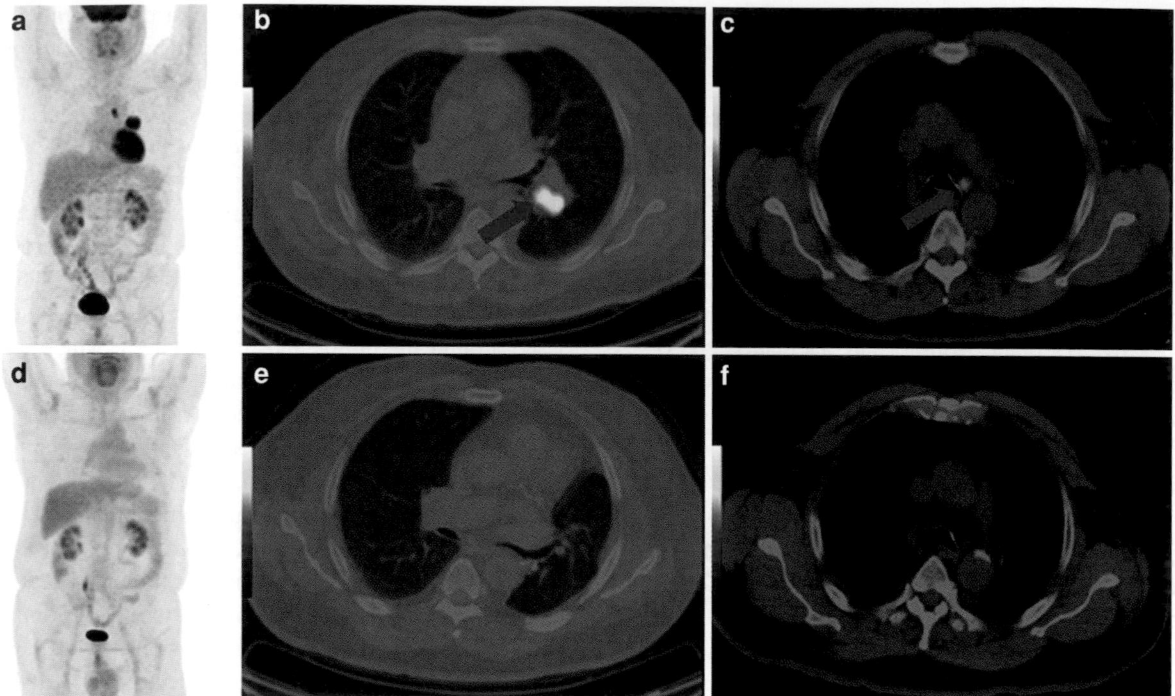

Fig. 1 Lung cancer 64-year-old man presented with incidental left lung nodule on CXR. Pretreatment PET/CT scan. Maximum intensity projection (**a**) and axial fused PET/CT (**b** and **c**) demonstrate FDG-avid left perihilar mass and metastatic 4L lymph node. The patient underwent two cycles of neoadjuvant chemotherapy (carboplatin and Taxol) followed by left-lower lobectomy and two more cycles of adjuvant chemotherapy. Post-therapy PET/CT maximum intensity projection (**d**) and axial fused PET/CT (**e** and **f**) demonstrate no evidence of FDG-avid persistent lung malignancy or metastatic lymph node

more responsive tumors. This may be due to therapy-induced blood flow alterations or vascular damage caused by the endothelial toxicity of chemotherapeutic agents (McDermott et al. 2007; Pickles et al. 2005; Tseng et al. 2004). These vascular delivery restrictions explain a reported chemotherapy-induced shift in the 18F-FDG metabolic rate-limiting step from the phosphorylation step to the influx step in some tumors (Czernin et al. 2007), which implies 18F-FDG PET becomes less sensitive to metabolic changes as chemotherapy progresses. Another plausible reason for minimal changes late in therapy is the possibility that the majority of chemosensitive cells could have been killed off by this time and that an influx of immune or stromal cells could mask 18F-FDG uptake changes in the tumor (McDermott et al. 2007).

4.2 Imaging of Cell Proliferation

Imaging cell proliferation of tumoral lesions is of much interest for both research and clinical purposes of oncology (Weber 2010). A high proliferation rate is general characteristic of most malignant tumors, while in benign neoplasms the fraction of cells in proliferation is comparatively small. In theory, imaging the rate of cell proliferation could provide a constructive tool for differentiating benign from malignant tumors. Chemotherapy and radiotherapy quickly diminish proliferation rates in responding tumors (Weber 2010) (Fig. 1). This effect usually heralds the reduction of tumor size in responding lesions. Therefore, imaging cellular proliferation could present an earlier report of therapeutic response than size measurements by anatomic imaging. Probably, one of the most important uses of cell proliferation imaging is to assess the response to treatment with novel targeted agents, such as protein kinase inhibitors, which have a predominantly cytostatic effect and theoretically do not lead to rapid tumor shrinkage. The beneficial effects of these therapeutic approaches may therefore be underestimated by anatomic criteria of CT and MRI, which depend on a significant reduction of tumor size within a few weeks of therapy. Proliferation imaging is of notable interest for further clinical development of such novel agents (Weber 2010).

Because of the theoretical advantages inherent to the technique, imaging of tumor proliferation with PET and SPECT has been studied with various probes and radiopharmaceuticals. In this context, thymidine and thymidine analogs have been in the center of attention, because these components are utilized by proliferating cells for DNA synthesis during the S-phase of cell cycle, but unlike other nucleosides required for DNA synthesis are not incorporated into RNA (Barwick et al. 2009). Radiolabeled thymidine has been used for years to study cell proliferation both in vitro and in vivo settings. 3′-deoxy-3′-18F-fluorothymidine (18F-FLT) which was first introduced by Shields et al. in 1998 for PET imaging, is by far the most extensively studied (Shields et al. 1998). Following intravenous injection, 18F-FLT enters the cell by active transporters (the expression of which may be upregulated in tumor cells) and to a lesser extent by passive diffusion (Barwick et al. 2009). However, after entrance into the cells, 18F-FLT is not incorporated into DNA and is trapped in the cytosol. Correlation of 18F-FLT flux with the rate of cell proliferation has been confirmed, using histopathologic markers of tumor cell proliferation, such as the Ki-67 labeling index, as the gold standard. Moreover, it has been confirmed that 18F-FLT uptake is significantly more specific than 18F-FDG uptake as an index of tumor proliferation and as a tool for cancer staging (Buck et al. 2003; Yap et al. 2006), with fewer false-positive findings in inflammatory lesions (Yamamoto et al. 2008; van Westreenen et al. 2005), although with false-positive findings because of the proliferation of lymphocytes in reactive lymph nodes (Troost et al. 2007). However, because of the lower tumor uptake of 18F-FLT as compared to 18F-FDG, the sensitivity of 18F-FLT PET is significantly lower than that of 18F-FDG PET.

Clinically, the simplest and most practical method of assessing FLT uptake is the SUV calculated from static PET images, typically acquired 40–90 min post-injection. More complex methods use dynamic images and kinetic modeling of tracer uptake, such as two compartmental models to estimate rate constants for FLT transport/retention in cells and overall flux of tracer into cells (Barwick et al. 2009). The most important limitation in these kinetic models is the timing of acquisition, as reliable measurements require 120 min of dynamic imaging (Muzi et al. 2005), which is considered too long for clinical applications.

4.2.1 18F-FLT PET in Clinical Practice

The feasibility of 18F-FLT PET studies of various tumors (including breast and lung cancer, and lymphoma) has been confirmed by numerous experiments. However, the magnitude of 18F-FLT uptake by tumor cells varies greatly, and consequently the best use of 18F-FLT PET as a valid measure of proliferative activity requires further investigation. In fact, there are problems with 18F-FLT PET that make it unlikely to have a dominant role in the initial diagnosis and staging of most cancers (probably except brain cancers) due to relatively low target-to-background ratios, remarkable interfering physiological activity in bone marrow, moderate 18F-FLT uptake in the liver, and also the interfering effects of renal excretion (Barwick et al. 2009). On the other hand, there is a general consensus that the most promising clinical application of 18F-FLT PET is monitoring tumor response to treatment. 18F-FLT uptake in untreated tumors is stable over time, with a test–retest reproducibility of less than 10 % for SUV measurements when patients were imaged twice within a week (Weber 2010), an advantage which is a prerequisite for assessment of response to treatment by a metabolic imaging modality. Experience with animal models has shown that 18F-FLT uptake reduces quickly in response to radiotherapy (Apisarnthanarax et al. 2006; Molthoff et al. 2007; Solit et al. 2007), chemotherapy (Barthel et al. 2003; Leyton et al. 2005; Lawrence et al. 2009), and other cancer treatment strategies such as protein kinase inhibitors (Waldherr et al. 2005; Wei et al. 2008; Ullrich et al. 2008; Brepoels et al. 2009). Also, preliminary clinical studies confirmed the potential of 18F-FLT PET for monitoring tumor response to therapy. Based on some (Apisarnthanarax et al. 2006; Solit et al. 2007; Barthel et al. 2003; Leyton et al. 2005; Ullrich et al. 2008) but not all of the available reports (Wei et al. 2008; Molthoff et al. 2007; Waldherr et al. 2005), reduction in 18F-FLT activity of the lesion better reflected the effects of therapy than did changes in 18F-FDG uptake. In patients with recurrent malignant brain neoplasms, tumor response on 18F-FLT PET after 1–2 weeks of treatment with irinotecan and bevacizumab correlated well with overall survival, while the competing imaging modality, MRI, was not a significant predictor of

Table 2 Studies utilizing FLT PET/CT for therapy response

Authors (Year)	Tumor type	No. of patients	Imaging protocol	Results	Conclusion
Herrmann et al. (2007)	High-grade nonHodgkin lymphoma	22	Baseline, as well as 1 and 6 weeks after R-CHOP/ CHOP, 2 days after rituximab	18F-FLT uptake decreased after R-CHOP/ CHOP by 77–85 %, but revealed no significant reduction after rituximab	18F-FLT PET seems to be promising for early evaluation of treatment effects in lymphoma
Leyton et al. (2005), Vera et al. (2011)	Non-small cell lung cancer	30	Three PET/CT scans were performed before and during (around dose 46 Gy, t46) radiotherapy with minimal intervals of 48 h between each PET/ CT scan	During radiotherapy, the largest reduction (an average of 53 %) in SUV_{max} was observed for 18F-FLT. The corresponding figures were 30 % for 18F-FDG and 7 % for F-MISO	This pattern of fast FLT response suggests that an earlier assessment (after the first fraction of radiotherapy) may be considered for further studies
Yue et al. (2010)	Esophageal squamous cell carcinoma	21	A pretreatment scan, followed by 1-3 scans after delivery of 2, 6, 10, 20, 30, 40, 50, or 60 Gy radiation to the tumor	Parameters reflecting 18F-FLT uptake in the tumor (i.e., SUV_{max} and proliferation target volume) decreased steadily	18F-FLT uptake can be used to monitor the biologic response of esophageal SCC to radiotherapy. Increased uptake of 18F-FLT after treatment interruptions may reflect accelerated repopulation. 18F-FLT PET/CT may have an advantage over 18F-FDG PET/CT in differentiating inflammation from tumor
Yang et al. (2010)	Non-small cell lung cancer	31	PET/CT images were compared with the pathology. Tumor cell proliferation was assessed by cyclin D1 immuno-histochemistry	Tumor SUV of FLT was significantly correlated with the cyclin D1 labeling index (as the marker of cell proliferation), but the SUV of 18F-FDG was not significantly correlated	Tumor FLT uptake correlates with tumor cell proliferation as indicated by the cyclin D1 labeling index, suggesting that further study is needed to evaluate the use of 18F-FLT PET/CT for the assessment of therapy response to anticancer drugs
Backes et al. (2009)	High-grade glioma	11	Compartmental modeling, automated extraction of an input function from 18F-FLT brain PET data, calculation of kinetic rate constants	A significant correlation between kinetic rate constants and the percentage of Ki-67-positive cells was observed	Kinetic modeling of 18F-FLT brain PET data using image-derived input functions extracted from human brain PET data provides information about the proliferative activity of brain tumors, which might have clinical relevance especially for monitoring of therapy response in clinical trials

survival (Chen et al. 2007). Pilot studies on breast cancer have also suggested that change in 18F-FLT uptake during treatment predicts later clinical response (Kenny et al. 2007; Weber 2010). Encouraging data has been reported for other cancers and treatment plans (Table 2). In patients with non–small cell lung cancer, the reduction of 18F-FLT uptake after 7 days of therapy with gefitinib was highly predictive of tumor response on CT at week 6 and of progression-free survival (Weber 2010; Sohn et al. 2008).

In some tumor types and forms of therapy, however, the correlation between early changes in 18F-FLT uptake and later clinical or histopathologic response has been less clear. In malignant lymphomas, treatment with rituximab did not result in early change in 18F-FLT uptake (Herrmann et al. 2007), although experimental data suggest that rituximab inhibits proliferation by interfering with cellular signaling (Weber 2010; Kheirallah et al. 2010). Thus, it was concluded that not all forms of growth inhibition may be captured by 18F-FLT PET. Conversely, tumor 18F-FLT uptake has been reported to change significantly in eventually nonresponding tumors. In patients with rectal cancer treated with neoadjuvant chemoradiation, 18F-FLT uptake significantly reduced at day 14 in all patients, with no difference between histopathologically responding and nonresponding lesions (Wieder et al. 2007), suggesting that inhibition of proliferation, although necessary, is not sufficient for a favorable response in some tumor types or some types of treatment. In such a case, the decrease in 18F-FLT uptake in histopathologic nonresponders may be because of treatment-induced growth arrest rather than cell death. This possibility could represent a limitation of 18F-FLT for monitoring of the response to treatment compared with 18F-FDG PET, meaning that complete growth arrest is not reflective of a sustained therapeutic effect (Barwick et al. 2009). Finally, a temporary rise in 18F-FLT uptake has been reported in lung cancer patients receiving chemoradiation (Weber 2010; Everitt et al. 2009). The evidence suggests that 18F-FLT uptake might be influenced by factors other than proliferation, such as altered vascular permeability or perfusion.

Another radiotracer for imaging cell proliferation is 18FMAU [1-(2′-deoxy-2′-fluoro-beta-D-arabinofuranosyl)thymine], which is a thymidine analog that can be phosphorylated and subsequently incorporated into DNA, and because of minimal marrow uptake and urinary excretion, appears to be promising for studying bone metastasis and the pelvic region (Nguyen and Aboagye 2010). Preliminary in vitro studies have demonstrated that the level of 18FMAU uptake is proportional to the level of DNA synthesis and the rate of tumor proliferation (Nishii et al. 2008; Sun et al. 2005). Further studies are needed to evaluate the potential of 18FMAU as a PET imaging tracer of cell proliferation and its utility in monitoring treatment (Nguyen and Aboagye 2010).

In summary, more research comparing 18F-FLT PET with 18F-FDG PET will be important to determine the complementary advantage of FLT PET in early response assessment, since 18F-FDG PET has been used successfully to monitor response in a variety of tumors (Weber 2010). Data to date are limited but encouraging and promising, and point toward an impending role as an early predictor of response to treatment and therapy monitoring, (Ullrich et al. 2008; Jensen et al. 2010; Rueger et al. 2010). In all cases, disease- and drug-specific effects must be considered when 18F FLT PET is used for treatment monitoring. Further research should also be facilitated by simplified synthesis of 18F-FLT PET with improved yields and an increasing commercial availability of the radiotracer (Barwick et al. 2009).

4.3 Imaging of Apoptosis

After several decades of debate, it is now widely acknowledged that effective therapy of tumors by radiation, chemotherapy or both, leads to iatrogenic induction of programmed cell death or the process of apoptosis. Given the central role of apoptosis, it would be useful to have a noninvasive imaging tool to serially detect and monitor this process in cancer patients undergoing conventional radiation and chemotherapy treatments (Blankenberg 2008a, b, 2009a, b; Belhocine and Blankenberg 2006; Strauss, H.W., et al., Translational imaging: imaging of apoptosis. Handb Exp Pharmacol 2008; Blankenberg 2008c; Blankenberg et al. 1999a, b, 2006; Belhocine et al. 2004; Ohtsuki et al. 1999; Vriens et al. 1998).

The most widely used in vivo imaging method involves a human protein with nanomolar affinity for cell membrane-bound anionic phospholipid phosphatidylserine called annexin V (Blankenberg 2008c). Radiolabeled annexin V has been used for both PET or SPECT studies of apoptosis in vivo. Annexin V (molecular weight almost 36,000) is an endogenous human protein that is widely distributed intracellularly, with high concentrations in the placenta and lower concentrations in endothelial cells, myocardium, kidneys, skeletal muscle, skin, red cells, platelets, and monocytes. Recent evidence shows that annexin V is a naturally occurring ligand specific for phospholipid phosphatidylserine. As apoptotic cells express sufficient phospholipid phosphatidylserine on their surface, theoretically it is feasible to use radiolabeled annexin V as a marker of apoptosis (Blankenberg 2008b, c).

Although there are numerous reports confirming the value of scintigraphic study of apoptosis using SPECT (including SPECT with ^{99m}Tc-BTAP-annexin-A5, ^{99m}Tc-HYNIC-annexin-A5, ^{99m}Tc-imino-annexin-A5, ^{99m}Tc-EC-annexin A5)), currently there are minimal published studies evaluating the efficacy of annexin V labeled with positron emitters in monitoring human cancer treatments. Most of the available reports are limited to small animal studies which seem to be promising. A small study using 18F-ML-10 (a novel molecular PET imaging agent for apoptosis) also shows promising output (Allen et al. 2009). Imaging applications for any of the apoptosis-directed PET imaging agents in clinic is unclear and warrants further investigations.

4.4 Hypoxia Imaging

Tumor hypoxia is a pathological state in which tumoral tissues lack enough oxygen for cells to metabolize normally. Hypoxia occurs when the tumor becomes large enough to disrupt the balance between oxygen supply and demand. More than 50 % of locally advanced solid tumors may exhibit hypoxic and/or anoxic tissue areas that are heterogeneously distributed within the tumor lesion (Sun 2010; Vaupel and Mayer 2007). Hypoxia is mainly due to rapid proliferation of tumor cells and vascular abnormalities of malignant lesions. Intratumoral vessels have significant structural abnormalities, which leads to perfusion-limited oxygen delivery. In solid tumors, hypoxia-induced proteome changes lead to cell cycle arrest, differentiation, apoptosis, and necrosis. At the same time it may promote tumor progression via mechanisms enabling tumoral cells to overcome nutritive deficiency, to escape from the hostile environment, and to favor unrestricted growth. Sustained hypoxia may also lead to cellular changes resulting in a more clinically aggressive phenotype (Sun 2010; Osinsky et al. 2009; Vaupel et al. 2004; Brat and Mapstone 2003; Sutherland 1998; Green and Giaccia 1998; Hockel et al. 1996). It has been demonstrated that the presence of hypoxic cells in solid tumors is associated with treatment failure following radiotherapy and chemoresistance (Matthews et al. 2001; Nordsmark et al. 2005). Thus, knowing the degree and extent of hypoxia prior to the initiation of treatment will be invaluable in treatment planning (Sun 2010; Fukumura and Jain 2007). Regarding these findings, it was hypothesized that measuring the intensity of lesion hypoxia might allow follow-up of cancer patients in the early stages of treatment, and prediction of drug resistance and radio-resistance. Subsequently, different techniques for measuring hypoxia have been developed. Invasive polarographic electrodes and immune-histochemical staining have been used extensively for the assessment of oxygenation and measuring pO2 in both human and animal tumors to provide an estimate of oxygen tension. The limitations inherent to these invasive techniques make clinical imaging modalities seem more useful. BOLD-MRI has been shown to be able to diagnose tumor hypoxia (Padhani 2010). The major disadvantage of BOLD-MRI is that the data provide the change of oxygen tension in vasculature, but not in the tissue. Furthermore, BOLD-MRI is not a quantitative method and can be easily affected by many factors such as flow effects, blood hematocrit, pH, and body temperature (Sun 2010; Mason 2006).

SPECT using single photon emitting radionuclides ligated with hypoxia-specific compounds has shown encouraging results, and there has been great interest in developing imaging agents using PET to noninvasively image hypoxia. The molecular markers for hypoxia imaging have been 2-nitroimidazoles and nucleoside conjugates labeled with different positron emitters (Table 3) (Sun 2010; Mees et al. 2009). These markers have maximum binding to severely hypoxic cells to form stable adducts that can be detected by PET scanner. They are rapidly re-oxidized and removed from the normal cells, and thus provide good demarcation between hypoxic and normoxia cells within the lesion (Sun 2010). Preliminary reports suggested that tumor imaging using hypoxia markers may be useful in the assessment of response to treatment (Wiedemann et al. 2010; Busk et al. 2009,2010; Lee et al.2009a, b; Wang et al. 1999,2008, 2009a, b; Dehdashti et al. 2000, 2008; Takai et al. 2007; Reischl et al. 2007; Dietz et al. 2007; Ito et al. 2006; Schwarz et al. 2004; Rajendran et al. 2002, 2003; Liu et al. 1999; Hustinx et al. 1999; Casciari et al. 1995; Yang et al. 1995), which is not yet confirmed by prospective clinical trials.

Until now, all imaging data from human studies have been collected from research protocols in academic settings, which show that imaging of hypoxia in a diagnostic setting has not yet become routine patient

Table 3 Molecular markers for hypoxia imaging

Molecular markers
Nitroimidazoles
Fluoromisonidazole (FMISO)
Fluoroetanidazole (FETA)
Fluoroerythronitroimidazole (FETNIM)
EF5
FAZA
Nucleoside conjugates
Iodoazomycin arabinoside (IAZA)
Cu(II)-diacetyl-bis(N 4-methylthiosemicarbazone) (Cu-ATSM)
Iodoazomycin galactopyranoside (IAZG)
Iodoazomycin galactoside
Positron emitters
^{18}F
^{124}I
$^{60/64}$Cu

management. Lec et al. found that 18F-FMISO incorporation during a course of platinum-based, intensity-modulated chemoradiotherapy is not encouraging and neither the presence nor the absence of hypoxia, as defined by positive 18F-FMISO findings on the mid-treatment PET scan, correlates with patient outcome. A recent study however suggests that 18F-FDG and 18F-MISO uptakes are significantly correlated before treatment in patients with non-small cell lung cancer (NSCLC) (F-MISO would complement 18F-FDG PET/CT before radiotherapy), while of less value during radiotherapy (Vera et al. 2011). Also, in one of the limited reports Takai et al. (Takai et al. 2007) found a correlation between tumor response to radiation and (Adams et al. 2010) FFRP-170 PET/CT imaging findings performed one month after the end of radiotherapy. Large-scale trials with frequent imaging during and after treatment are needed to assess the feasibility and accuracy of this approach.

4.5 Imaging of Amino Acid and Protein Metabolism

Although it is well known that the amino acid transport system plays a critical role in the regulation of cellular proliferation, the details of its function to promote tumor cell proliferation have not been clearly elucidated. Amino acid tracers such as O-[18F]-fluoroethyl-L-tyrosine and O-[18F]-fluoromethyl-L-tyrosine, as well as F-alpha-methyl tyrosine (18F-FMT), are transported into cells, but are not metabolized for protein synthesis. Hence, their efficacy in tumor imaging has been widely studied (Kaira et al. 2010; Pauleit et al. 2005; Inoue et al. 1998a, b, 2001; Tomiyoshi et al. 1999; Aoyagi et al. 1999; Mehrkens et al. 2008; Kubota et al. 2006; Weckesser et al. 2005; Pauleit et al. 2004). Experimental studies with labeled amino acid tracers have suggested that these tracers may be suited to assess treatment efficacy (Pauleit et al. 2005; Yamaura et al. 2006).

Clinical studies have shown that 18F-FMT uptake within tumor lesion correlates with the expression of L-type amino acid transporter 1 (Kaira et al. 2010). Therefore, it has been hypothesized that 18F-FMT might be an alternative to 18F-FDG for the assessment of therapeutic response. However, just a few clinical studies have been performed to verify this point (Kaira et al. 2010; Chesnay et al. 2003). In one of these reports 18F-FMT was used to assess therapy response in lung cancer. Agreement of therapeutic response evaluated by RECIST (Response Evaluation Criteria in Solid Tumors) was noted in 56 % of patients evaluated with 18F-FDG PET and in 89 % of patients evaluated with 18F-FMT PET. In patients with partial response, partial metabolic response was observed in 89 % by 18F-FDG PET and in 100 % by 18F-FMT PET. Based on this evidence, 18F-FMT might be a promising PET tracer for monitoring response to chemoradiotherapy; further assessment in large samples of patients with different cancers is warranted (Kaira et al. 2010). In another report, 11C-Methionine PET estimation of response in hypopharyngeal cancer was performed before and after the first course of chemotherapy, using MRI as the gold standard. A sensitivity of 83 % and specificity of 86 % were achieved (Chesnay et al. 2003). As with all of these interesting new methods, further investigation is necessary.

5 Clinical Applications

5.1 Lung Cancer

Effective from January 28, 2005, Medicare in the United States covers 18F-FDG PET for monitoring response to treatment of non-small cell lung cancer

(NSCLC), when a change in therapy is anticipated (Fig. 1). Lung cancer is the first cancer in which monitoring of treatment using 18F-FDG PET has established its critical clinical role in daily practice of oncology. The critical role of PET in these settings is emphasized by the fact that almost 170,000 people are diagnosed with lung cancer just in the United States each year (Erdi et al. 2000). The tremendous growth in non-surgical management of early primary lung cancer in recent years, and the availability of different therapeutic options far beyond conventional radiation therapy, emphasize the need for effective tools to assess the response to treatment early after or even during the course of such therapies (Eradat et al. 2011). A recent comprehensive review reported by Langer confirms that due to improved care and less exposure to futile treatments, personalized medicine using PET may be cost-effective, the strongest evidence for which is still in the staging of NSCLC (Langer 2010).

Also, aggregated data collected by Hicks on the use of 18F-FDG PET in the evaluation of response to treatment strongly indicate that a reduction in the lesion 18F-FDG uptake, however it is measured and at whatever time after treatment it is recorded, is more likely to be associated with both a pathologic response and improved survival than is a lack of change (Hicks 2009). Numerous studies on this issue support this hypothesis.

The positive and negative predictive values of 18F-FDG PET in assessing the therapeutic response 2 weeks after the completion of preoperative chemoradiotherapy was reported to be 80 and 55 %, respectively. The low negative predictive value has been attributed to be the fact that the complete pathologic response rate in the studied population was only 31 % (Ryu et al. 2002). Using the cutoff of a post-treatment SUV equal to 3.0, the sensitivity for residual disease was 88 % (Ryu et al. 2002). Subsequent studies were more encouraging, as they showed a nearly linear correlation between the change in the SUV_{max} and the percentage of nonviable tumor in the resected tissue (Cerfolio et al. 2004) as well as a correlation between the residual rate of glucose metabolism, as estimated by 18F-FDG kinetics, and the pathologic tumor response (Choi et al. 2002). Larger samples resulted in an accuracy of 96 %, when a reduction of greater than 80 % in the SUV_{max} was the criteria for detecting a pathologic response (Cerfolio et al. 2004). Generally, post-treatment SUV_{max} of the lesions of pathologic responders are significantly lower than nonresponders (Yamamoto et al. 2006; Pottgen et al. 2006). These studies suggest that to assess the pathologic response of mediastinal nodes, a residual SUV_{max} of 4.0 provides the best discrimination between responders and nonresponders (Pottgen et al. 2006). Prognostic stratification to validate performance of 18F-FDG PET in response assessment also supports the reliability of 18F-FDG PET for these purposes. A metabolic response to chemoradiation, as assessed by visual interpretation of 18F-FDG PET, is also much more powerfully correlated with survival than the response on CT (Vansteenkiste et al. 1998; Manus 2003). A reduction of 45–55 % in the SUV_{max} of the primary tumor as a cutoff indicates that patients with a more marked metabolic response have a survival rate of 83 % at 16 months; the rate for patients with smaller reductions is just 43 % (Pottgen et al. 2006).

Patients with persistent major mediastinal nodal involvement on 18F-FDG PET experience a 5-year overall survival rate of 0 % (Dooms et al. 2008). Shiraishi et al suggested a cutoff value of 0.6 for the SUV ratio and found that such a ratio predicts the pathological tumor response with significantly higher accuracy than the size ratio obtained from CT images (Shiraishi et al. 2010). Recently, delta SUV has been proposed as a reliable measure of tumor response. The percentage change of pretreatment and mid-treatment SUV_{max} was significantly different in responders compared to nonresponders (62 vs 34 %). In this report, the 1-year survival rates of the responders and nonresponders were 68.0 % and 38.1 %, respectively (Zhang et al. 2010). Similarly, it has been reported that a reduction of more than 20 % in SUV_{max} at week 3 is associated with longer progression-free survival (de Langen et al. 2011). A reduction in the SUV of greater than 50 % between the first and third weeks predicted survival for more than 6 months, whereas a reduction of less than 50 % led to death within 6 months. Generally, it has been shown that following successful treatment, changes might be observed in the SUV as early as 1 week after the initiation of treatment (Nahmias et al. 2007).

In the assessment of the response to treatment, PET/CT is not only more accurate than CT (83 vs 60 %) but also more accurate than mediastinoscopy (83 vs 60 %) with a low sensitivity for mediastinoscopy (29 %)

(De Leyn et al. 2006). Another major limitation of mediastinoscopy is that up to 60 % of patients have an incomplete procedure due to fibrosis and adhesions (De Leyn et al. 2006; Rankin 2008). Although 18F-FDG PET appears to be a reliable modality to assess the response in both the primary lesions and metastases, it is less accurate for the mediastinal nodes, with a 20 % false negative and 25 % false positive rate. Therefore, 18F-FDG positive nodes should undergo biopsy and histologic evaluation prior to definitive surgery (Rankin 2008).

The reliability of PET/CT for the assessment of response to treatment has been validated not only for chemotherapy and radiotherapy, but also for radiofrequency ablation procedures. However, Eradat et al. in their comprehensive review have stated that 1 week after ablation is too soon to detect treatment response by 18F-FDG PET (Eradat et al. 2011). In fact, post-ablation inflammation may obscure subcentimeter residual tissue, and so it is usually delayed until 2 months (Okuma et al. 2006). However, during the intermediate phase (1 week to 2 months), a reduction of less than 60 % of uptake relative to pretreatment value is an indicator of persistent disease (Eradat et al. 2011).

Although most of the available information, both from human and animal experiments (McKinley et al. 2011) is encouraging, there are also a few reports that are not so encouraging. A retrospective study of Memorial Sloan-Kettering Cancer Center on 56 patients found that PET overstaged nodal status in 33 % of the patients (Akhurst et al. 2002). Also, Port et al. reported that a 50 % reduction in the SUV_{max} is a poor predictor of a major pathologic response (Port et al. 2004). In another study, with 18F-FDG PET performed between 1 and 13 days after the last dose of chemotherapy and surgery within a few weeks of the PET study, no significant difference in survival was apparent. In this report, an exceptionally unusual finding for any therapeutic monitoring trial comparing anatomic and metabolic responses was the presence of more anatomic responses than metabolic responses. More interestingly, survival was actually longer in patients without a metabolic response on PET than in those with a response, although with no statistical significance (Hicks 2009) (Tanvetyanon et al. 2008). The explanation for such a marked discordance with a significant number of therapeutic monitoring studies for non-small cell lung cancers, and also the literature comparing metabolic and morphologic responses across a broad range of malignancies is not obvious. Hicks in his comprehensive review suggested that perhaps the use of only the lesion with the most intense uptake for analysis was the problem (Hicks 2009).

5.1.1 Limitations

In the case of chemotherapy, acquisition of an 18F-FDG PET scan too soon after the last dose of treatment would tend to overestimate the response (Tanvetyanon et al. 2008). Also, in the case of 18F-FDG PET for response monitoring after radiotherapy, 18F-FDG uptake in inflamed normal tissues must be considered (Hicks 2009). Kong et al. using serial imaging during and after radiotherapy showed that inflammatory 18F-FDG uptake in normal tissues increases in the first few months after treatment rather than occurring early during radiotherapy (Kong et al. 2007). This could significantly impair interpretation and assignment of appropriate regions of interest for semiquantitative analysis if inflammatory changes or reactive lymphadenopathy are not seen by pattern recognition. However, these delayed changes need not prevent an experienced interpreter from correctly evaluating the treatment response visually (Hicks 2009), because the common foci of abnormal 18F-FDG uptake are generally well recognized by experienced readers (Wang et al. 2007). On the other hand, a positive relationship between 18F-FDG uptake in normal tissues and the response to treatment has been proposed (Hicks et al. 2004).

5.2 Breast Cancer

Since the development of neoadjuvant chemotherapy protocols, PET has been proved to be the most sensitive and accurate imaging modality for early therapy response assessment and treatment monitoring of breast cancers. Both quantitative and/or semi-quantitative PET studies yield priceless information on breast malignancies regarding prognosis and response to chemo-hormone-therapy, in a timely fashion (Baum and Przetak 2001) (Fig. 2). For breast cancer molecular imaging, several tumor targets are candidates for development of tumor-specific tracers. To target general phenomena one can visualize the tumor cell glucose metabolism or DNA synthesis, which are

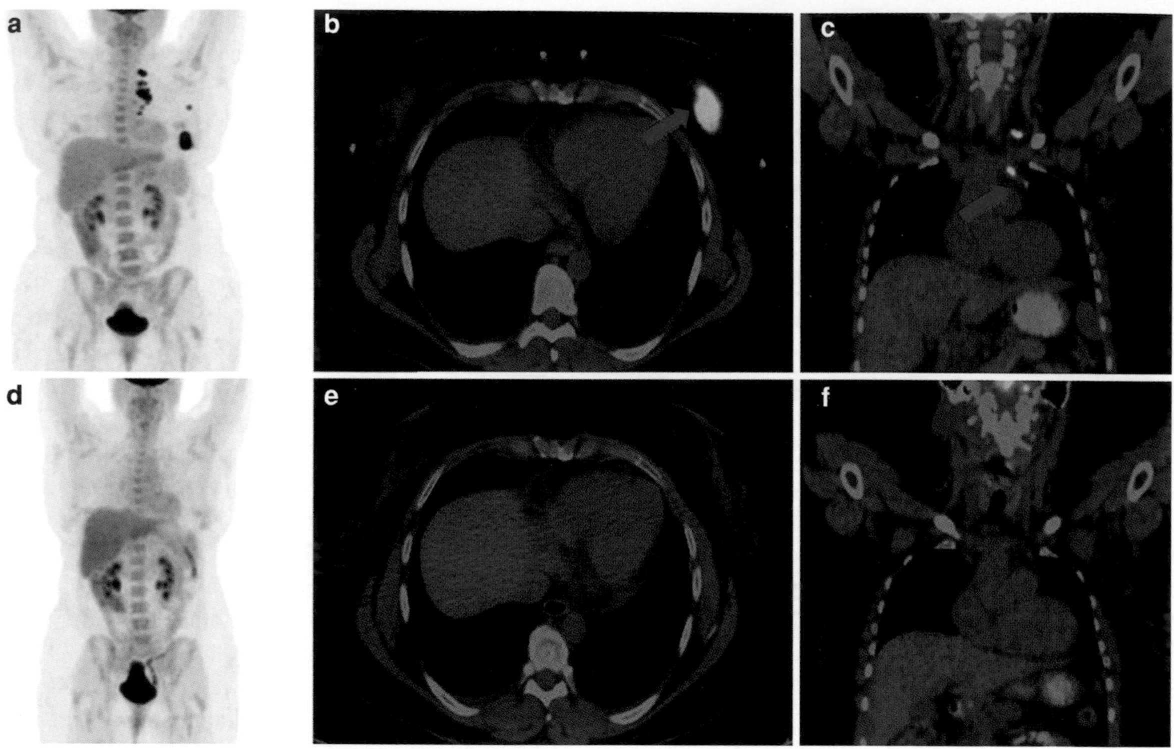

Fig. 2 Breast cancer 46-year-old woman presented with self-palpated left breast nodule, which was biopsied, compatible with triple positive ductal carcinoma. Staging PET/CT scan maximum intensity projection (**a**) and fused PET/CT (**b** and **c**) demonstrate FDG-avid left breast mass with metastatic mediastinal, left axillary and supraclavicular lymphadenopathy. The patient received combined chemotherapy with Taxol and Herceptin for 12 weeks. Post-therapy PET/CT maximum intensity projection (**d**) and fused PET/CT (**e** and **f**) demonstrate no evidence of persistent FDG-avid lesion

both augmented in tumor cells compared to normal cells. Most breast cancer cells express hormone receptors, making these receptors interesting targets for molecular imaging. Also, receptors located at the tumor cell membrane, such as human epidermal growth factor receptor 2 (HER2), epidermal growth factor receptor (EGFR), insulin-like growth factor-1 receptor (IGF-1R) and platelet-derived growth factor β receptor (PDGF-βR), may be of interest for such purposes. In addition, tumor cells excrete growth factors, such as vascular endothelial growth factor (VEGF) and transforming growth factor β (TGF-β), in the microenvironment of breast cancers and theoretically are tracer target candidates. Finally, all targets involved in the processes of angiogenesis (VEGF-receptors, $\alpha V\beta 3$ integrin, fibronectin, endostatin) and hypoxia can be considered as imaging targets, since both processes are key players in tumor growth that are generally not present in normal breast tissue (Munnink 2009).

Seventeen years ago, Wahl et al. reported on changes in tumor metabolic activity in women with locally advanced primary breast cancer who had received a combination of primary chemotherapy and hormone therapy. Tumor 18F-FDG uptake promptly decreased in 8 patients, with subsequent partial or complete pathologic responses, whereas tumors in three nonresponders did not show a significant reduction in 18F-FDG uptake (Wahl et al. 1993). Later studies confirmed a more pronounced reduction in 18F-FDG SUV after the first and second cycles of primary chemotherapy in patients showing a histopathologic response than in nonresponders (Avril et al. 2009). In the neoadjuvant setting, in patients with a histological total or near-total therapeutic effect, reduction in 18F-FDG uptake shows an increasing pattern after each cycle of chemotherapy. The average reductions of 18F-FDG uptake after 1, 2, 3, and 6 cycles have been reported to be 59.6, 78.7, 86.3 and 90.2 %, respectively. In patients with no or less than 50 % therapeutic response histologically, 18F-FDG uptake is only reduced to an average of 53.2 % following 6 cycles of treatment. Regarding these features, the sensitivity, specificity, and negative predictive value of 18F-FDG PET are 61, 96, and 68 % after one course of chemotherapy, 89, 95, and 85 % after 2 courses, and 88, 73, and 83 % after 3 courses, respectively. The same parameters with ultrasound are 64, 43, and 55 %, and with mammography 31, 56, and 45 %. It has been concluded that pathologic response to neoadjuvant chemotherapy in stage II and III breast cancer can be predicted accurately by 18F-FDG PET soon after 2 courses of chemotherapy. Assessment of tumor response with ultrasonography or mammography is never significant, whatever the cutoff (Rousseau et al. 2006; de Vries et al. 2009).

These conclusions have been confirmed by the same observations of other groups. With 18F-FDG PET at baseline and after the first and second chemotherapy cycle, none of the patients with low baseline SUV (< 3.0) experienced a histopathological response to chemotherapy, defined as minimal residual disease. In patients with a baseline 18F-FDG SUV greater than 3.0, histopathological responders show an average reduction of 51 % in 18F-FDG uptake, while nonresponders show an average decrease of 37 %. A threshold of 45 % decrease in SUV correctly identifies most of responders, and histopathologic nonresponders are identified with a negative predictive value of 90 %. Similar results can be found after the second cycle, using a threshold of 55 % relative reduction in SUV. Thus, the level of 18F-FDG uptake values at baseline and after each cycle can be used to predict the response to treatment. Moreover, the relative changes in SUV after the first and second cycles are strong predictors of response to chemotherapy. Therefore, 18F-FDG PET may be helpful for individual treatment stratification and planning in breast cancer (Schwarz-Dose et al. 2009).

Based on current documentation, 18F-FDG PET response monitoring is likely to be most effective for tumors above a minimum pre-therapy size (approximately 3 cm in diameter) and for the most metabolically active tumor types (e.g., invasive ductal carcinomas) (McDermott et al. 2007). Table 4 shows a brief review on the available reports on this issue.

The pattern of metabolic changes in hormonal treatments seems to be somewhat different. Dehdashti and his colleagues have proved the predictive value of increased metabolic activity, or metabolic flare, detected by 18F-FDG PET in response to hormonal treatment for tumor response and overall survival (Mortimer et al. 2001, 2003; Dehdashti et al. 1997, 1999). Such a flare phenomenon has not been observed following chemotherapy regimens (Pons et al. 2009).

In conclusion, although 18F-FDG PET is not yet recommended as a routine assessment of the response to treatment, the information on its role and accuracy is increasing. The application of 18F-FDG PET in the assessment of the response to therapy can be of value, especially in further treatment planning soon after a few courses of chemotherapy. Generally, the most prudent time to monitor chemotherapy response using 18F-FDG PET is between the end of the first cycle and the midpoint of chemotherapy, which is a compromise between avoiding the early phase where tumor 18F-FDG uptake falls rapidly and minimizing the patient's exposure to chemotherapeutic regimens (McDermott et al. 2007; Escalona et al. 2010).

Limited experience with 18F-FLT PET has also been reported (Dittmann et al. 2009; Kenny et al. 2005, 2007; Smyczek-Gargya et al. 2004). A strong correlation has been shown between the percentage reduction in FLT tumor uptake 1 or 2 weeks following initiation of chemotherapy and late CT size changes. Right after docetaxel or doxorubicin treatment, FLT uptake corresponds to the induced reduction of tumor cell proliferation (Dittmann et al. 2009). Overall, 18F-FLT PET is not regarded as a routine staging tool for breast cancer, but it may play a role in prediction or monitoring of response to therapy, possibilities that warrant further study (Dittmann et al. 2009; Kenny et al. 2005, 2007; Smyczek-Gargya et al. 2004). Similarly, limited reports are available on using Methionine PET for monitoring of response to the treatment. It has been shown that Methionine uptake clearly diminishes in breast cancer metastases after successful therapy. Accordingly, it has been suggested that Methionine PET may be feasible in predicting the early response to therapy in advanced breast cancer. However, the results of these limited preliminary experiences come from a rather small group of patients with different oncological medications. Further studies are needed to confirm the predictive value of this technique in breast cancer (Lindholm et al. 1996, 2009; Huovinen et al. 1993).

Table 4 A brief review of the currently available reports concerning response monitoring of breast cancer using 18F-FDG PET

Authors (Years)	Number of patients	Design	Major findings	Conclusion
Smith, et al. (2000)	30	Dynamic PET immediately before the first, second and fifth doses and after the last dose. Semi-quantitative dose uptake ratio [DUR] and influx constant were calculated	The mean reduction in DUR after the first pulse of chemotherapy is significantly greater in lesions that achieve a partial or complete pathologic response. PET after a single pulse of chemotherapy can predict complete pathologic response with a sensitivity of 90 % and specificity of 74 %	18F-FDG PET imaging of primary and metastatic breast cancer after a single pulse of chemotherapy may be of value in the prediction of pathologic treatment response
McDermott, et al. (2007)	96	PET data were acquired before the first and second cycles, at the midpoint and at the endpoint of neoadjuvant chemotherapy	Only tumors with an initial tumor to background ratio of greater than 5 showed a difference between response categories. Mean SUV at the midpoint of therapy identifies 77 % of low responding tumors and 100 % of high responding tumors. ROC area is 0.93	18F-FDG PET is efficacious for predicting the pathologic response of most primary breast tumors throughout the duration of neoadjuvant therapy. However, PET is ineffective for tumors with low image contrast on pre-therapy scans
Berriolo-Riedinger, et al. (2007)	47	Tumor uptake of 18F-FDG evaluation before and after the first course of neoadjuvant chemotherapy	A SUV reduction of 60 % predicts the pathologically proven complete response (pCR) with an accuracy of 87 %	18F-FDG SUV reduction after the first cycle of chemotherapy is a powerful predictive factor for a pCR
Schelling et al. (2000)	22	Quantification of regional 18F-FDG uptake of the breast acquired after the first and second courses of chemotherapy as compared to the baseline scan	As early as after the first course of chemotherapy, all responders were correctly identified (sensitivity 100 %, specificity 85 %) by a SUV reduction below 55 % of the baseline scan. At this threshold, histopathologic response could be predicted with an accuracy of 88 % and 91 % after the first and second courses of therapy, respectively	18F-FDG PET differentiates responders from nonresponders early in the course of therapy, improves patient management by avoiding ineffective chemotherapy and supporting the decision to continue dose-intensive preoperative chemotherapy in responding patients
Kim et al. (2004)	50	Reduction rate (RR) of peak standardized uptake values were compared with pathological response	When -88 % of RR was used as threshold value for differentiation between pathological partial response (pPR) and pathological complete response (pCR), the area under the curve (AUC) was 0.788 (sensitivity and specificity: 100 % and 56.5 %, respectively). with -79 % of RR, the AUC was 0.838 (sensitivity and specificity: 85.2 and 82.6 %, respectively)	The study suggested "a possible predictive value of 18F-FDG PET for the assessment of the pathological response of primary breast cancer after neo-adjuvant chemotherapy"

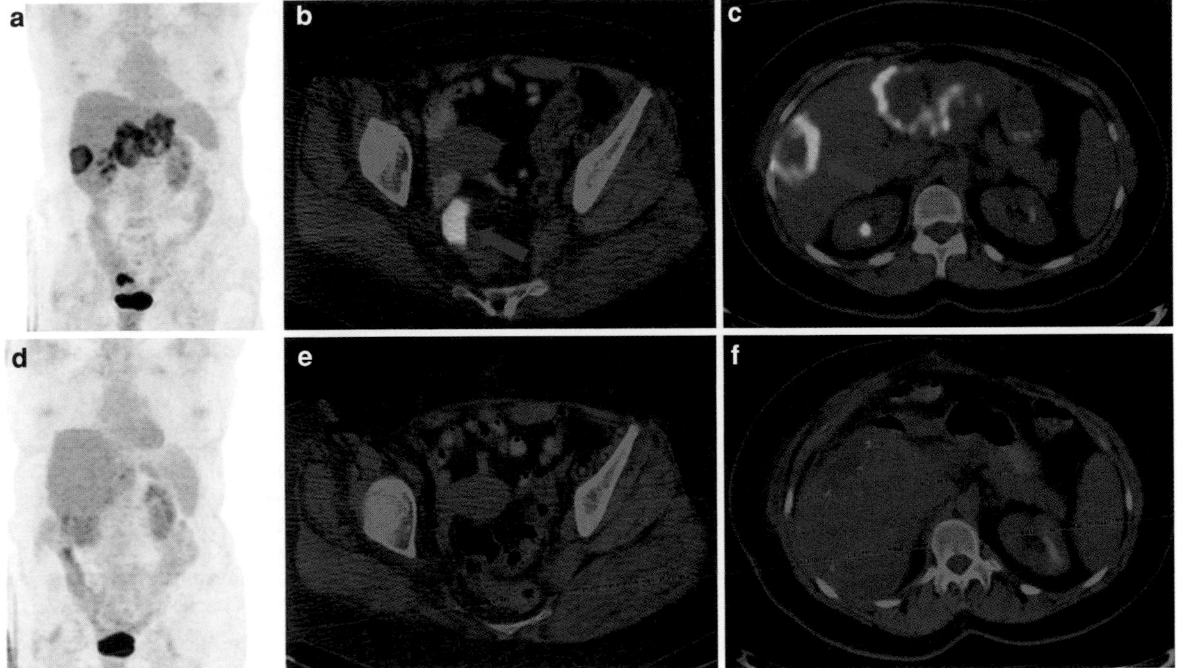

Fig. 3 Colorectal cancer 54-year-old woman experiencing diffuse abdominal pain and hepatic abnormalities on ultrasound. Pretreatment PET/CT scan maximum intensity projection (**a**) and fused PET/CT (**b** and **c**) show FDG-avid sigmoidal mass and hepatic lesions. The patient received 3 cycles of neoadjuvant XELOX chemotherapy, followed by partial colectomy and left hepatectomy. The treatment was completed with right hepatic lesions radio frequency ablation and 3 cycles of adjuvant chemotherapy. Post-therapy PET/CT maximum intensity projection (**d**) and axial fused PET/CT (**e** and **f**) demonstrate no evidence of persistent FDG-avid disease

5.3 Colorectal Cancer

Some colorectal cancer primary or metastatic lesions do not respond to chemotherapy well. In these cases early identification of nonresponders might allow the use of other regimens (de Geus-Oei et al. 2009; Bender et al. 1999). 18F-FDG PET has emerged as a promising diagnostic modality, not only for staging and re-staging of colorectal cancer (Fig. 3), but also as predictive of response to therapy and a promising tool for early monitoring of treatment (Wiering et al. 2008). A recent systematic review by de Geus-Oei et al. has covered almost all available documents in the field. The authors concluded that use in clinical practice and systematic inclusion in therapeutic trials is warranted to explore the potential of 18F-FDG PET for response monitoring in advanced colorectal cancer, in monitoring the effects of local ablative therapies, preoperative radiotherapy, and multimodality treatment response evaluation in primary rectal cancer (de Geus-Oei et al. 2009). More recently, Vriens et al. found no relationship between changes in dynamic contrast-enhanced MRI parameters and overall survival and progression-free survival, while change in glucose metabolic rate as detected by 18F-FDG PET was able to predict overall survival, after correction for confounders. These interesting and promising reports have increased utilization of PET imaging in patients with colorectal cancers (Pawlik et al. 2009).

PET provides a valuable tool to differentiate and compare the effects of different therapeutic approaches. Janssen et al., applied sequential 18F-FDG PET/CT scans both prior to treatment and after the first week of treatment and showed that for the patients referred for pre-operative radiochemotherapy, significant reductions of SUV_{mean} and SUV_{max} within the tumor are found after the first week of treatment, while radiotherapy alone did not result in significant changes in the metabolic activity of the tumor, despite the higher applied radiation dose (Janssen et al. 2010).

Table 5 A brief review of studies investigating the role of PET in the evaluation of response to chemotherapy of colorectal cancers

Author (Year)	No. of Patients studied	Protocol	Results
Findlay et al. (1996)	20	18F-FDG PET before and at 1–2 and 4–5 weeks on treatment	Pretreatment target/lesion (T:L) ratios and SUVs did not correlate with tumor response, although response is associated with lower 1-2- week (1.8 vs. 2.2) and 4-5 week (1.4 vs. 2.3) T:L ratios. Responding lesions had a greater reduction in metabolism (67 % v 99 %). The 4- to 5-week T:L ratio was able to discriminate response from nonresponse both in a lesion-by-lesion and overall patient response assessment (sensitivity 100 %; specificity 90 and 75 %, respectively)
Bender et al. (1999)	10 patients with documented nonresectable liver metastases	Prior and 72 h after a single infusion of 5-Fluorouracil and folinic acid. Follow up for at least 6 months	All metastases responding to therapy exerted a significant decrease of 18F-FDG uptake (−22 ± 10 %), metastases showing a short-term effect had a slightly diminished, and progressing metastases an enhanced 18F-FDG uptake (13 ± 17 %)
Dimitrakopoulou-Strauss et al. (2003)	28 patients (total of 55 metastases)	Quantitative dynamic 18F-FDG PET	The median SUV as measured in the tumor lesions prior to onset to FOLFOX was 3.15, in comparison with 2.68 SUV after the first cycle and 2.61 SUV after the second cycle, leading to the conclusion that quantitative, dynamic 18F-FDG PET should be used preferentially for monitoring patients with metastatic colorectal cancer receiving chemotherapy
Dimitrakopoulou-Strauss et al. (2004)	25 cases with metastatic colorectal cancer	PET before the onset of FOLFOX therapy and after completion of the first and fourth cycles	SUV provided a correct classification rate ranging from 62–69 %, regarding the short- and long-term survival groups
de Geus-Oei et al. (2008)	50	Dynamic 18F-FDG PET was carried out before and at 2 and 6 months after the start of treatment	The progression-free survival and overall survival analysis showed a significant predictive value at broad ranges of delta-MRGlu (metabolic rate of glucose) and delta-SUV cut-off levels
Bystrom et al. (2009)	51	18F-FDG PET was carried out before treatment and after two cycles	There was a strong correlation between metabolic response (changes in SUV) and objective response, with a sensitivity of 77 % and a specificity of 76 %. There was no significant correlation between metabolic response and time to progression or overall survival ($P = 0.1$)
Zhu et al. (2010)	35	18F-FDG PET scans were obtained at baseline and after completion of the second cycle	18F-FDG PET showed a significant decrease in SUV_{max} after 2 cycles of treatment. Change in SUV_{max} was a significant predictor of progression-free survival and overall survival
Shamim et al. (2011)	32	Retrospective	In responders, baseline and follow-up mean SUV_{max} were 11.8 ± 10.1 and 3.7 ± 4.1, respectively (significant decrease). Among nonresponders, baseline and follow-up mean SUV_{max} were 8.1 ± 5.2 and 14.1 ± 9.0, respectively (significant increase)

5.3.1 Assessment of Response to Chemotherapy

Generally the extent of chemotherapy-induced changes in tumor glucose metabolism is highly predictive of patient outcome and long-term survival. In fact, based on the available evidence (Table 5), the use of 18F-FDG PET for therapy monitoring seems clinically feasible (de Geus-Oei et al. 2008). Chemotherapy-sensitive lesions show a reduction in metabolic rate even after a single course of chemotherapy, which is indicative of the outcome after an anticipated therapy cycle (Bender et al. 1999). Specifically, cytotoxic chemotherapy does not alter dynamic contrast-enhanced MRI-derived properties of tumor vasculature, but decreases glucose consumption of tumor cells, which emphasizes the advantages of PET over the competing methods of anatomical imaging in patients with colorectal cancer (Vriens et al. 2009).

One of the major concerns in therapy monitoring with 18F-FDG PET is the fact that chemotherapy-induced normalization of the metabolic rate of glucose in liver metastases of colorectal cancer does not always indicate a complete pathologic response (de Geus-Oei et al. 2009). It has been found that, despite the absence of detectable 18F-FDG uptake above the background, viable tumor cells could still be found in up to 85 % of the lesions. This observation led to the advice that currently, curative resection of liver metastases in patients with liver metastases of colorectal carcinoma should not be deferred on the basis of 18F-FDG PET findings (Tan et al. 2007). As an explanation, it was speculated that "a reduction in the number of viable tumor cells below the limit of detection may be an important reason why lesions are not seen by 18F-FDG PET following treatment and the relatively high level of 18F-FDG uptake in normal hepatic parenchyma makes it more difficult to detect lesions with a partial metabolic response resulting in uptake only slightly greater than that of the normal liver" (de Geus-Oei et al. 2009). The effect of chemotherapy on tumor 18F-FDG uptake is another explanation, as chemotherapeutic agents may reduce 18F-FDG uptake by altering the glucose metabolism, decreasing the activity of the key glycolytic enzyme hexokinase (de Geus-Oei et al. 2009; Akhurst et al. 2005). As evidence, Glazer et al. reported a negative predictive value of 13.3 %, a positive predictive value of 94.3 %, sensitivity of 89.9 %, specificity of 22.2 %, and overall accuracy of 85.5 % for 18F-FDG PET in colorectal cancer patients undergoing chemotherapy and ablation therapy for liver metastasis. The disappointing features led the authors to conclude that 18F-FDG PET within 4 weeks of chemotherapy is not a reliable test for response evaluation of colorectal hepatic metastases. The high rate of false-negative cases (likely due to metabolic inhibition caused by chemotherapy) indicates that physicians should not use PET in patients recently completing chemotherapy; in fact, they must undergo the appropriate oncologic hepatic operation based on the high probability of viable malignant lesion" (Glazer et al. 2010).

Technically, some authors have recommended that a combination of kinetic parameters from the baseline scan and mid-treatment scans provides the best results for classification into short- and long-term survival classes and suggested that quantitative dynamic 18F-FDG PET should be used preferentially for chemotherapy response monitoring (Dimitrakopoulou-Strauss et al. 2004). However, based on more recent data, simplified methods (SUV measurement without the need for complex dynamic imaging protocols) seem to be sufficiently reliable (de Geus-Oei et al. 2008). It has been emphasized that none of the currently available normalization methods show any statistical advantage over the other. Therefore, simplifying the methods for analysis of 18F-FDG PET data can facilitate incorporation of 18F-FDG PET in clinical treatment-response monitoring and may raise its application in future trials (Vriens et al. 2009). Also, non-complex approaches are advantageous over a full kinetic analysis as they will improve patient compliance, which is an important characteristic of successful clinical trials (de Geus-Oei et al. 2009). Another advantage of SUV measurements is that they can be calculated from static whole-body 18F-FDG PET images, which depict all metastases. In dynamic scans, in contrast, only one axial field of view (usually 15–20 cm) can be imaged during data acquisition. As metastatic foci in different parts of the body may respond differently to chemotherapy, this will pose a remarkable shortcoming to kinetic analysis, making it more logical to rely on SUV analysis over kinetic analysis (de Geus-Oei et al. 2009).

5.3.2 Local Ablative Techniques

Assessment of the efficacy of local ablative techniques (including microwave tumor coagulation, laser-induced thermotherapy, injection of ethyl alcohol, cryosurgical ablation or cryotherapy (CSA), and radiofrequency ablation (RFA)) is another area of strength for PET in colorectal cancer. In this circumstance, anatomical imaging techniques encounter remarkable limitations, which are partly due to the rim-like increase in contrast enhancement that occurs immediately after the procedure, resembling peripheral hyperperfusion. Such a peripheral contrast enhancement may lead to inadequate detection of residual tumor by CT or MRI, delayed diagnosis of treatment failure or confusion between incomplete local ablative treatment and the occurrence of new metastases in regions adjacent to the treatment site (de Geus-Oei et al. 2009; Antoch et al. 2005; Aschoff et al. 2000). Feasibility of 18F-FDG PET to identify residual tumor very early after local ablative treatments has been confirmed by several studies (de Geus-Oei et al. 2009; Langenhoff et al. 2002). Even some groups have stated that PET/CT performed within 24 h after radiofrequency ablation can effectively detect whether residual tumor exists, which may improve the efficacy of the therapeutic strategy and can guide further treatment (Liu et al. 2010). Langenhoff et al. found that 18F-FDG PET performed early after local ablation provides valuable information about the efficacy of treatment by differentiating post-treatment changes from residual or recurrent malignant lesions. Results from18F-FDG PET became negative in almost 90 % of lesions within 3 weeks following local ablative therapy, meaning that 18F-FDG-accumulating liver metastases became photopenic with a negative predictive value of 100 % during the follow-up (de Geus-Oei et al. 2009; Langenhoff et al. 2002). In most of those patients with positive post-treatment 18F-FDG PET, local recurrence was identified on CT during the mean follow-up of 16 months. In all cases, 18F-FDG PET detected recurrence considerably earlier than CT (3.8 vs. 8.5 months) (de Geus-Oei et al. 2009; Langenhoff et al. 2002). The negative predictive value of 18F-FDG PET of 100 % (with positive predictive value of 88 %) is also confirmed by the study of Joosten et al. (Joosten et al. 2005). Moreover, the superiority of PET over CT has been confirmed by Veit et al. who found accuracy of 68 % for PET vs. 47 % for CT. The authors concluded that dual-modality PET/CT simplifies guidance for reinterventions and that a follow-up scan soon after radiofrequency is ideal to shorten the time to a possible reintervention. The authors recommended that a follow-up scan should be done as soon as 2 days after ablation, before tissue regeneration takes place. Such a strategy was recommended because tissue regeneration might cause rim-like tracer distribution at the ablative margin; in contrast, viable tumor residue results in an area of focally increased 18F-FDG uptake (de Geus-Oei et al. 2009; Veit et al. 2006). Similar promising results have been reported by other groups, performing 18F-FDG PET 1–4 weeks after local ablative treatment. The evidence all together suggests that 18F-FDG PET is accurate in monitoring the local effect of local ablation techniques as it recognizes incomplete tumor ablation early, even when it is not detectable by CT (de Geus-Oei et al. 2009; Joosten et al. 2005; Veit et al. 2006; Donckier et al. 2003). In conclusion, 18F-FDG PET, while still under evaluation, presents promise for the routine assessment of response of unresectable liver metastases to ablative interventions in the near future.

5.3.3 Radiotherapy and Multimodality Treatment Response Monitoring in Primary Rectal Cancer

As patients with locally advanced rectal cancer are at the highest risk for failure to respond to local treatment, preoperative radiotherapy is usually required to achieve a radical resection and improve the local control rate (Wong et al 2007). As for the widely discussed shortcomings of the histopathologic approaches, clearly the need for reliable noninvasive methods suitable for the prediction of responses, especially complete pathologic remission, has been emphasized. The remarkably low accuracy of mainly anatomically based imaging modalities, such as CT, MRI, and endorectal ultrasound–ranging (from only 30–60 %–in these settings) leads to demand for imaging modalities that provide a combination of functional data and morphologic information, most importantly PET/CT (de Geus-Oei et al. 2009). The comprehensive review of Vriens et al. on the almost 20 available reports confirms the remarkable interest in applying PET to radiotherapy and multimodality treatment response monitoring in primary rectal cancer (Vriens et al.2009). This systematic review in conjunction with more recently reported supporting evidence (De Ridder et al. 2009, 2010; Avallone et al. 2009) confirms that PET is probably a promising alternative approach to current standard methods of therapy assessment in these settings (conventional histopathologic analysis, measuring the extent of the residual tumor) (de Geus-Oei et al. 2009), making it possible to identify nonresponders and any clinically relevant consequences during the course of chemoradiation.

Since the first studies of Engenhart et al. (Haberkorn et al. 1991; Engenhart et al. 1992), there have been multiple reports, most of which confirm a remarkable reduction in 18F-FDG uptake 2–3 weeks after radiotherapy. This reduction correlates significantly with the reduction in tumor cell burden and cell death (Schiepers et al. 1999). Using 18F-FDG PET it is possible to discriminate successful treatments from unsuccessful as early as 2 weeks after radiotherapy. The accuracy of this approach has been reported to be 80–100 %, depending on the applied cutoff value of SUV reduction after treatment (de Geus-Oei et al. 2009; Janssen et al. 2010; Vriens et al.2009; Schiepers et al. 1999). In fact, lack of consensus about the optimal cutoff value of delta SUV is one of the major limitations of the available reports on practical application of 18F-FDG in routine clinical settings. Although most of the studies have used cutoff values of more than 40 % reduction, these discordant results call for systematic investigations of the best cut-off value for treatment response evaluation with 18F-FDG PET. The lack of agreement is partly due to confounding radiotherapy-induced effects on 18F-FDG uptake. About 25 % of 18F-FDG uptake occurs in surrounding tissue such as macrophages, neutrophils, fibroblasts, and granulation tissue. There is also a short-lived but reversible decrease in glucose metabolism in the affected tumor cells(de Geus-Oei et al. 2009; Kubota et al. 1992; Larson 1994; Amthauer et al. 2004). These concerns have led to the recommendation that 18F-FDG PET studies should be delayed until 60 days after radiotherapy (Haberkorn et al. 1991), a long interval which is not clinically acceptable in the neoadjuvant setting (de Geus-Oei et al. 2009). Clearly, further work is needed to ascertain the exact sequence of time-dependent radiobiologic effects of neoadjuvant multimodality treatment in order to set a standard timing of PET imaging in the assessment of response to therapy.

5.3.4 Conclusion

At present, there is a growing body of data that semi-quantitative assessment of therapy-induced changes in colorectal cancer FDG PET avidity may predict early tumor response and patient outcome. Treatment plans might be changed. For example, nonresponders metabolic imaging approach allows identifying those patients requiring additional therapeutic interventions or palliative care. On the other hand, for those with a satisfactory metabolic response, a cost-saving strategy could avoid expensive diagnostic procedures during the follow-up and, more importantly, reducing the risk of overtreating. In any case, as even a partial metabolic response may be an indication for continuing treatment, the advantage of metabolic imaging over conventional anatomical modalities may be clinically relevant. Published data (although heterogeneous with respect to the methods of PET quantification, the evaluation interval, the metabolic response criteria, and the clinical endpoints) indicate that 18F-FDG PET has a high predictive value in the therapeutic management of patients with colorectal cancer. This technique could be an asset for improving patient care by decreasing the side effects, costs, and effort associated with ineffective futile treatments in nonresponders (Wiering et al. 2008).

6 Lymphoma

6.1 Non-Hodgkin Lymphoma

Although lymphomas are very chemosensitive, almost 50 % of patients with aggressive non-Hodgkin lymphoma (NHL) do not respond to the standard first-line treatment, which consists of six cycles of doxorubicin, vincristine, prednisolone, and cyclophosphamide (CHOP), recently complemented with rituximab (Moulin-Romsee et al. 2008). This fact emphasizes the importance of early evaluation of the response to treatment, to provide clinicians with the information required for early modification or adjustment of treatment and therapy.

In this era, 18F-FDG PET has provided a very useful tool for therapy planning and monitoring of NHL (Spaepen and Mortelmans 2001) (Fig. 4). Treatment monitoring with 18F-FDG PET probably has the highest impact on the management of malignant lymphomas; several studies have confirmed that patients with metabolically active residual masses after the end of chemotherapy have a poorer outcome and survival compared to those with metabolically inactive residual masses (Pons et al. 2009). There is

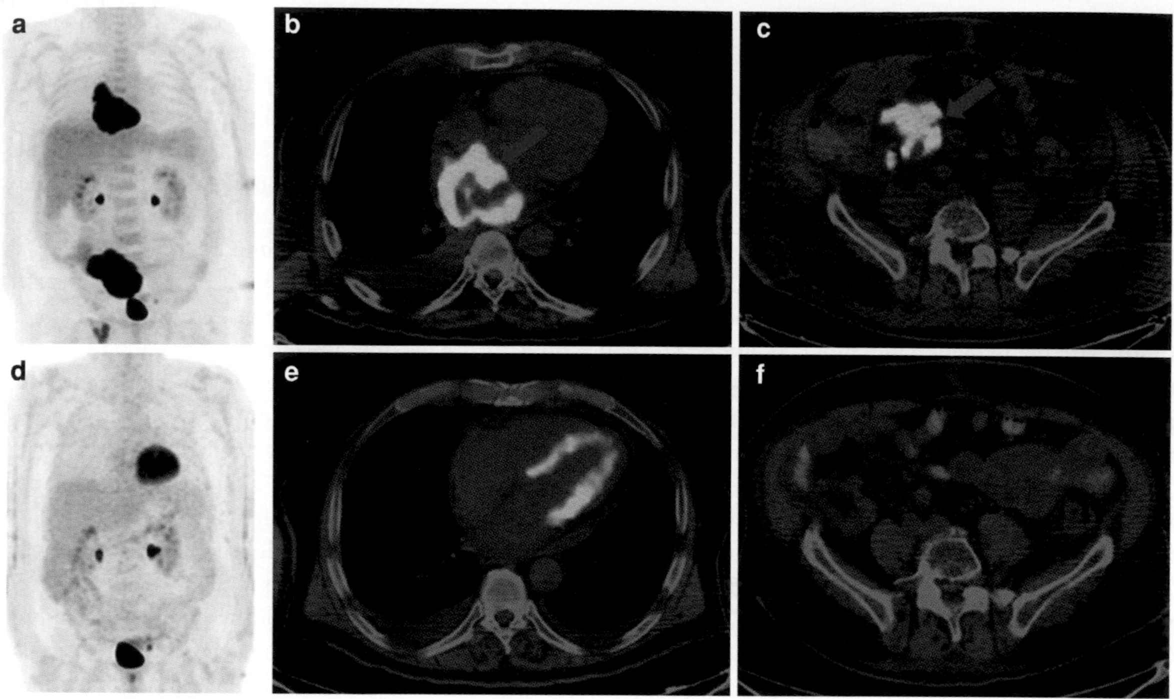

Fig. 4 Diffuse large B cell non Hodgkin lymphoma with atrial involvement 71-year-old man originally presented with fatigue, shortness of breath and vague chest pain. Pretreatment PET/CT scan maximum intensity projection (**a**) and axial fused PET/CT (**b** and **c**) show FDG-avid lobulated atrial and mesenteric masses with abnormal FDG uptake in the right acetabulum. The patient received 6 cycles of R-CHOP chemotherapy and intrathecal prophylaxis. Three week mid-therapy PET/CT maximum intensity projection (**d**) and axial fused PET/CT (**e** and **f**) demonstrate complete resolution of all FDG-avid disease

no doubt that 18F-FDG PET is more accurate than CT and its accuracy is high enough that it is currently the standard method of remission assessment, either in addition to CT, or with PET/CT to replace CT. The reported sensitivity and specificity for detecting residual disease in aggressive NHL is remarkably high, at 72 and 100 %, respectively (Juweid et al. 2007). According to the current criteria, a patient is considered to be in complete remission even when a residual CT mass is present, provided the mass has changed from being PET-positive to PET-negative (Cheson et al. 2007b). It has been shown that changes in 18F-FDG uptake can closely follow changes in tumor viability and hence clinical PET scanning can be used to monitor response to treatment over a short time span (Barrington and Carr 1995). Regarding the strong supporting evidence, 18F-FDG PET seems to be the ideal tool for the evaluation of treatment response (Spaepen and Mortelmans 2001). The accuracy of 18F-FDG PET versus CT/MRI is 84 versus 50 % for evaluation of treatment response (Isohashi et al. 2008). In evaluating response to treatment at pathologic sites with discrepant findings between 18F-FDG PET and CT/MRI, the frequency of accurate diagnosis by 18F-FDG PET (76 %) is higher than that of CT or MRI (24 %) (Isohashi et al. 2008).

In the application of PET for the purpose of response assessment in the setting of NHL, the pathologic type of the tumor is a major factor. For some NHL types such as diffuse large B cell lymphoma (DLBCL), the interim 18F-FDG PET is unquestionably able to predict outcome, but for some other types concerns remain. For example, although 18F-FDG PET appears useful in identifying residual disease in DLBCL, the value of 18F-FDG PET in primary mediastinal B cell lymphoma (PMBL), a subtype of DLBCL, as well as AIDS-related lymphomas is not as clear. A recent study on newly diagnosed, HIV-negative patients with either PMBL or mediastinal gray zone lymphoma (MGZL) indicated that while the negative predictive value of post-treatment 18F-FDG PET is high (95 %), the positive predictive value is low (62.5 %). The positive predictive value is remarkably lower for PMBL than MGZL (25 % vs. 100 %). Furthermore, positive post-treatment 18F-FDG PET is not closely correlated with residual viable tumor in PMBL. The high a priori likelihood of cure in these patients combined with a relatively small sample size of the study are thought to explain these findings (Dunleavy et al. 2010).

The same concern about the accuracy of 18F-FDG PET studies in the evaluation of the response to treatment applies to HIV-associated DLBCL. In a recent study on newly diagnosed patients with HIV-associated DLBCL evaluated with interim 18F-FDG PET, the negative predictive value was reported to be 91 %, while the positive predictive value was disappointingly low (15 %). In this population, the potential for confounding disease processes associated with high FDG-avidity is likely to have contributed to the low positive predictive value. This emphasizes the importance of interpreting 18F-FDG PET in the context of an individual patient's clinical setting, but also the difficulty that confronts the profession in defining a unifying definition of PET response and the accompanying prognostic implications of any given PET finding (Dunleavy et al. 2010).

Generally, it is accepted that the results of early or post-treatment response assessment using 18F-FDG PET can be applied to guide therapeutic decisions, known as response-adapted treatment planning, particularly in certain lymphomas such as Hodgkin disease and DLBCL (Dunleavy et al. 2010). In fact, the value of 18F-FDG PET in the acute management and evaluation of response to treatment of lymphoma has been confirmed with numerous studies and therefore is widely used investigationally (Dunleavy et al. 2010). Although it has been mentioned that currently 18F-FDG PET for monitoring treatment should only be used in a clinical trial or as part of a prospective registry (Juweid et al. 2007), there is considerable interest in the use of 18F-FDG PET to assess early response to treatment in the clinical setting. Three observational studies involving almost 300 patients with aggressive NHL suggest that visually assessed interim 18F-FDG PET can identify response early during chemotherapy, and that interim PET can predict outcome in DLBCL (Townsend et al. 2004; Czernin et al. 2007; Weber 2005). In all three studies, a statistically significant difference in progression-free and overall survival between the PET-positive and PET-negative groups was found. Furthermore, mid-treatment 18F-FDG PET was reported to be a stronger prognostic factor for progression-free and overall survival than the international prognostic index (Dunleavy et al. 2010).

Based on the available data, NHL patients with persistent 18F-FDG uptake after three cycles are unlikely to gain a complete remission and continuing chemotherapy is useless. Investigating the costs and benefits for the use of PET in this early treatment setting shows a substantial cost savings if management of NHL patients is based on a mid-treatment 18F-FDG PET scan. Applying such an approach in clinical practice and with an 18F-FDG PET price of €700 (US $917) and CHOP price (per cycle) of €1,829 (US $2400), a cost saving of €1,879 (US $2460) per patient is achieved. The 18F-FDG PET price can increase up to €2,580 (US $3380) and the cost for one cycle of CHOP can diminish to €500 (US $655) before cost savings are nil (Moulin-Romsee et al. 2008).

According to Bishton et al., 18F-FDG PET can stratify patients into risk groups for relapse. Furthermore, 18F-FDG PET scan status at 3 months may predict extended event-free survival more accurately than CT (Bishton et al. 2008). Also, PET response assessment is promising in predicting which NHL patients are likely to benefit from radioimmunotherapy such as 131I-Rituximab (Bishton et al. 2008). Almost 85–90 % of NHL patients with a negative interim PET achieved have maintained a continuous complete response (Zinzani et al. 2010; Thomas et al. 2010), which indicates that mid-treatment PET represents a significant step forward in helping physicians make crucial decisions on further treatment of patients with NHL (Zinzani et al. 2010). Incorporation of pre-therapy prognosis can improve predictive utility (Zinzani et al. 2010; Thomas et al. 2010).

Residual visceral damage post therapy does not necessarily lead to significant 18F-FDG uptake and the infrequent incidence of inflammatory reactions as a consequence of chemotherapy need not discourage the clinicians from imaging early after treatment (Barrington and Carr 1995). This conclusion has been confirmed: It has been shown that standard chemotherapy causes rapid decrease of tumor metabolic activity as early as 1 week after treatment, which continues to decline during therapy (Wu et al. 2010). Also, it has been confirmed that the diagnostic accuracy of PET/CT is equal to or even superior to that of volumetric MRI for early treatment response evaluation of aggressive NHL (Wu et al. 2010).

The optimal time after initiating treatment for evaluation of the response to treatment is also a matter of debate. The reduction of SUV from baseline to post-therapy PET/CT has been reported to be on average 72.9 % in those PET/CT studies done after 2 cycles of chemotherapy and 79.8 % in studies done after 4 cycles of chemotherapy. However, the difference is not statistically or clinically significant (Iagaru et al. 2008). In the report of Wu et al., the reduction of SUV from baseline to post-therapy PET/CT was an average of 60 % in those PET/CT studies done after 1 week of chemotherapy and another 59 % in studies done after 3 cycles of chemotherapy, giving a total decrease of 83 %. These figures closely parallel tumor volume, as assessed by volumetric MRI, which shows that both volumetric MRI and PET/CT are valuable tools for early treatment response evaluation of aggressive NHL with equivalent diagnostic efficacy. Also, during the course of the treatment, the tumor volume on MRI correlated with the active tumor volume on fused PET/CT images in the same region of interest, which emphasizes the reliability of volumetric assessment of PET/CT images (Wu et al. 2010).

6.1.1 Recommended Protocol

As mentioned earlier, the main limitation in the wide clinical application of interim 18F-FDG PET is the lack of standardized imaging protocols and reporting criteria, and unproven reproducibility of interpretation. Using existing response criteria, the reproducibility of 18F-FDG PET interpretation has been moderate, with one study reporting only 68–71 % agreement between expert nuclear medicine clinicians (Horning et al. 2010). Therefore, recommendations for the application of 18F-FDG PET have been published. Generally, use of attenuation-corrected PET is strongly encouraged (Juweid et al. 2007). Based on the expert consensus advice, 18F-FDG PET after completion of treatment should be performed at least 3 weeks, and preferably at 6 to 8 weeks, after chemotherapy or chemo-immunotherapy, and 8 to 12 weeks following radiation or chemo-radiotherapy. Visual analysis alone is adequate for interpreting 18F-FDG PET findings as positive or negative when assessing response to treatment. Mediastinal blood pool activity is recommended as the reference background activity to define 18F-FDG PET positivity for a residual mass 2 cm or larger in greatest transverse diameter, regardless of its location. A smaller residual mass or a normal sized lymph node (i.e, less than 1×1 cm in diameter) should be considered positive if its activity is above that of the surrounding background (Juweid et al. 2007). Specific criteria for defining 18F-FDG PET positivity in the liver, spleen, lung, and bone marrow have also been proposed.

6.2 Hodgkin Disease

The value of mid-treatment 18F-FDG PET is also confirmed for Hodgkin disease (HD) (Furth et al. 2010; Zaucha et al. 2009; Markova et al. 2008, 2009a, b; Eich et al. 2008a, b; Krochmalczyk et al. 2008). It is recommended to use 18F-FDG PET scanning after 4 cycles of BEACOPP regimen (PET-4). A high negative predictive value of PET-4 in HD patients treated with BEACOPP has been reported, with no progression or relapse for PET negative cases (Markova et al. 2008, 2009; Eich et al. 2008a).

In advanced-stage HD, radiotherapy has frequently been administered following combination chemotherapy to treat residual masses and sites of initial bulky disease (Dunleavy et al. 2010; Jost et al. 2005). Based on the available evidence, the negative predictive value of 18F-FDG PET may be sufficiently high that it could be used to spare some patients from unnecessary radiotherapy (Dunleavy et al. 2010). The negative predictive value in patients who underwent post-chemotherapy 18F-FDG PET is 94 %, with progression-free survival rates of 96 and 86 % for PET-negative and PET-positive patients, respectively (Dunleavy et al. 2010) (Fig. 5). However, the only randomized trial to date has raised concerns regarding the appropriateness of omitting radiotherapy just on the basis of PET negativity (Picardi et al. 2007). In this study, 160 patients with advanced-stage HD, who were PET-negative following induction chemotherapy were randomly divided into 2 groups: one to receive radiotherapy to the initial bulky site and the other followed but not treated. After a median follow-up of 40 months, histological analysis detected remnant/residual or recurrent tumor in 14 % of patients of the second group, but in only 4 % of the first group, suggesting a benefit for consolidation radiotherapy (Picardi et al. 2007). On the other hand, a PET-based treatment algorithm has been successfully employed at the BC Cancer Agency for patients with

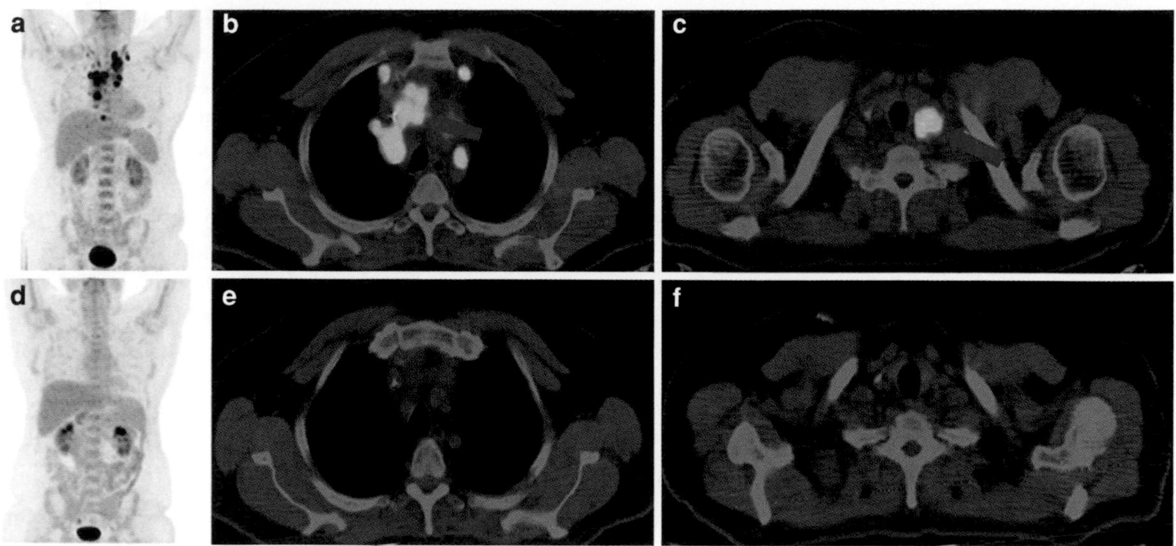

Fig. 5 Hodgkin lymphoma 50-year-old man presented with flu-like symptoms and swollen supraclavicular lymph nodes. Pretreatment PET/CT scan maximum intensity projection (**a**) and axial fused PET/CT (**b** and **c**) show multiple FDG-avid lymph nodes in supraclavicular, mediastinal, and internal mammary stations. The patient was treated with 6 cycles of ABVD. Post-therapy PET/CT maximum intensity projection (**d**) and axial fused PET/CT (**e** and **f**) demonstrate no evidence of persistent FDG-avid disease

advanced-stage HL or DLBCL to limit the number of patients undergoing potentially unnecessary radiotherapy. In the HL algorithm, patients receive 6 cycles of ABVD, followed by a 18F-FDG PET in patients with a residual mass $\geq$ 2 cm. Patients who are PET-negative receive no further therapy, while PET-positive patients receive consolidative radiotherapy. An initial review of this ongoing experience demonstrated that in 40 patients with a negative PET who were spared radiation therapy, the 2-year PFS was 91 % (Savage et al. 2007).

7 Brain Tumors

Assessment of response to therapy in both clinical and investigational neuro-oncology settings nearly always relies on contrast (gadolinium)-enhanced T1-weighted MRI. However, as described comprehensively by Dhermain et al., MRI suffers from remarkable shortcomings for this purpose: MRI is mainly influenced by vascular leakage, which makes it impossible to provide a specific measure of tumor size and activity (Dhermain et al. 2010). Hence, in some cases, changes in enhancement do not correlate well with response to treatment. Pseudoprogression (in which an increase in contrast uptake does not reflect tumor progression) and pseudoresponse (in which a decrease in contrast enhancement does not reflect tumor regression) are well-known difficulties with MRI in the assessment of response to treatment of gliomas, especially in the setting of anti-angiogenic therapies (Dhermain et al. 2010; Taal et al. 2008; Brandes et al. 2008; de Wit et al. 2004; Brandsma et al. 2008; Batchelor et al. 2007).

To overcome these shortcomings, PET has been actively tested in noninvasive assessment of glioma using various radiotracers. In fact, PET seems to provide a reliable alternative for the assessment of glioma response to treatment. 18F-FDG (a widely available radiotracer, but with the disadvantage of high uptake in normal brain), 11C-Met (which has much lower uptake by normal brain tissue, but requires an on-site cyclotron), and 18F-FLT or 18F-FET (low uptake by the normal brain tissue, but relatively expensive) are the most extensively studied radiotracers for monitoring response to treatment (Alexiou et al. 2010). Although initially it was claimed that the amount of 18F-FDG uptake strongly correlates with response to therapy in gliomas (a decrease in 18F-FDG uptake indicates a positive response) (van der Hiel et al. 2001; Chen et al. 2004;

Riemann et al. 2004), based on extensive studies and experience, currently 18F-FDG is considered unsuitable for detection of residual tumor after treatment. One of the main causes is the high cortical background activity. Also, a possible transient increase of 18F-FDG uptake in the initial phase is observed, which is most likely caused by infiltration of macrophages. Regarding this initial increased uptake, the effects of radiotherapy and chemotherapy only appear on 18F-FDG PET after a few weeks of treatment (Dhermain et al. 2010; Charnley et al. 2006; Ozsunar et al. 2010; Brock et al. 2000; Kim et al. 2005; Van Laere et al. 2005). Sensitivity and specificity of 18F-FDG PET for the detection of recurrent tumor compared to radiation necrosis has been reported to be 75 and 81 %, respectively (Chao et al. 2001). It seems that 18F-FDG PET has only negative but not positive predictive value for therapy assessment (Wurker et al. 1996). Because of the development of improved PET for detection of amino acids and 18F-FLT, centers with access to these radiotracers prefer not to use 18F-FDG PET in the assessment of treatment response of gliomas (Dhermain et al. 2010; Jacobs et al. 2005).

11C-Met PET and 18F-FLT PET are promising for following the effects of radiotherapy and chemotherapy, with higher interobserver agreement in image readings and interpretations (100 % for MET as compared to 73 % for 18F-FDG) (Van Laere et al. 2005). These radiotracers show a reduction of relative radiotracer uptake following successful treatment. 11C-Met PET and 18F-FET PET can detect response as soon as 2 weeks (Dhermain et al. 2010; Herholz et al. 2003; Galldiks et al. 2006; Wyss et al. 2009; Tsuyuguchi et al. 2004), much more reliably than MRI (Chen et al. 2007). In fact, deactivation of amino acid transport seems to be an early sign of chemotherapy response (Dhermain et al. 2010). 11C-methionine PET can differentiate between recurrent tumor and radiation necrosis with the detection of recurrent tumor with a sensitivity of 75 % and a specificity of 75 % (Dhermain et al. 2010). Providing quantitative values, the ratio of 11C-Met uptake of the tumor compared with uptake in the contralateral background frontal-lobe gray matter is the most informative index for discrimination of tumor recurrence and radiation necrosis, with a cutoff value of 1.58 to achieve the best accuracy (Terakawa et al. 2008).

18F-FET PET has been shown to be equivalently promising in the assessment of response after radiotherapy, radiosurgery, and multimodal treatment such as radioimmunotherapy (Dhermain et al. 2010), providing 92.9 % specificity and 100 % sensitivity, while the specificity of conventional MRI alone is only 50 %. It has been concluded that for patients with gliomas undergoing multimodal treatment or various forms of irradiation, conventional follow-up with MRI is insufficient to distinguish between benign side effects of therapy and tumor recurrence and 18F-FET PET is a more powerful tool to improve the differential diagnosis in these settings (Rachinger et al. 2005). After radioimmunotherapy, a cutoff tumor-to-background ratio of 2.4 for 18F-FET uptake allows the best differentiation between recurrence and reactive changes, providing sensitivity of 82 % and specificity of 100 % (Popperl et al. 2006). Further studies are needed to clarify the precise pharmacokinetics of 18F-FLT and 18F-FET and their role in the assessment of the response to treatment of gliomas, because the blood–brain barrier likely affects their uptake (Bradbury et al. 2008; Gerstner and Batchelor 2010).

Keeping in mind all the advantages and disadvantages of the available modalities, it has been recommended that morphological MRI should be considered as the basis of brain tumor response to therapy assessment; however, because the specificity of MRI post treatment is low, MRI should be combined with PET (Dhermain et al. 2010). Development of scanners that combine PET and MRI in a single unit could provide better assessment of response to treatment of glioma.

8 Ovarian Cancer

Despite the clinical absence of tumor and normalization of CA-125 levels following initial therapeutic intervention, 36–73 % of patients are found to have persistent ovarian cancer at the second-look laparotomy (Rose et al. 2001; Grigsby 2009). The predictive value of abdominal pelvic CT scanning in ovarian cancer patients who have completed chemotherapy is highly variable and even when combined with a normalization of initially elevated CA-125 levels, the predictive value of CT has been reported to be disappointingly low (Rose et al. 1996). The use of other tumor markers has not increased the sensitivity for persistent disease (Rose et al. 2001). Although an invasive operative procedure, second-look laparotomy remains the most sensitive and reliable method for determining the tumor status of patients with ovarian cancer who have had a complete clinical response following primary chemotherapy. There are advantages inherent to metabolic imaging, and 18F-FDG PET has been used before second-look surgery and the findings compared to the pathologic results, as a possible alternative approach. PET only (not integrated PET/CT) demonstrated 10 % sensitivity and 42 % specificity, even though technical modifications including bladder activity dilution, intravenous hydration with diuretic administration, and mechanical bowel preparations were used to reduce background activity (Rose et al. 2001). On the other hand, PET/CT has a more promising sensitivity and specificity of 78 and 75 %, respectively, for visualizing lesions prior to second-look surgery, when the lesions were more than 5 mm (Sironi et al. 2004). The superiority of PET/CT over PET alone is not surprising, because co-registered functional and anatomical information has been shown to be superior in detecting primary and metastatic tumors compared to single imaging procedures (Siegel and Dehdashti 2005).

As a tool for monitoring treatment of ovarian cancers, sequential 18F-FDG PET predicted patient outcome as early as after the first cycle of neoadjuvant chemotherapy and is more accurate than clinical or histopathologic response criteria, including alteration of tumor marker CA125. In fact, 18F-FDG PET/CT appears to be a promising tool for early prediction of response to chemotherapy (Baum and Przetak 2001; Avril et al. 2005). A significant correlation exists between 18F-FDG PET/CT metabolic response after the first and third cycle of chemotherapy and overall survival. By using a threshold for reduction in SUV from baseline of 20 % after the first cycle, median overall survival has been reported to be 38.3 months in metabolic responders compared with 23.1 months in metabolic nonresponders. At a threshold of 55 % reduction of SUV after the third cycle, median overall survival has been reported to be 38.9 months in metabolic responders compared with 19.7 months in nonresponders. The importance of 18F-FDG PET/CT findings is emphasized by the fact that there is no correlation between clinical response criteria or CA125 response criteria and overall survival. Also, there is only a weak correlation between histopathologic response criteria and overall survival (Avril et al. 2005). It has been shown that 18F-FDG PET/CT-derived parameters, including SUV and percentage change, have the potential to predict response to chemotherapy or chemoradiotherapy in patients with advanced gynecologic cancer, including uterine and ovarian cancers. When an arbitrary SUV of 3.8 is taken as the cutoff for differentiating between responders and nonresponders after therapy, 18F-FDG PET/CT shows a sensitivity of 90 %, a specificity of 63.6 %, and an accuracy of 76.2 %. When an arbitrary percentage change of 65 % is taken as the cutoff, 18F-FDG PET/CT shows the respective values of 90, 81.8, and 85.7 % (Nishiyama et al. 2008). As an alternative radiopharmaceutical, early response to therapy has been successfully monitored by quantitative PET using Cu-64-DOTA-trastuzumab. This approach may be valuable in monitoring the therapeutic response in HER-2-positive cancer patients (Niu et al. 2009).

9 Cancer of Cervix

18F-FDG PET has been used in the assessment of cervical cancer patients after the completion of treatment (Schwarz et al. 2009). At Washington University in St. Louis, 18F-FDG PET has been used for more than 10 years to assess response to chemoradiation for patients with carcinoma of the cervix (Schwarz et al. 2009). Schwarz et al. reported their experience on 378 patients, in which they divided the patients into 3 categories based on post-treatment 18F-FDG PET results: Complete metabolic response–absence of abnormal 18F-FDG uptake at sites of abnormal 18F-FDG uptake noted on the pretreatment 18F-FDG PET study; partial metabolic response–any persistent abnormal 18F-FDG uptake at the known sites; and progressive metabolic disease– new sites of abnormally increased 18F-FDG uptake. They found that post-treatment metabolic response is predictive of both cause-specific and progression-free survival after chemoradiation for cancer of cervix (Schwarz et al. 2009; Grigsby et al. 2004; Schwarz et al. 2007; Lin et al. 2006). The 3-year progression-free survival rates according to metabolic response in patients with complete metabolic response, partial metabolic response, and progressive disease were 78, 33, and 0 %, respectively (Lin et al. 2006). Investigators believe that in the future, FDG PET may be used to guide early interventions for patients with less than complete metabolic response. However, the current evidence comes from only a few institutions, and it is important to confirm the reproducibility of the results across imaging centers (Lin et al. 2006).

The same group has applied 18F-FDG PET during radiation therapy to obtain an early readout of tumor metabolic response. According to them, treatment

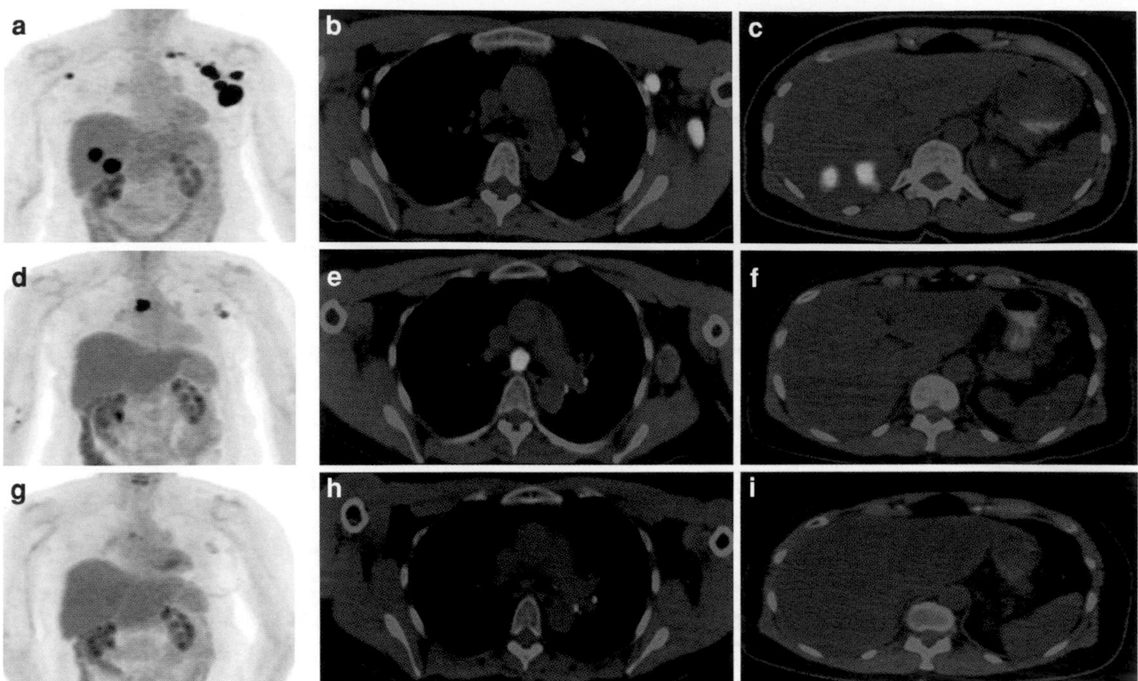

Fig. 6 Melanoma 50-year-old woman presented with enlarged left axillary nodes. Pretreatment PET/CT scan maximum intensity projection (**a**) and axial fused PET/CT (**b** and **c**) show multiple FDG-avid lymph nodes in supraclavicular and axillary stations with two FDG-avid hepatic metastases. The patient received chemotherapy followed by 32 months of anti-PD-1 antibody. One year after therapy PET/CT scan maximum intensity projection (**d**) and axial fused PET/CT (**e** and **f**) show very good treatment response for all initial lesions but in the interval developed a new FDG-avid subcarinal node. The patient was restarted on anti-PD-1 antibody treatment. One year after reinitiated therapy PET/CT scan maximum intensity projection (**g**) and axial fused PET/CT (**h** and **i**) demonstrate near resolution of FDG-avid subcarinal node without new FDG-avid disease

regimens (including radiation dose with or without chemotherapy drugs) could be modified, based on 18F-FDG PET in the therapy planning and monitoring. Despite promising preliminary data on the use of 18F-FDG PET during radiation therapy for primary tumors, the authors did not suggest an optimal time for performing 18F-FDG PET during therapy (Lin et al. 2006). Also recently, Olsen et al. showed that even among women whose squamous cell carcinoma antigen normalized at the completion of radiotherapy, almost 40 % had persistent or new disease on post-treatment 18F-FDG PET/CT, affirming the importance of post-treatment 18F-FDG PET/CT evaluation (Olsen et al. 2010).

Unlike radiation or chemoradiation therapy, the use of 18F-FDG PET to monitor response to chemotherapy alone or neoadjuvant chemotherapy with planned surgical resection is still investigational, and the available reports are limited to case reports and case series (Dose et al. 2000; Yoshida et al. 2004). These findings should be interpreted with caution because of the very small sample size and a nontraditional approach to treatment planning (Lin et al. 2006).

10 Melanoma

Melanoma is the most aggressive cutaneous malignancy with an increasing rate of incidence in the recent decades (Petrescu et al. 2010). Adjuvant treatment in advanced stages of the disease (including chemotherapy, unspecific immunotherapy and interferon) often offer poor results, and hence just expose the patients to the adverse effects of chemotherapy with no clinical beneficial effect (Petrescu et al. 2010). In fact, despite all new knowledge and technological progress, advanced-stage melanoma management still remains an unsolved problem. Preliminary evidence suggests that PET/CT can be considered as a valuable tool to prevent futile treatments in these settings and provide a guide for the management of melanoma patients (Hofman et al. 2007; Yoshimoto et al. 2007). However, much research is needed before this is included in routine clinical practice (Nicol et al. 2008).

There is a statistically significant agreement between 18F-FDG PET/CT and CT regarding response to chemotherapy. There is a clear trend to longer survival of PET/CT responders as compared to PET/CT nonresponders, with a remarkably better 1-year survival of 80 % compared to 40 % (Fig. 6). There is a significantly longer progression-free survival of PET/CT responders compared with PET/CT nonresponders. As chemotherapy response assessment with serum S-100B tumor marker fails to show correlation with survival, 18F-FDG PET/CT may present a promising tool (Strobel et al. 2008). Strobel et al. also reached to the same conclusion. They stated that in a third of melanoma patients with metastases, the S-100B tumor marker is not suitable for therapy assessment and in these cases, imaging techniques remain necessary. In this subset of patients, 18F-FDG PET/CT can be used for response assessment (Strobel et al. 2007). In many clinical trials, CT remains the modality of choice for the assessment of the response to treatment in patients with stage IV melanoma. The main advantage of 18F-FDG PET/CT over CT is that this method provides the combination of morphological and metabolic information. The accuracy of 18F-FDG PET/CT for M staging is significantly higher than that of PET alone and CT alone (98 vs. 93 and 84 %) (Reinhardt et al. 2002). The criteria for accurate therapy response assessment using PET/CT are yet to be defined, but it has been stated that measurements such as total lesion glycolysis (delta TLG) may not be better than the simpler and more reproducible SUV_{max} measurements for interpretation of the results (Strobel et al. 2007).

As 18F-FDG is relatively nonspecific for melanoma, new melanoma-directed PET/CT radiopharmaceuticals should become available. As neuroendocrine tumors (carcinoids, pheochromocytoma, neuroblastoma, medullary thyroid cancer, microcytoma, carotid glomus tumors, and melanoma) show increased levels of L-DOPA decarboxylase, they also show a high uptake of 18F-DOPA (Caroli et al. 2010; Dimitrakopoulou-Strauss et al. 2001). It is possible that 18F-DOPA may provide a suitable target for PET imaging of melanoma patients, particularly for patients with negative 18F-FDG findings (Dimitrakopoulou-Strauss et al. 2001).

PET has also been applied for choroidal melanoma with promising results (Finger and Chin 2011). Following a cohort of 217 patients diagnosed with uveal melanoma and eligible for ophthalmic plaque brachytherapy, it was shown that treatment-related diminished SUV may correlate to both local control and loss of ability of choroidal melanoma to metastasize over time (Finger and Chin 2011). It was concluded that PET/CT imaging can be used to assess choroidal melanomas for their response to treatment. Larger studies to prove this possible application are highly warranted.

11 Head and Neck Tumors

Based on the available evidence, PET provides a valuable tool to assess the response to treatment of head and neck cancers (Ceulemans et al. 2010; Gupta et al. 2010; Kikuchi et al. 2010; Passero et al. 2010; Farrag et al. 2010; Bussink et al. 2010; Schoder et al. 2009; Andrade et al. 2006; Nam et al. 2005; Yao et al. 2004; Kostakoglu and Goldsmith 2004; Sakamoto et al. 1998) (Fig. 7). A negative PET scan on combined 18F-FDG PET/CT after chemoradiotherapy is a powerful predictor of outcome, not only in conventional chemoradiotherapy regimens (Passero et al. 2010), but also in those treated with novel targeted anticancer therapeutics such as epidermal growth factor receptor tyrosine kinase inhibitors (e.g. Erlotinib) (Vergez et al. 2010). Geets et al. showed that the tumor volumes based on mid-treatment 18F-FDG PET are significantly smaller than those from anatomical imaging modalities, which results in a 15–40 % reduction of the irradiated volume compared with the pretreatment CT-scan. The authors suggested that weekly 18F-FDG PET monitoring during radiotherapy could be used to modify or reduce the treated volume of pharyngolaryngeal tumors (Geets et al. 2007).

A remarkable number of studies have concentrated on the optimal interval after treatment to perform PET/CT (Bussink et al. 2010; Greven et al. 2001). Greven et al. found that specificity and sensitivity of 18F-FDG PET for detection of residual or recurrent tumor at 1 month is 95 and 59 %, respectively (Greven et al. 2001). At 4 months, specificity remains

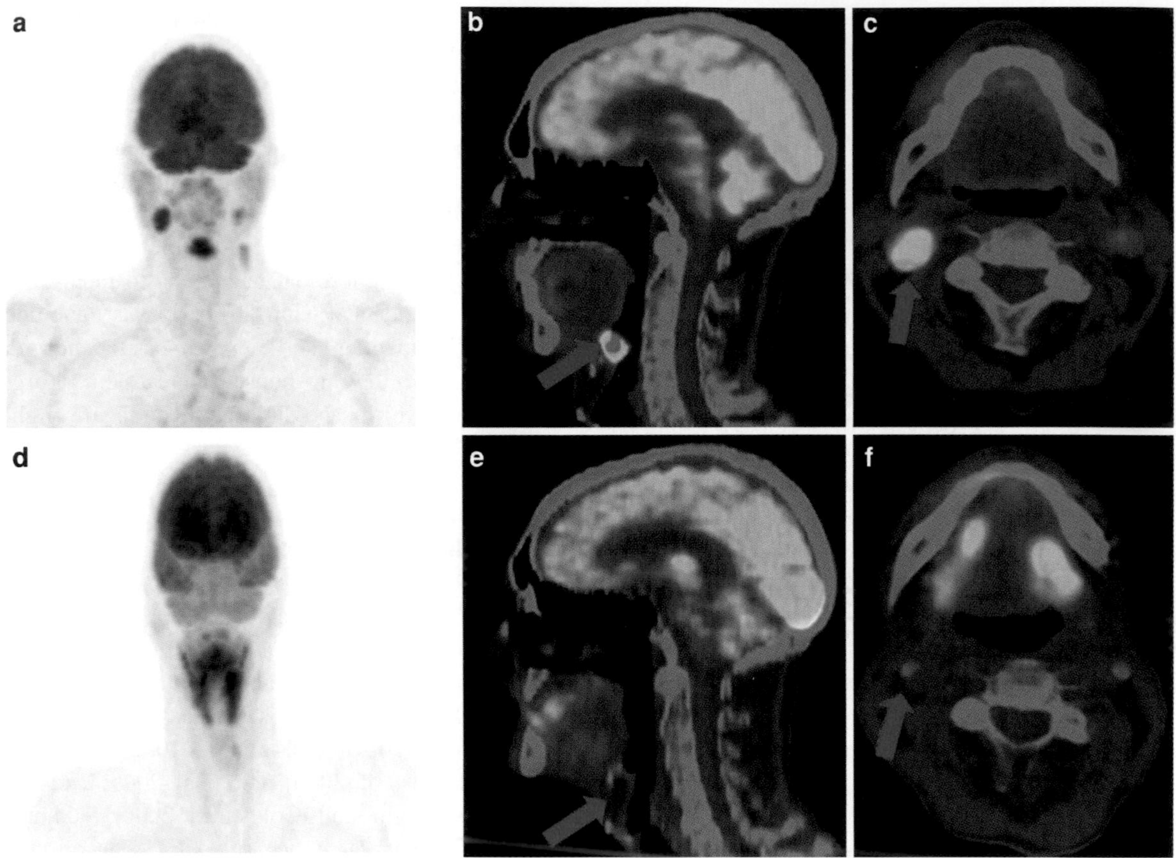

Fig. 7 Head and neck cancer 68-year-old man presented with dysphagia and odynophagia. Pretreatment PET/CT scan maximum intensity projection (**a**), sagittal fused PET/CT image (**b**), and axial fused PET/CT (**c**) demonstrate a vallecular FDG-avid mass with bilateral level IIA metastatic lymph nodes. The patient received cisplatin-based concurrent chemoradiation therapy (total dose of 70 Gy in 35 fractions). The post-therapy PET/CT maximum intensity projection (**d**), sagittal fused PET/CT image (**e**), and axial fused PET/CT (**f**) demonstrate no evidence of FDG-avid persistent disease

high at 90 %, but sensitivity improves to 100 %. Therefore, the optimum time to assess the response to treatment is between 1 and 4 months (Greven et al. 2001). Andrade et al. also showed that all false-negative and false-positive 18F-FDG PET/CT results occur between 4 and 8 weeks after treatment (Andrade et al. 2006). In contrast to PET studies of 4 months after radiotherapy, the sensitivity of PET study at the end of week 4 is low. Therefore, evaluation of the tumor response with 18F-FDG PET at 4 months after radiotherapy completion cannot be replaced by 18F-FDG PET during radiotherapy (Ceulemans et al. 2010). Finally, Isles et al. recommended an interval of at least 10 weeks between completion of treatment and 18F-FDG PET. In their meta-analysis, the pooled sensitivity and specificity of PET for detecting residual or recurrent head and neck squamous cell carcinoma in 27 studies were 94 % [95 % CI, 87–97 %] and 82 % (95 % CI, 76–86 %), respectively. Positive and negative predictive values were also high, at the level of 75 % (95 % CI, 68–82 %) and 95 % (95 % CI, 92–97 %), respectively. The authors proposed a protocol for the application of PET/CT in post-treatment surveillance of patients with head and neck cancers (Isles et al. 2008). In our clinical practice, we recommend an interval of 12 weeks after completion of radiation therapy to decrease the inflammatory uptake and false positive FDG PET/CT studies.

Although 18F-FDG PET/CT will remain the major clinical tool for monitoring treatment in head and neck cancers, other PET radiotracers have also been investigated for identifying response to treatment (Schoder et al. 2009; Heuveling et al. 2011). Hypoxia

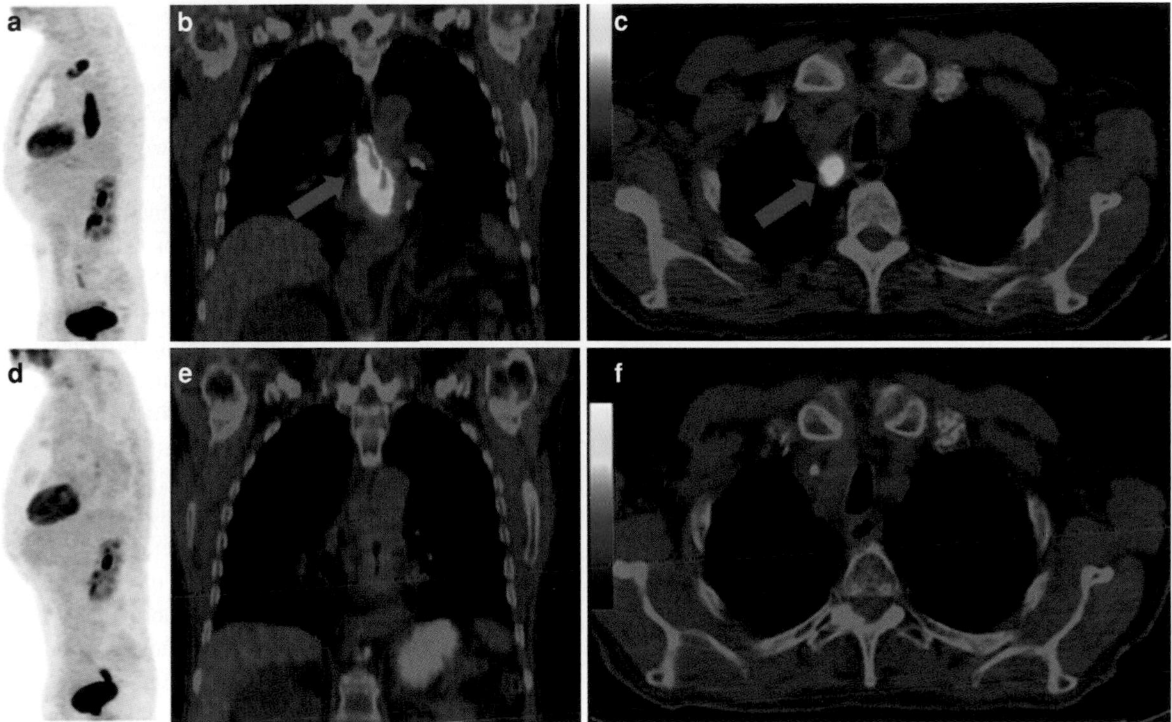

Fig. 8 Esophageal cancer 79-year-old man presented with increasing fatigue, decreased hematocrit,and positive occult blood testing. Pretreatment PET/CT scan maximum intensity projection (**a**) and fused PET/CT (**b** and **c**) demonstrate FDG-avid mid-to-distal esophageal mass with upper paraesophageal lymph nodes. He was treated with two cycles of neoadjuvant FOLFOX chemotherapy followed by concurrent chemoradiotherapy of the mediastinum (total of 41 Gy in 23 fractions) with additional esophageal boost (90 Gy in 5 fractions). Post therapy PET/CT maximum intensity projection (**d**) and fused PET/CT (**e** and **f**) demonstrate no evidence of persistent FDG-avid lesion

imaging using 18F-FMISO incorporation during a course of platinum-based, intensity-modulated chemoradiotherapy was not promising, as neither the presence nor the absence of hypoxia on the mid-treatment PET scan correlated with patient outcome Lee et al. (2009c). Although hypoxia imaging using 18F-FAZA in animal models was promising (Solomon et al. 2005), no human study is available. In contrast, 18F-FLT tumor cell proliferation imaging seems to be successful for this purpose, with highly reproducible results. 18F-FLT uptake changes greatly early after start of treatment (Bussink et al. 2010). A reduction of 20–25 % in SUV_{max}, which has been shown to be greater than reproducibility error or temporal fluctuation, has been considered as treatment related (de Langen et al. 2009). Based on Troost et al., after five daily 2 Gy fractions of radiotherapy, a more than twofold decrease of 18F-FLT uptake in tumors is achieved, which increases to a fourfold reduction at the fourth week post treatment (Troost et al. 2010). However, the authors stated that quantification of tracer uptake reduction is not always straightforward: in oropharyngeal tumors, radiotherapy leads to an increase in tracer uptake in the tonsillar region, probably due to proliferation of inflammatory cells, which limits the accuracy of the response using 18F-FLT PET (Troost et al. 2010).

In conclusion, PET is highly accurate in the assessment of the response to treatment of head and neck cancers. It is less sensitive early after treatment but reaches a high accuracy within 10 weeks following the completion of treatment. PET may significantly reduce the necessity for check endoscopies and planned neck dissections in the treatment monitoring of patients with head and neck cancers. Reduction in signal intensity, which is a clear indication of cellular response to treatment, largely precedes changes in tumor volume, as seen in static anatomical imaging methods, and can help to redirect treatment.

12 Esophageal Cancers

Although single-center studies have provided promising results, prospective randomized multicenter trials will have to be performed to address the applicability of 18F-FDG PET/CT in assessing the response of patients with esophageal cancer and monitoring of treatment (Krause et al. 2009). Similar to other tumors, it has been emphasized that PET/CT, by combining volumetric and metabolic data, may be even more accurate for assessing histopathologic tumor response in patients with esophageal cancer (Krause et al. 2009) (Fig. 8). In assessing the tumor response after completion of therapy, residual 18F-FDG uptake after treatment or any changes in 18F-FDG uptake between pretreatment and posttherapy scan are correlated to postoperative histopathologic response and/or patient survival (Krause et al. 2009). It has been emphasized that 18F-FDG uptake in patients responding to therapy should decrease to the background level, and any residual 18F-FDG accumulation indicates viable tumor tissue in most cases. According to Krause et al. it is not necessary to perform a quantitative analysis on 18F-FDG PET/CT studies (Krause et al. 2009).

Tumor response can be assessed early during the course of chemotherapy or chemoradiotherapy. For such a purpose, the first mid-treatment scan is performed 2–4 weeks after initiation of the first therapy cycle. Metabolic activity in the tumor tissue most probably will be reduced in responders, but at the time of the early mid-treatment scan there will still be a considerable number of viable tumor cells, leading to significant remnant 18F-FDG uptake (Krause et al. 2009). In this setting, a reduction of more than 35 % in baseline SUV_{mean} allows prediction of clinical response with a sensitivity and specificity of 93 and 95 %, respectively (Weber et al. 2001). These features have been confirmed by Wieder et al. who reported the respective sensitivity and specificity of 93 % and 88 %, keeping a reduction of more than 30 % in baseline SUV as the cutoff point (Wieder et al. 2004). As expected, higher cutoff values (e.g. 40 % reduction in SUV) result in lower sensitivity (Krause et al. 2009). In fact, although 18F-FDG PET currently seems to be the best imaging modality for the assessment of response to therapy in patients with esophageal cancer, there is no currently available guideline or consensus for the optimal timing of 18F-FDG PET in these settings (Kim et al. 2009). These results are encouraging regarding the high sensitivities and specificities, given that no other imaging modality or surrogate marker is currently available to provide a more accurate early prediction of response to therapy. One should remember that if radiotherapy is included in the treatment plan, non-specific 18F-FDG accumulation in inflammatory lesions may cause overestimation of 18F-FDG uptake due to radiation-mediated inflammatory processes, which may persist from weeks to months, potentially influencing the assessment of changes in glucose metabolism for the purpose of response to therapy assessment (Rosenberg et al. 2009).

The MUNICON study prospectively evaluated the feasibility and potential effect on prognosis of administering PET-response-guided chemotherapy to patients with locally advanced adenocarcinoma of the esophagus and the esophagogastric junction: metabolic responders (after 2 weeks of induction chemotherapy) continued to receive chemotherapy for a maximum of 12 weeks before undergoing surgery, while metabolic nonresponders discontinued chemotherapy only after 2 weeks and tumors were immediately resected. Such an approach seems a promising path to personalized treatment for patients with esophageal cancer. After a median follow-up of 2.3 years, median overall survival was not reached in metabolic responders, while median overall survival was 25.8 months in nonresponders (hazard ratio: 2.13 [1-14-3.99]). Median event-free survival was 29.7 months in metabolic responders and 14.1 months in nonresponders (hazard ratio: 2.18 [1-32-3.62]). Major histological remissions (< 10 % residual tumor) were noted in 58 % of metabolic responders, but none of the metabolic nonresponders (Lordick et al. 2007). This study confirmed the feasibility of a PET-guided treatment algorithm and is a step toward treatment based on individual tumor biology. (Lordick et al. 2007).

13 Conclusion

PET is becoming established as a reliable and clinically useful technique for treatment monitoring of cancers. There is now a considerable amount of evidence that PET, PET/CT provide accurate assessment of tumor response to chemotherapy and chemoradiotherapy. This has been extensively confirmed for NSCLC, malignant lymphomas and breast cancer, and a variety of other solid tumors. Available data show that 18F-FDG PET/CT predicts response to treatment very effectively with sensitivity, specificity, and accuracy of 83–100 %, 85–94 %, and 88–91 % in breast cancer, and 90, 100, and 96 % in lung cancer. Based on current knowledge, PET/CT not only evaluates response to treatment, but can also help to define significant time points of progression.

PET is currently poised to become a necessary tool for treatment monitoring in oncologic settings. The need for further studies remains and it is likely that more well-designed and large clinical studies on PET/CT will expand its approved clinical indications in this context. It is crucial to follow a strict protocol for image acquisition, reconstruction, and data analysis in order to obtain robust and reproducible quantitative data from 18F-FDG PET scans. There are encouraging data that quantitative assessment 18F-FDG PET images facilitate prediction of tumor response early in the course of therapy. Currently, the majority of PET/CT studies for the purpose of prediction of response to treatment and therapy monitoring, use 18F-FDG as the tracer; however, the changing demand to assess tumor angiogenesis, cell proliferation, tumor hypoxia, and receptors has led to development of specific tracers, which should find great clinical acceptance in the near future.

References

Adams MC et al (2010) A systematic review of the factors affecting accuracy of SUV measurements. AJR Am J Roentgenol 195(2):310–320

Akhurst T et al (2002) An initial experience with FDG-PET in the imaging of residual disease after induction therapy for lung cancer. Ann Thorac Surg 73(1):259–264 discussion 264-6

Akhurst T et al (2005) Recent chemotherapy reduces the sensitivity of [18F]fluorodeoxyglucose positron emission tomography in the detection of colorectal metastases. J Clin Oncol 23(34):8713–8716

Alexiou GA et al (2010) Assessment of glioma proliferation using imaging modalities. J Clin Neurosci 17(10):1233–1238

Allen AM et al (2009) Early prediction of radiation response of brain metastases with [F-18]-ML-10: a novel molecular PET imaging agent for apoptosis. Int J Radiat Oncol Biol Phys 75(3):S44

Allen-Auerbach M, Weber WA (2009) Measuring Response with FDG-PET: Methodological Aspects. Oncologist 14(4):369–377

Amthauer H et al (2004) Response prediction by FDG-PET after neoadjuvant radiochemotherapy and combined regional hyperthermia of rectal cancer: correlation with endorectal ultrasound and histopathology. Eur J Nucl Med Mol Imaging 31(6):811–819

Andrade RS et al (2006) Posttreatment assessment of response using FDG-PET/CT for patients treated with definitive radiation therapy for head and neck cancers. Int J Radiat Oncol Biol Phys 65(5):1315–1322

Antoch G et al (2005) Assessment of liver tissue after radiofrequency ablation: findings with different imaging procedures. J Nucl Med 46(3):520–525

Aoyagi K et al (1999) Detection of malignant tumors with whole-boby PET using F-18 alpha-methyl tyrosine: comparison with whole-body FDG PET. J Nucl Med 40(5):229p

Apisarnthanarax S et al (2006) Early detection of chemoradioresponse in esophageal carcinoma by 3 '-deoxy-3 '-H-3-fluorothymidine using preclinical tumor models. Clin Cancer Res 12(15):4590–4597

Aschoff AJ et al (2000) Thermal lesion conspicuity following interstitial radiofrequency thermal tumor ablation in humans: a comparison of STIR, turbo spin-echo T2-weighted, and contrast-enhanced T1-weighted MR images at 0.2 T. J Magn Reson Imaging 12(4):584–589

Avallone A et al (2009) Circulating endothelial cells (CECs) and FDG-PET for early prediction of response in high-risk locally advanced rectal cancer (HR-LARC) patients (pts) treated with two different schedules of bevacizumab (BEV) in combination with preoperative chemo-radiotherapy (CT-RT). EJC Suppl 7(2):358–358

Avril N et al (2005) Prediction of response to neoadjuvant chemotherapy by sequential F-18-fluorodeoxyglucose positron emission tomography in patients with advanced-stage ovarian cancer. J Clin Oncol 23(30):7445–7453

Avril N, Sassen S, Roylance R (2009) Response to therapy in breast cancer. J Nucl Med 50(Suppl 1):55S–63S

Backes H et al (2009) Noninvasive quantification of (18)F-FLT human brain PET for the assessment of tumour proliferation in patients with high-grade glioma. Eur J Nucl Med Mol Imaging 36(12):1960–1967

Barrington SF, Carr R (1995) Staging of Burkitt's lymphoma and response to treatment monitored by PET scanning. Clin Oncol (R Coll Radiol) 7(5):334–335

Barthel H et al (2003) 3 '-deoxy-3 '-[F-18]fluorothymidine as a new marker for monitoring tumor response to antiproliferative therapy in vivo with positron emission tomography. Cancer Res 63(13):3791–3798

Barwick T et al (2009) Molecular PET and PET/CT imaging of tumour cell proliferation using F-18 fluoro-L-thymidine: a comprehensive evaluation. Nucl Med Commun 30(12):908–917

Batchelor TT et al (2007) AZD2171, a pan-VEGF receptor tyrosine kinase inhibitor, normalizes tumor vasculature and alleviates edema in glioblastoma patients. Cancer Cell 11(1):83–95

Baum RP, Przetak C (2001) Evaluation of therapy response in breast and ovarian cancer patients by positron emission tomography (PET). Q J Nucl Med 45(3):257–268

Belhocine TZ, Blankenberg FG (2006) The imaging of apoptosis with the radiolabelled annexin A5: a new tool in translational research. Curr Clin Pharmacol 1(2):129–137

Belhocine T et al (2004) The imaging of apoptosis with the radiolabeled annexin V: optimal timing for clinical feasibility. Technol Cancer Res Treat 3(1):23–32

Bender H et al (1999) Possible role of FDG-PET in the early prediction of therapy outcome in liver metastases of colorectal cancer. Hybridoma 18(1):87–91

Berriolo-Riedinger A et al (2007) [F-18]FDG-PET predicts complete pathological response of breast cancer to neoadjuvant chemotherapy. Eur J Nucl Med Mol Imaging 34(12): 1915–1924

Bishton MJ et al (2008) A prospective study of the separate predictive capabilities of 18[F]-FDG-PET and molecular response in patients with relapsed indolent non-Hodgkin's lymphoma following treatment with iodine-131-rituximab radio-immunotherapy. Haematologica 93(5):789–790

Blankenberg FG (2008a) Monitoring of treatment-induced apoptosis in oncology with PET and SPECT. Curr Pharm Des 14(28):2974–2982

Blankenberg FG (2008b) In vivo imaging of apoptosis. Cancer Biol Ther 7(10):1525–1532

Blankenberg FG (2008c) In vivo detection of apoptosis. J Nucl Med 49(Suppl 2):81S–95S

Blankenberg FG (2009a) Imaging the molecular signatures of apoptosis and injury with radiolabeled annexin V. Proc Am Thorac Soc 6(5):469–476

Blankenberg FG (2009b) Apoptosis imaging: anti-cancer agents in medicinal chemistry. Anticancer Agents Med Chem 9(9):944–951

Blankenberg F, Ohtsuki K, Strauss HW (1999a) Dying a thousand deaths. Radionuclide imaging of apoptosis. Q J Nucl Med 43(2):170–176

Blankenberg FG et al (1999b) Imaging of apoptosis (programmed cell death) with 99 mTc annexin V. J Nucl Med 40(1):184–191

Blankenberg FG et al (2006) Radiolabeling of HYNIC-annexin V with technetium-99 m for in vivo imaging of apoptosis. Nat Protoc 1(1):108–110

Boellaard R et al (2008) The Netherlands protocol for standardisation and quantification of FDG whole body PET studies in multi-centre trials. Eur J Nucl Med Mol Imaging 35(12):2320–2333

Bradbury MS et al (2008) Dynamic small-animal PET Imaging of tumor proliferation with 3 '-Deoxy-3 '-F-18-fluorothymidine in a genetically engineered mouse model of high-grade gliomas. J Nucl Med 49(3):422–429

Brandes AA et al (2008) MGMT promoter methylation status can predict the incidence and outcome of pseudoprogression after concomitant radiochemotherapy in newly diagnosed glioblastoma patients. J Clin Oncol 26(13):2192–2197

Brandsma D et al (2008) Clinical features, mechanisms, and management of pseudoprogression in malignant gliomas. Lancet Oncol 9(5):453–461

Brat DJ, Mapstone TB (2003) Malignant glioma physiology: cellular response to hypoxia and its role in tumor progression. Ann Intern Med 138(8):659–668

Brepoels L et al (2009) F-18-FDG and F-18-FLT uptake early after cyclophosphamide and mTOR Inhibition in an experimental lymphoma model. J Nucl Med 50(7):1102–1109

Brock CS et al (2000) Early evaluation of tumour metabolic response using [F-18]fluorodeoxyglucose and positron emission tomography: a pilot study following the phase II chemotherapy schedule for temozolomide in recurrent high-grade gliomas. Br J Cancer 82(3):608–615

Buyse M et al (2000) Relation between tumour response to first-line chemotherapy and survival in advanced colorectal cancer: a meta-analysis. Lancet 356(9227):373–378

Buck AK et al (2003) Imaging proliferation in lung tumors with PET: 18F-FLT versus 18F-FDG. J Nucl Med 44(9):1426–1431

Busk M et al (2009) Can hypoxia-PET map hypoxic cell density heterogeneity accurately in an animal tumor model at a clinically obtainable image contrast? Radiother Oncol 92(3):429–436

Busk M et al (2010) Assessing hypoxia in animal tumor models based on pharmocokinetic analysis of dynamic FAZA PET. Acta Oncol 49(7):922–933

Bussink J et al (2010) PET-CT for response assessment and treatment adaptation in head and neck cancer. Lancet Oncol 11(7):661–669

Bystrom P et al (2009) Early prediction of response to first-line chemotherapy by sequential [F-18]-2-fluoro-2-deoxy-D-glucose positron emission tomography in patients with advanced colorectal cancer. Ann Oncol 20(6):1057–1061

Caroli P et al (2010) Non-FDG PET in the practice of oncology. Indian J Cancer 47(2):120–125

Casciari JJ, Graham MM, Rasey JS (1995) A modeling approach for quantifying tumor hypoxia with [F-18] fluoromisonidazole pet time-activity data. Med Phys 22(7):1127–1139

Cerfolio RJ et al (2004) Repeat FDG-PET after neoadjuvant therapy is a predictor of pathologic response in patients with non-small cell lung cancer. Ann Thorac Surg 78(6): 1903–1909

Ceulemans G et al (2010) Can 18-FDG-PET During Radiotherapy Replace Post-Therapy Scanning for Detection/ Demonstration of Tumor Response in Head-and-Neck Cancer? Int J Radiat Oncol Biol Phys 81(4):938–942

Chao ST et al (2001) The sensitivity and specificity of FDG PET in distinguishing recurrent brain tumor from radionecrosis in patients treated with stereotactic radiosurgery. Int J Cancer 96(3):191–197

Charnley N et al (2006) Early change in glucose metabolic rate measured using FDG-PET in patients with high-grade glioma predicts response to temozolomide but not temozolomide plus radiotherapy. Int J Radiat Oncol Biol Phys 66(2):331–338

Chen YR et al (2004) Value of 18F-FDG PET imaging in diagnosing tumor residue of intracranial glioma after surgery and radiotherapy. Ai Zheng 23(10):1210–1212

Chen W et al (2007) Predicting treatment response of malignant gliomas to bevacizumab and irinotecan by imaging proliferation with [F-18] fluorothymidine positron emission tomography: a pilot study. J Clin Oncol 25(30):4714–4721

Chesnay E et al (2003) Early response to chemotherapy in hypopharyngeal cancer: Assessment with C-11-methionine PET, correlation with morphologic response, and clinical outcome. J Nucl Med 44(4):526–532

Cheson BD (2007a) The International Harmonization Project for response criteria in lymphoma clinical trials. Hematol Oncol Clin North Am 21(5):841–854

Cheson BD et al (2007b) Revised response criteria for malignant lymphoma. J Clin Oncol 25(5):579–586

Choi NC et al (2002) Dose-response relationship between probability of pathologic tumor control and glucose metabolic rate measured with FDG pet after preoperative chemoradiotherapy in locally advanced non-small-cell lung cancer. Int J Radiat Oncol Biol Phys 54(4):1024–1035

Czernin J, Allen-Auerbach M, Schelbert HR (2007) Improvements in cancer staging with PET/CT: literature-based evidence as of September 2006. J Nucl Med 48(Suppl 1):78S–88S
de Geus-Oei LF et al (2008) Chemotherapy response evaluation with FDG-PET in patients with colorectal cancer. Ann Oncol 19(2):348–352
de Geus-Oei LF et al (2009) Monitoring and predicting response to therapy with 18F-FDG PET in colorectal cancer: a systematic review. J Nucl Med 50(Suppl 1):43S–54S
de Langen AJ et al (2009) Reproducibility of quantitative F-18-3'-deoxy-3'-fluorothymidine measurements using positron emission tomography. Eur J Nucl Med Mol Imaging 36(3): 389–395
de Langen AJ et al (2011) Monitoring Response to Antiangiogenic Therapy in Non-Small Cell Lung Cancer Using Imaging Markers Derived from PET and Dynamic Contrast-Enhanced MRI. J Nucl Med 52(1):48–55
De Leyn P et al (2006) Prospective comparative study of integrated positron emission tomography-computed tomography scan compared with remediastinoscopy in the assessment of residual mediastinal lymph node disease after induction chemotherapy for mediastinoscopy proven stage IIIA-N2 non-small-cell lung cancer: A Leuven lung cancer group study. J Clin Oncol 24(21):3333–3339
De Ridder M et al (2009) Prediction of response to neo-adjuvant radiotherapy in patients with locally advanced rectal cancer by means of sequential 18F-FDG-PET. EJC Suppl 7(4):15–15
De Ridder M et al (2010) Prediction of response to neo-adjuvant radiotherapy in patients with locally advanced rectal cancer by means of sequential 18f-Fdg-Pet. Ann Oncol 21:I55–I55
de Vries E et al (2009) Molecular imaging of breast cancer. Breast 18:S8–S9
de Wit MCY et al (2004) Immediate post-radiotherapy changes in malignant glioma can mimic tumor progression. Neurology 63(3):535–537
Dehdashti F, Flanagan FL, Siegel BA (1997) PET assessment of metabolic flare in advanced breast cancer. Radiology 205:340–340
Dehdashti F et al (1999) Positron emission tomographic assessment of "metabolic flare" to predict response of metastatic breast cancer to antiestrogen therapy. Eur J Nucl Med 26(1):51–56
Dehdashti F et al (2000) Evaluation of tumor hypoxia with Cu-60 ATSM and PET. J Nucl Med 41(5):34p
Dehdashti F et al (2008) Assessing tumor hypoxia in cervical cancer by PET with Cu-60-labeled diacetyl-bis(N-4-methylthiosemicarbazone). J Nucl Med 49(2):201–205
Delgado-Bolton RC, Delgado JLC (2009) Positron emission tomography (PET) in the evaluation of response to therapy in non-small cell lung cancer. Curr Cancer Ther Rev 5:20–27
Dhermain FG et al (2010) Advanced MRI and PET imaging for assessment of treatment response in patients with gliomas. Lancet Neurology 9(9):906–920
Dietz D et al (2007) Tumor hypoxia predicts response to neoadjuvant chemoradiation therapy in rectal cancer: results of a pilot study of the novel hypoxia-detecting 60Cu-ATSM PET scan. Dis Colon Rectum 50(5):780
Dimitrakopoulou-Strauss A, Strauss LG, Burger C (2001) Quantitative PET studies in pretreated melanoma patients: A comparison of 6-[F-18] fluoro-L-dopa with F-18-FDG and O-15-water using compartment and noncompartment analysis. J Nucl Med 42(2):248–256
Dimitrakopoulou-Strauss A, Strauss LG, Rudi J (2003) PET-FDG as predictor of therapy response in patients with colorectal carcinoma. Q J Nucl Med 47(1):8–13
Dimitrakopoulou-Strauss A et al (2004) Prognostic aspects of 18F-FDG PET kinetics in patients with metastatic colorectal carcinoma receiving FOLFOX chemotherapy. J Nucl Med 45(9):1480–1487
Dittmann H et al (2009) 3'-Deoxy-3'-[(18)F]fluorothymidine (FLT) uptake in breast cancer cells as a measure of proliferation after doxorubicin and docetaxel treatment. Nucl Med Biol 36(2):163–169
Donckier V et al (2003) [F-18] fluorodeoxyglucose positron emission tomography as a tool for early recognition of incomplete tumor destruction after radiofrequency ablation for liver metastases. J Surg Oncol 84(4):215–223
Dooms C et al (2008) Prognostic stratification of stage IIIA-N2 non-small-cell lung cancer after induction chemotherapy: a model based on the combination of morphometric-pathologic response in mediastinal nodes and primary tumor response on serial 18-fluoro-2-deoxy-glucose positron emission tomography. J Clin Oncol 26(7):1128–1134
Dose J, Hemminger GE, Bohuslavizki KH (2000) Therapy monitoring using FDG-PET in metastatic cervical cancer. Lancet Oncol 1:106
Dunleavy K et al (2010) The value of positron emission tomography in prognosis and response assessment in non-Hodgkin lymphoma. Leuk Lymphoma 51(Suppl 1):28–33
Eich HT et al (2008a) Response-adapted therapy using FDG-PET after BEACOPP-chemotherapy in advanced stage Hodgkin's lymphoma—An interim analysis of the German Hodgkin Study Group (GHSG) trial HD15. Int J Radiat Oncol Biol Phys 72(1):S471–S471
Eich HT et al (2008b) FDG-PET for treatment response assessment in advanced stage Hodgkin Lymphoma - report on the 2nd interim analysis of GHSG trial HD15. Strahlenther Onkol 184:11–11
Eisenhauer EA et al (2009) New response evaluation criteria in solid tumours: revised RECIST guideline (version 1.1). Eur J Cancer 45(2):228–247
Engenhart R et al (1992) Therapy monitoring of presacral recurrences after high-dose irradiation: value of PET, CT, CEA and pain score. Strahlenther Onkol 168(4):203–212
Eradat J et al (2011) Evaluation of treatment response after nonoperative therapy for early-stage non-small cell lung carcinoma. Cancer J 17(1):38–48
Erdi YE et al (2000) Use of PET to monitor the response of lung cancer to radiation treatment. Eur J Nucl Med 27(7): 861–866
Escalona S et al (2010) A systematic review of FDG-PET in breast cancer. Med Oncol 27(1):114–129
Everitt S et al (2009) Imaging cellular proliferation during chemo-radiotherapy: a pilot study of serial F-18-Flt positron emission tomography/computed tomography imaging for non-small-cell lung cancer. Int J Radiat Oncol Biol Phys 75(4):1098–1104

Farrag A et al (2010) Can 18F-FDG-PET response during radiotherapy be used as a predictive factor for the outcome of head and neck cancer patients? Nucl Med Commun 31(6):495–501

Findlay M et al (1996) Noninvasive monitoring of tumor metabolism using fluorodeoxyglucose and positron emission tomography in colorectal cancer liver metastases: correlation with tumor response to fluorouracil. J Clin Oncol 14(3):700–708

Finger PT, Chin KJ (2011) [(18)F]Fluorodeoxyglucose positron emission tomography/computed tomography (PET/CT) physiologic imaging of choroidal melanoma: before and after ophthalmic plaque radiation therapy. Int J Radiat Oncol Biol Phys 79(1):137–142

Fukumura D, Jain RK (2007) Tumor microvasculature and microenvironment: targets for anti-angiogenesis and normalization. Microvasc Res 74(2–3):72–84

Furth C et al (2010) Evaluation of interim-PET for response assessment in pediatric Hodgkin lymphoma—Results for dedicated assessment criteria in a blinded, dual-center read. Eur J Nucl Med Mol Imaging 37:S213–S213

Galldiks N et al (2006) Use of C-11-methionine PET to monitor the effects of temozolomide chemotherapy in malignant gliomas. Eur J Nucl Med Mol Imaging 33(5):516–524

Geets X et al (2007) Adaptive biological image-guided IMRT with anatomic and functional imaging in pharyngo-laryngeal tumors: Impact on target volume delineation and dose distribution using helical tomotherapy. Radiother Oncol 85(1):105–115

Gerstner ER, Batchelor TT (2010) Imaging and response criteria in gliomas. Curr Opin Oncol 22(6):598–603

Glazer ES et al (2010) Effectiveness of positron emission tomography for predicting chemotherapy response in colorectal cancer liver metastases. Arch Surg 145(4):340–345 discussion 345

Green SL, Giaccia AJ (1998) Tumor hypoxia and the cell cycle: implications for malignant progression and response to therapy. Cancer J Sci Am 4(4):218–223

Greven KM et al (2001) Serial positron emission tomography scans following radiation therapy of patients with head and neck cancer. Head Neck-J Sci Special Head Neck 23(11): 942–946

Grigsby PW (2009) Role of PET in gynecologic malignancy. Curr Opin Oncol 21(5):420–424

Grigsby PW et al (2004) Posttherapy [F-18] fluorodeoxyglucose positron emission tomography in carcinoma of the cervix: response and outcome. J Clin Oncol 22(11):2167–2171

Gupta T et al (2010) Diagnostic performance of response assessment FDG-PET/CT in patients with head and neck squamous cell carcinoma treated with high-precision definitive (chemo)radiation. Radiother Oncol 97(2):194–199

Haberkorn U et al (1991) Pet studies of fluorodeoxyglucose metabolism in patients with recurrent colorectal tumors receiving radiotherapy. J Nucl Med 32(8):1485–1490

Herholz K, Kracht LW, Heiss WD (2003) Monitoring the effect of chemotherapy in a mixed glioma by C-11-methionine PET. J Neuroimaging 13(3):269–271

Heron DE et al (2008) PET-CT in radiation oncology - The impact on diagnosis, treatment planning, and assessment of treatment response. Am J Clin Oncol-Cancer Clin Trials 31(4):352–362

Herrmann K et al (2007) Early response assessment using 3 '-Deoxy-3 '-[F-18]fluorothymidine-positron emission tomography in high-grade non-Hodgkin's lymphoma. Clin Cancer Res 13(12):3552–3558

Heuveling DA, de Bree R, van Dongen GA (2011) The potential role of non-FDG-PET in the management of head and neck cancer. Oral Oncol 47(1):2–7

Hicks RJ et al (2004) Early FDG-PET imaging after radical radiotherapy for non-small-cell lung cancer: inflammatory changes in normal tissues correlate with tumor response and do not confound therapeutic response evaluation. Int J Radiat Oncol Biol Phys 60(2):412–418

Hicks RJ (2009) Role of 18F-FDG PET in assessment of response in non-small cell lung cancer. J Nucl Med 50(Suppl 1): 31S–42S

Hockel M et al (1996) Association between tumor hypoxia and malignant progression in advanced cancer of the uterine cervix. Cancer Res 56(19):4509–4515

Hofman MS et al (2007) Assessing response to chemotherapy in metastatic melanoma with FDG PET: early experience. Nucl Med Commun 28(12):902–906

Horning SJ et al (2010) Interim positron emission tomography scans in diffuse large B-cell lymphoma: an independent expert nuclear medicine evaluation of the Eastern cooperative oncology group E3404 study. Blood 115(4):775–777

Huovinen R et al (1993) Carbon-11-Methionine and Pet in Evaluation of Treatment Response of Breast-Cancer. Br J Cancer 67(4):787–791

Hustinx R et al (1999) Non-invasive assessment of tumor hypoxia with the 2-nitroimidazole F-18-EF1 and PET. J Nucl Med 40(5):99p–99p

Iagaru A et al (2008) (18)F-FDG-PET/CT evaluation of response to treatment in lymphoma: when is the optimal time for the first re-evaluation scan? Hell J Nucl Med 11(3):153–156

Inoue T et al (1998a) Biodistribution studies on L-3-[fluorine-18]fluoro-alpha-methyl tyrosine: A potential tumor-detecting agent. J Nucl Med 39(4):663–667

Inoue T et al (1998b) Preliminary clinical study of PET with F-18 alpha methyl tyrosine (FMT) in patients with brain tumor. J Nucl Med 39(5):53p–53p

Inoue T et al (2001) Detection of malignant tumors: whole-body PET with fluorine 18 alpha-methyl tyrosine versus FDG—preliminary study. Radiology 220(1):54–62

Isles MG, McConkey C, Mehanna HM (2008) A systematic review and meta-analysis of the role of positron emission tomography in the follow up of head and neck squamous cell carcinoma following radiotherapy or chemoradiotherapy. Clin Otolaryngol 33(3):210–222

Isohashi K et al (2008) 18F-FDG-PET in patients with malignant lymphoma having long-term follow-up: staging and restaging, and evaluation of treatment response and recurrence. Ann Nucl Med 22(9):795–802

Ito M et al (2006) PET and planar imaging of tumor hypoxia with labeled metronidazole. Acad Radiol 13(5):598–609

Jacobs AH et al (2005) F-18-fluoro-L-thymidine and C-11-methylmethionine as markers of increased transport and proliferation in brain tumors. J Nucl Med 46(12):1948–1958

Janssen MHM et al (2010) Evaluation of early metabolic responses in rectal cancer during combined radiochemotherapy or radiotherapy alone: sequential FDG-PET-CT findings. Radiother Oncol 94(2):151–155

Jensen MM et al (2010) Early detection of response to experimental chemotherapeutic Top216 with [18F]FLT and [18F]FDG PET in human ovary cancer xenografts in mice. PLoS One 5(9):e12965

Joosten J et al (2005) Cryosurgery and radiofrequency ablation for unresectable colorectal liver metastases. Eur J Surg Oncol 31(10):1152–1159

Jost LM, Stahel RA, Force EGT (2005) ESMO minimum clinical recommendations for diagnosis, treatment and follow-up of Hodgkin's disease. Ann Oncol 16:54–55

Juweid ME et al (2007) Use of positron emission tomography for response assessment of lymphoma: consensus of the imaging subcommittee of international harmonization project in lymphoma. J Clin Oncol 25(5):571–578

Kaira K et al (2010) Assessment of therapy response in lung cancer with (1)F-alpha-methyl tyrosine PET. AJR Am J Roentgenol 195(5):1204–1211

Kenny LM et al (2005) Quantification of cellular proliferation in tumor and normal tissues of patients with breast cancer by [18F]fluorothymidine positron emission tomography imaging: evaluation of analytical methods. Cancer Res 65(21): 10104–10112

Kenny L et al (2007) Imaging early changes in proliferation at 1 week post chemotherapy: a pilot study in breast cancer patients with 3 '-deoxy-3 '-[F-18]fluorothymidine positron emission tomography. Eur J Nucl Med Mol Imaging 34(9):1339–1347

Kheirallah S et al (2010) Rituximab inhibits B-cell receptor signaling. Blood 115(5):985–994

Kikuchi M et al (2010) Sequential FDG-PET/CT after Neoadjuvant Chemotherapy is a Predictor of Histopathologic Response in Patients with Head and Neck Squamous Cell Carcinoma. Mol Imaging Biol 13(2):368–377

Kim SJ et al (2004) Predictive value of [F-18]FDG PET for pathological response of breast cancer to neo-adjuvant chemotherapy. Ann Oncol 15(9):1352–1357

Kim S et al (2005) 11C-methionine PET as a prognostic marker in patients with glioma: comparison with 18F-FDG PET. Eur J Nucl Med Mol Imaging 32(1):52–59

Kim TJ et al (2009) Multimodality assessment of esophageal cancer: preoperative staging and monitoring of response to therapy. Radiographics 29(2):403–421

Kong FMS et al (2007) A pilot study of [F-18] fluorodeoxyglucose positron emission tomography scans during and after radiation-based therapy in patients with non-small-cell lung cancer. J Clin Oncol 25(21):3116–3123

Kostakoglu L, Goldsmith SJ (2004) PET in the assessment of therapy response in patients with carcinoma of the head and neck and of the esophagus. J Nucl Med 45(1):56–68

Krak NC et al (2005) Effects of ROI definition and reconstruction method on quantitative outcome and applicability in a response monitoring trial. Eur J Nucl Med Mol Imaging 32(3):294–301

Krause BJ et al (2009) 18F-FDG PET and 18F-FDG PET/CT for assessing response to therapy in esophageal cancer. J Nucl Med 50(Suppl 1):89S–96S

Krochmalczyk D et al (2008) Pet guided beacopp de-escalation in advanced hodgkin lymphoma patients with a good response after the second chemotherapy cycle. Ann Oncol 19:250–250

Kubota R et al (1992) Intratumoral distribution of fluorine-18-fluorodeoxyglucose in vivo: high accumulation in macrophages and granulation tissues studied by microautoradiography. J Nucl Med 33(11):1972–1980

Kubota K et al (2006) Whole body tumor imaging with O-[C-11] methyl-L-tyrosine and PET: Comparison wiht FDG. Eur J Nucl Med Mol Imaging 33:S201–S201

Langenhoff BS et al (2002) Efficacy of fluorine-18-deoxyglucose positron emission tomography in detecting tumor recurrence after local ablative therapy for liver metastases: a prospective study. J Clin Oncol 20(22):4453–4458

Langer A (2010) A systematic review of PET and PET/CT in oncology: a way to personalize cancer treatment in a cost-effective manner? BMC Health Serv Res 10:283

Larson SM (1994) Cancer or inflammation? a Holy Grail for nuclear medicine. J Nucl Med 35(10):1653–1655

Larson SM, Schwartz LH (2006) F-18-FDG PET as a candidate for "Qualified Biomarker": Functional assessment of treatment response in oncology. J Nucl Med 47(6):901–903

Larson SM et al (1999) Tumor treatment response based on visual and quantitative changes in global tumor glycolysis using PET-FDG imaging. The visual response score and the change in total lesion glycolysis. Clin Positron Imaging 2(3):159–171

Lawrence J et al (2009) Use of 3'-Deoxy-3'-[18f]Fluorothymidine Pet/Ct for Evaluating Response to Cytotoxic Chemotherapy in Dogs with Non-Hodgkin's Lymphoma. Vet Radiol Ultrasound 50(6):660–668

Lee N et al (2009a) Correlation of dynamic contrast enhanced magnetic resonance imaging (DCE MRI) with (18)f-fluoromisonidazole positron emission and computed tomography (F-18-FMISO PET/CT) in assessing tumor hypoxia in a series of head and neck cancer (HNC) patients with nodal metastases. J Clin Oncol 27(15)::6083

Lee N et al (2009b) Correlation of F-18-Fluoromisonidazole Positron Emission and Computed Tomography (F-18-FMISO PET/CT) with Dynamic Contrast Enhanced Magnetic Resonance Imaging (DCE MRI) in Assessing Tumor Hypoxia in Head and Neck Cancer(HNC) Patients with Nodal Metastases. Int J Radiat Oncol Biol Phys 75(3):S176–S176

Lee N et al (2009c) Prospective trial incorporating Pre-/Mid-treatment [F-18]-Misonidazole positron emission tomography for head-and-neck cancer patients undergoing concurrent chemoradiotherapy. Int J Radiat Oncol Biol Phys 75(1): 101–108

Leyton J et al (2005) Early detection of tumor response to chemotherapy by 3'-deoxy-3'-[18F]fluorothymidine positron emission tomography: the effect of cisplatin on a fibrosarcoma tumor model in vivo. Cancer Res 65(10):4202–4210

Lin LL et al (2006) FDG-PET imaging for the assessment of physiologic volume response during radiotherapy in cervix cancer. Int J Radiat Oncol Biol Phys 65(1):177–181

Lindholm P et al (1996) Evaluation of early response to therapy in advanced breast cancer by 11C-methionine PET. J Nucl Med 37(5):1145–1145

Lindholm P et al (2009) Preliminary study of carbon-11 methionine PET in the evaluation of early response to therapy in advanced breast cancer. Nucl Med Commun 30(1):30–36

Liu RS et al (1999) Pitfalls of [F-18]FMISO PET in evaluation of tumor hypoxia after radiation therapy: false positive results caused by radiation necrosis. J Nucl Med 40(5):60p–61p

Liu ZY et al (2010) Early PET/CT after radiofrequency ablation in colorectal cancer liver metastases: is it useful? Chin Med J (Engl) 123(13):1690–1694

Lonsdale MN, Beyer T (2010) Dual-modality PET/CT instrumentation-Today and tomorrow. Eur J Radiol 73(3):452–460

Lordick F et al (2007) PET to assess early metabolic response and to guide treatment of adenocarcinoma of the oesophagogastric junction: The MUNICON phase II trial. Lancet Oncol 8(9):797–805

Manus Mac (2003) M.P., et al., Positron emission tomography is superior to computed tomography scanning for response-assessment after radical radiotherapy or chemoradiotherapy in patients with non-small-cell lung cancer. J Clin Oncol 21(7):1285–1292

Markova J et al (2008) FDG-PET for assessment of early therapy response after 4 cycles of chemotherapy in advanced stage Hodgkin lymphoma. Ann Oncol 19:135–135

Markova J et al (2009a) Early and late response assessment with Fdg-Pet after Beacopp-based Chemotherapy in advanced-Stage Hodgkin Lymphoma patients has a high negative predictive value. Haematologica-the Hematology J 94:33–33

Markova J et al (2009b) FDG-PET for assessment of early treatment response after four cycles of chemotherapy in patients with advanced-stage Hodgkin's lymphoma has a high negative predictive value. Ann Oncol 20(7):1270–1274

Mason RP (2006) Non-invasive assessment of kidney oxygenation: a role for BOLD MRI. Kidney Int 70(1):9–11

Matthews NE et al (2001) Nitric oxide-mediated regulation of chemosensitivity in cancer cells. J Natl Cancer Inst 93(24): 1879–1885

McDermott GM et al (2007) Monitoring primary breast cancer throughout chemotherapy using FDG-PET. Breast Cancer Res Treat 102(1):75–84

McKinley ET et al (2011) 18FDG-PET predicts pharmacodynamic response to OSI-906, a dual IGF-1R/IR inhibitor, in preclinical mouse models of lung cancer. Clin Cancer Res 17(10):3332–3340

Mees G et al (2009) Molecular imaging of hypoxia with radiolabelled agents. Eur J Nucl Med Mol Imaging 36(10): 1674–1686

Mehrkens JH et al (2008) The positive predictive value of O-(2-[F-18]fluoroethyl)-L-tyrosine (FET) PET in the diagnosis of a glioma recurrence after multimodal treatment. J Neurooncol 88(1):27–35

Molthoff CF et al (2007) Monitoring response to radiotherapy in human squamous cell cancer bearing nude mice: comparison of 2'-deoxy-2'-[18F]fluoro-D-glucose (FDG) and 3'-[18F]fluoro-3'-deoxythymidine (FLT). Mol Imag Biol 9(6):340–347

Mortimer JE et al (2001) Metabolic flare: indicator of hormone responsiveness in advanced breast cancer. J Clin Oncol 19(11):2797–2803

Mortimer JE et al (2003) Metabolic flare by positron emission tomography (PET) predicts for response to tamoxifen more accurately than her-2 status in advanced postmenopausal ER plus breast cancer. Breast Cancer Res Treat 82:S104–S104

Moulin-Romsee G et al (2008) Non-Hodgkin lymphoma: retrospective study on the cost-effectiveness of early treatment response assessment by FDG-PET. Eur J Nucl Med Mol Imaging 35(6):1074–1080

Muzi M et al (2005) Kinetic modeling of 3 '-deoxy-3 '-fluorothymidine in somatic tumors mathematical studies. J Nucl Med 46(2):371–380

Nahmias C et al (2007) Time course of early response to chemotherapy in non-small cell lung cancer patients with 18F-FDG PET/CT. J Nucl Med 48(5):744–751

Nam SY et al (2005) Early evaluation of the response to radiotherapy of patients with squamous cell carcinoma of the head and neck using 18FDG-PET. Oral Oncol 41(4):390–395

Nguyen Q, Aboagye EO (2010) Imaging the life and death of tumors in living subjects: Preclinical PET imaging of proliferation and apoptosis. Integ Biol 2(10):483–495

Nicol I et al (2008) Role of FDG PET-CT in cutaneous melanoma. Bull Cancer 95(11):1089–1101

Nishii R et al (2008) Evaluation of 2'-deoxy-2'-[18F]fluoro-5-methyl-1-beta-L: -arabinofuranosyluracil ([18F]-L: -FMAU) as a PET imaging agent for cellular proliferation: comparison with [18F]-D: -FMAU and [18F]FLT. Eur J Nucl Med Mol Imaging 35(5):990–998

Nishiyama Y et al (2008) Monitoring the neoadjuvant therapy response in gynecological cancer patients using FDG PET. Eur J Nucl Med Mol Imaging 35(2):287–295

Niu G et al (2009) Monitoring therapeutic response of human ovarian cancer to 17-DMAG by noninvasive PET imaging with Cu-64-DOTA-trastuzumab. Eur J Nucl Med Mol Imaging 36(9):1510–1519

Nordsmark M et al (2005) Prognostic value of tumor oxygenation in 397 head and neck tumors after primary radiation therapy. An international multi-center study. Radiother Oncol 77(1):18–24

Ohtsuki K et al (1999) Technetium-99 m HYNIC-annexin V: a potential radiopharmaceutical for the in-vivo detection of apoptosis. Eur J Nucl Med 26(10):1251–1258

Okuma T et al (2006) Fluorine-18-fluorodeoxyglucose positron emission tomography for assessment of patients with unresectable recurrent or metastatic lung cancers after CT-guided radiofrequency ablation: preliminary results. Ann Nucl Med 20(2):115–121

Olsen JR et al (2010) Prognostic utility of squamous cell carcinoma antigen in carcinoma of the cervix: association with pre- and posttreatment FDG-PET. Int J Radiat Oncol Biol Phys 8:772–7771

Ott K et al (2003) Prediction of response to preoperative chemotherapy in gastric carcinoma by metabolic imaging: results of a prospective trial. J Clin Oncol 21(24):4604–4610

Osinsky S, Zavelevich M, Vaupel P (2009) Tumor hypoxia and malignant progression. Exp Oncol 31(2):80–86

Oude Munnink TH, et al (2009) Molecular imaging of breast cancer. Breast 18 (Suppl 3):S66–73

Ozsunar Y et al (2010) Glioma recurrence versus radiation necrosis? A pilot comparison of arterial spin-labeled, dynamic susceptibility contrast enhanced MRI, and FDG-PET imaging. Academic Radiology 17(3):282–290

Padhani A (2010) Science to practice: what does mr oxygenation imaging tell us about human breast cancer hypoxia? Radiology 254(1):1–3

Passero VA et al (2010a) Response assessment by combined PET-CT scan versus CT scan alone using RECIST in patients with locally advanced head and neck cancer treated with chemoradiotherapy. Ann Oncol 21(11):2278–2283

Passero VA et al (2010b) Response assessment by combined PET-CT scan versus CT scan alone using RECIST in

patients with locally advanced head and neck cancer treated with chemoradiotherapy. Ann Oncol 21(11):2278–2283
Pauleit D et al (2004) PET with O-(2-[F-18]fluoroethyl)-L-tyrosine (FET) in peripheral tumors. Eur J Nucl Med Mol Imaging 31:S340–S341
Pauleit D et al (2005) PET with O-(2-F-18-fluoroethyl)-L-tyro sine in peripheral tumors: First clinical results. J Nucl Med 46(3):411–416
Pawlik TM et al (2009) Trends in nontherapeutic laparotomy rates in patients undergoing surgical therapy for hepatic colorectal metastases. Ann Surg Oncol 16(2):371–378
Petrescu I et al (2010) Diagnosis and treatment protocols of cutaneous melanoma: latest approach 2010. Chirurgia (Bucur) 105(5):637–643
Picardi M et al (2007) Randomized comparison of consolidation radiation versus observation in bulky Hodgkin's lymphoma with post-chemotherapy negative positron emission tomography scans. Leuk Lymphoma 48(9):1721–1727
Pickles MD et al (2005) Role of dynamic contrast enhanced MRI in monitoring early response of locally advanced breast cancer to neoadjuvant chemotherapy. Breast Cancer Res Treat 91(1):1–10
Pons F, Duch J, Fuster D (2009) Breast cancer therapy: the role of PET-CT in decision making. Q J Nucl Med Mol Imaging 53(2):210–223
Popperl G et al (2006) Serial O-(2-[(18)F]fluoroethyl)-L: -tyrosine PET for monitoring the effects of intracavitary radioimmunotherapy in patients with malignant glioma. Eur J Nucl Med Mol Imaging 33(7):792–800
Port JL et al (2004) Positron emission tomography scanning poorly predicts response to preoperative chemotherapy in non-small cell lung cancer. Ann Thorac Surg 77(1):254–259 discussion 259
Pottgen C et al (2006) Value of F-18-fluoro-2-deoxy-D-glucose-positron emission tomography/computed tomography in non-small-cell lung cancer for prediction of pathologic response and times to relapse after neoadjuvant chemoradiotherapy. Clin Cancer Res 12(1):97–106
Rachinger W et al (2005) Positron emission tomography with O-(2-[F-18]fluoroethyl)-L-tyrosine versus magnetic resonance imaging in the diagnosis of recurrent gliomas. Neurosurgery 57(3):505–511
Rajendran JG et al (2002) (FMISO)-F-18 PET hypoxia imaging in head and neck cancer: Heterogeneity in hypoxia—Primary tumor vs lymph nodal metastases. J Nucl Med 43(5):73p–74p
Rajendran JG et al (2003) F-18 FMISO PET tumor hypoxia imaging: Investigating the tumor volume-hypoxia connection. J Nucl Med 44(5):376p–376p
Rankin, S., PET/CT for staging and monitoring non small cell lung cancer. Cancer Imaging, 2008. 8 Spec No A: p. S27-31
Reinhardt MJ et al (2002) Value of tumour marker S-100B in melanoma patients: a comparison to 18F-FDG PET and clinical data. Nuklearmedizin 41(3):143–147
Reischl G et al (2007) Imaging of tumor hypoxia with [I-124] IAZA in comparison with [F-18] FMISO and [F-18]FAZA - first small animal PET results. J Pharm Pharm Sci 10(2):203–211
Riemann B et al (2004) Early effects of irradiation on [(123)I]-IMT and [(18)F]-FDG uptake in rat C6 glioma cells. Strahlenther Onkol 180(7):434–441
Rose PG et al (1996) The impact of CA-125 on the sensitivity of abdominal pelvic CT scan before second-look laparotomy in advanced ovarian carcinoma. Int J Gynecol Cancer 6(3):213–218
Rose PG et al (2001a) Positive emission tomography for evaluating a complete clinical response in patients with ovarian or peritoneal carcinoma: correlation with second-look laparotomy. Gynecol Oncol 82(1):17–21
Rose PG et al (2001b) Positive emission tomography for evaluating a complete clinical response in patients with ovarian or peritoneal carcinoma: Correlation with second-look laparotomy. Gynecol Oncol 82(1):17–21
Rosenberg R et al (2009) The predictive value of metabolic response to preoperative radiochemotherapy in locally advanced rectal cancer measured by PET/CT. Int J Colorectal Dis 24(2):191–200
Rousseau C et al (2006) Monitoring of early response to neoadjuvant chemotherapy in stage II and III breast cancer by [F-18]fluorodeoxyglucose positron emission tomography. J Clin Oncol 24(34):5366–5372
Rueger MA et al (2010) [(18)F]FLT PET for Non-Invasive Monitoring of Early Response to Gene Therapy in Experimental Gliomas. Mol Imaging Biol 13:547–557
Ryu JS et al (2002) FDG-PET in staging and restaging non-small cell lung cancer after neoadjuvant chemoradiotherapy: correlation with histopathology. Lung Cancer 35(2): 179–187
Saquib N et al (2007) Weight gain and recovery of pre-cancer weight after breast cancer treatments: evidence from the women's healthy eating and living (WHEL) study. Breast Cancer Res Treat 105(2):177–186
Sakamoto H et al (1998) Monitoring of response to radiotherapy with fluorine-18 deoxyglucose PET of head and neck squamous cell carcinomas. Acta Otolaryngol Suppl 538:254–260
Savage KJ et al (2007) FDG-PET guided consolidative radiotherapy in patients with advanced stage Hodgkin lymphoma with residual abnormalities on post chemotherapy CT scan. Blood 110(11):70a
Schelling M et al (2000) Positron emission tomography using [F-18]fluorodeoxyglucose for monitoring primary chemotherapy in breast cancer. J Clin Oncol 18(8):1689–1695
Schiepers C et al (1999) The effect of preoperative radiation therapy on glucose utilization and cell kinetics in patients with primary rectal carcinoma. Cancer 85(4):803–811
Schoder H et al (2009) PET monitoring of therapy response in head and neck squamous cell carcinoma. J Nucl Med 50(Suppl 1):74S–88S
Schwarz J et al (2004) Oncologic imaging of tumor hypoxia by Cu-ATSM and correlating findings on Cu-ATSM PET scans to cellular markers that may predict for radiation response. Int J Radiat Oncol Biol Phys 60(1):S305–S306
Schwarz JK et al (2007) Association of posttherapy positron emission tomography with tumor response and survival in cervical carcinoma. JAMA 298(19):2289–2295
Schwarz JK et al (2009) The role of 18F-FDG PET in assessing therapy response in cancer of the cervix and ovaries. J Nucl Med 50(Suppl 1):64S–73S
Schwarz-Dose J et al (2009) Monitoring primary systemic therapy of large and locally advanced breast cancer by using sequential positron emission tomography imaging with [F-18] Fluorodeoxyglucose. J Clin Oncol 27(4):535–541

Shamim SA et al (2011) FDG PET/CT evaluation of treatment response in patients with recurrent colorectal cancer. Clin Nucl Med 36(1):11–16

Shields AF et al (1998) Imaging proliferation in vivo with [F-18]FLT and positron emission tomography. Nat Med 4(11): 1334–1336

Shiraishi K et al (2010) Repeat FDG-PET for Predicting Pathological Tumor Response and Prognosis after Neoadjuvant Treatment in Nonsmall Cell Lung Cancer: Comparison with Computed Tomography. Ann Thorac Cardiovasc Surg 16(6):394–400

Siegel BA, Dehdashti F (2005) Oncologic PET/CT: current status and controversies. Eur Radiol 15:D127–D132

Sironi S et al (2004) Integrated FDG PET/CT in patients with persistent ovarian cancer: Correlation with histologic findings. Radiology 233(2):433–440

Smith IC et al (2000) Positron emission tomography using [F-18]-fluorodeoxy-D-glucose to predict the pathologic response of breast cancer to primary chemotherapy. J Clin Oncol 18(8):1676–1688

Smyczek-Gargya B et al (2004) PET with [18F]fluorothymidine for imaging of primary breast cancer: a pilot study. Eur J Nucl Med Mol Imaging 31(5):720–724

Sohn HJ et al (2008) [F-18] Fluorothymidine Positron Emission Tomography before and 7 Days after Gefitinib Treatment Predicts Response in Patients with Advanced Adenocarcinoma of the Lung. Clin Cancer Res 14(22):7423–7429

Solit DB et al (2007) 3'-deoxy-3'-[F-18]fluorothymidine positron emission tomography is a sensitive method for imaging the response of BRAF-dependent tumors to MEK inhibition. Cancer Res 67(23):11463–11469

Solomon B et al (2005) Modulation of intratumoral hypoxia by the epidermal growth factor receptor inhibitor gefitinib detected using small animal PET imaging. Mol Cancer Ther 4(9):1417–1422

Spaepen K, Mortelmans L (2001) Evaluation of treatment response in patients with lymphoma using [18F]FDG-PET: differences between non-Hodgkin's lymphoma and Hodgkin's disease. Q J Nucl Med 45(3):269–273

Strauss, H.W., et al., Translational imaging: imaging of apoptosis. Handb Exp Pharmacol, 2008(185 Pt 2): p. 259–275

Strobel K et al (2007) S-100B and FDG-PET/CT in therapy response assessment of melanoma patients. Dermatology 215(3):192–201

Strobel K et al (2008) Chemotherapy response assessment in stage IV melanoma patients-comparison of 18F-FDG-PET/CT, CT, brain MRI, and tumormarker S-100B. Eur J Nucl Med Mol Imaging 35(10):1786–1795

Sun HH et al (2005) Imaging DNA synthesis with [F-18]FMAU and positron emission tomography in patients with cancer. Eur J Nucl Med Mol Imaging 32(1):15–22

Sun X et al. (2010) Tumor hypoxia imaging. Mol Imaging Biol 13:399–410

Sutherland RM (1998) Tumor hypoxia and gene expression–implications for malignant progression and therapy. Acta Oncol 37(6):567–574

Taal W et al (2008) Incidence of early pseudo-progression in a cohort of malignant glioma patients treated with chemoirradiation with temozolomide. Cancer 113(2):405–410

Takai Y et al (2007) [(18)]FFRP-170: A novel hypoxia maker for PET: Initial clinical data for the usefulness and the correlation between tumor response to radiotherapy and [(18)]FFRP-170 uptake. EJC Suppl 5(4):135–135

Tan MCB et al (2007) Chemotherapy-induced normalization of FDG uptake by colorectal liver metastases does not usually indicate complete pathologic response. J Gastrointest Surg 11(9):1112–1119

Tanvetyanon T et al (2008) Computed tomography response, but not positron emission tomography scan response, predicts survival after neoadjuvant chemotherapy for resectable non-small-cell lung cancer. J Clin Oncol 26(28):4610–4616

Terakawa Y et al (2008) Diagnostic accuracy of C-11-methionine PET for differentiation of recurrent brain tumors from radiation necrosis after radiotherapy. J Nucl Med 49(5):694–699

Thomas A et al (2010) 18-Fluoro-deoxyglucose positron emission tomography report interpretation as predictor of outcome in diffuse large B-cell lymphoma including analysis of 'indeterminate' reports. Leuk Lymphoma 51(3):439–446

Tomiyoshi K et al (1999) Metabolic studies of [F-18-alpha-methyl]tyrosine in mice bearing colorectal carcinoma LS-180. Anticancer Drugs 10(3):329–336

Townsend DW et al (2004) PET/CT today and tomorrow. J Nucl Med 45:4S–14S

Troost EG et al (2007) 18F-FLT PET does not discriminate between reactive and metastatic lymph nodes in primary head and neck cancer patients. J Nucl Med 48(5):726–735

Troost EGC et al (2010) F-18-FLT PET/CT for early response monitoring and dose escalation in oropharyngeal tumors. J Nucl Med 51(6):866–874

Tseng J et al (2004) F-18-FDG kinetics in locally advanced breast cancer: Correlation with tumor blood flow and changes in response to neoadjuvant chemotherapy. J Nucl Med 45(11):1829–1837

Tsuyuguchi N et al (2004) Methionine positron emission tomography for differentiation of recurrent brain tumor and radiation necrosis after stereotactic radiosurgery–in malignant glioma. Ann Nucl Med 18(4):291–296

Ullrich RT et al (2008) Early detection of erlotinib treatment response in NSCLC by 3'-deoxy-3'-[F]-fluoro-L-thymidine ([F]FLT) positron emission tomography (PET). PLoS One 3(12):e3908

van Westreenen HL et al (2005) Comparison of 18F-FLT PET and 18F-FDG PET in esophageal cancer. J Nucl Med 46(3):400–404

van der Hiel B, Pauwels EK, Stokkel MP (2001) Positron emission tomography with 2-[18F]-fluoro-2-deoxy-D-glucose in oncology. Part IIIa: Therapy response monitoring in breast cancer, lymphoma and gliomas. J Cancer Res Clin Oncol 127(5):269–277

Van Laere K et al (2005) Direct comparison of 18F-FDG and 11C-methionine PET in suspected recurrence of glioma: sensitivity, inter-observer variability and prognostic value. Eur J Nucl Med Mol Imaging 32(1):39–51

Vansteenkiste JF et al (1998) Potential use of FDG-PET scan after induction chemotherapy in surgically staged IIIa-N-2 non-small-cell lung cancer: A prospective pilot study. Ann Oncol 9(11):1193–1198

Vaupel P, Mayer A (2007) Hypoxia in cancer: significance and impact on clinical outcome. Cancer Metastasis Rev 26(2): 225–239

Vaupel P, Mayer A, Hockel M (2004) Tumor hypoxia and malignant progression. Methods Enzymol 381:335–354

Veit P et al (2006) Detection of residual tumor after radiofrequency ablation of liver metastasis with dual-modality PET/CT: initial results. Eur Radiol 16(1):80–87

Vera P et al (2011) Simultaneous positron emission tomography (PET) assessment of metabolism with (18)F-fluoro-2-deoxy-D-glucose (FDG), proliferation with (18)F-fluorothymidine (FLT), and hypoxia with (18)fluoro-misonidazole (F-miso) before and during radiotherapy in patients with non-small-cell lung cancer (NSCLC): A pilot study. Radiother Oncol 98(1):109–116

Vergez S et al (2010) Preclinical and clinical evidence that deoxy-2-[F-18]fluoro-D-glucose positron emission tomography with computed tomography is a reliable tool for the detection of early molecular responses to erlotinib in head and neck cancer. Clin Cancer Res 16(17):4434–4445

Vriens PW et al (1998) The use of technetium Tc 99 m annexin V for in vivo imaging of apoptosis during cardiac allograft rejection. J Thorac Cardiovasc Surg 116(5):844–853

Vriens D et al (2009a) Chemotherapy response monitoring of colorectal liver metastases by dynamic Gd-DTPA-enhanced MRI perfusion parameters and F-18-FDG PET metabolic rate. J Nucl Med 50(11):1777–1784

Vriens D et al (2009b) Evaluation of different normalization procedures for the calculation of the standardized uptake value in therapy response monitoring studies. Nucl Med Commun 30(7):550–557

Vriens D et al (2009c) Tailoring therapy in colorectal cancer by PET-CT. Q J Nucl Med Mol Imaging 53(2):224–244

Wahl RL et al (1993) Metabolic monitoring of breast-cancer chemohormonotherapy using positron emission tomography—initial evaluation. J Clin Oncol 11(11):2101–2111

Wahl RL et al (2009) From RECIST to PERCIST: Evolving Considerations for PET response criteria in solid tumors. J Nucl Med 50(Suppl 1):122S–150S

Waldherr C et al (2005) Monitoring antiproliferative responses to kinase inhibitor therapy in mice with 3'-deoxy-3'-18F-fluorothymidine PET. J Nucl Med 46(1):114–120

Wang HE et al (1999) Biological characterization of three diastereomers of [F-18]4-fluoro-1-(2 '-nitro-1 '-imidazolyl)-2,3-dihydroxybutane as PET agents for tumor hypoxia evaluation. J Nucl Med 40(5):311p

Wang G et al (2007) How do oncologists deal with incidental abnormalities on whole-body fluorine-18 fluorodeoxyglucose PET/CT? Cancer 109(1):117–124

Wang L et al (2008) PET study demonstrates radiation dependent changes on tumor hypoxia and proliferation during the course of radiotherapy in a lung cancer xenograft model. Int J Radiat Oncol Biol Phys 72(1):S30–S30

Wang WL et al (2009a) Impact of attenuation and scatter correction in estimating tumor hypoxia-related kinetic parameters for FMISO dynamic animal-PET imaging. 2008 IEEE Nuclear Science Symposium and Medical Imaging Conference (2008 Nss/Mic), Vols 1–9, 2009: pp 4500–4505

Wang WL et al (2009b) Evaluation of a compartmental model for estimating tumor hypoxia via FMISO dynamic PET imaging. Phys Med Biol 54(10):3083–3099

Weber WA et al (2001) Prediction of response to preoperative chemotherapy in adenocarcinomas of the esophagogastric junction by metabolic imaging. J Clin Oncol 19(12):3058–3065

Weber WA (2005) PET for response assessment in oncology: radiotherapy and chemotherapy. Br J Radiol 78:42–49

Weber WA (2006) Positron emission tomography as an imaging biomarker. J Clin Oncol 24(20):3282–3292

Weber WA (2010) Monitoring tumor response to therapy with 18F-FLT PET. J Nucl Med 51(6):841–844

Weckesser M et al (2005) O-(2-[F-18]fluorethyl)-L-tyrosine PET in the clinical evaluation of primary brain tumours. Eur J Nucl Med Mol Imaging 32(4):422–429

Wei LH et al (2008) Changes in tumor metabolism as readout for mammalian target of rapamycin kinase inhibition by rapamycin in glioblastoma. Clin Cancer Res 14(11):3416–3426

Wieder HA et al (2004) Time course of tumor metabolic activity during chemoradiotherapy of esophageal squamous cell carcinoma and response to treatment. J Clin Oncol 22(5):900–908

Wieder HA et al (2007) PET imaging with [F-18]3 '-deoxy-3 '-fluorothymidine for prediction of response to neoadjuvant treatment in patients with rectal cancer. Eur J Nucl Med Mol Imaging 34(6):878–883

Wiedemann N et al (2010) Dynamics of tumor hypoxia in patients undergoing radiochemotherapy for head and neck cancer evaluated with serial F-18 fluoromisonidazole PET. Int J Radiat Oncol Biol Phys 78(3):S703–S703

Wiering B et al (2008) Controversies in the management of colorectal liver metastases: role of PET and PET/CT. Dig Surg 25(6):413–420

Wong RK et al (2007) Pre-operative radiotherapy and curative surgery for the management of localized rectal carcinoma. Cochrane Database Syst Rev 2:CD002102

Wu X et al (2010) Early treatment response evaluation in patients with diffuse large B-cell lymphoma-A pilot study comparing volumetric MRI and PET/CT. Mol Imaging Biol 13(4):785–792

Wurker M et al (1996) Glucose consumption and methionine uptake in low-grade gliomas after iodine-125 brachytherapy. Eur J Nucl Med 23(5):583–586

Wyss M et al (2009) Early metabolic responses in temozolomide treated low-grade glioma patients. J Neurooncol 95(1):87–93

Yamamoto Y et al (2006) Correlation of FDG-PET findings with histopathology in the assessment of response to induction chemoradiotherapy in non-small cell lung cancer. Eur J Nucl Med Mol Imaging 33(2):140–147

Yamamoto Y et al (2008) Comparison of (18)F-FLT PET and (18)F-FDG PET for preoperative staging in non-small cell lung cancer. Eur J Nucl Med Mol Imaging 35(2):236–245

Yamaura G et al (2006) O-[F-18]fluoromethyl-L-tyrosine is a potential tracer for monitoring tumour response to chemotherapy using PET: an initial comparative in vivo study with deoxyglucose and thymidine. Eur J Nucl Med Mol Imaging 33(10):1134–1139

Yang DJ et al (1995) Development of F-18 labeled fluoroerythronitroimidizole as a pet agent for imaging tumor hypoxia. Radiology 194(3):795–800

Yang W et al (2010) Imaging of proliferation with 18F-FLT PET/CT versus 18F-FDG PET/CT in non-small-cell lung cancer. Eur J Nucl Med Mol Imaging 37(7):1291–1299

Yao M et al (2004) Value of FDG PET in assessment of treatment response and surveillance in head-and-neck cancer patients after intensity modulated radiation treatment: a preliminary report. Int J Radiat Oncol Biol Phys 60(5):1410–1418

Yap CS et al (2006) Evaluation of thoracic tumors with 18F-fluorothymidine and 18F-fluorodeoxyglucose-positron emission tomography. Chest 129(2):393–401

Yoshida Y et al (2004) Metabolic monitoring of advanced uterine cervical cancer neoadjuvant chemotherapy by using [F-18]-Fluorodeoxyglucose positron emission tomography: preliminary results in three patients. Gynecol Oncol 95(3):597–602

Yoshimoto Y et al (2007) Defining regional infusion treatment strategies for extremity melanoma: comparative analysis of melphalan and temozolomide as regional chemotherapeutic agents. Mol Cancer Ther 6(5):1492–1500

Yue J et al (2010) Measuring tumor cell proliferation with 18F-FLT PET during radiotherapy of esophageal squamous cell carcinoma: a pilot clinical study. J Nucl Med 51(4):528–534

Zaucha J et al (2009) The role of PET for interim response assessment in patients with Hodgkin's lymphoma. Wspolczesna Onkologia-Contemporary Oncology 13(4):161–166

Zhang HQ et al (2010) Prognostic value of (18)F-fluorodeoxyglucose uptake in patients with non-small cell lung cancer treated by concurrent chemoradiotherapy. Zhonghua Zhong Liu Za Zhi 32(8):603–606

Zhu AX et al (2010) Efficacy and safety of gemcitabine, oxaliplatin, and bevacizumab in advanced biliary-tract cancers and correlation of changes in 18-fluorodeoxyglucose PET with clinical outcome: a phase 2 study. Lancet Oncol 11(1):48–54

Zinzani PL et al (2010) Midtreatment (18)F-fluorodeoxyglucose positron-emission tomography in aggressive non-Hodgkin lymphoma. Cancer 117(5):1010–1018

Metastatic Disease

Patrick J. Peller

Contents

P. J. Peller (✉)
Department of Radiology,
Mayo Clinic, 200 1st Street SW,
Rochester, MN 55905, USA
e-mail: Peller.patrick@mayo.edu

Abstract

This chapter reviews PET/PET identification of metastatic disease, the main cause of cancer deaths. More than one-third of newly diagnosed cancer patients have metastases detectable by PET/CT. There are three major pathways by which tumor cells disseminate: blood borne, lymphatic spread, and by seeding body cavities. The primary tumor location and histology in large part determines the most common route and frequency of metastasis. Increased FDG uptake in metastases permits identification on PET/CT. Cancer of unknown primary site is a relatively common clinical entity, resulting from a wide variety of primary sites. PET/CT identification of the primary tumor allows for focused therapy and potentially improved survival.

1 Key Points

Metastatic disease, and not the primary tumor, kills the majority of cancer patients. Tumor cells detach from the primary tumor and some enter into adjacent capillaries, lymphatics, or cavities. The strength of FDG PET imaging is the ability to detect metastatic disease in lymph nodes too small to identify by size criteria and to exclude cancer in uninvolved enlarged nodes. Hematogenous dissemination can be via the local venous system producing metastases in the drainage region of the primary tumor and to distant sites. The lungs, liver, bones, brain, and adrenal glands are the most common sites of blood borne metastases. PET/CT readily detects metastasis, except in the brain. PET/CT can be very helpful in evaluating patients with cancer of unknown primary.

P. Peller et al. (eds.), *PET-CT and PET-MRI in Oncology*, Medical Radiology. Diagnostic Imaging,
DOI: 10.1007/174_2012_622, © Springer-Verlag Berlin Heidelberg 2012

2 Introduction

Metastatic disease is the cause of death in more than 90 % of cancer patients. Uncontrolled growth, local invasion, and metastasis are the hallmarks of a malignancy. Tumor hypoxia and diminished nutrients produce genetic alterations, which enhance the likelihood of metastases. It is the ability to spread beyond the original primary site that makes cancer lethal. Metastasis is a very complex and inefficient process in which few of the cells that leave the primary tumor site actually reach and grow at a new site. Successful metastasis requires the tumor cell to have the ability to proliferate in a foreign environment and usually induce angiogenesis. The distribution of metastatic disease is not random and significant observed patterns are important to recognize (Gupta and Massague 2006; Chiang and Massagué 2008).

Cancer cells disseminate by three major pathways: blood borne, via the lymphatic system, and seeding a body cavity. Lymphatic and hematogenous routes are not mutually exclusive, as numerous interconnections are present between the lymphatic and vascular systems. The majority of tumor staging systems use the tumor, node, and metastasis (TNM) scheme. The real value of the TNM system is as an indicator of the cancer's potential to metastasize and to ensure that any local intervention encompasses all known tumor (Chiang and Massagué 2008).

3 Lymphatic Metastasis

Although tumor dissemination through the lymphatic system is common, the prevalence of nodal disease differs according to the histology of the primary tumor. For example, lymph node metastases are very frequent in patients with squamous cell head and neck cancers but are uncommon in soft tissue sarcomas. The rapid growth of many malignancies results not only in local invasion but tumor cells detaching and entering adjacent small lymphatic vessels. The tumor cells float in the lymph and are filtered out by lymph nodes. Most tumor cells are destroyed by the immune system but a few survive and grow. Nodal involvement is an adverse prognostic feature in the majority of cancers. Imaging is frequently employed to evaluate nodal stage prior treatment but histologic examination remains the gold standard. Cancer specific classifications are used in the node portion of the TNM staging system.

CT remains the most widely used imaging modality for nodal staging. Nodal size is the most widely used criteria for differentiating malignant from nonmalignant nodes. Other CT criteria include shape, contour, number and clustering of normal sized nodes. Conventional imaging with CT or MRI is limited in the detection of nodal metastases because pathologic nodes are often considered solely on the basis of size criteria and up to 40 % of metastases occur in small nodes. The specificity of conventional imaging can also be limiting—as low as 39 % for CT and 48 % for MRI of the neck nodes (Teknos et al. 2001; Schöder et al. 2004).

FDG PET detection of nodal metastasis is based on the increased activity exhibited by nodes infiltrated with tumor cells. In most studies, PET imaging has been shown to be more sensitive and specific than CT for the detection of nodal metastases. In head and neck cancer, the sensitivity of FDG PET imaging for the staging of cervical lymph nodes is between 67–91 %, and the specificity is between 80–100 % in published studies (Ng et al. 2005; Branstetter et al. 2005; Schöder et al. 2006). The sensitivity for metastases 4 mm or smaller is only 17–23 % but the positive predictive value is greater than 99 %. The sensitivity rises to 93–95 % for nodes 10 mm or larger (Kitajima et al. 2008). PET studies have also demonstrated that the absence of ^{18}FDG uptake in enlarged nodes identified at CT is highly indicative of lack of metastatic involvement (Kim et al. 2006; Jeon et al. 2010). The strength of PET imaging is the ability to detect nodal disease in lymph nodes too small to identify by size criteria and to exclude enlarged nodes not involved with tumor (Fig. 1).

4 Hematogenous Metastasis

Tumor cells detach from the primary tumor and some intravasate into adjacent capillaries or lymphatics. Both routes ultimately can lead to the venous circulation. Blood sampling from patients with the most common forms of carcinomas have yielded viable tumor cells.

Hematogenous dissemination via the local venous system explains the presence of metastases in the drainage region of the primary tumor. Remote hematogenous metastases result when cancer cells pass through the venous system into the arterial blood supply. The sites of hematogenous metastatic disease are determined both by blood flow and tissue-specific factors (Allard et al. 2004).

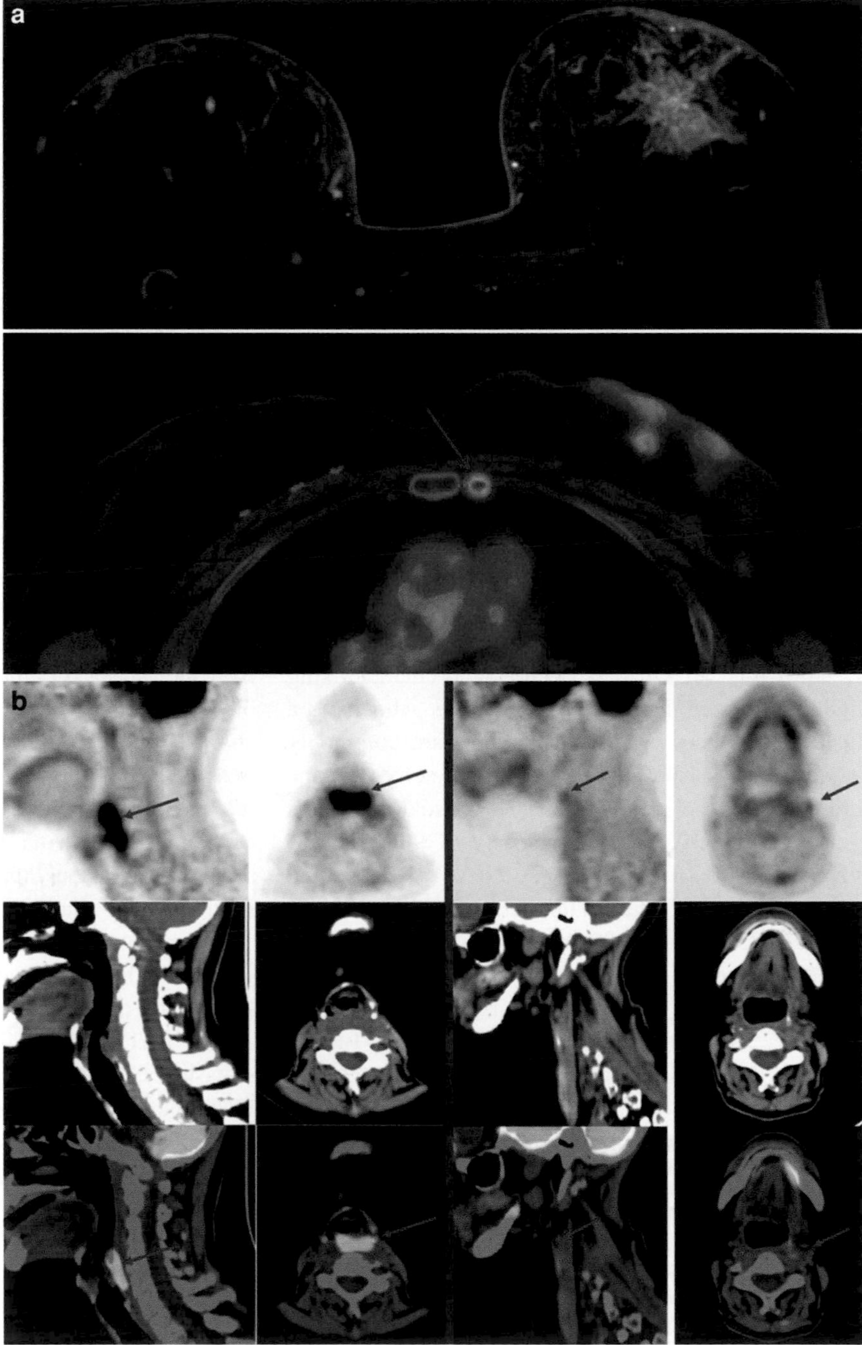

Fig. 1 **a** The intense FDG uptake on PET/CT identified a 5 mm internal mammary nodal metastasis (*arrow*), confirmed by cytology from a US-guided fine needle biopsy in this 46-year-old woman with locally advanced left breast cancer. **b** The moderate activity in a single 7 mm nodal metastasis (*arrow*) on dedicated PET/CT of the neck was confirmed at surgery in this 48-year-old man with laryngeal cancer and a clinically N0 neck

4.1 Lung

Lung metastases are common in patients with malignancies. Autopsy series have demonstrated that pulmonary metastases are present in 20–54 % of all patients who die of cancer. Most pulmonary metastases arise from common tumors, such as breast, colorectal, prostate, bronchial, head and neck, and renal cancers. Detection of pulmonary metastases is crucial for the patients with cancer. Typically pulmonary metastases are multiple, vary in size from 2 to 20 mm, and are located in the outer third of the lungs, especially in the subpleural regions of the lower zones. Nodules smaller than 2 cm are often round and have smooth margins. Solitary pulmonary metastases are uncommon, accounting less than 10 % of all solitary nodules (Hirakata et al. 1993).

Multidetector CT is the modality of choice for the detection of pulmonary metastases, but as most initial lung metastases are less than 5 mm in size, the sensitivity has a wide range, 53–84 %. The patterns of metastatic lung disease vary among tumors, but solid nodules predominate. Other patterns include ground glass attenuation, lobulated nodules, branching configuration, calcification, and cavitation.

Adenocarcinomas most frequently produce atypical pulmonary metastases. Pleural metastases can manifest as effusions, pleural thickening, nodules or masses (Davis 1991; Chang et al. 1979; Christie-Large et al. 2008).

The FDG uptake of pulmonary metastases is typically moderate to intense. The detected activity is impacted by the partial volume effect due to the size of the nodule and the amount of respiratory motion. Despite this, PET/CT is accurate at characterizing nodules greater than 7 mm in patients who have a history of cancer. Malignant nodules are commonly diagnosed by visual comparison to the activity in the blood within the great vessels. This visual method is generally effective, with sensitivity of 96 %, specificity of 83 %, PPV of 84 %, NPV of 96 %, and accuracy of 89 % (Bar-Shalom et al. 2008; De Wever et al. 2007; Yi et al. 2006; Mavi et al. 2005) (Fig. 1a).

Lymphangitic spread of tumor cells is common within the lung and is present in 35 % of the autopsies of patients with solid tumors. Breast, stomach, pancreas, lung, and prostate cancer most commonly develop lymphangitic spread into the lungs and associated pleural involvement is frequent. The malignant cells migrate through the interlobular septa. Edema and a desmoplastic type reaction produce interstitial thickening. CT shows thickened interlobular septa and bronchovascular markings of irregular contour. Often a nodular component from intraparenchymal extension is associated with lymphangitic carcinomatosis. Pleural effusions are present in 30–50 % of patients and hilar lymphadenopathy in 20–40 % (Meziane et al. 1988). Diffused FDG uptake is seen in areas of lymphangitic spread associated with the areas of interstitial thickening. The pleural and hilar nodes typically have greater activity than the parenchymal disease (Acikgoz et al. 2006) (Fig. 2b).

4.2 Liver

The liver is the most common site of hematogenous metastasis. The dual blood supply and the high concentration of the humeral factors appear to promote tumor cell growth. The liver is well protected as the sinusoids are heavily lined with tissue macrophages, which have significant tumorcidal activity. The liver is the most common site of metastatic disease for epithelial tumors, especially colon, breast, lung, pancreas, and stomach. Autopsy series suggests liver metastases are present in more than 70 % of cancer patients at their time of death. Most liver metastases are multiple; in 77 % of patients both lobes are involved and in only 10 % of cases is the metastasis solitary. Early detection and correct identification of liver metastases is extremely important in the cancer patient for appropriate staging and intervention when needed (Lise et al. 1991).

CT is frequently employed to evaluate possible liver metastases. On multiphase contrast CT, the dual blood supply of the liver impacts the enhancement characteristics of metastases, as compared with normal liver parenchyma. On CT, the majority of liver metastases are hypovascular in comparison with surrounding parenchyma; therefore, on nonenhanced CT scans, most lesions appear either hypoattenuating or isoattenuating relative to the surrounding parenchyma. The accuracy of CT in the detection of metastases varies with the technique used, the underlying primary lesion, and the degree of vascularity.

On PET/CT the detection of individual liver metastases depends on their size and the degree of FDG uptake in the tumor. The detection rate for liver metastases smaller than 8 mm is generally better for triple phase CT and MRI than for FDG PET. In a meta-analysis of patients with colorectal cancer, Niekel et al. 2010 concluded that PET/CT has the highest sensitivity (mean 96.8 %) for identification of liver metastases on a per-patient basis, but MRI had the highest sensitivity (mean 87.3 %) on a per-lesion basis. Despite the high sensitivity, integrated PET/CT maintained a specificity of 96.2 %. Kinkel et al. 2002 compared US, CT, MRI, and FDG PET for the detection of liver metastases from colorectal, gastric, and esophageal cancers and found that PET is the most sensitive noninvasive imaging modality for the diagnosis of liver metastases and has equivalent specificity (Rohren et al. 2002; Badiee et al. 2008) (Fig. 3).

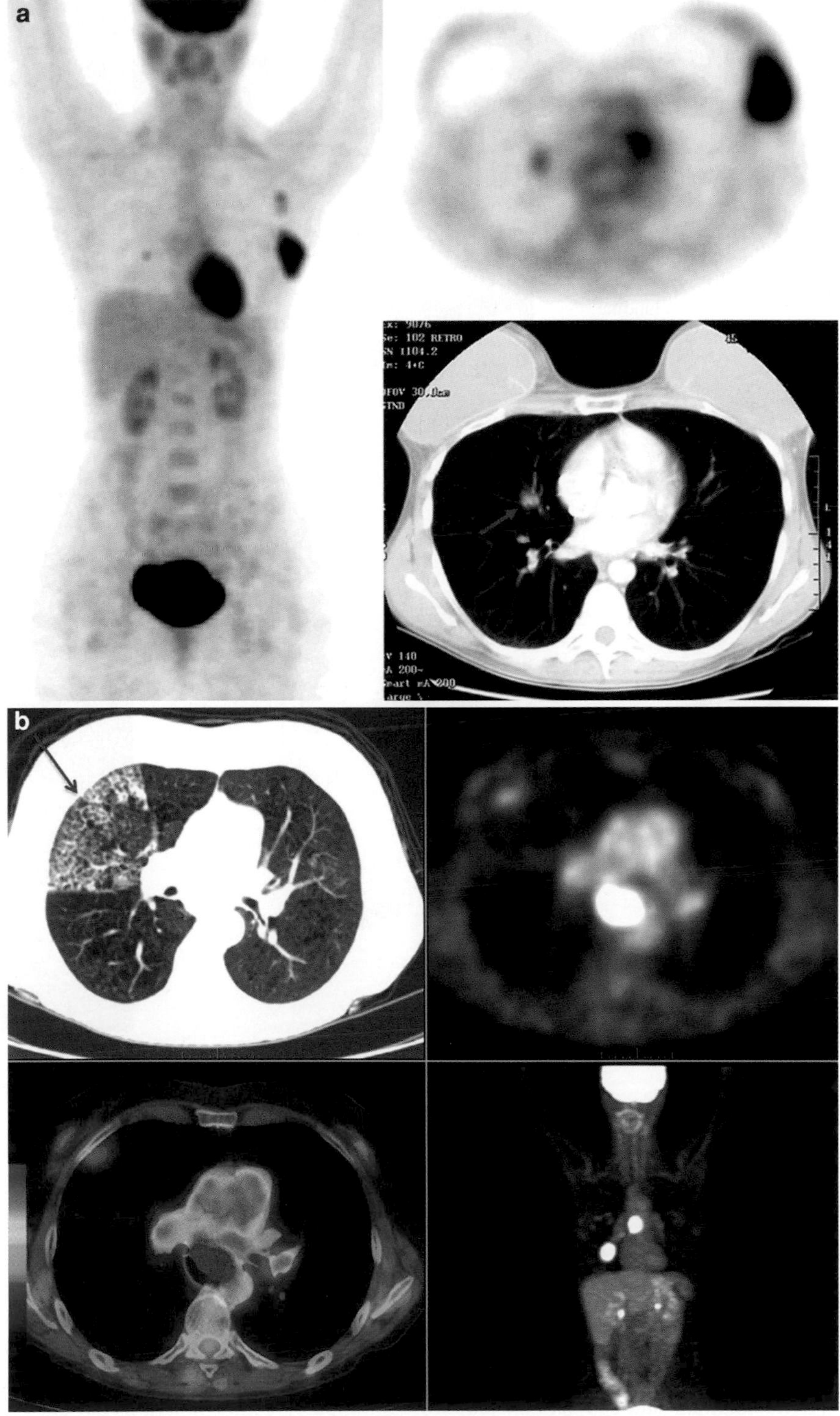

Fig. 2 **a** Staging PET/CT shows intense FDG accumulation in both axillary nodes and an unsuspected right lung nodule (*arrow*) in this 41-year-old woman with breast implants who discovered a palpable left breast mass. CT-guided needle biopsy of the lung nodule yielded metastatic breast cancer. **b** PET/CT shows intense pleural activity adjacent to a region of thickened, nodular interlobular septa with mild activity (*arrow*) due to lymphangitic spread in the right lung. There is also intense uptake in subcarinal nodal metastases and primary right lung adenocarcinoma in this 78-year-old man undergoing staging

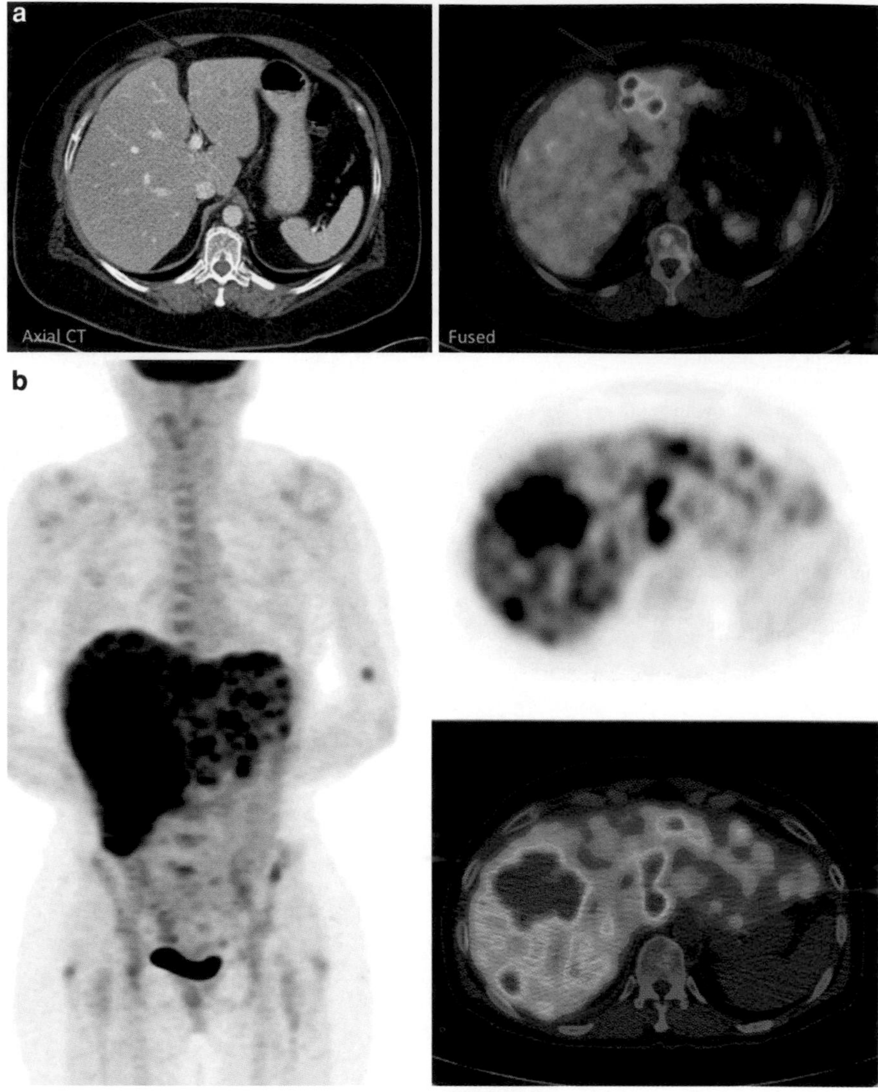

Fig. 3 **a** PET/CT identified 3 hypermetabolic metastases (*arrow*) after the CT suggested metastases in the left lobe of the liver in this 49-year-old woman with a history of endometrial cancer. Biopsy confirmation led to an interventional ablation. **b** PET/CT shows the preferential liver metastases often observed with metastatic uveal melanoma, as in this 59-year-old man

4.3 Brain

Brain metastases can arise from any hematogenously disseminated malignancy but the majority of brain metastases originate from lung cancer, breast cancer, renal cell carcinoma, and melanoma. About 10 % of cancer patients develop brain metastases. Most brain metastases occur late in the natural history of malignant disease. Imaging for asymptomatic brain metastases is undertaken only in selected patients where the risk is high and the treatment strategy is impacted. Most commonly, this is performed in both non-small cell and small cell lung cancer patients with planned treatment for curative intent and in patients with non-seminomatous testicular cancer (Wen and Loeffler 1999; Hochstenbag et al. 2000).

Most patients with a known primary tumor undergo CT or MRI brain imaging when neurologic signs and symptoms of brain metastasis arise. Contrast-enhanced CT scanning is used widely because of its accessibility. Gadolinium-enhanced MRI is the most sensitive modality for detecting brain metastases (Akeson et al. 1995).

FDG PET/CT has low sensitivity for brain metastases due to the high background activity in the white and especially the gray matter. When whole-body FDG PET is used in cancer staging, intracerebral metastases may appear as hyper- or hypometabolic foci relative to adjacent brain. For the identification of cerebral metastases FDG PET has a sensitivity of 75 % and a specificity of 83 %. Around 32–40 % of cerebral metastases seen on MRI imaging will not be detected

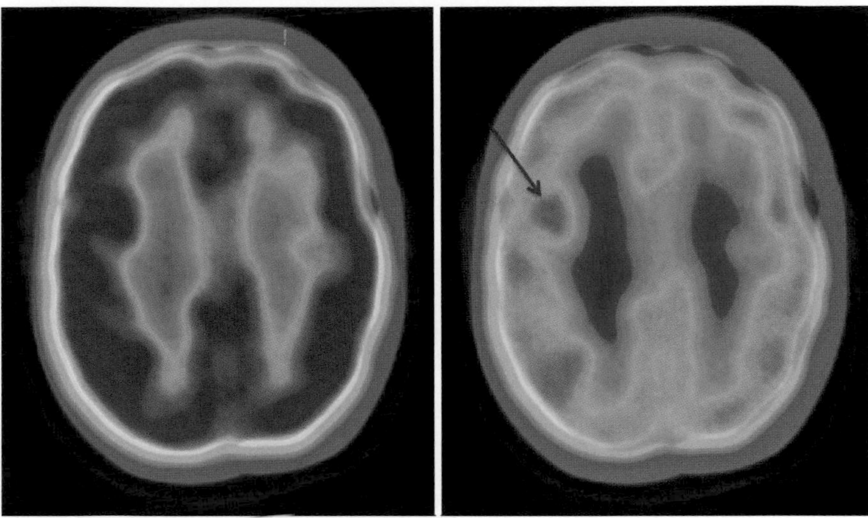

Fig. 4 The right cortical metastasis (*arrow*) is visible on PET/CT once the intensity of the FDG is scaled down to match the brain in this is 39-year-old man with a history of a melanoma resected from his back 3 years prior

on FDG PET (Griffeth et al. 1993; Rohren et al. 2003; Kitajima et al. 2008). The intensity of whole-body FDG PET images must be decreased when reviewing the brain to improve detection of metastasis (Fig. 4).

4.4 Adrenal

The adrenal glands, despite their small size, represent the fourth most common site of metastatic disease after lungs, liver, and bone. At autopsy, adrenal metastases are found in approximately 27 % of patients with cancer. The most common malignancies producing adrenal metastases are: breast, lung, melanoma, gastrointestinal, and kidney. Adrenal metastases are typically asymptomatic and are often incidentally detected on CT. Confirmation of adrenal metastasis has an important impact on staging, typically indicating stage IV disease (Ctvrtlík et al. 2009; Johnson et al. 2009).

PET/CT can be used to characterize adrenal masses by comparing the activity in the adrenal mass to that of the liver. Those adrenal nodules equal to or greater than the liver are likely malignant. Using the liver as an internal standard, PET/CT imaging has a sensitivity of 83–100 %, a specificity of 85–97 %, a PPV of 67–87 %, and an NPV of 93–100 % for the characterization of adrenal lesions. On PET/CT 3–10 % of benign adrenal lesions will demonstrate increased FDG accumulation. Some authors have proposed a cutoff SUV of 3.1, which has yielded a similar sensitivity of 98.5 % and a specificity of 92 % for characterization of malignant adrenal lesions (Metser et al. 2006; Blake et al. 2006; Boland et al. 2009) (Fig. 5).

4.5 Bone

Bone metastases are quite common in patients with cancer and over 50 % of people who die of cancer in the USA each year are thought to have bone involvement. The majority of bone metastases have been present for a considerable length of time before symptoms develop. Pain is the most frequent presenting manifestation of a bone metastasis. Breast, lung, prostate, renal cell, and colorectal cancers are the most common cause of bony metastases. In adults, more than 90 % of all osseous metastases are found in the axial and proximal appendicular skeleton where there is residual red marrow. Bone metastases are often multiple at the time of diagnosis (Salmon and Kilpatrick 2000; Coleman 2001; Mundy 2002).

Bone scintigraphy is an effective screening tool for detecting metastatic bone deposits by the increased osteoblastic activity they induce. Bone scan abnormalities reflect the bony reparative response around a metastasis, an indirect marker of tumor. FDG accumulates within the tumor and can help in identifying bone metastases at an early stage before host reactions to the osteoblasts occur. PET/CT excels in identifying tumor deposits prior to changes on CT. There is high FDG uptake in lytic or mixed lytic and sclerotic bone lesion. Sclerotic metastases are sometimes only visible on the CT component of the PET/CT and can be better visualized on

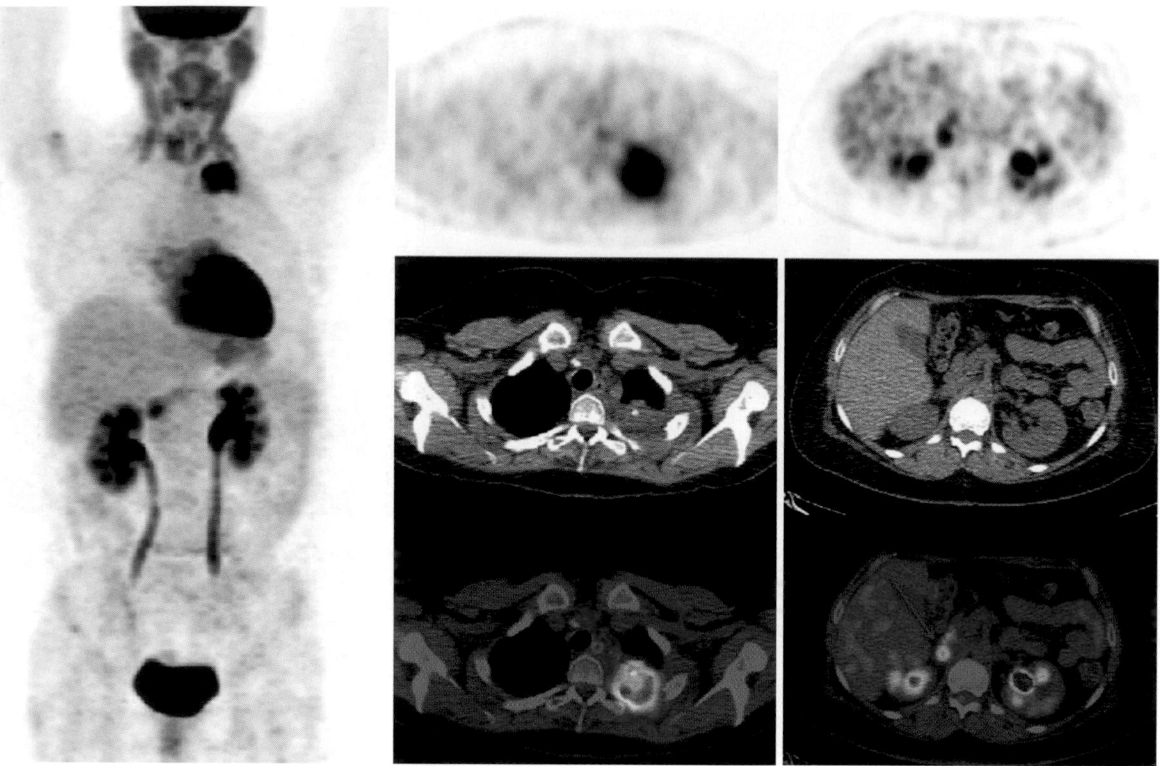

Fig. 5 PET/CT demonstrates an isolated hypermetabolic 1 cm right adrenal nodule (*arrow*) in this 68-year-old man who presented for staging of his left apical lung cancer. No mediastinal nodal disease was identified but cytology from a fine needle aspiration confirmed metastasis in the adrenal gland

bone scan. PET/CT is more sensitive and specific for bony metastases prior to treatment of most common carcinomas, except prostate cancer. ^{18}F-Fluoride PET is very sensitive for the detection of both lytic and sclerotic bone lesions, but like TcMDP, ^{18}F is not tumor specific. ^{18}F PET is more likely to detect skeletal metastases from tumors that typically have low FDG activity, whereas FDG PET is more likely to detect bone marrow metastases. Improved specificity is seen when the ^{18}F PET scan is interpreted with a fused CT exam. Lesions that measure less than 3 mm have limited detectability on PET (Cook et al. 1998; Uematsu et al. 2005; Even-Sapir 2005; Even-Sapir et al. 2006; Grant et al. 2008) (Fig. 6).

5 Cavitary Metastasis

The pleural, peritoneal, and pericardial cavities are potential spaces containing a very small amount of glycoprotein rich fluid, which facilitates motion with minimal friction. Tumors in direct contact shed cancer cells into these spaces. Hematogenous seeding of the pleural, peritoneal, and pericardial cavities is a less common route. Cancer cells entering these cavities can spread widely over the surfaces but often do not invade the parenchyma of the organs. Lung, breast, ovarian, and gastric cancers, and lymphoma most commonly cause pleural metastasis. The presence of metastatic pleural disease is an ominous sign; the average life expectancy is 5–16 months. The detection of peritoneal metastases is essential in the staging and restaging of gastrointestinal and gynecologic malignancies (Matthay et al. 1990; Sahn 1988).

On FDG PET/CT, pleural spread can present as hypermetabolism along the pleural surface or as focal FDG-avid nodules. The finding of increased FDG uptake greater than mediastinal blood pool activity that conforms to the pleural cavity is highly suggestive of a malignant effusion with a sensitivity of 95–100 %, specificity 67–71 %, and PPV 63–95 % (Erasmus et al. 2000; Bunyaviroch and Coleman 2006).

The findings on PET imaging which suggest the diagnosis of peritoneal carcinomatosis include: (1) hypermetabolism outlining abdominal organs,

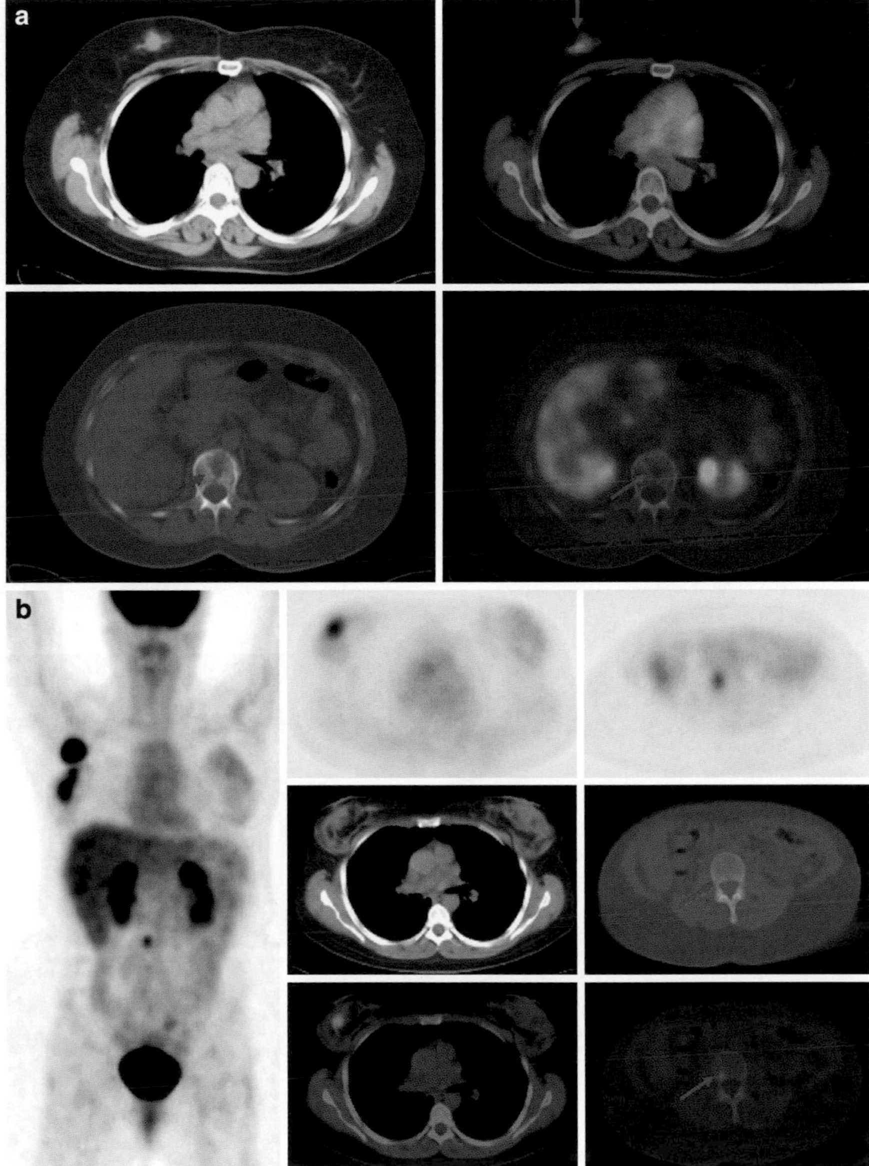

Fig. 6 **a** PET/CT shows intense FDG uptake in a predominantly lytic spine lesion (*arrow*) of this 61-year-old woman who presented for staging of right breast cancer. MRI of the spine identified a similar lesion. **b** This hypermetabolic L1 lesion on FDG PET has no corresponding CT abnormality (*arrow*) in this 37-year-old woman with right breast cancer and palpable right axillary nodes. Neoadjuvant chemotherapy produced resolution of L1 uptake and mild sclerosis, typical of metastasis

especially the liver capsule, and ascending or descending colon; (2) uniform low-grade tracer uptake throughout the abdomen obscuring the normal discrete visceral outlines of the bowel and liver; and (3) focal nodular areas of tracer uptake, especially in the Pouch of Douglas, right paracolic gutter, and around the right lower quadrant. FDG PET has a reported sensitivity of 71 % and specificity of 100 % for the detection of peritoneal carcinomatosis. Multidetector CT integrated with FDG PET improves the ability to detect peritoneal deposits (Schröder et al. 1999; Turlakow et al. 2003) (Fig. 7).

6 Rare Routes of Metastasis

6.1 Perineural

Neoplastic invasion of nerves is difficult, as the tumor cells must traverse the dense connective tissue of the epineurium. Although entry through the nerve sheath is difficult, once inside tumor cells are in a privileged growth environment. Involvement of the peripheral nerves with cancer is uncommon and usually associated

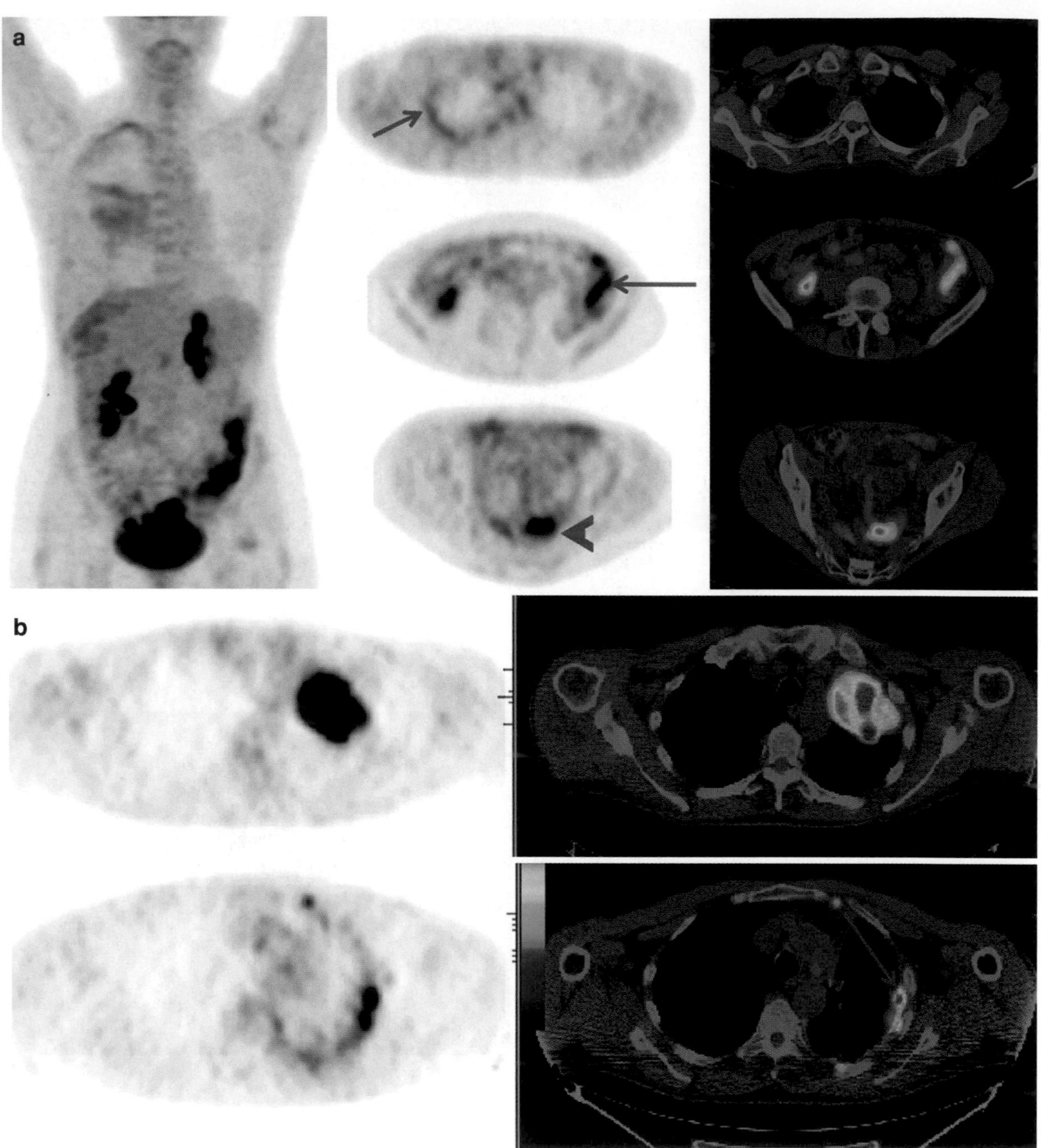

Fig. 7 **a** This 49-year-old woman presented with a right pleural effusion and pleural fluid sampling suggested malignant cells. PET/CT showed diffuse increased activity along the right pleural surface (*short arrow*) and left peritoneal hypermetabolism typical of carcinomatosis (*long arrow*). The intensely FDG-avid left pelvic mass was the patient's ovarian cancer primary (*arrowhead*). **b** The hypermetabolic nodule along the left pleural represents spread of the patient's known lung cancer

with lymphoproliferative malignancies. The perineural pathway of distant tumor spread is a feature in head and neck, pancreatic, colorectal, prostate, gastric, breast, and biliary cancers. The reason certain tumors are neurotropic is unknown, but it is a marker of poor outcome. Perineural metastasis spread is an increasingly recognized route of cancer metastasis on PET/CT (Liebig et al. 2009) (Fig. 8a).

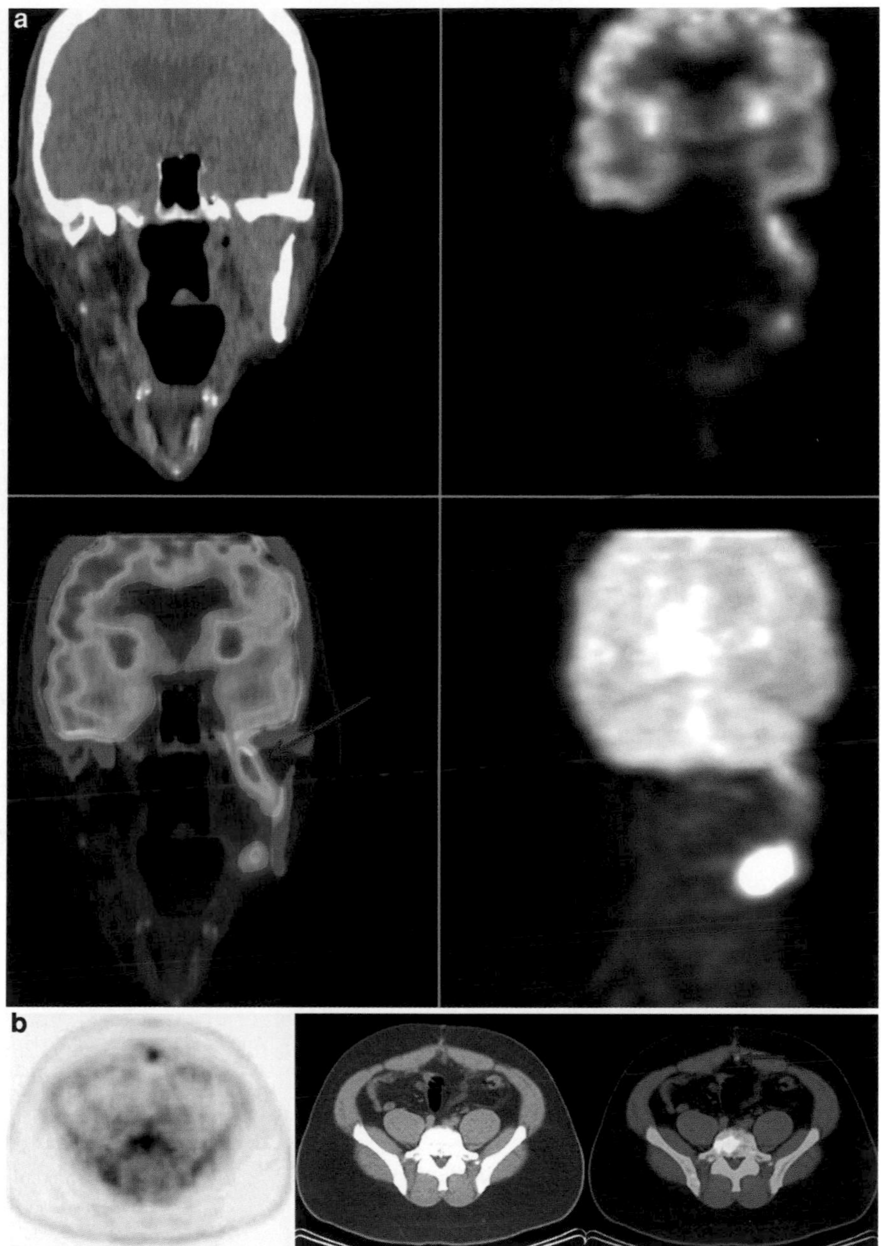

Fig. 8 **a** The intensely FDG-avid left mandibular squamous cell carcinoma extends along a branch of the left facial nerve (*arrow*). **b** Three years after a laparoscopic colon cancer resection, restaging PET/CT identified an 8 mm hypermetabolic nodule near the umbilicus. Resection confirmed an isolated colon cancer implantation metastasis

6.2 Transfer

Transfer or implantation metastasis results from the mechanical carriage of fragments of tumor cells. The cancer cells can be carried on biopsy needles, surgical instruments, and drainage tubes. Implanted tissues that harbor primary or metastatic cancer cells can take hold in a new host aided by immunosuppressive treatment given to the host. Transfer or implantation metastases are increasing in frequency with the greater application of endoscopic and laparoscopic surgeries. Transfer metastasis can be recognized readily on PET/CT (Fig. 8b).

7 Cancer of Unknown Primary

About 2–9 % of patients present with cancer of unknown primary (CUP) site. Typically the histology is not specific for a primary site. CUP is a heterogeneous group of malignancies, but all exhibit aggressive

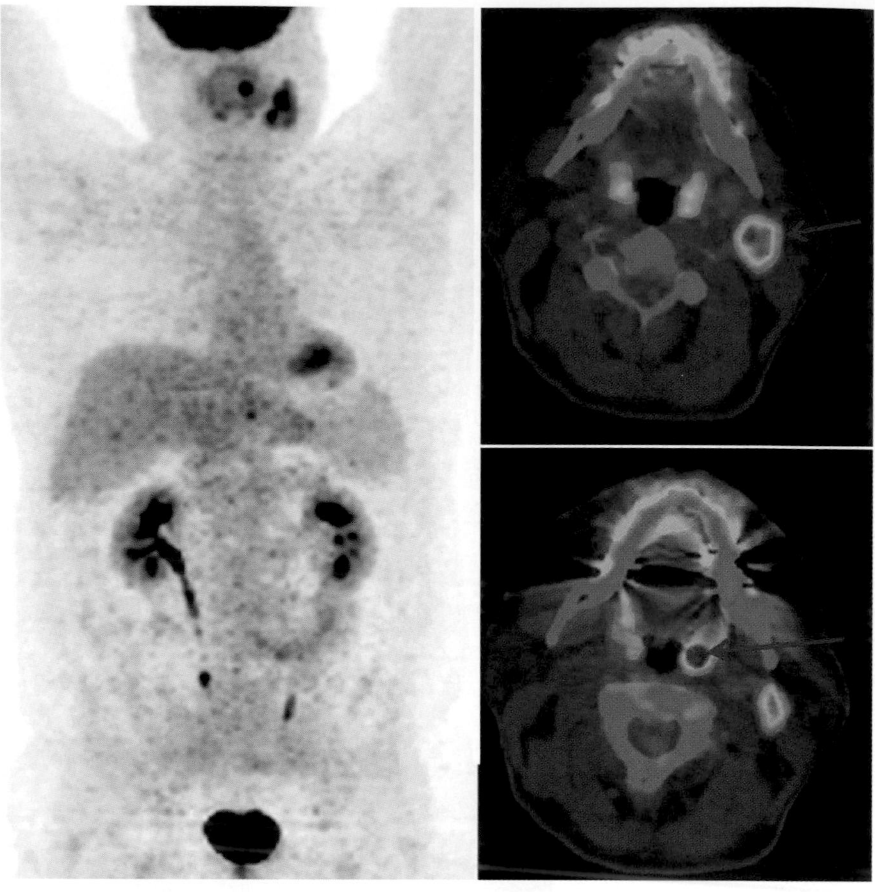

Fig. 9 This 57-year-old smoker presented with a left neck mass. Cytology from a fine needle aspiration biopsy showed squamous cell carcinoma but no primary tumor was identified on initial staging. PET/CT showed a hypermetabolic left tonsilar primary cancer (*long arrow*) and intense uptake in the left neck nodes (*short arrow*)

biologic and clinical behavior (Pavlidis and Fizazi 2009). The median survival is 6–10 months, but if the primary is identified and treated, the median survival is 23 months. For patients with neck node presentations, the 5-year survival is 100 % versus 58 % otherwise (Raber et al. 1991; Muir 1995; Haas et al. 2002; Pavlidis and Fizazi 2009).

FDG PET/CT has been shown to identify the primary tumor in about 24–57 % of patients with negative conventional imaging results. A meta-analysis has shown PET imaging to locate the primary in 37 % of patients. The pooled sensitivity was 84 % and specificity 84 % for the detection of the primary tumor. The PET findings changed therapy in 18.2–60 % of patients. The most common false positive locations were the lungs and oropharynx and the most common site of missed cancer was the breast. An added benefit of FDG PET imaging is the identification of additional sites of distant metastatic disease in 31 % of patients (Jeong et al. 2002; Delgado-Bolton et al. 2003; Gutzeit et al. 2005; Kwee and Kwee 2009) (Fig. 9).

References

Acikgoz G, Kim SM, Houseni M et al (2006) Pulmonary lymphangitic carcinomatosis (PLC): spectrum of FDG-PET findings. Clin Nucl Med 31(11):673–678

Akeson P, Larsson EM, Kristoffersen DT (1995) Brain metastases–comparison of gadodiamide injection-enhanced MR imaging at standard and high dose, contrast-enhanced CT and non-contrast-enhanced MR imaging. Acta Radiol 36(3):300–6

Allard WJ, Matera J, Miller MC et al (2004) Tumor cells circulate in the peripheral blood of all major carcinomas but not in healthy subjects or patients with nonmalignant diseases. Clin Cancer Res 10:6897–6904

Badiee S, Franc BL, Webb EM, Chu B, Hawkins RA, Coakley F (2008) Role of IV iodinated contrast material in 18F-FDG PET/CT of liver metastases. AJR Am J Roentgenol 191:1436–1439

Bar-Shalom R, Kagna O, Israel O, Guralnik L (2008) Noninvasive diagnosis of solitary pulmonary lesions in cancer patients based on 2-fluoro-2-deoxy-D-glucose avidity on positron emission tomography/computed tomography. Cancer 113:3213

Blake MA, Slattery JM, Kalra MK, Halpern EF, Fischman AJ, Mueller PR, Boland GW (2006) Adrenal lesions: characterization with fused PET/CT image in patients with proved or suspected malignancy—initial experience. Radiology 238(3):970–977

Boland GW, Blake MA, Holalkere NS, Hahn PF (2009) PET/CT for the characterization of adrenal masses in patients with cancer: qualitative versus quantitative accuracy in 150 consecutive patients. AJR Am J Roentgenol 192:956–962

Branstetter BF 4th, Blodgett TM, Zimmer LA et al (2005) Head and neck malignancy: is PET/CT more accurate than PET or CT alone? Radiology 235:580–586

Bunyaviroch T, Coleman RE (2006) PET evaluation of lung cancer. J Nucl Med 47:451–469

Chang AE, Schaner EG, Conkle DM et al (1979) Evaluation of computed tomography in the detection of pulmonary metastases: a prospective study. Cancer 43:913–916

Chiang AC, Massagué J (2008) Molecular basis of metastasis. N Engl J Med 359:2814–2823

Christie-Large M, James SL, Tiessen L, Davies AM, Grimer RJ (2008) Imaging strategy for detecting lung metastases at presentation in patients with soft tissue sarcomas. Eur J Cancer 44:1841–1845

Coleman RE (2001) Metastatic bone disease: clinical features, pathophysiology and treatment strategies. Cancer Treat Rev 27:165

Cook GJ, Houston S, Rubens R, Maisey MN, Fogelman I (1998) Detection of bone metastases in breast cancer by 18FDG PET: differing metabolic activity in osteoblastic and osteolytic lesions. J Clin Oncol 16:3375–3379

Ctvrtlík F, Herman M, Student V, Tichá V, Minarík J (2009) Differential diagnosis of incidentally detected adrenal masses revealed on routine abdominal CT. Eur J Radiol 69:243–252

Davis SD (1991) CT evaluation for pulmonary metastases in patients with extrathoracic malignancy. Radiology 180:1–12

De Wever W, Meylaerts L, De Ceuninck L, Stroobants S, Verschakelen JA (2007) Additional value of integrated PET-CT in the detection and characterization of lung metastases: correlation with CT alone and PET alone. Eur Radiol 17(2):467–473

Delgado-Bolton RC, Fernández-Pérez C, González-Maté A, Carreras JL (2003) Meta-analysis of the performance of 18F-FDG PET in primary tumor detection in unknown primary tumors. J Nucl Med 44:1301–1314

Erasmus JJ, McAdams HP, Rossi SE et al (2000) FDG PET of pleural effusions in patients with non-small cell lung cancer. AJR Am J Roentgenol 175:245–249

Even-Sapir E, Metser U, Mishani E, Lievshitz G, Lerman H, Leibovitch I (2006) The detection of bone metastases in patients with high-risk prostate cancer: 99mTc-MDP Planar bone scintigraphy, single- and multi-field-of-view SPECT, 18F-fluoride PET, and 18F-fluoride PET/CT. J Nucl Med 47:287–297

Even-Sapir E (2005) Imaging of malignant bone involvement by morphologic, scintigraphic, and hybrid modalities. J Nucl Med 46:1356–1367

Grant FD, Fahey FH, Packard AB, Davis RT, Alavi A, Treves ST (2008) Skeletal PET with 18F-fluoride: applying new technology to an old tracer. J Nucl Med 49:68–78

Griffeth LK, Rich KM, Dehdashti F et al (1993) Brain metastases from non-central nervous system tumors: evaluation with PET. Radiology 186:37–44

Gupta GP, Massague J (2006) Cancer metastasis: building a framework. Cell 127:679–695

Gutzeit A, Antoch G, Kühl H et al (2005) Unknown primary tumors: detection with dual-modality PET/CT–initial experience. Radiology 234:227–234

Haas I, Hoffmann TK, Engers R, Ganzer U (2002) Diagnostic strategies in cervical carcinoma of an unknown primary (CUP). Eur Arch Otorhinolaryngol 259:325–333

Hirakata K, Nakata H, Haratake J (1993) Appearance of pulmonary metastases on high-resolution CT scans: comparison with histopathologic findings from autopsy specimens. AJR Am J Roentgenol 161:37–43

Hochstenbag MM, Twijnstra A, Wilmink JT (2000) Asymptomatic brain metastases (BM) in small cell lung cancer (SCLC): MR-imaging is useful at initial diagnosis. J Neurooncol 48:243–248

Jeon TY, Lee KS, Yi CA et al (2010) Incremental value of PET/CT over CT for mediastinal nodal staging of non-small cell lung cancer: comparison between patients with and without idiopathic pulmonary fibrosis. AJR Am J Roentgenol 195:370–376

Jeong HJ, Chung JK, Kim YK et al (2002) Usefulness of whole-body (18)F-FDG PET in patients with suspected metastatic brain tumors. J Nucl Med 43:1432–1437

Johnson PT, Horton KM, Fishman EK (2009) Adrenal mass imaging with multidetector CT: pathologic conditions, pearls, and pitfalls. Radiographics 29:1333–1351

Kim BT, Lee KS, Shim SS et al (2006) Stage T1 non-small cell lung cancer: preoperative mediastinal nodal staging with integrated FDG PET/CT—a prospective study. Radiology 241:501–509

Kinkel K, Lu Y, Both M (2002) Detection of hepatic metastases from cancers of the gastrointestinal tract by using noninvasive imaging methods (US, CT, MR imaging, PET): a meta-analysis. Radiology 224:748–756

Kitajima K, Murakami K, Yamasaki E et al (2008a) Accuracy of 18F-FDG PET/CT in detecting pelvic and paraaortic lymph node metastasis in patients with endometrial cancer. AJR Am J Roentgenol 190:1652–1658

Kitajima K, Nakamoto Y, Okizuka H, Onishi Y, Senda M, Suganuma N et al (2008b) Accuracy of whole-body FDG-PET/CT for detecting brain metastases from non-central nervous system tumors. Ann Nucl Med 22:595–602

Kwee TC, Kwee RM (2009) Combined FDG-PET/CT for the detection of unknown primary tumors: systematic review and meta-analysis. Eur Radiol 19:731–744

Liebig C, Ayala G, Wilks JA, Berger DH, Albo D (2009) Perineural invasion in cancer: a review of the literature. Cancer 115:3379–3391

Lise M, Da Pian PP, Nitti D (1991) Colorectal metastases to the liver: present results and future strategies. J Surg Oncol Suppl 2:69–73

Matthay RA, Coppage L, Shaw C, Filderman AE (1990) Malignancies metastatic to the pleura. Invest Radiol 25:601–619

Mavi A, Lakhani P, Zhuang H (2005) Fluorodeoxyglucose-PET in characterizing solitary pulmonary nodules, assessing pleural diseases, and the initial staging, restaging, therapy planning, and monitoring response of ung cancer. Radiol Clin North Am 43:1–21

Metser U, Miller E, Lerman H, Lievshitz G, Avital S, Even-Sapir E (2006) 18F-FDG PET/CT in the evaluation of adrenal masses. J Nucl Med 47:32–37

Meziane MA, Hruban RH, Zerhouni EA et al (1988) High resolution CT of the lung parenchyma with pathologic correlation. Radiographics 8:27–54

Muir C (1995) Cancer of unknown primary site. Cancer 75(1 Suppl):353–356

Mundy GR (2002) Metastasis to bone: causes, consequences and therapeutic opportunities. Nat Rev Cancer 2:584

Ng SH, Yen TC, Liao CT, Chang JT, Chan SC, Ko SF, Wang HM, Wong HF (2005) 18F-FDG PET and CT/MRI in oral cavity squamous cell carcinoma: a prospective study of 124 patients with histologic correlation. J Nucl Med 46:1136–1143

Niekel MC, Bipat S, Stoker J (2010) Imaging for colorectal liver metastases-a meta-analysis. Ann Oncol 21(S1):37

Pavlidis N, Fizazi K (2009) Carcinoma of unknown primary (CUP). Crit Rev Oncol Hematol 69:271–278

Raber MN, Faintuch J, Abbruzzese JL, Sumrall C, Frost P (1991) Continuous infusion 5-fluorouracil, etoposide and cis-diamminedichloroplatinum in patients with metastatic carcinoma of unknown primary origin. Ann Oncol 2:519–520

Rohren EM, Provenzale JM, Barboriak DP, Coleman RE (2003) Screening for cerebral metastases with FDG PET in patients undergoing whole-body staging of non-central nervous system malignancy. Radiology 226:181–187

Rohren EM, Paulson EK, Hagge R et al (2002) The role of F-18 FDG positron emission tomography in preoperative assessment of the liver in patients being considered for curative resection of hepatic metastases from colorectal cancer. Clin Nucl Med 27:550–555

Salmon JM, Kilpatrick SE (2000) Pathology of skeletal metastases. Orthop Clin North Am 31:537–44, Oct

Schöder H, Carlson DL, Kraus DH et al (2006) 18F-FDG PET/CT for detecting nodal metastases in patients with oral cancer staged N0 by clinical examination and CT/MRI. J Nucl Med 47:755–762

Schöder H, Yeung HW, Gonen M, Kraus D, Larson SM (2004) Head and neck cancer: clinical usefulness and accuracy of PET/CT image fusion. Radiology 231:65–72

Schröder W, Zimny M, Rudlowski C, Büll U, Rath W (1999) The role of 18F-fluoro-deoxyglucose positron emission tomography (18F-FDG PET) in diagnosis of ovarian cancer. Int J Gynecol Cancer 9:117–122

Sahn SA (1988) State of the art. Pleura Am Rev Respir Dis 138:184–234

Teknos TN, Rosenthal EL, Lee D, Taylor R, Marn CS (2001) Positron emission tomography in the evaluation of stage III and IV head and neck cancer. Head Neck 23:1056–1060

Turlakow A, Yeung HW, Salmon AS, Macapinlac HA, Larson SM (2003) Peritoneal carcinomatosis: role of (18)F-FDG PET. J Nucl Med 44:1407–1412

Uematsu T, Yuen S, Yukisawa S, Aramaki T, Morimoto N, Endo M, Furukawa H, Uchida Y, Watanabe J (2005) Comparison of FDG PET and SPECT for detection of bone metastases in breast cancer. AJR Am J Roentgenol 184:1266–1273

Wen PY, Loeffler JS (1999) Management of brain metastases. Oncology (Williston Park) Jul, 13(7):941–54, 957–61; discussion 961–2, 9

Yi CA, Lee KS, Kim BT et al (2006) Tissue characterization of solitary pulmonary nodule: comparative study between helical dynamic CT and integrated PET/CT. J Nucl Med 47:443–449

Radiotherapy Planning

Minh Tam Truong and Rathan M. Subramaniam

Contents

M. T. Truong (✉)
Boston University School of Medicine,
Boston, MA, USA
e-mail: minh-tam.truong@bmc.org

M. T. Truong · R. M. Subramaniam
Department of Radiation Oncology,
Boston Medical Center, Boston, MA, USA

M. T. Truong
Harvard Medical School, Boston, MA, USA

Abstract

Advances in radiotherapy planning and delivery in the past decade, including the increased use of three-dimensional conformal radiotherapy and intensity-modulated radiotherapy (IMRT), have made accurate tumor volume delineation critical for radiotherapy planning, particularly since IMRT results in sharp dose gradients between normal tissue and the tumor. As a result, with the simultaneous rapid growth of PET/CT utilization, integration of PET/CT into radiotherapy planning has been important for accurate and consistent tumor volume delineation, improved identification of nodal and distant metastatic disease and assessing response to radiotherapy. Determining the optimal method of using PET/CT for tumor volume delineation with different methods of volumetric segmentation is currently being studied. Experimental studies with novel PET tracers and applications of PET to adaptive radiotherapy planning based on PET/CT response are also being carried out. PET/CT is an important imaging modality for radiotherapy planning in many solid tumors.

1 Introduction

External beam radiotherapy is one of the main treatment modalities for treating cancer and benign tumors. During radiotherapy treatment, the patient is immobilized in the optimal position for delivering radiation beams to the tumor target while minimizing radiation to the adjacent normal tissue. Therapeutic radiation usually delivers high energy megavoltage

P. Peller et al. (eds.), *PET-CT and PET-MRI in Oncology*, Medical Radiology. Diagnostic Imaging,
DOI: 10.1007/174_2012_580,

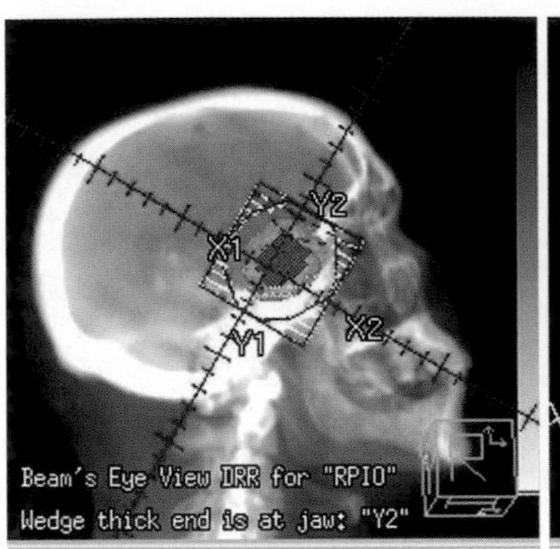

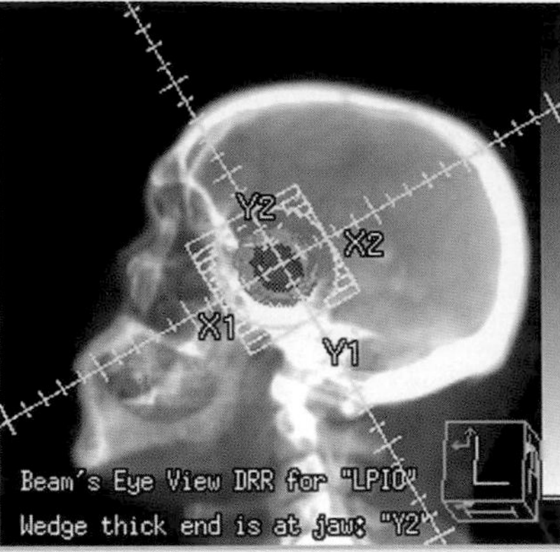

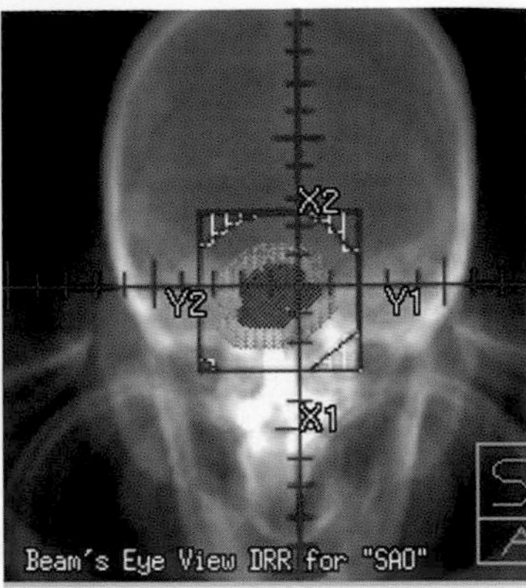

Fig. 1 An example of 3D conformal radiotherapy using CT planning with a three field plan targeting a pituitary macroadenoma. Each beam is shaped with a multileaf collimator to conform to the shape of the tumor. The center of the graticule represents the treatment isocenter

photon beams (in the energy range of 4–18 MV), or less commonly electron or proton beams. The radiation beams are shaped or collimated to conform to the shape of the target and multiple beams may be used to focus on the target to reduce the dose to the normal tissue (Fig. 1). Based on radiobiological principles, radiation treatments are often fractionated to maximize the therapeutic ratio in order to increase the probability of sterilizing the tumor cells while allowing normal tissues to repair during the course of treatment and minimizing late injury to the normal tissue (Hall 2000).

2 Simulation and Immobilization

A typical course of radiotherapy requires reproducing the same configuration of radiation beams and immobilizing the patient in the same treatment position for daily treatments ranging from 1 to 35 treatments, over one to several weeks. To achieve this aim, simulation is an essential part of the treatment planning, process to accurately identify the tumor and adjacent organs, design the optimal beam arrangement or configuration, to calculate the dose distribution to the target and avoidance structures, and to reproduce the same treatment over multiple fractions.

The patient is initially immobilized in the treatment position using an immobilization device to allow daily reproducibility. In head and neck cancer or brain tumors, a custom thermoplastic mask is used to immobilize the head and neck (Fig. 2), in the chest or abdomen, a custom-made polystyrene bead vacuum mold may be used to immobilize the patient. A treatment isocenter is placed in or near the vicinity of the tumor mass, and all beams are referenced to the treatment isocenter (Fig. 1). Lasers mounted on the walls of the treatment room and in the simulator room are used to align the patient and reproduce the same setup defined in the simulator (Fig. 3). Surface landmarks on the patient, usually tattoos or marks made on the immobilization device (triangulation points) are used with the lasers to correctly position the patient to the treatment isocenter each day.

3 PET/CT Simulation

A PET/CT for radiation treatment planning is performed on a flat bed with the same immobilization devices to be used for the treatment setup. The scan may be performed in conjunction with a diagnostic whole body scan or as a separate limited examination in the intended treatment region. At our institution, a non-contrast CT simulation for isocenter placement and fabrication of any custom immobilization devices is performed prior to the PET/CT scan. The patient then undergoes a dedicated contrast-enhanced PET/CT scan. The PET/CT scanner is equipped with alignment lasers similar to the CT simulation suite. After fasting, the patient is injected with a standard dose of 10–15 mCi of 18-FDG. The PET/CT is then performed with CT sections of 1.25 cm (Subramaniam et al. 2010).

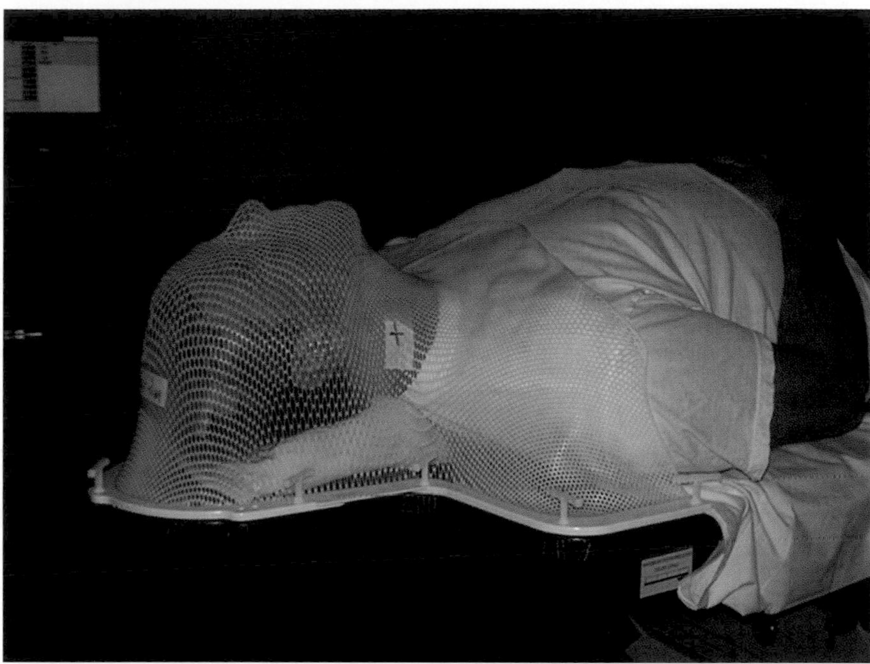

Fig. 2 A custom thermoplastic mask to immobilize a patient with head and neck cancer in the treatment position

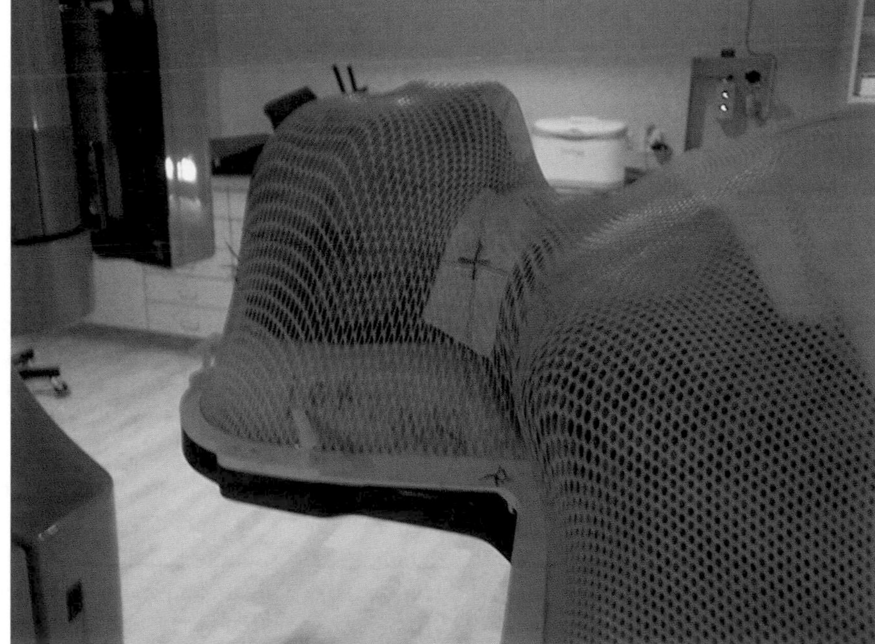

Fig. 3 Lasers mounted on the walls of the treatment room are used to align the patient on a daily basis using triangulation points on the patient's mask

4 Treatment Planning

4.1 2D Radiotherapy to 3D Conformal Radiotherapy

Traditionally, two-dimensional kilovoltage X-rays were used for simulation, the tumor was often wired or hand drawn onto the X-ray film and X-rays were taken with a fluoroscopy unit. The location of the tumor was based on clinical examination and treatment margins around the tumor were large to account for variations in the daily setup and also potential microscopic disease. As a result larger radiation portals were often used and large areas of normal tissue were irradiated. However, with the emergence of CT and its integration into the simulation process, treatment planning has been revolutionized over the past 10–15 years. With CT, the concept of virtual simulation has emerged, in which the patient undergoes a treatment planning CT in the treatment position. Radiotherapy planning is performed using the planning CT data set as the virtual patient. This has greatly improved the accuracy of treatment planning while also improving patient comfort by minimizing the duration of the simulation. Three-dimensional conformal radiotherapy (3DCRT) has evolved as a result of CT simulation. The tumor and normal organs are drawn on each axial slice of the CT data set. Beam arrangements are designed by the physician and/or physicist using specialized radiation treatment planning software. All dose calculations with CT planning are based on Hounsfield units, representing the density of the tissue. Dose distributions can be visualized on each axial CT slice and a digital reconstructed radiograph of each beam can be reconstructed from the CT data set to generate a beam's eye view of the target (Fig. 1). Furthermore, the beam can be accurately shaped using multileaf collimators in the linear accelerator to conform to the shape of the tumor as defined by CT. The dose to the tumor and normal tissues can be analyzed using dose-volume histograms; manual adjustments of the plan can be performed based on the information provided by the dose-volume histogram or dose distributions seen on the axial CTs. Traditional field 2D and 3DCRT design uses forward planning where the physician and physicist decide on the ideal beam arrangement based on their experience and training.

4.2 Target Volume Definition

Standards for target volume definition for radiotherapy planning have been determined by the International Commission of Radiation Units and Measurements (ICRU) in reports 50 and 62 (1993, 1999). Initial target definition includes defining the gross tumor volume (GTV), which is the gross demonstrable extent and location of the tumor, and a clinical target volume, which is defined by the GTV and any other tissue with presumed tumor. This includes regions of potential microscopic spread of tumor. A planning target volume includes the clinical target volume and a margin for setup error, which includes patient motion and setup uncertainties.

In ICRU Report 62, an internal target volume, was defined that describes an internal margin added to the clinical target volume to account for internal physiological movement, such as breathing, which can alter the position, shape, and size of the clinical target volume.

4.3 Intensity-Modulated Radiotherapy

Intensity-modulated radiotherapy (IMRT) is an advanced form of three-dimensional radiotherapy which incorporates computerized radiation beam delivery and computer-generated algorithms to optimize beam arrangements and modulation of the radiation intensity within each beam. For IMRT, the beam optimization is done by inverse planning in which the computer performs hundreds to thousands of iterations (Xia and Ling 2004). In contrast, 3DCRT uses uniform beam intensities and forward planning with the physicist and radiation oncologist making manual adjustments to optimize beam arrangements based on their experience and knowledge of areas at risk for tumor spread. The advantage of IMRT is the ability to better spare normal tissue while still delivering high doses to the tumor, which could not have been achieved by conventional 3DCRT, particularly for concave target volumes adjacent to critical structures such as the spinal cord. In head and neck cancer, the parotid gland cannot be spared by conventional 2D or 3DCRT using opposed lateral beams. With IMRT, it is possible to spare the parotid glands with a mean dose of less than 30 Gy while delivering 70 Gy to an adjacent head and neck tumor. IMRT also allows dose escalation in the treatment of prostate cancer while minimizing the dose to the adjacent rectum and bladder.

For IMRT, the radiation oncologist is required to contour the tumor and all normal organs at risk in the treatment region. As a result, a detailed knowledge of normal tissue anatomy is critical to accurately delineate normal tissues as avoidance structures. The radiation oncologist defines the organs at risk, and then proposes radiation dose limits to the normal tissues to minimize the risk of radiation-induced toxicity. In the IMRT treatment planning process, failure to contour an avoidance structure can result in "hot spots", or high doses of radiation inadvertently delivered to the structure causing radiation-induced toxicity.

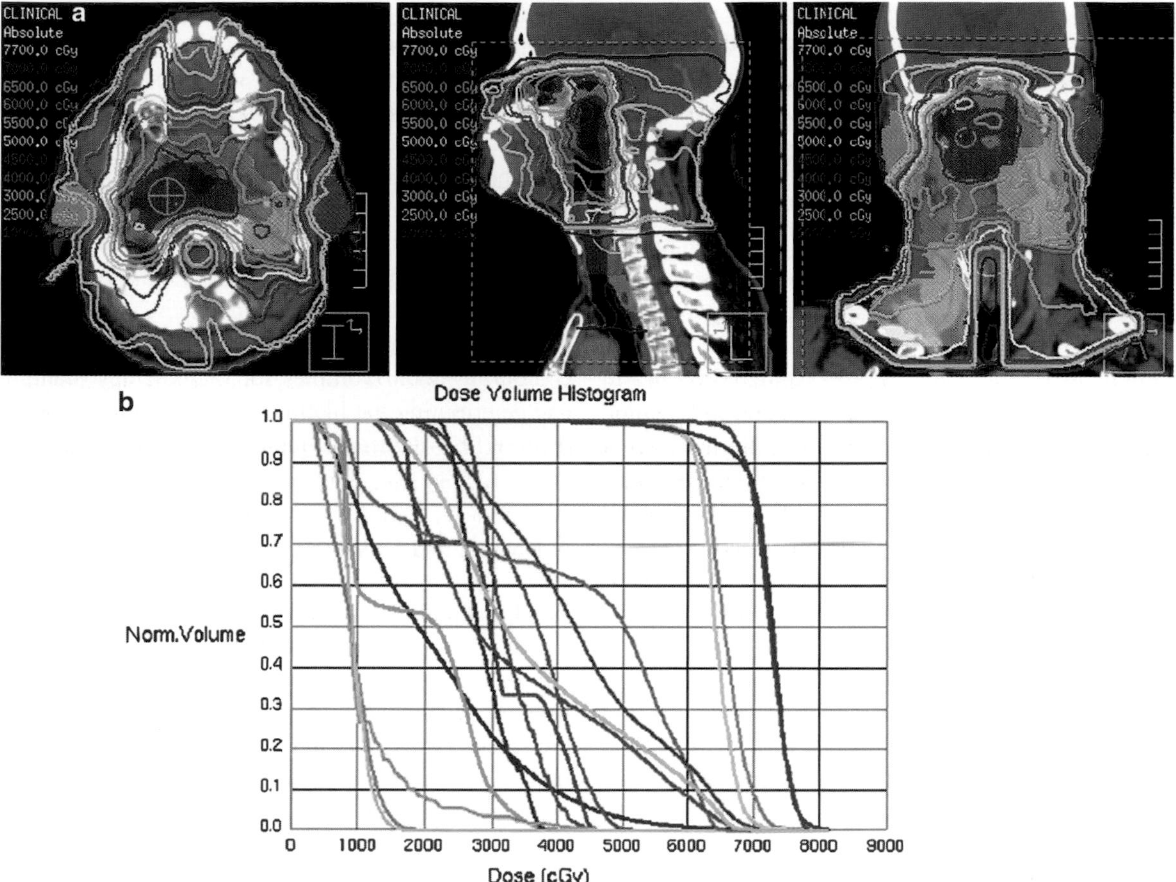

Fig. 4 **a** An example of beam arrangements and isodoses for a head and neck IMRT plan in a patient with locally advanced nasopharyngeal cancer. Bilateral parotid glands, oral cavity and spinal cord are being spared. Superior IMRT field is matched to a low anterior neck field (anterior photon field). **b** Corresponding dose-volume histogram of a head and neck cancer patient treated with intensity modulated radiotherapy

The advantage of IMRT is that the prescribed radiation dose can be precisely shaped to the target volume with rapid dose falloff to spare the adjacent normal tissue, and minimizing the risk of normal tissue toxicity. With such steep dose gradients between the planning target volumes and the normal tissues, accurate tumor delineation is particularly important to minimize the risk of under-dosing the tumor.

IMRT is significantly more labor-intensive for the physician and physicist, since contour delineation of tumor and multiple normal structures, planning optimization, quality assurance testing, and beam delivery is significantly more time-consuming and complicated than 3DCRT. Figure 4 demonstrates an example of IMRT for a locally advanced head and neck cancer.

4.4 Stereotactic Body Radiotherapy

Stereotactic body radiotherapy (SBRT) is a specialized form of conformal radiotherapy using the principles of stereotactic radiosurgery which have been used for many decades to treat intracranial and skull-based conditions, applied extracranially to numerous body sites. SBRT allows highly focused delivery of radiation to extracranial sites using stereotactic localization of the target. The main applications of SBRT include inoperable early stage lung cancers, oligometastases of the spine and liver, pancreatic, and recurrent head and neck cancer (Truong et al. 2009). The advantage of SBRT is the ability to escalate the radiation dose to the tumor, while sparing maximum normal tissue to minimize toxicity. SBRT is typically delivered in 1–5 fractions. Fractionated SBRT can target potentially larger tumor volumes than single fraction treatment as fractionation allows sparing of the normal tissues. Frameless radiosurgery systems rely on real-time imaged guided systems to ensure accurate localization and compensate for patient external motion and internal tumor motion, while delivering high precision stereotactic radiosurgery or SBRT without the use of an invasive stereotactic frame (Adler et al. 1999). Planning target volumes used in SBRT are minimal (0–5 mm) compared to 3DCRT and IMRT, because stereotactic localization of the target and real-time imaging minimize setup uncertainties. Hence target definition for SBRT is critical to minimize marginal tumor miss, or to avoid unnecessarily large volumes, as higher doses are used and normal tissue irradiation should be kept a minimum. Figure 5a, b shows an example of PET/CT used for SBRT for a liver metastasis.

5 Integration of PET/CT into Radiotherapy Planning

As radiation planning and treatment delivery have become more sophisticated by improving dose conformality around the tumor, reducing treatment margins and sparing more normal tissue, accurate target definition has become critically important. Biologic imaging such as PET/CT have improved diagnosis and staging, and integration of PET/CT imaging into radiotherapy planning has been rapidly adopted in clinical practice. PET/CT gives the radiation oncologist a biologic imaging tool for defining the tumor volume in addition to anatomic imaging, in an attempt to improve the accuracy of tumor contouring.

One of the questions regarding incorporating PET/CT into treatment planning is whether PET/CT improves the accuracy of target definition over CT or MRI alone. Many different contouring methods are available for use with PET imaging to define the tumor volume, such as visual determination, SUV criteria, and various SUV segmentation methods. Determining which SUV criteria distinguishes between benign or inflammatory changes versus malignancy is important; the wrong criteria can potentially confound the use of PET/CT in radiotherapy planning. Furthermore, physiologically normal tissue FDG uptake can also make determination of the tumor more difficult for the inexperienced user. In a study by Murakami et al. (2007) of 23 patients with head and neck carcinoma, nodal lesions detected by PET/CT were correlated with pathology. The SUV_{max} overlapped in lymph nodes less than 15 mm diameter for both pathologically positive and negative nodes. Using a size-based SUV_{max} cutoff of 1.9, 2.5 and 3.0 for lymph nodes <10, 10–15, and >15 mm respectively, PET/CT yielded a sensitivity of 79% and specificity of 99% for nodal staging. This information is important when contouring nodal volumes for radiotherapy planning and determining the likelihood of pathologic involvement of PET-detected lymph nodes.

5.1 Image Fusion

The CT simulation scan is the primary image set on which all dose calculations are based. The PET, PET/CT, or MRI scans are secondary image sets that are fused or registered to the radiation planning CT. The secondary image sets are used to improve visualization of the target and sometimes the normal tissues to aid target definition and accurately contour avoidance structures. The two image sets are fused or co-registered. The accuracy of the registration is usually checked visually or measured by the physicist and radiation oncologist, and contours can be drawn on either image set. Fusion can be performed manually or automatically depending on the planning software. Manual fusion methods include a multiple point system overlay. Points are chosen by the physician or physicist in three dimensions of specific anatomic points on each scan and then the software shifts the secondary image set to the primary image to achieve the best registration. Alternatively, anatomic contours are identified and the software manipulates the secondary image set to match the primary image set based on the contours. Both systems use rigid fusion where there is no spatial manipulation of either image set. Figure 6 shows an example of rigid fusion, with the patient in the treatment planning position during the PET/CT scan to minimize an inaccuracy in the overlay of images.

Deformable (non-rigid) registration of image sets may be performed using specialized software when two image sets show different anatomic positions, such that accurate fusion at one axial level may result

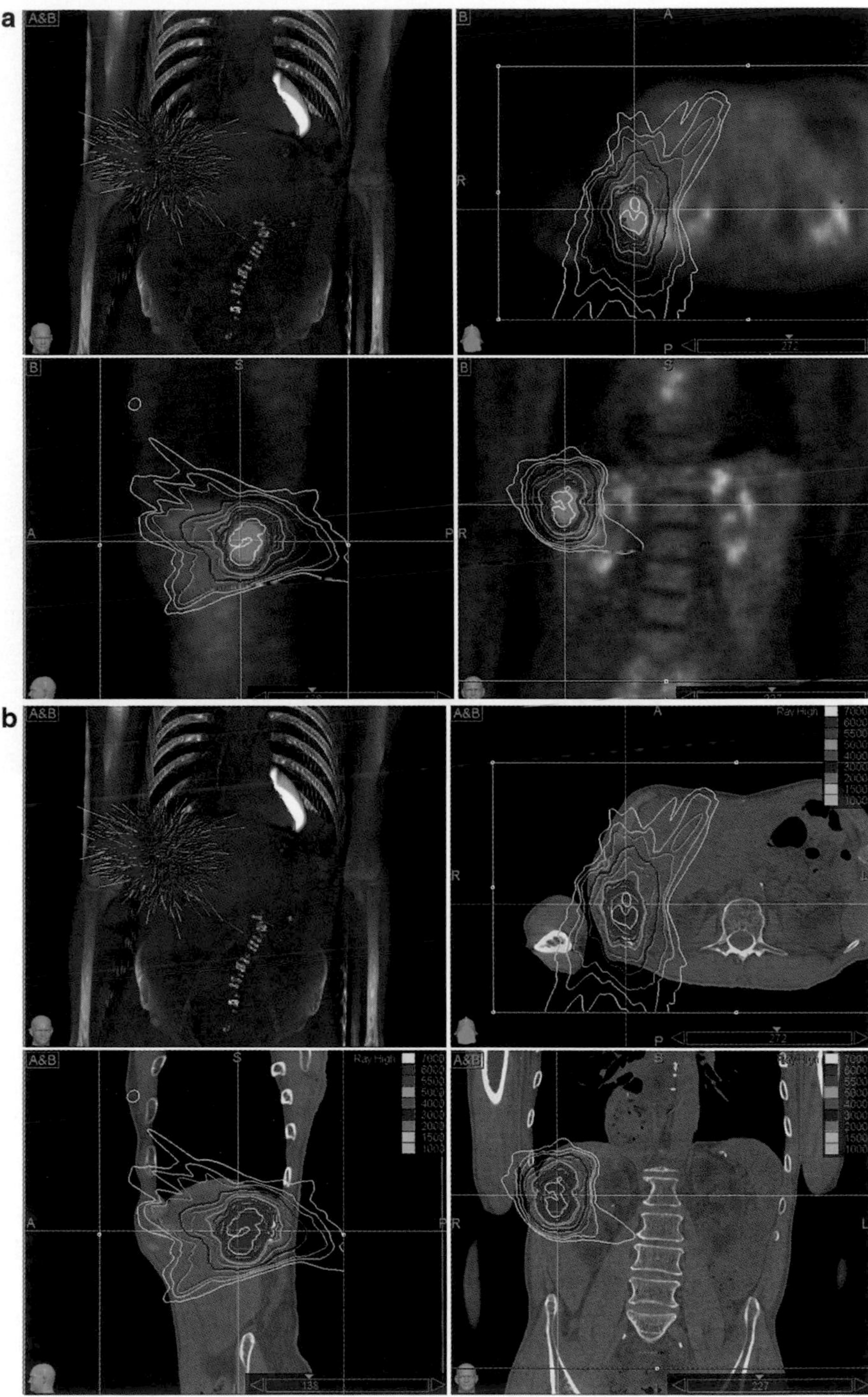

Fig. 5 **a** An example of SBRT for a liver metastasis using PET and PET/CT for the gross tumor volume definition. The beam configuration is shown in the *top left hand corner* and the isodose distributions are shown in axial (*top right*), sagittal (*bottom left*) and coronal planes (*bottom right*). **b**

in significant fusion error cranially or caudally. For example, if a patient's neck is flexed during the diagnostic PET/CT scan, but extended during the CT simulation, rigid fusion of the PET scan to the CT simulation scan can result in significant error. Deformable registration can overcome positional variation by deforming the second scan to match the primary image set. Deformable registration can greatly improve the utility of a diagnostic PET scan not performed in treatment position, which is useful when the PET/CT scan cannot be repeated. Figure 7 demonstrates deformable registration of a diagnostic

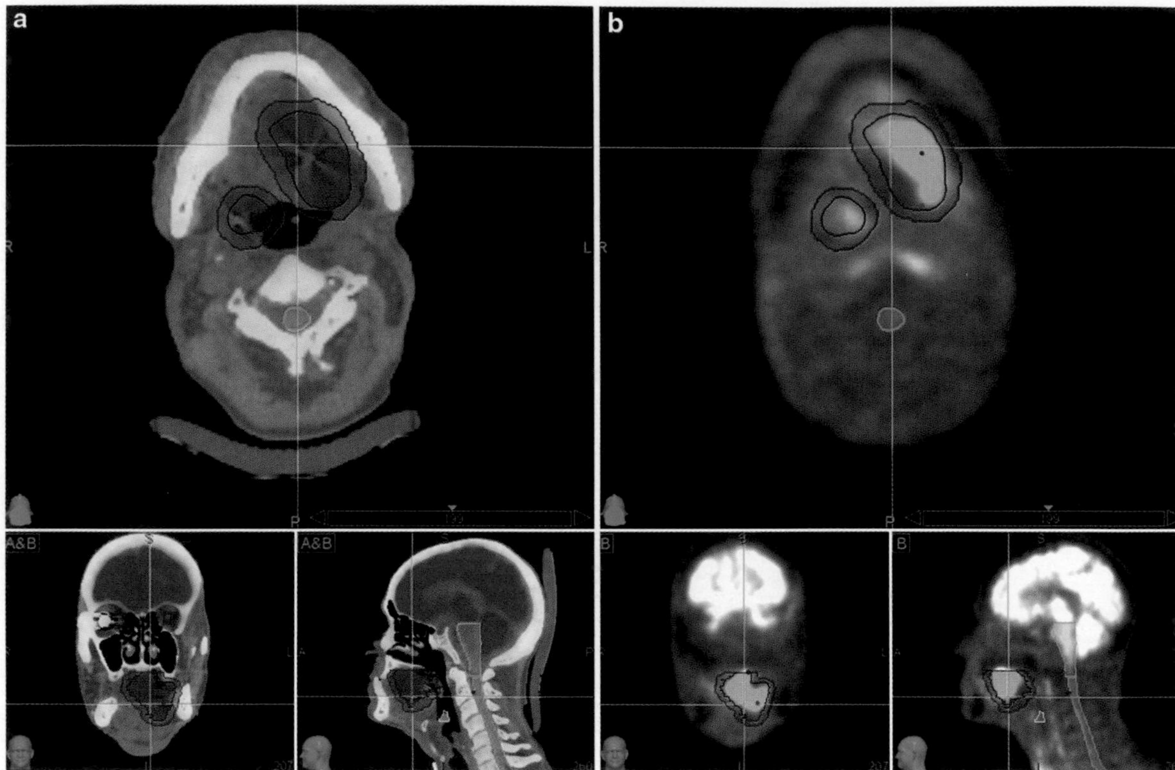

Fig. 6 **a** An example of PET/CT in a head and neck cancer patient in the treatment position before undergoing stereotactic body re-irradiation using cyberknife radiosurgery. **b** shows the PET component and the GTV (in *blue*) and PTV (in *red*) contours

pre-operative PET/CT to the post-operative CT simulation scan in a head and neck cancer patient. The PET/CT assists in localizing the tumor bed after surgical resection. Hwang et al. (2009) demonstrated in a study of 12 head and neck cancer patients that it was possible to co-register a PET or PET/CT acquired in diagnostic position using rigid registration, although they cautioned against its use in the neck for nodal target volumes. They found PET/CT more accurate than PET alone. The registration error was measured at 3.2 mm for the brain and 8.4 mm for the spinal cord using a diagnostic PET/CT. Deformable registration improved the accuracy with errors ranging from 1.1 to 5.4 mm.

In a study by Ireland et al. (2007) PET/CT was acquired in five head and neck cancer patients in both diagnostic and treatment planning positions and co-registered with the planning CT using both rigid and non-rigid (deformable) registration. They found significantly larger registration errors for rigid registration when using the treatment position PET/CT of 4.96 mm compared to 2.77 mm for deformable registration, ($p = 0.001$). Interestingly, when using the diagnostic planning PET/CT, they found greater accuracy with deformable registration compared to the treatment position PET/CT using rigid registration. This study suggests that deformable registration of the PET/CT is more accurate for treatment planning even when the PET/CT is acquired in diagnostic position.

5.2 Effect of PET/CT on Gross Tumor Volume Definition

In the past decade, there has been intense interest and rapidly increasing utilization of PET/CT imaging in radiotherapy treatment planning for multiple cancer sites. Many single institution studies have examined the impact of PET and/or PET/CT on GTV delineation for radiotherapy planning. Due to the significant number of publications on this topic, we will review the literature by primary cancer site.

Studies to determine whether using PET or PET/CT for target volume delineation of the GTV increases

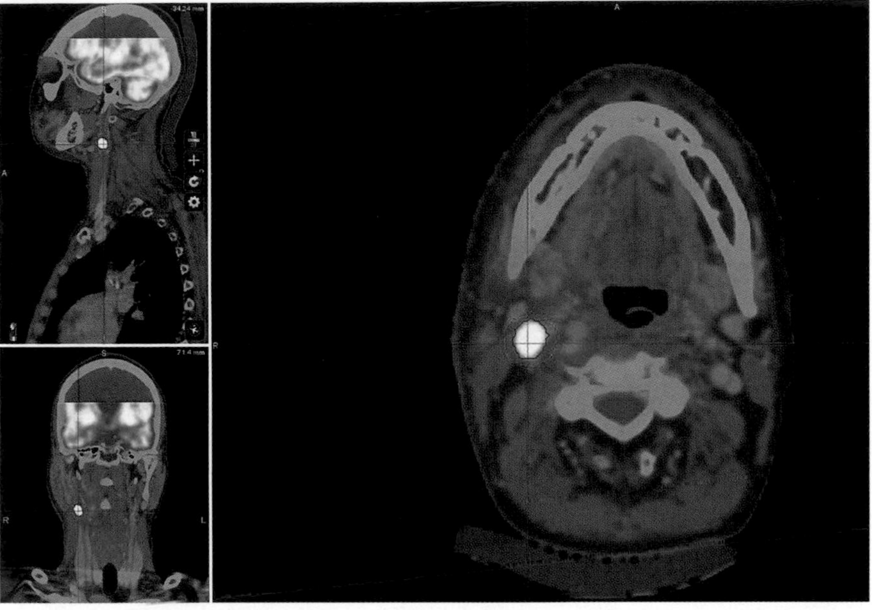

Fig. 7 Deformable registration of a diagnostic PET/CT in a head and neck cancer patient to the CT simulation scan in the treatment position with thermoplastic immobilization to localize a level II PET-avid node

or reduces target volumes have produced conflicting results, since most of the studies are non-randomized and include few patients. Studies do show however, that PET/CT is superior to PET or CT alone for diagnostic performance and initial staging (Ishikita et al. 2010). PET/CT also appears to improve the consistency of contouring for both intraobserver and interobserver variability (Riegel et al. 2006). New multidisciplinary contouring protocols involving radiology and radiation oncology should be developed to improve interobserver variability of PET/CT drawn contours (Berson et al. 2009).

5.3 PET/CT Planning for Head and Neck Cancer

Major published series examining PET imaging in radiotherapy planning for head and neck cancer are described in Table 1. Studies have examined the relative value of PET compared to other imaging modalities including CT and MRI for target delineation of the GTV. In a study by Daisne et al., diagnostic CT, MRI, and PET/CT were correlated to pathological surgical specimens in nine patients with pharyngeal and laryngeal cancer. In this study, the PET/CT tumor volumes were smaller than CT- and MRI-based volumes. PET/CT correlated most accurately to the surgical specimen, although none of the imaging studies were able to determine the superficial extension of the tumor (Daisne et al. 2004).

In a study of 25 head and neck cancer patients El-Bassiouni et al. (2007) found that the CT-based GTVs were larger than the PET-based GTV in 72% of cases, and smaller in 28%. A few studies have demonstrated larger GTVs with PET/CT than with CT (Igdem et al.; Scarfone et al. 2004), but most series generally have found smaller GTVs for the primary tumor when using PET/CT compared to CT alone (Geets et al. 2006; Guido et al. 2009; Heron et al. 2004; Paulino et al. 2005).

The discrepancies between these studies may depend on multiple factors including inter- and intraobserver variability (Riegel et al. 2006; Berson et al. 2009), segmentation methods, tumor site, and histology.

Schniagl et al. (2007) studied five different segmentation methods for PET target volume definition in 78 head and neck cancer patients, including visual determination, applying a fixed SUV threshold of 2.5, using a fixed threshold of 40 and 50% of the maximum signal intensity, and applying an adaptive threshold based on the signal to background ratio. In this study, using an SUV threshold of 2.5 failed to identify the GTV in most of the cases, as the PET-defined GTV was too large compared to the CT-defined GTV.

The other automated segmentation methods using 40 and 50% threshold produced volumes smaller than the CT based GTVs. The 50% threshold and the adaptive threshold technique appeared to

Table 1 Summary of studies exploring the role of PET/CT for GTV delineation in radiation treatment planning for tumors of Head and Neck

First author, year	Institution	Patient number	Imaging Technique	Impact of PET on GTV	Conclusion
Ashamalla et al. (2007)	Cornell University, New York, NY	25	CT versus PET-CT	≥ 25% volume modification seen in 68% with PET-CT	Used ABC (anatomic biologic contouring) halo method Increase in concordance between observers with PET-CT
Berson et al. (2009)	St. Vincent's Comprehensive Cancer Center, New York, NY	16	CT, PET-CT	Mean GTV increased in 25% of users Mean GTV decreased in 75% of users	Omit this one, confusing paper
Breen et al. (2007)	University of Toronto, Toronto, Canada	10	CT, Contrast-enhanced CT, PET-CT in treatment position	Non contrast CT volumes larger than PET CT PET decreases GTV	Contrast-enhanced CT was most consistent; PET-CT less reliable than contrast-enhanced CT. PET-CT to primary site GTV delineation of head and neck cancers does not change the volume of the GTV. An FDG-PET may demonstrate differences in neck node delineation
Ciernik et al. (2003)	University of Zurich, Zurich, Switzerland	12	CT. PET-CT, CT, and a FDG-PET were obtained in treatment position in an integrated PET/CT scanner, and coregistered images were used for treatment planning	GTV increased by 25% or more because of PET in 17% of cases with head-and-neck (2/12) GTV reduction ≥ 25% in 4 of 12 patients	The GTV changes were 32% (±11%). The corresponding change in PTV was 20% (±5%) Integrated PET/CT for treatment planning for three-dimensional conformal radiation therapy improves the standardization of volume delineation compared with that of CT alone. PET/CT has the potential for reducing the risk for geographic misses
Daisne et al. (2004)	Université Catholique de Louvain, Brussels, Belgium	29	CT, MRI, FDG-PET Volumes were coregistered by using a semiautomated rigid method based on surface segmentation (no for treatment planning, all diagnostic scans)	For oropharyngeal tumors and for laryngeal or hypopharyngeal tumors, no significant difference (P _ .99) was observed between average GTVs delineated at CT (32.0 and 21.4 cm^3, respectively) or MR imaging (27.9 and 21.4 cm^3, respectively), whereas average GTVs at PET were smaller (20.3 [P _ .10] and 16.4 cm^3 [P _ .01], respectively). GTVs from surgical specimens were significantly smaller (12.6 cm^3, P _ .06)	Compared with GTVs at CT and MR imaging, GTVs at FDG PET were smaller. In 9 patients for whom a surgical specimen was available, PET was found to be the most accurate modality. However, no modality managed to depict superficial tumor extension

(continued)

Table 1 (continued)

First author, year	Institution	Patient number	Imaging Technique	Impact of PET on GTV	Conclusion
Deantonio et al. (2008)	University of Piemonte Orientale , Novara, Italy	22	CT, PET, PET-CT in treatment planning position	PET-GTV was smaller than CT-GTVPET/CT-GTV (26 cc), was significantly greater than CT-GTV ($p < 0.0001$)	PET changed staging in 22 %
Dizendorf et al. (2003)	University Hospital, Zurich, Switzerland	55 (202 total)	CT, PET-CT	A change in radiation volume was necessary in 12 patients (6%): head and neck tumors, 2%; gynecologic tumors, 11%; breast cancer, 4%; lung cancer, 4%; malignant lymphomas, 13%; and gastrointestinal tumors, 11%	The results of this study show that 18F-FDG PET has a major impact on the management of patients for radiation therapy, influencing both the stage and the management in 27% of patients
El-bassiouni et al. (2007)	University of Zurich, Zurich, Switzerland	25	CT, PET-CT	The GTVCT was larger ($p = 0.0022$) than the GTVPET in 18 cases (72%) and smaller in 7 cases (28%)	PET signal threshold is optimal in PET-based radiotherapy treatment planning
Gardner et al. (2009)	Centre René Huguenin, Saint-Cloud, France	35	MRI, PET-CT	GTV, the CT InterObserverVariability (IOV) was higher (mean, 4.22 mL) than the MRI IOV (mean, 3.28 mL; $p < .0007$). PET-CT changed the treatment design in 6 of 21 patients	Diagnostic imaging performed in the treatment position can improve the accuracy of radiotherapy planning in case of intracranial tumor extension, heavy dental work, or contraindication for contrast-enhanced CT, but not in the absence of these conditions—not such a great study on PET
Geets et al. (2006)	Université Catholique de Louvain, Brussels, Belgium	18	MRI, FDG-PET Contrast-enhanced CT	Pretreatment FDG-PET were significantly smaller than those based on pretreatment CT GTVPET,0 Gy were significantly smaller than GTVCT,0 Gy. This difference translated into significant (pZ0.001) differences in the prophylactic CTV (72.7G11.3 ml versus 97.7G14.8 ml) and in the prophylactic PTV (139.6G16.7 ml versus 180.4G22.5 ml) delineation	Reduction in GTV results in greater normal tissue sparing

(continued)

Table 1 (continued)

First author, year	Institution	Patient number	Imaging Technique	Impact of PET on GTV	Conclusion
Guido et al. (2009)	Policlinico S. Orsola, Bologna, Italy	38	Contrast-enhanced CT PET-CT	In 35 (92%) of 38 cases, the CT-based GTVs were larger than the PET/CT-based GTVs $p < 0.05$	GTVs, but not planning target volumes, were significantly changed by the implementation of combined PET/CT
Heron et al. (2004)	University of Pittsburgh School of Medicine, Pittsburgh, PA	21	CT, PET-CT simulation in treatment position	Positron emission tomography demonstrated the primary in all cases, whereas CT did not find the primary in 3 cases. In 8 patients, additional areas of disease were seen only in PET. The average ratio of GTVc/GTVp was 3.1 Volumes for the primaries were significantly larger on CT than on PET (p _ 0.002) but not for nodal regions (p _ 0.5)	Hybrid PET-CT simulation is feasible and provides valuable information that results in greater delineation of normal tissues from tumor bearing areas at high risk for recurrence
Hwang et al. (2009)	University of California, San Francisco, San Francisco, CA	12	CT, PET, PET-CT in non-treatment position	Registration accuracy was better with PET/CT than with PET alone	It is possible to incorporate PETand/or PET/CTacquired in diagnostic positions into the treatment planning. Precautions must be taken, particularly when delineating tumor volumes in the neck. Acquisition of PET/CT in the treatment-planning position would be the ideal method to minimize registration errors
Igdem et al. (2010)	Istanbul Bilim University, Istanbul, Turkey	26	CT, PET-CT	PET/CT volumes were larger than our CT-based volumes. Major changes (_25%) in GTV delineation were observed in 44% of patients. In 16% of cases, PET/CT detected incidental second primaries and metastatic disease, changing the treatment strategy from curative to palliative. PET/CT-based target volumes (mean = 35.5 cm^3) were significantly larger compared with CT-based volumes (mean 26.5 cm^3) (*P*= 0.004). The mean change in GTV was 20%	Integrating functional imaging with FDG-PET/CT into the radiotherapy planning process resulted in major changes in a significant proportion of our patients. An interdisciplinary approach between imaging and radiation oncology departments is essential in defining the target volumes

(continued)

Table 1 (continued)

First author, year	Institution	Patient number	Imaging Technique	Impact of PET on GTV	Conclusion
Ireland et al. (2007)	University of Sheffield, Sheffield, United Kingdom	5	CT, PET-CT In diagnostic and treatment position, rigid and non-rigid co-registration	GTV not studied REMOVE: study on registration	Nonrigid registration provides a more accurate registration of head and neck PET/CT to treatment planning CT than rigid registration. In addition, nonrigid registration of PET/CT acquired with patients in a standardized, diagnostic position can provide images registered to planning CT with greater accuracy than a rigid registration of PET/CT images acquired in treatment position. This may allow greater flexibility in the timing of PET/CT for head and neck cancer patients due to undergo radiotherapy
Ishikita et al. (2010)	Gunma University Graduate School of Medicine, Maebashi, Japan	40 (primary H&N) 129 (relapse H&N)	PET, PET-CT		PET CT is better than PET alone
Koshy et al. (2005)	Emory Clinic and Emory University, Atlanta, Georgia	36	CT, PET-CT diagnostic	PET-CT altered the TNM score in 13 patients (36.1%) and the AJCC stage in 5 patients (13.9%). PET-CT altered GTV by visual determination rather than SUV. RT volume and dose were altered in 5 patients (14%) and 4 patients (11%), respectively	PET-CT fusion may have a significant impact on staging and determination of RT treatment volume and dose
Kruser et al. (2009)	University of Wisconsin, Madison, WI	25	CT, PET-CT		No information
Murakami et al. (2007)	Kumamoto University Hospital, Kumamoto Japan	23	FDG-PET-CT		Is this study relevant? Remove but add into an other section

(continued)

Table 1 (continued)

First author, year	Institution	Patient number	Imaging Technique	Impact of PET on GTV	Conclusion
Newbold et al. (2008)	The Royal Marsden NHS Foundation Trust, London, UK	18	CT, PET, PET-CT	The PET/CT identified a primary site of disease in 5/9 (55.6%) of the cases presenting as unknown primaries. The combined primary and nodal GTV (GTVp+n) was increased by 74% with PET CT	18FDG-PET revealed disease lying outside the conventional target volume, either extending a known area or highlighting a previously unknown area of disease, including the primary tumor
Nishioka et al. (2002)	Hokkaido University, Sapporo, Japan	21	CT, MRI, FDG-PET, FDG-PET/MRI/CT	GTV volumes for primary tumors were not changed by image fusion in 19 cases (89%). Normal tissue sparing was more easily performed based on clearer GTV and CTV determination on the fusion images using 18FDG-PET and MRI/CT, parotid sparing achieved in 71% of patients with fusion imaging	Image fusion between 18FDG-PET and MRI/CT was useful in GTV and CTV determination in conformal RT and facilitates sparing of normal tissues
Paulino et al. (2005)	Emory Clinic and Emory University, Atlanta, GA	40	CT, PET-CT in treatment position	The PET-GTV was smaller, the same size, and larger than the CT-GTV in 30 (75%), 3 (8%), and 7 (18%) cases respectively	The PET-GTV was larger than the CT-GTV in 18% of cases. In approximately 25% of patients with intact head-and-neck cancer treated using IMRT, the volume of PET-GTV is underdosed when the CT-GTV is used for IMRT planning
Paulsen et al. (2006)	University of Tuebingen, Germany	11	PET-CT		Only 8 patients have PET scans
Rahn et al. (1998)	Johann-Wolfgang-Goethe-Universität Frankfurt	34	PET	In all cases, changes of treatment strategy or target volume were necessary	Especially in patients with recurrent disease and patients with advanced tumor stages, FDG-PET is able to give clinically relevant information compared to conventional staging procedures. Therefore, in these group of patients an FDG-PET study prior to radiotherapy planning should be considered
Riegel et al. (2006)	St. Vincent's Comprehensive Cancer Center, New York, NY	16	CT, PET-CT	Significant differences between PET and PET/CT GTVs were seen and inter-observer variability of PET/CT and CT contoured GTVs	Significant differences in GTV delineation were found between multiple observers contouring on PET/CT fusion

(continued)

Table 1 (continued)

First author, year	Institution	Patient number	Imaging Technique	Impact of PET on GTV	Conclusion
Rothschild et al. (2007)	University of Zurich, Zurich, Switzerland	45	PET-CT	PET/CT and treatment with IMRT improved cure rates compared to patients without PET/CT and IMRT	Is this study relevant?
Scarfone et al. (2004)	Vanderbilt University Medical Center, Nashville, Tennessee	6	CT, PET-CT	CT GTV was modified in all remaining patients based on 18F-FDG PET data. The resulting PET/CT GTV was larger than the original CT volume by an average of 15%. In 5 cases, 18F-FDG PET identified active lymph nodes that corresponded to lymph nodes contoured on CT. The pathologically enlarged CT lymph nodes were modified to create final lymph node volumes in 3 of 5 cases. In one of 6 patients, 18F-FDG–avid lymph nodes were not identified as pathologic on CT	Inclusion of 18F-FDG PET data resulted in modified target volumes in radiotherapy planning for HNC. PET and CT data acquired on separate, dedicated scanners may be coregistered for therapy planning; however, dual-acquisition PET/CT systems may be considered to reduce the need for reregistrations
Schinagl et al. (2007)	Radboud University Nijmegen Medical Centre, Nijmegen, The Netherlands	78	CT, PET	GTV method of applying an isocontour of a standardized uptake value of 2.5 failed to provide successful delineation in 45% of cases. For the other PET delineation methods, volume and shape of the GTV were influenced heavily by the choice of segmentation tool. On average, all threshold-based PET-GTVs were smaller than on CT. Nevertheless, PET frequently detected significant tumor extension outside the GTV delineated on CT (15–34%of PET volume)	Choice of segmentation tool for target-volume definition of head and neck cancer based on FDGPET images is not trivial because it influences both volume and shape of the resulting GTV. With adequate delineation, PET may add significantly to CT- and physical examination–based GTV definition
Schwartz et al. (2005)	University of Washington, Seattle, Washington	20	Contrast-enhanced CT PET-CT	FDG-avid disease with 0.5 cm margins to dose escalate to 74.9 Gy	Used PET-CT to reduce theoretical IMRT volumes, by eliminating elective nodal volumes and potentially dose escalate while improving normal tissue sparing, although did not comment on impact of PET/CT on GTV

(continued)

Table 1 (continued)

First author, year	Institution	Patient number	Imaging Technique	Impact of PET on GTV	Conclusion
Schwartz et al. (2005)	University of Washington, Seattle, Washington	20	CT, PET-CT	FDG-PET/CT detected 17 of 17 heminecks and 26 of 27 nodal zones histologically positive by dissection (100% and 96% sensitivity, respectively). The nodal level staging sensitivity and specificity for FDG-PET/CT was 96% (26 of 27) and 98.5% (68 of 69), respectively. FDG-PET/CT correctly detected nodal disease in 2 patients considered to have node-negative disease by CT alone	FDG-PET/CT is superior to CT alone for geographic localization of diseased neck node levels
Soto et al. (2008)	University of Michigan, Ann Arbor, MI	61	CT, PET-CT, MRI	Correlated PET GTV with locoregional failure (LRF). For patients with an LRF, 100% (9/9) of failures were in-field. Of the in-field failures, one of nine, 11% was outside the PET GTV, but within the CT and physical examination GTV. All failures occurred in the high dose PTV prescribed to 70Gy. In addition, they were noted to map within the CT/MRI abnormality, including the recurrence which mapped outside the PET-defined GTV	Advocate use of PET defined GTV as an important, but not exclusive, role in defining the GTV
Vernon et al. (2008)	Medical College of Wisconsin, Milwaukee, WI	42	PET-CT	The maximum standard uptake volume (SUV) of primary tumor, adenopathy, or both on PET did not correlate with recurrence, with mean values of 12.0 for treatment failures versus 11.7 for all patients	A high level of disease control combined with favorable toxicity profiles was achieved in a cohort of HNC patients receiving PET/CT fusion guided radiotherapy plus/minus chemotherapy. Maximum SUV of primary tumor and/or adenopathy was not predictive of risk of disease recurrence

(continued)

Table 1 (continued)

First author, year	Institution	Patient number	Imaging Technique	Impact of PET on GTV	Conclusion
Wang et al. (2006)	Medical College of Wisconsin, Milwaukee, WI	28	CT, PET-CT	PET/CT resulted in CT-based staging changes in 16 of 28 (57%) patients. Volume analysis revealed that the PET/CT-based gross target volumes (GTVs) were significantly different from those contoured from the CT scans alone in 14 of 16 patients. Abnormal PET areas with SUV _ 2.5 in primary tumor site and lymph nodes were included in the GTV after a joint review of diagnostic PET/CT with an experienced head-and-neck radiologist	
Wong et al. (1996)	Guy's and St. Thomas Hospitals, London, UK	30	CT, MRI, FDG-PET	For primary tumors CT-PET-FDG (97%) and MR-PET-FDG (100%) delineated the tumor more accurately than CT (69%) or MR (40%) alone. Similarly, CT-PET-FDG (98%) and MR-PET FDG (100%) were better than CT (70%) and MR alone (80%) in identifying tumor invasion of specific anatomical structures. Management was altered in 7 of 30 patients	registered CT/MR-PET-FDG images provide additional clinically relevant information over CT/MR alone
Zheng et al. (2006)	Southern Medical University, Guangzhou, People's Republic of China	33 (29)	CT versus PET-CT	For the remaining 29 patients, GTV based on FDG-PET was smaller than GTV based on CT in 24 (82.8%) cases and was greater in 5 (17.2%) cases, respectively	Use of FDG-PET was found to influence the salvage treatment decision making for locally persistent NPC by identifying patients who were not likely to benefit from additional treatment and by improving accuracy of GTV definition in salvage treatment planning

show similar overlapping volumes. However, the two latter segmentation techniques were not equivalent, and geographic similarity was less than 90% in 26 of 73 cases. Another limitation of automatic segmentation methods with PET-defined GTVs is that there may be significant background activity due to physiologic uptake in the normal musculature in the head and neck, and normal structures could be inadvertently contoured.

In a series of eight head and neck cancer patients, Ford et al. (2006) used an automatic segmentation technique set at progressively higher thresholds, and those tumor volumes were compared to CT-based GTVs contoured by a physician. The study found that PET-based contours were sensitive to the threshold contouring level, and that a 5% change in threshold contour level could translate to a 200% increase in volume. Whether using a threshold technique of 50%, visualization, or other segmentation technique, PET-defined GTVs should be used as a complementary contouring tool in addition to other imaging modalities and clinical exam. The exclusive use of PET/CT scanning for target delineation may underestimate the tumor if regions of the tumor are necrotic or lack metabolic activity. Hence, there is still potential inaccuracy when defining the GTV using PET/CT imaging for radiotherapy planning alone, and so it is important to integrate diagnostic information, including contrast-enhanced CT, MRI, surgical, and clinical examination findings into the final GTV for radiation planning (Wong et al. 2002).

While studies have shown that PET/CT can alter target definition, the impact of PET/CT radiotherapy planning on cure rates after radiotherapy remains to be determined. In a study by Vernon et al. (2008) 42 head and neck cancer patients who received PET/CT fusion-guided radiotherapy planning showed a high rate of disease control and favorable toxicity profiles. PET/CT radiotherapy planning is now being incorporated into multi-institutional randomized trials; we await these results to determine the long-term impact of PET/CT in radiotherapy planning.

5.4 PET/CT Planning for Lung Cancer

Major published series examining PET imaging in radiotherapy planning for lung cancer are described in Table 2. In lung cancer, PET/CT is an important tool in the diagnostic workup and staging for both small-cell and non small-cell lung cancer. Radiotherapy advances for non small-cell lung cancer, include reduction of treatment volumes by reducing or eliminating elective nodal irradiation, dose escalation of the GTV with IMRT or SBRT, 4DCT, and respiratory gated radiotherapy. All these techniques rely on accurate tumor volume delineation. In lung cancer, primary tumor volume delineation can be confounded by adjacent lung collapse or consolidation, in which case the edge of the tumor cannot be determined by contrast CT alone. Furthermore, the volume of normal lung that is irradiated, and the dose, significantly effect lung toxicity including pneumonitis and lung fibrosis. Radiation oncologists use dose-volume histograms to analyze the mean lung dose and the volume of the lung that is receiving low doses of radiation at 5 and 20 Gy, as these parameters correlate with toxicity risk. Multiple studies examining the role of PET in radiotherapy planning show similar results. These studies show that PET significantly changes the staging and treatment plan in up to two-thirds of cases, often upstaging the patients by revealing regional lymph node metastases or distant metastases. The radiotherapy planning volume was altered by PET/CT in the majority of cases, but not with CT-based volumes; PET/CT is particularly helpful in distinguishing tumor from lung atelectasis and in reducing the target volumes in these patients. However, when PET detects nodal disease, the planning target volumes are usually increased, with increases in the mean lung dose, V20, esophageal, or cardiac dose (Igdem et al.; Bradley et al. 2004; Erdi et al. 2002; Deniaud-Alexandre et al. 2005; De Ruysscher et al. 2005; Ciernik et al. 2003; Ceresoli et al. 2007; Gondi et al. 2007; Grills et al. 2007; Kalff et al. 2001; Mac Manus et al. 2001; Mah et al. 2002; Messa et al. 2005). Four-dimensional PET/CT can improve the detection and delineation of small lung tumors by controlling for respiratory motion. Respiratory gated PET/CT scans show smaller diameter lesions than non-gated images, and may improve tumor detection as respiratory motion can decrease detection and degrade image quality (Larson et al. 2005).

How to determine which threshold should be used for delineating the PET GTV for accurate target volume definition for lung cancer is not clear. In a study by Biehl et al. (2006) 40 and 20% thresholds underestimated the CT-based GTV for 80 and 70% of

Table 2 Summary of studies exploring the role of PET/CT in radiation treatment planning for tumors of Lung

First author, year	Institution	Patient number	Imaging Technique	Change in GTV	Conclusion
Ashamalla et al. (2005)	Cornell University, Brooklyn, NY	19	CT versus PET-CT	≥ 25% volume modification seen in 52% of cases (10/19)	Position emission tomography/CT-based radiation treatment planning is a useful tool resulting in modification of GTV in 52% and improvement of inter-observer variability up to 84%. The use of PET/CT-based ABC can potentially replace the use of GTV. The anatomic biologic halo can be used for delineation of volumes
Biehl et al. (2006)	Washington University School of Medicine, St. Louis, Missouri	20	CT versus PET-CT	The PETGTV at the 40 and 20% thresholds underestimated the CTGTV for 16 of 20 and 14 of 20 lesions, respectively	No single threshold delineating the PETGTV provides accurate volume definition, compared with that provided by the CTGTV, for the majority of NSCLCs. The strong correlation of the optimal threshold with the CTGTV warrants further investigation
Bradley et al. (2004)	Washington University School of Medicine, St. Louis, Missouri	26	CT versus PET-CT	Of these 24 patients, PET clearly altered the GTV in 14 patients. PET helped to delineate tumor within regions of atelectasis in 3 patients, reducing the GTV for each. PET increased the GTV in 11 patients	Radiation targeting with fused FDG-PET and CT images resulted in alterations in radiation therapy planning in over 50% of patients by comparison with CT targeting. The increasing availability of integrated PET/CT units will facilitate the use of this technology for radiation treatment planning. A confirmatory multicenter, cooperative group trial is planned within the Radiation Therapy Oncology Group
Brianzoni et al. (2005)	S. Lucia Hospital, Macerata, ASUR Marche, Italy	24 (28 including lumphoma) Satudy sample 25 (includes lymphoma)	CT versus PET-CT	In 14 of the aforementioned 25 cases (56%), the PET information did not significantly change the GTV or CTV. In 5/11 cases, the target volume was decreased. In the other 6/11 cases, the target volume was increased	FDG-PET is a highly sensitive imaging modality that offers better visualisation of local and locoregional tumor extension. This study confirmed that coregistration of CT data and FDG-PET images may lead to significant modifications of RT planning and patient management
Caldwell et al. (2001)	Sunnybrook and Women's College Health Sciences Centre, Toronto, Canada	30	CT versus PET-CT	The mean ratios of largest to smallest GTV were 2.31 and 1.56 for CT only and for CT/FDG coregistered data, respectively. The addition of PET reduced this ratio in 23 of 30 cases and increased it in 7	High-observer variability in CT-based definition of the GTV can occur. A more consistent definition of the GTV can often be obtained if coregistered FDG-hybrid PET images are used

(continued)

Table 2 (continued)

First author, year	Institution	Patient number	Imaging Technique	Change in GTV	Conclusion
Ceresoli et al. (2007)	Istituto Clinico Humanitas, Rozzano, Milan, Italy	21	CT versus PET-CT	In 7/18 (39%) patients treated with radical radiotherapy, a significant (> or =25%) change in volume between GTVCT and GTVPET/CT was observed	Our study suggests that [18F]-fluorodeoxyglucose-PET should be integrated in no-ENI techniques, as it improves target volume delineation without a major increase in predicted toxicity
Ciernik et al. (2003)	University of Zurich, Zurich, Switzerland	6	CT versus PET-CT	The GTV increased by 25% or more because of PET in 17% of cases with lung cancer (1/6).The GTV was reduced >25% in 67% with lung cancer (4/6)	Integrated PET/CT for treatment planning for three-dimensional conformal radiation therapy improves the standardization of volume delineation compared with that of CT alone. PET/CT has the potential for reducing the risk for geographic misses, to minimize the dose of ionizing radiation applied to non-target organs, and to change the current practice to three-dimensional conformal radiation therapy planning by taking into account the metabolic and biologic features of cancer. The impact on treatment outcome remains to be demonstrated
De Ruysscher et al. (2005)	MAASTRO Clinic, Maastricht, The Netherlands	21	CT versus PET-CT	Two-thirds of the radiotherapy plans changed with incorporation of the PET-CT data. In 2 patients, the radiotherapy fields became larger because of the PET-CT information, in 12 patients, they became smaller, and in 7 patients, they remained the same	The use of a combined dedicated PET-CT-simulator reduced radiation exposure of the esophagus and the lung, and thus allowed significant radiation dose escalation while respecting all relevant normal tissue constraints
Deniaud-Alexandre et al. (2005)	Tenon Hospital A.P.-H.P., Paris, France	101	CT versus PET-CT	The gross tumor volume (GTV) was decreased by CT-PET image fusion in 21 patients (23%) and was increased in 24 patients (26%). The GTV reduction was >25% in 7 patients because CT-PET image fusion reduced the pulmonary GTV in 6 patients (3 patients with atelectasis) and the mediastinal nodal GTV in 1 patient. The GTV increase was >25% in 14 patients owing to an increase in the pulmonary GTV in 11 patients (4 patients with atelectasis) and detection of occult mediastinal lymph node involvement in 3 patients	The results of our study have confirmed that integrated hybrid PET/CT in the treatment position and coregistered images have an impact on treatment planning and management of non–small-cell lung cancer. However, FDG images using dedicated PET scanners and respiration-gated acquisition protocols could improve the PET-CT image coregistration. Furthermore, the impact on treatment outcome remains to be demonstrated

(continued)

Table 2 (continued)

First author, year	Institution	Patient number	Imaging Technique	Change in GTV	Conclusion
Dizendorf et al. (2003)	University Hospital, Zurich, Switzerland	26 (202 total)	CT, PET-CT	A change radiation volume was necessary in 12 patients (6%): head and neck tumors, 2%; gynecologic tumors, 11%; breast cancer, 4%; lung cancer, 4%; malignant lymphomas, 13%; and gastrointestinal tumors, 11%	The results of this study show that 18F-FDG PET has a major impact on the management of patients for radiation therapy, influencing both the stage and the management
Erdi et al. (2002)	Memorial Sloan-Kettering Cancer Center, New York, NY	11	CT, PET-CT	In 7 out of 11 cases, we found an increase in PTV volume (average increase of 19%) to incorporate distant nodal disease. In other 4 patients PTV was decreased to an average of 18%	The incorporation of PET data improves definition of the primary lesion by including positive lymph nodes into the PTV. Thus, the PET data reduces the likelihood of geographic misses and hopefully improves the chance of achieving local control
Fox et al. (2005)	Memorial Sloan-Kettering Cancer Center, New York, NY	19	CT, PET-CT	Not clear	Registration of FDG-PET and planning CT images results in greater consistency in tumor volume delineation
Giraud et al. (2001)	Institut Curie, Paris, France	12	CT versus PET-CT	Tumor volume irradiated at the 95% isodose (V95) was increased by 22% and 8% for 2 patients, respectively, and was decreased by an average of 59% for 3 patients after fusion. No difference in terms of Vl20 and V95 was observed for the other 7 patients	We have validated CT and FDG-CDET lung image fusion to facilitate determination of lung cancer volumes, which improved the accuracy of 3D-CRT
Gondi et al. (2007)	University of Wisconsin, Madison, WI	14	CT versus PET-CT	In 12 of the 14 (85.7%) NSCLC patients, the addition of the FDG-PET data led to the definition of a smaller GTV	The incorporation of a hybrid FDG-PET/CT scanner had an impact on the radiotherapy planning of esophageal cancer and NSCLC. In future studies, we recommend adoption of a conformality index for a more comprehensive comparison of newer treatment planning imaging modalities to conventional options
Grills et al. (2007)	William Beaumont Hospital, Royal Oak, MI	21	CT versus PET-CT	For the primary tumor GTV, the Set 1 (CT) volume was larger than the Set 2 (PET) volume in 48%, smaller in 33%, and equal in 19%	Computed tomography and PET are complementary and should be obtained in the treatment position and fused to define the GTV for NSCLC. Although the quantitative absolute target volume is sometimes similar, the qualitative target locations can be substantially different, leading to underdosage of the target when planning is done using CT alone without PET fusion

(continued)

Table 2 (continued)

First author, year	Institution	Patient number	Imaging Technique	Change in GTV	Conclusion
Hanna et al. (2009)	University of Belfast, Belfast, Northern Ireland, United Kingdom	28	CT, PET-CT	The median of the mean percentage of volume change from GTVCT to GTVFUSED was _5.21% for the induction chemotherapy group and 18.88% for the RT-alone group. Using the Mann-Whitney U test, this was significantly different (p = .001)	PET-CT RT planning scan, in addition to a staging PET-CT scan, reduces inter-observer variability in GTV definition for NSCLC. The GTV size with PET-CT compared with CT in the RT-alone group increased and was reduced in the induction chemotherapy group
Herbert et al. (1996)	Duke University Medical Center, Durham, NC	20	CXR, CT, PET	Six of seven well-demarcated tumors showed increased uptake of 18FDG correlating with the CT/CXR tumor volume. Twelve poorly demarcated tumors demonstrated increased 18FDG uptake. In 7 of 12, the CT/CXR abnormality correlated with changes on PET scan. In 3 of 12, CT/CXR abnormalities were larger than on PET, whereas in 2 of 12, abnormalities on PET extended outside the region of CT/CXR changes. The 13th patient in the poorly demarcated category had diffuse carcinoma in situ at the surgical margin that demonstrates increased 18FDG uptake, but was not visible by CT/CXR	18FDG PET may be useful for delineation of lung cancer volumes that are poorly defined by CXR and/or CT scan. The value of PET in differentiating tumor from fibrosis after radiotherapy for lung cancer remains to be established
Igdem et al. (2010)	Istanbul Bilim University, Istanbul, Turkey	13	CT, PET-CT	The mean PET/CT-based GTV was 94.2 cm^3 (range 9.8–257 cm^3), with CT 89.2 cm^3 (range 4.1–300.7 cm^3). The difference was not statistically significant. In 3 patients, an enlargement in GTV greater than 25% was observed and in only 1 patient a reduction of _25%	Integrating functional imaging with FDG-PET/CT into the radiotherapy planning process resulted in major changes in a significant proportion of our patients. An interdisciplinary approach between imaging and radiation oncology departments is essential in defining the target volumes
Kalff et al. (2001)	Peter MacCallum Cancer Institute, Melbourne, Victoria, Australia	105	CT, PET	Not clear	FDG PET scanning changed or influenced management decisions in 70 patients (67%) with NSCLC. Patients were frequently spared unnecessary treatment, and management was more appropriately targeted
Kiffer et al. (1998)	Austin and Repatriation Medical Centre, Melbourne, Australia	15	CT, PET	From a qualitative viewpoint, by analyzing the respective coronal PET scans, diagnostic images and simulator films of each of the 15 patients, it was readily appreciated that 4 patients (26.7%) had abnormal mediastinal nodal PET activity which had been regarded as normal on diagnostic CT	Of 15 patients analyzed, 26.7% (4 patients) would have had their RT volume influenced by PET findings, highlighting the potential value of PET in treatment planning

(continued)

Table 2 (continued)

First author, year	Institution	Patient number	Imaging Technique	Change in GTV	Conclusion
Kruser et al. (2009)	University of Wisconsin, Madison, WI	38	CT, PET-CT	Full article?	Hybrid PET/CT imaging at the time of treatment planning may be highly informative and an economical manner in which to obtain PET imaging, with the dual goals of staging and treatment planning
Mac Manus et al. (2007)	Peter MacCallum Cancer Centre, Melbourne, Australia	10	CT, PET-CT	The PTV derived from CT scans alone ranged from 230.5 to 1034.3 cm3 and on average were not significantly different from those planned using CT/PET images (P = 0.322). However, this gives a misleading impression of the effect of PET. In three cases, the volume of PTV was more than 10% greater for the PET-assisted plan (average increase in volume 124 cc) compared with that of the CT-alone plan. In 6 patients, the PET/CT PTV was smaller by 10% or more (average 18 8 cc). In one case (patient D), the absolute volumes were almost identical, but they occupied significantly different anatomic locations	Use of coregistered PET/CT images significantly altered treatment plans in a majority of cases. This method could be used in routine practice at centers without access to a combined PET/CT scanner
Mac Manus et al. (2001)	Peter MacCallum Cancer Centre, Melbourne, Australia	153	CT, PET	For 22 of 102 patients who received radical radiotherapy after PET, there was a significant increase in the target volume because of the inclusion of structures previously considered uninvolved by tumor. In 16 patients, the target volume was significantly reduced because of PET, because areas of lung consolidation with low FDG uptake were excluded from the treatment volume or because uninvolved lymph node groups were not treated. In three cases, primary tumors were visualized on PET that were unapparent or unrecognized on CT	Positron emission tomography-assisted staging detected unsuspected metastasis in 20%, strongly influenced choice of treatment strategy, frequently impacted RT planning, and was a powerful predictor of survival. Potential impact of FDG-PET is even greater in radical RT candidates with NSCLC than in surgical candidates

(continued)

Table 2 (continued)

First author, year	Institution	Patient number	Imaging Technique	Change in GTV	Conclusion
Mah et al. (2002)	Toronto-Sunnybrook Regional Cancer Centre, Toronto, Canada	30	CT, PET-CT	The effect of FDG-PET on target definition varied with the physician, leading to a reduction in PTV in 24–70% of cases and an increase in 30–76% of cases	The coregistration of planning CT and FDG-PET images made significant alterations to patient management and to the PTV. Ultimately, changes to the PTV resulted in changes to the radiation treatment plans for the majority of cases. Where possible, we would recommend that FDG-PET data be integrated into treatment planning of non-small-cell lung carcinoma, particularly for three-dimensional conformal techniques
Messa et al. (2005)	University of Milano-Bicocca, Milan, Italy	21	CT, PET-CT	3 patients were shifted to palliative radiotherapy for metastatic disease or very large tumor size, showed by [18F]FDG-PET. Of the remaining 18 patients a CTV change, after inclusion of PET/CT data, was observed in 10/18 cases (55%): larger in 7/18 (range 33-279%) and smaller in 3/18 patients (range 26-34%), mainly due to inclusion or exclusion of lymph-nodal disease and to better definition of tumor extent. CTV changes smaller than 25% occurred in the remaining 8/18 patients	[18F]FDG-PET and CT images co-registration in radiotherapy treatment planning led to a change in CTV definition in the majority of our patients, which may significantly modify management and radiation treatment modality in these patients
Munley et al. (1999)	Duke Uni6ersity Medical Center, Durham, NC	139	CT, SPECT, PET	PET appears to be useful for target localization; resulting in a modification of CT-based treatment fields in 34% of cases. The PET data resulted in an increase in field size since the treatment planner typically designed the treatment fields from the union of the CT and PET abnormalities	Nuclear medicine imaging techniques appear to be a potentially valuable tool during radiotherapy treatment planning for patients with lung cancer. The utilization of accurate nuclear medicine image reconstruction techniques and TCT may improve the treatment planning process
Nestle et al. (1999)	Saarland University Medical Center Homburg/Saar, Germany	34	CT, PET (4 methods)	In 12/34 cases, the shape and/or size of the portals were changed, primarily (*n* 5 10) the size of the fields was reduced	In this retrospective analysis, the information provided by FDG-PET would have contributed to a substantial reduction of the size of radiotherapy portals. This applies particularly for patients with tumor-associated dys- or atelectasis

(continued)

Table 2 (continued)

First author, year	Institution	Patient number	Imaging Technique	Change in GTV	Conclusion
Nestle et al. (2005)	Saarland University Medical Center Homburg/Saar, Germany	25	CT, PET-CT	We found substantial differences between the four methods of up to 41% of the GTVvis. The volumes increased significantly from GTV40 (mean 53.6 mL) _ GTVbg (94.7mL) _ GTVvis (157.7 mL) and GTV2.5 (164.6 mL). The volumes increased significantly from GTV40 (mean 53.6 mL) _ GTVbg (94.7mL) _ GTVvis (157.7 mL) and GTV2.5 (164.6 mL). In inhomogeneous lesions, GTV40 led to visually inadequate tumor coverage in 3 of 8 patients, whereas GTVbg led to intermediate, more satisfactory volumes. In contrast to all other GTVs, GTV40 did not correlate with the GTVCT	The different techniques of tumor contour definition by (18)F-FDG PET in radiotherapy planning lead to substantially different volumes, especially in patients with inhomogeneous tumors. Here, the GTV(40) does not appear to be suitable for target volume delineation. More complex methods, such as system-specific contrast-oriented algorithms for contour definition, should be further evaluated with special respect to patient data
Paulsen et al. (2006)	University of Tuebingen, Germany	16	PET-CT	In 23 PET/CT examinations performed solely for radiation treatment planning, target volume was modified in 44%	Despite the low number of patients and an expected bias of selection, the first results are encouraging to perform more extended and detailed trials of this technology in radiotherapy planning. Whether PET/CT is superior to PET alone is part of ongoing investigations
Pfannenberg et al. (2007)	Eberhard-Karls-University, Tübingen, Germany	50	PET-CT (contrast and non-contrast)	Relevant? Compares two pet-ct types.s In 63% of tumor sites, CE PET/CT altered lesion delineation in comparison to LD PET/CT	In patients with advanced NSCLC, contrast-enhanced CT as part of the PET/CT protocol more accurately assessed the TNM stage in 8% of patients compared with non-contrast PET/CT. However, for planning of 3D conformal radiotherapy and non-conventional surgery, contrast-enhanced PET/CT protocols are indispensable owing to their superiority in precisely defining the tumor extent
Schmucking et al. (2003)	Klinik fur Nuklearmedizin, Bad Berka, Germany	27	CT, PET-CT	Metabolic radiation treatment planning by PET led to smaller planning target volumes (PTVs) for radiation therapy (between 3 and 21% in 25/27 patients), resulting in a reduction of dose exposure to healthy tissue. In 2 patients, PET-PTV was larger than CT-based PTV, since PET detected lymph node metastases smaller than 1 cm	FDG-PET provides clinically important information; changes therapeutic management, can predict noninvasively effectiveness of chemotherapy, and may lead to better tumor control with less radiation-induced toxicity

(continued)

Table 2 (continued)

First author, year	Institution	Patient number	Imaging Technique	Change in GTV	Conclusion
Song et al. (2006)	Memorial Sloan-Kettering Cancer Center, New York, NY	5	CT, PET-CT	The PET-defined GTV, PETGTV, was consistently larger than the CT-defined GTV, CT-GTV, for all three cases. The differences between PETGTV and CT-GTV were 30.26, 74.65, and 13.13 cm3 for patient Nos. 1, 2, and 3, respectively. In terms of percentage, the differences were 70.2, 31.98, and 86.15%, respectively	The objectives of the study were to investigate the inter-modality variation in gross tumor volume delineation defined by two imaging modalities for lung cancer: CT and 18FDG-PET/CT and its dosimetric implications in intensity modulated radiation therapy (IMRT)
Steenbakkers et al. (2006)	The Netherlands Cancer Institute, Amsterdam, The Netherlands	22	CT, PET-CT	Compared with the first phase (CT only), the mean delineated volume of all delineated GTVs of the second phase (matched CT–FDG-PET) was reduced from 69 cm^3 to 62 cm^3 (p _ 0.041, paired Student's t-test). This volume difference was mainly due to the separation of tumor from atelectasis in 3 patients by the second phase	For high-precision radiotherapy, the delineation of lung target volumes using only CT introduces too great a variability among radiation oncologists. Implementing matched CT-FDG-PET and adapted delineation protocol and software reduced observer variation in lung cancer delineation significantly with respect to CT only. However, the remaining observer variation was still large compared with other geometric uncertainties (setup variation and organ motion)
Stroom et al. (2007)	Netherlands Cancer Institute–Antoni van Leeuwenhoek Hospital, Amsterdam, The Netherlands	5	CT, PET	Compared to GET-Path - In 4 of 5 patients, the GTVCT was, on average, 4 cm3 (_53%) too large. In contrast, for 1 patient (with lymphangitis carcinomatosa), the GTVCT was 16 cm^3 (_40%) too small. The GTVPET was too small for 1 patient and large/equal to path in 3 patients. One subject did not have PET	Our results have shown that pathology-correlated lung imaging is feasible and can be used to improve target definition. Ignoring deformations of the lung might result in underestimation of the microscopic spread
Subedi et al. (2009)	Leeds Teaching Hospitals NHS Trust, Leeds, United Kingdom	161	CT, PET-CT	Relevant?	Addition of PET-CT to comprehensive evaluation of lung cancer can have significant clinical impact. There is marked improvement in staging the disease. Patients were frequently spared unnecessary treatment, and management was more appropriately targeted. PET permits reduction in the number of thoracotomies performed for non-resectable disease with predicted reduction in the morbidity rate and cost associated with unnecessary interventions

(continued)

Table 2 (continued)

First author, year	Institution	Patient number	Imaging Technique	Change in GTV	Conclusion
van Baardwijk et al. (2007)	University Hospital Maastricht, Maastricht, The Netherlands	33	PET-CT	The edited auto-contour of the primary tumor (GTV-1auto) (median, 31.8 cm^3) was smaller than the manually contoured GTV-1 (median, 34.6 cm3; z _ _3.36, p _0.001)	Source-to-background ratio-based auto-delineation showed a good correlation with pathology, decreased the delineated volumes of the GTVs, and reduced the inter-observer variability. Auto-contouring may further improve the quality of target delineation in NSCLC patients
van Der Wel et al. (2005)	University Hospital Maastricht, Maastricht, The Netherlands	21	CT, PET-CT	Of the 21 RT plans, 14 (67%; 95% confidence interval 43–85%) changed with incorporation of the PET data. In 11 patients, the radiation fields decreased with CT-PET planning and in 3 patients, they increased. In 2 patients, in whom the CT-PET–determined GTV was larger than the CTdetermined GTV, no change occurred in the radiation fields. In 7 patients, no changes occurred	In this group of clinical CT Stage N2-N3 NSCLC patients, use of FDG-PET scanning information in radiotherapy planning reduced the radiation exposure of the esophagus and lung, and thus allowed significant radiation dose escalation while respecting all relevant normal tissue constraints. This, together with a reduced risk of geographic misses using PET-CT, led to an estimated increase in TCP from 13 to 18%. The results of this modeling study support clinical trials investigating incorporation of FDG-PET information in CT-based radiotherapy planning
Vanuytsel et al. (2000)	University Hospital Gasthuisberg, Leuven, Belgium	73	CT, PET-CT	The CT de®ned volume was identical to the PET-CT de®ned volume in 28 patients leaving 45 patients (62%) in whom the additional acquisition of PET data changed treatment volumes. In 16 patients (22%), the PET-CT de®ned volume was larger than the CT volume. In 29 patients (40%), the PET-CT de®ned volume was smaller than the CT de®ned Volume Form 45, Thus, in all, PET data resulted in a correct change of volume in 36 patients (49%), an inappropriate change in 2 patients (3%) and an insuf®cient change in 7 patients (10%)	In patients with NSCLC considered for curative radiation treatment, assessment of locoregional LN tumor extension by PET will improve tumor coverage, and in selected patients, will reduce the volume of normal tissues irradiated, and thus toxicity. This subgroup of patients could then become candidates for treatment intensification

(continued)

Table 2 (continued)

First author, year	Institution	Patient number	Imaging Technique	Change in GTV	Conclusion
Wu et al. (2009)	University of Toronto, Toronto, Canada	31	CT, PET	The correlation coefficient of the GTVCT1 was the best (r = 0.87). The median MDof GTVPET changed from 5.72cm to 2.67cm as the PET thresholds increased. The correlation coefficient of the GTVPET compared with the pathologic finding ranged from 0.51 to 0.77. The correlation coefficient of GTV50 was the best (r = 0.77)	Compared with the MD of GTV(PET), the MD of GTV(CT) had better correlation with the pathologic MD. The GTV(CT1) and GTV(50) had the best correlation with the pathologic results
Yu et al. (2009a)	Shandong Cancer Hospital and Institute, Jinan, China	15	PET	Not clear	This study evaluated the use of GTV(path) as a criterion for determining the optimal cutoff SUV for NSCLC target volume delineation. Confirmatory studies including more cases are being performed
Yu et al. (2009c)	Shandong University, Jinan, China	52	CT, PET, PET-CT	No significant differences were observed among the tumor sizes measured by three images and pathological method. Compared with pathological measurement, CT size at X, Y, Z axis was larger, whereas combined 18F-FDG PET/CT and 18F-FDG PET size were smaller. Combined 18F-FDG PET/CT size was more similar to the pathological size than that of 18F-FDG PET or CT. Results of linear regressions showed that integrated 18F-FDG PET/CT was the most accurate modality in measuring the size of cancer	18F-FDG PET/CT correlates more faithfully with pathological findings than 18F-FDG PET or CT. Integrated 18F-FDG PET/CT is an effective tool to define the target of GTV in radiotherapy
Zasadny et al. (1998)	University of Michigan Medical Center, Ann Arbor, MI	7	CT, PET	Mean tumor volume was 187 +- 189 cm3. Tumor volume determined by means of PET and CT was strongly correlated (r = 0.98, P <0.001, N=8) in the patients with untreated tumors	Tumor volume determination by FDG-PET was strongly correlated with tumor volumes determined by anatomic imaging with CT. FDG-PET appears comparable to CT in measuring untreated tumor volumes of this size. FDG-PET may be superior to anatomic techniques in assessing metabolically active tumor volume, and warrants further study in this role

lesions respectively, and the authors concluded that no single threshold criteria for delineating PET/GTV provided accurate target volume definition. Other studies have used an SUV of 2.5.

In a study by Yu et al. 2009a of 15 patients with non small-cell lung cancer, pathologic correlation to PET/CT was studied to determine the optimal SUV cutoff criteria. The optimal threshold or optimal absolute SUV was defined as the value at which the PET GTV was the same as the pathologic GTV. The optimal threshold SUV was 31% +/− 11% and the absolute SUV was 3.0 +/− 1.6. The optimal threshold was inversely proportional to the pathological GTV and tumor diameter. The absolute SUV did not significantly correlate with the pathologic GTV or tumor diameter (Yu et al. 2009b).

5.5 PET/CT Planning for Gastrointestinal Malignancies

Major published series examining PET imaging in radiotherapy planning for gastrointestinal malignancies are described in Table 3. FDG PET/CT is part of the standard workup of a number of gastrointestinal malignancies including esophageal, gastric, rectal, and anal carcinoma. In esophageal carcinoma, using PET/CT for radiotherapy planning appears to improve target volume definition over CT alone. It also allows better normal tissue sparing of the heart and lungs, and potentially reduces the risk of marginal tumor miss, and several studies have shown modification of treatment plans when using PET/CT compared to CT alone (Moureau-Zabotto et al. 2005; Muijs et al. 2009; Leong et al. 2006; Schreurs et al. 2010). In a contrary report by Shimizu et al. (2009) PET/CT correlated with surgical specimens did not improve the detection of occult subclinical lymph node metastases, and the authors concluded that PET/CT should not be used for clinical target volume definition when 1 cm margins are used. However, typically for definitive radiotherapy, long craniocaudal margins of 3–5 cm are still used for defining clinical target volumes, as submucosal spread and occult periesophageal metastases are still encompassed in the radiotherapy field.

In gastrointestinal malignancies, endoscopic staging is particularly important to determine treatment strategy. In a study by Konski et al. (2005) 25 patients with esophageal cancer were evaluated with PET and endoscopic ultrasound and with the CT simulation. The length of the tumor measured by endoscopic ultrasound was compared to the CT- and PET-defined (using a SUV of 2.5) tumor length. The tumors were significantly longer on CT compared with PET ($p = 0.0063$). PET correlated better with the EUS tumor length than CT. EUS also detected more periesophageal and celiac lymphadenopathy than PET and CT. The SUV of the esophageal tumors was higher in patients with periesophageal lymphadenopathy identified on PET scans. These results suggest that integration of PET and endoscopic ultrasound can significantly aid GTV delineation in patients with esophageal carcinoma compared to CT alone. In a study by Gondi et al. (2007) 16 patients with esophageal cancer underwent PET/CT radiotherapy planning scans. The PET GTV margin was defined by standardizing the liver PET activity in all images. They compared the CT and PET/CT GTVs quantitatively by using a conformality index, defined as the ratio of the two GTVs to their union. The mean index of conformality was 0.46 (range 0.13–0.80). In 62.5% of patients PET data led to the definition of a smaller GTV.

6 Novel PET Tracers and Therapy Planning

Over the past decade, many novel PET tracers have entered experimental clinical imaging, and they may play a role in radiotherapy planning in the future. These novel PET tracers allow imaging of various tumor pathways in tumor biology, including proliferation, hypoxia, protein synthesis, receptor, and gene expression. ^{11}C-methionine, an amino acid derivative, allows delineation of brain tumors and metastasis contours (Matsuo et al. 2009). ^{11}C and ^{18}F choline derivatives are promising PET tracers for prostate cancer imaging (Pinkawa et al. 2011). Hypoxic tumor cells are radio resistant, and it would be useful to identify the hypoxic component of the tumors in vivo, which could be experimentally treated with a higher dose than the rest of the tumor. Dose painting with hypoxic PET tracers such as ^{18}F -FMISO, ^{18}F -FAZA, and Cu_{64}-ATSM is potentially valuable for radiotherapy planning (Dirix et al. 2009). ^{18}F fluorothymidine (FLT) is a surrogate marker for thymidine

Table 3 Summary of studies exploring the role of PET/CT in radiation treatment planning for tumors of the gastrointestinal tract

First author, year	Institution	Patient number	Imaging Technique	Change in GTV	Conclusion
Anderson et al. (2007)	Emory University School of Medicine, Atlanta, GA	23 (20 rectal, 3 anal ca)	CT versus PET-CT	Mean PET-GTV was smaller than the mean CT-GTV (91.7 vs. 99.6 cm^3) In 4 of 23 patients (17%; one anal canal tumor and three rectal tumors), integration of the PET volume with the planning volumes resulted in a change in the PTV. 26% of patients (6 of 23) experienced a change in the radiation treatment-planning process. Changes included increasing field sizes because traditional fields would have cut through a contoured PET tumor volume or changing a treatment course from definitive to palliative because of the detection of distant metastases	Variation in volume was significant, with 17 and 26% of patients requiring a change in treatment fields and patient management, respectively. Positron emission tomography can change the management for anorectal tumors by early detection of metastatic disease or disease outside standard radiation fields
Bassi et al. (2008)	University of Piemonte Orientale, Novara, Italy	25 rectal cancer pts	CT versus PET-CT	The PET/CT-GTVand PET/CT-CTV were significantly greater than the CT-GTV ($p = 0.00013$) and CT-CTV ($p = 0.00002$), respectively. The mean difference between PET/CT-GTV and CT-GTV was 25.4% and between PET/CT-CTV and CT-CTV was 4.1%	Imaging with PET/CT for preoperative radiotherapy of rectal cancer may lead to a change in staging and target volume delineation. Stage variation was observed in 12% of cases and a change of treatment intent in 4%. The GTVand CTV changed significantly, with a mean increase in size of 25 and 4%, respectively
Ciernik et al. (2005)	Zurich University Hospital, Zurich, Switzerland	11 rectal ca	CT versus PET-CT	Immediate treatment volume definition based on the choice of a single-tumor volume–derived PET-voxel resulted in a tumor volume that strongly correlated with the CT-derived GTV (r2 _ 0.84; $p < 0.01$) and the volume as assessed on subsequent anatomic-pathologic analysis (r2 _ 0.77; $p < 0.01$). In providing sufficient extension margins from the CT-derived GTV and the PET-derived GTV, to PTV, respectively, the correlation of the CT-derived and PET-derived PTV was sufficiently accurate for PTV definition for external-beam therapy (r2 _ 0.96; $p < 0.01$	Automated segmentation of the PET signal from rectal cancer may allow immediate and sufficiently accurate definition of a preliminary working PTV for preoperative RT. If required, correction for anatomic precision and geometric resolution may be applied in a second step. Computed PET-based target-volume definition could be useful for the definition of standardized simultaneous internal-boost volumes for intensity modulated radiation therapy (IMRT) based on biologic target volumes

(continued)

Table 3 (continued)

First author, year	Institution	Patient number	Imaging Technique	Change in GTV	Conclusion
Ciernik et al. (2003)	University of Zurich, Zurich, Switzerland	21 (pelvic i.e. includes 8 gyn cases, 6 rectal, 8 anal ca)	CT versus PET-CT	The GTV increased by 25% or more because of PET in 33% (7/21) in cancer of the pelvis. The GTV was reduced >25% in 19% with cancer of the pelvis (4/21)	Integrated PET/CT for treatment planning for three-dimensional conformal radiation therapy improves the standardization of volume delineation compared with that of CT alone. PET/CT has the potential for reducing the risk for geographic misses, to minimize the dose of ionizing radiation applied to non-target organs, and to change the current practice to three-dimensional conformal radiation therapy planning by taking into account the metabolic and biologic features of cancer. The impact on treatment outcome remains to be demonstrated
Dizendorf et al. (2003)	University Hospital, Zurich, Switzerland	18 GIT (202 total)	CT, PET-CT	A change in radiation volume was necessary in 12 patients (6%): head and neck tumors, 2%; gynecologic tumors, 11%; breast cancer, 4%; lung cancer, 4%; malignant lymphomas, 13%; and gastrointestinal tumors, 11%	The results of this study show that 18F-FDG PET has a major impact on the management of patients for radiation therapy, influencing both the stage and the management in 27% of patients
Gondi et al. (2007)	University of Wisconsin, Madison, WI	16 eso	CT, PET-CT	In 10 of the 16 (62.5%) esophageal cancer patients, and in 12 of the 14 (85.7%) NSCLC patients, the addition of the FDG-PET data led to the definition of a smaller GTV	The incorporation of a hybrid FDG-PET/CT scanner had an impact on the radiotherapy planning of esophageal cancer and NSCLC. In future studies, we recommend adoption of a conformality index for a more comprehensive comparison of newer treatment planning imaging modalities to conventional options
Han et al. (2010)	Shandong Cancer Hospital and Institute, Jinan, China	22 eso	CT, FLT PET-CT FDG PET-CT	The mean ± standard deviation pathologic gross tumor length was 4.94 ± 2.21 cm. On FLT PET/CT, the length of the standardized uptake value 1.4 was 4.91 ± 2.43 cm. On FDG PET/CT, the length of the standardized uptake value 2.5 was 5.10 ± 2.18 cm, both of which seemed more approximate to the pathologic gross tumor length	The incorporation of PET data improves definition of the primary lesion by including positive lymph nodes into the PTV. Thus, the PET data reduces the likelihood of geographic misses and hopefully improves the chance of achieving local control

(continued)

Table 3 (continued)

First author, year	Institution	Patient number	Imaging Technique	Change in GTV	Conclusion
Hong et al. (2008)	Massachusetts General Hospital, Boston, MA	19 eso	CT, PET-CT	Comparing CT-based gross tumor volumes (GTVs) with manually defined PET/CT-based GTVs, use of PET changed volumes for 21 of 25 (84%) patients: 12 patients (48%) exhibited minor differences, whereas for 9 patients (36%), the differences were major. For 4 (16%) patients, the major difference was due to discrepancy in celiac or distant mediastinal lymph node involvement Use of automated PET volumes changed the manual PET length in 14 patients (56%): 8 minor and 6 major	The use of PET/CT in treatment planning for esophageal cancer can affect target definition. Two PET-based techniques can also produce significantly different tumor volumes in a large percentage of patients. Further investigations to clarify the optimal use of PET/CT data in treatment planning are warranted
Igdem et al. (2010)	Istanbul Bilim University, Istanbul, Turkey	2 eso 1 rectal	CT, PET-CT	Relevant?	Integrating functional imaging with FDG-PET/CT into the radiotherapy planning process resulted in major changes in a significant proportion of our patients. An interdisciplinary approach between imaging and radiation oncology departments is essential in defining the target volumes
Konski et al. (2005)	Fox Chase Cancer Center, Philadelphia, PA	25 eso	CT, PET-CT	The mean length of the cancer was 5.4 cm (95% Confidence interval [CI], 4.4–6.4 cm) as determined by PET scan, 6.7 cm (95% CI, 5.6 –7.9 cm) as determined by CT scan, and 5.1 cm (95% CI, 4.0–6.1 cm) for the 22 patients who underwent endoscopy. The length as determined by PET scan correlated better with endoscopy than with CT scans as determined by Pearson correlation coefficients (r _0.67 and r _ 0.61 day, respectively). The length of the tumors was significantly longer as measured by CT scans compared with PET scans,regardless of the SUV (p _ 0.0063). No significant difference was noted between the length of tumor in the measurements by PET and EUS	Endoscopic ultrasound and PET scans can add additional information to aid the radiation oncologist's ability to precisely identify the GTV in patients with esophageal carcinoma

(continued)

Table 3 (continued)

First author, year	Institution	Patient number	Imaging Technique	Change in GTV	Conclusion
Krengli et al. (2010)	University of Piemonte Orientale, Novara, Italy	27 anal ca	CT, PET-CT	Based on PET/CT imaging, GTV and CTV contours changed in 15/27 (55.6%) and in 10/27 cases (37.0%) respectively. PET-GTV and PET-CTV resulted significantly smaller than CT-GTV (p = 1.2x10-4) and CT-CTV (p = 2.9x10-4). PET/CT-GTV and PET/CT-CTV, that were used for clinical purposes, were significantly greater than CT-GTV (p = 6x10-5) and CT-CTV (p = 6x10-5)	FDG-PET/CT has a potential relevant impact in staging and target volume delineation of the carcinoma of the anal canal. Clinical stage variation occurred in 18.5% of cases with change of treatment intent in 3.7%. The GTV and the CTV changed in shape and in size based on PET/CT imaging
Kruser et al. (2009)	University of Wisconsin, Madison, WI	9 eso	CT, PET-CT	Full article?	Hybrid PET/CT imaging at the time of treatment planning may be highly informative and an economical manner in which to obtain PET imaging, with the dual goals of staging and treatment planning
Leong et al. (2006)	University of Melbourne, Melbourne, Australia	21 eso	CT, PET-CT	16 patients proceeded to the radiotherapy planning phase of the study and received definitive chemoradiation planned with the PET/CT data set. The GTV based on CT information alone excluded PET-avid disease in 11 patients (69%), and in 5 patients (31%) this would have resulted in a geographic miss of gross tumor. The discordance between CT and PET/CT was due mainly to differences in defining the longitudinal extent of disease in the esophagus. The cranial extent of the primary tumor as defined by CT versus PET/CT differed in 75% of cases, while the caudal extent differed in 81%	This study demonstrates that if combined PET/CT is used for radiotherapy treatment planning, there may be alterations to the delineation of tumor volumes when compared to CT alone, with the potential to avoid a geographic miss of tumor
Moureau-zabotto et al. (2005)	Hôpital Tenon, Paris, France	34 eso	CT, PET	The gross tumor volume (GTV) was decreased by CT and FDG image fusion in 12 patients (35%) and increased in 7 patients (21%). The GTV reduction was >25% in 4 patients owing to a reduction in the length of the esophageal tumor. The GTV increase was >25% with FDG-PET in 2 patients owing to the detection of occult mediastinal lymph node involvement in 1 patient and an increased length of the esophageal tumor in 1 patient	In our study, CT and FDG-PET image fusion appeared to have an impact on treatment planning and management of esophageal carcinoma. The affect on treatment outcome remains to be demonstrated

(continued)

Table 3 (continued)

First author, year	Institution	Patient number	Imaging Technique	Change in GTV	Conclusion
Muijs et al. (2009)	University of Groningen, The Netherlands	21 eso	CT, PET-CT	The addition of PET led to the modification of CT-TV with at least 10% in 12 of 21 patients (57%) (reduction in 9, enlargement in 3). PET/CT-TV was inadequately covered by the CT-based treatment plan in 8 patients (36%)	This study demonstrated that TV s based on CT might exclude PET-avid disease. Consequences are under dosing and thereby possibly ineffective treatment. Moreover, the addition of PET in radiation planning might result in clinical important changes in NTCP
Paskeviciute et al. (2009)	University Hospital Munster, Germany	36 rectal	CT, PET-CT	PET/CT-GTVs were smaller than CT-GTVs ($p < 0.05$). PET/CT imaging resulted in a change of overall management for 3 patients (8 %). In 16 of 35 patients (46 %), PET/CT resulted in a need for modification of the usual target volumes (CT-PTV) because of detection of a geographic miss	FDG-PET/CT had significant impact on radiotherapy planning and overall treatment of patients with LARC
Patel et al. (2007)	Stanford University School of Medicine, Stanford, CA	6 rectal	CT, FLT PET-CT FDG PET-CT	An inter-observer similarity index (SI), ranging from a value of 0 for complete disagreement to 1 for complete agreement of contoured voxels, was calculated for each set of volumes. For primary gross tumor volume (GTVp), the difference in estimated SI between CT and FDG was modest (CT SI = 0.77 versus FDG SI = 0.81), but statistically significant ($p = 0.013$). The SI difference between CT and FLT for GTVp was also slight (FLT SI = 0.80) and marginally non-significant ($s < 0.082$)	Boost target volumes in rectal cancer based on combined PET/CT results in lower inter-observer variability compared with CT alone, particularly for nodal disease. The use of FDG and FLT did not appear to be different from this perspective
Schreurs et al. (2010)	University Medical Center Groningen, Groningen, The Netherlands	28-eso	CT, PET-CT	In 11 out of 28 patients (39%), FDG-PET information led to an increase in the GTV-pt (mean increase: 13.3 cm^3; range: 0.1– 33.1 cm^3) and in 17 patients (61%) to a decrease (mean decrease: 4.3 cm^3; range: 0.3–9.4 cm^3)	Combining FDG-PET and CT may improve target volume definition with less geographic misses, but without significant effects on inter-observer variability in esophageal cancer

(continued)

Table 3 (continued)

First author, year	Institution	Patient number	Imaging Technique	Change in GTV	Conclusion
Shimizu et al. (2009)	Hokkaido University, Sapporo, Japan	20-eso	CT, EUS, PET-CT	Not clear	The detection rate of subclinical lymph node metastasis did not improve with the use of PET-CT, for either the cervical and supraclavicular, mediastinal, or abdominal regions. It is not recommended to use FDG-PET or PET-CT alone as a diagnostic tool to determine CTV if pathologically involved lymphatic regions are to be included in the CTV in the treatment protocol. The accuracy of PETCT must be further improved in order to better detect positive nodes and improve the definition of the CTV
Steffen et al. (2009)	Universitätsmedizin Berlin, Berlin, Germany	19 (25 sessions) Liver metastases from rectal ca	PET-CT (contrast and non-contrast)	An increased CTV was observed in 15 cases and a decrease in 6; in 4 cases, the CT-CTV and PET/CT-CTV were equal	Retrospective implementation of fluorodeoxyglucose-PET for CTV specification for CT-guided brachytherapy for colorectal liver metastases revealed a significant change in the CTVs. Additional PET-positive tumor regions with incomplete dose coverage could explain unexpected early local progression
Tonkopi et al. (2010)	Anderson Cancer Center, Houston, TX	48 colorectal cancer patients with metastasis in the liver and 52 esophageal cancer patients	CT, PET-CT	Relevant?	ACT was effective in improving registration between the CT and PET data in PET/CT for the colorectal and esophageal cancer patients
Vesprini et al. (2008)	University of Toronto, Toronto, Canada	10 gastro-eso ca	CT, PET-CT	The addition of FDG-PET imaging decreased the median standard deviation for tumor length from 10 mm (range 8.1e33.3, mean 12.4 mm) for computed tomography alone to 8 mm (range 4.4e18.1, mean 8.1 mm) for PETeCT (P[0.02). There was significantly less intra-observer variability in all measures when PETeCT was used. The median standard deviation in length improved from 5.3 to 1.8 mm, the median standard deviation in volume improved from 4.5 to 3 cm^3 and the median observer agreement index improved from 76.2 to 78.7% when computed tomography alone was compared with PETeCT. The corresponding P values were 0.001, 0.033 and 0.022, respectively	The addition of FDG-PET to computed tomography-based planning for the identification of primary tumor GTV in patients with gastro-esophageal carcinoma decreases both inter-observer and intra-observer variability

(continued)

Table 3 (continued)

First author, year	Institution	Patient number	Imaging Technique	Change in GTV	Conclusion
Vrieze et al. (2004)	University Hospital Gasthuisberg, Leuven, Belgium	30 eso	CT, PET-CT	In 14 of the 30 patients (47%) discordances were found in detection of the pathological lymph nodes between CT/EUS and FDGPET. In 8 patients, 9 lymph node regions were found with pathologic nodes on conventional imaging only. In three of these patients the influence of FDG-PET findings would have led to a decrease in the irradiated volume. In 6 patients, 8 lymph node regions were found with a normal CT/EUS and pathologic nodes on FDG-PET. In three of these patients (10%) the influence of the FDG-PET would have led to enlargement of the irradiated volume	The chance of a false negative result on FGD-PET is not negligible; therefore, the irradiated volume should not be reduced based on a negative-FDG-PET in a region with suspect nodes on other investigations. However, due to the high specificity of FDG-PET enlarging the irradiated volume based on a positive-FDG-PET in a region without suspected lymph nodes on CT and/or EUS should be considered. This indicates a role for FDG-PET in radiotherapy planning for esophageal cancer
Yu et al. (2009b)	Fudan University, Shanghai, China	16 eso	CT, PET-CT	Lengths of GTVs were recorded as LCT, L20%, L40%, L2.5, L40%M, and Lpath, respectively. The former five GTVs/lengths were compared with GTVpath/Lpath. Mean GTVCT, GTV20%, GTV40%, GTV2.5, GTV40%M and GTVpath were 29.16 ± 18.56, 18.75 ± 12.37, 12.52 ± 8.08, 22.69 ± 14.84, 9.18 ± 5.96 and 28.16 ± 17.02 cm^3	The SUVbgd + 20%(SUVmax(slice) _ SUVbgd) method optimally estimated gross tumor length, but only reached an unsatisfactory CI for GTV. Due to possible motion factor enveloped in PET images and lack of histopathologic transverse reference, the information from both PET and CT should be referred to complementarily when delineating GTV
Zhong et al. (2009)	Tianjin Medical University Cancer Hospital and Institute, Tianjin, China	36 eso	CT, PET-CT	The length of tumors on PET scan were measured and recorded as Lengthvis, Length2.5, and Length40, respectively, and compared with the length of gross tumor in the resected specimen (Lengthgross). The mean Lengthvis ($p = 0.123$) and Length2.5 ($p = 0.957$) were not significantly different from Lengthgross, and Length2.5 seems more approximate to Lengthgross. The mean Length40 was significantly shorter than Lengthgross ($p < 0.001$)	The optimal PET method to estimate the length of gross tumor varies with tumor length and SUVmax; an SUV cutoff of 2.5 provided the closest estimation in this study

kinase activity and thus proliferation, which may provide additional information about the proliferative capacity or aggressiveness of tumor cells (Han et al. 2010).

In a study by Dali Han et al. (2010) 22 esophageal patients underwent FLT PET and FDG PET and the results were correlated with pathological examination. The FDG PET used an SUV of 2.5, and FLT PET used an SUV of 1.4 as the best estimate to determine the pathologic length of the tumor. When comparing FLT PET- to FDG PET-defined tumor volumes, using a 7-field IMRT plan, potential improvements in normal tissue dosimetry to the lungs and the heart were demonstrated with the FLT PET-defined GTVs. A recent study investigated the feasibility of boosting the radiation dose to areas of FMISO avidity within FDG-avid tumor volumes. Regions of elevated FMISO uptake within the PET/CT GTV were targeted for an IMRT boost. The heterogeneous distribution of FMISO in the GTV indicated variable levels of hypoxia. It was possible to escalate the dose in the FMISO-avid GTV regions to 84 Gy in all 10 head and neck cancer patients and in one patient to 105 Gy without exceeding the normal tissue tolerance (Lee et al. 2008).

7 Conclusions

Use of PET/CT in radiotherapy planning has gained momentum at numerous sites, including head and neck cancer, lung cancer, gastrointestinal malignancies, and other cancer sites. Overall, PET/CT appears to change the GTV when compared to a CT-defined GTV. Pathologic correlative studies seem to show that PET/CT is more accurate compared to CT alone or MRI for numerous sites. However, in current clinical practice, most would use PET/CT as a complementary exam in addition to other imaging modalities and clinical examination, particularly for heterogeneous or necrotic tumors with low FDG avidity. Determining the ideal method for accurate tumor contour delineation is subjected to much clinical investigation. PET/CT minimizes the intra- and inter-user variability in contouring target volumes and improves radiotherapy planning, regardless of the method of volumetric segmentation. Novel PET tracers provide in vivo tumor biologic information that may be useful in treatment planning in the future.

References

Adler JR Jr, Murphy MJ, Chang SD, Hancock SL (1999) Image-guided robotic radiosurgery. Neurosurgery 44(6):1299–1306 (discussion 306–307)

Anderson C, Koshy M et al (2007) PET-CT fusion in radiation management of patients with anorectal tumors. Int J Radiat Oncol Biol Phys 69(1):155–162

Ashamalla H, Guirgius A et al (2007) The impact of positron emission tomography/computed tomography in edge delineation of gross tumor volume for head and neck cancers. Int J Radiat Oncol Biol Phys 68(2):388–395

Ashamalla H, Rafla S et al (2005) The contribution of integrated PET/CT to the evolving definition of treatment volumes in radiation treatment planning in lung cancer. Int J Radiat Oncol Biol Phys 63(4):1016–1023

Bassi MC, Turri L et al (2008) FDG-PET/CT imaging for staging and target volume delineation in preoperative conformal radiotherapy of rectal cancer. Int J Radiat Oncol Biol Phys 70(5):1423–1426

Berson AM, Stein NF et al (2009) Variability of gross tumor volume delineation in head-and-neck cancer using PET/CT fusion, Part II: the impact of a contouring protocol. Med Dosim 34(1):30–35

Biehl KJ, Kong F-M, Dehdashti F et al (2006) 18F-FDG PET definition of gross tumor volume for radiotherapy of non-small cell lung cancer: is a single standardized uptake value threshold approach appropriate? J Nucl Med 47(11):1808–1812

Bradley J, Thorstad WL, Mutic S et al (2004) Impact of FDG-PET on radiation therapy volume delineation in non-small-cell lung cancer. Int J Radiat Oncol Biol Phys 59(1):78–86

Brianzoni E, Rossi G et al (2005) Radiotherapy planning: PET/CT scanner performances in the definition of gross tumour volume and clinical target volume. Eur J Nucl Med Mol Imaging 32(12):1392–1399

Breen SL, Publicover J et al (2007) Intraobserver and interobserver variability in GTV delineation on FDG-PET-CT images of head and neck cancers. Int J Radiat Oncol Biol Phys 68(3):763–770

Caldwell CB, Mah K et al (2001) Observer variation in contouring gross tumor volume in patients with poorly defined non-small-cell lung tumors on CT: the impact of 18FDG-hybrid PET fusion. Int J Radiat Oncol Biol Phys 51(4):923–931

Ceresoli GL, Cattaneo GM, Castellone P et al (2007) Role of computed tomography and [18F] fluorodeoxyglucose positron emission tomography image fusion in conformal radiotherapy of non-small cell lung cancer: a comparison with standard techniques with and without elective nodal irradiation. Tumori 93(1):88–96

Ciernik IF, Dizendorf E et al (2003) Radiation treatment planning with an integrated positron emission and computer tomography (PET/CT): a feasibility study. Int J Radiat Oncol Biol Phys 57(3):853–863

Ciernik IF, Huser M et al (2005) Automated functional image-guided radiation treatment planning for rectal cancer. Int J Radiat Oncol Biol Phys 62(3):893–900

Daisne JF, Duprez T et al (2004) Tumor volume in pharyngolaryngeal squamous cell carcinoma: comparison at CT, MR imaging, and FDG PET and validation with surgical specimen. Radiology 233(1):93–100

Day E, Betler J et al (2009) A region growing method for tumor volume segmentation on PET images for rectal and anal cancer patients. Med Phys 36(10):4349–4358

Deantonio L, Beldi D et al (2008) FDG-PET/CT imaging for staging and radiotherapy treatment planning of head and neck carcinoma. Radiat Oncol 3:29

Deniaud-Alexandre E, Touboul E, Lerouge D et al (2005) Impact of computed tomography and 18F-deoxyglucose coincidence detection emission tomography image fusion for optimization of conformal radiotherapy in non-small-cell lung cancer. Int J Radiat Oncol Biol Phys 63(5):1432–1441

De Ruysscher D, Wanders S, Minken A et al (2005) Effects of radiotherapy planning with a dedicated combined PET-CT-simulator of patients with non-small cell lung cancer on dose limiting normal tissues and radiation dose-escalation: a planning study. Radiother Oncol 77(1):5–10

Dirix P, Vandecaveye V, De Keyzer F, Stroobants S, Hermans R, Nuyts S (2009) Dose painting in radiotherapy for head and neck squamous cell carcinoma: value of repeated functional imaging with (18)F-FDG PET, (18)F-fluoromisonidazole PET, diffusion-weighted MRI, and dynamic contrast-enhanced MRI. J Nucl Med 50(7):1020–1027

Dizendorf EV, Baumert BG et al (2003) Impact of whole-body 18F-FDG PET on staging and managing patients for radiation therapy. J Nucl Med 44(1):24–29

El-Bassiouni M, Ciernik IF et al (2007) [18FDG] PET-CT-based intensity-modulated radiotherapy treatment planning of head and neck cancer. Int J Radiat Oncol Biol Phys 69(1):286–293

Erdi YE, Rosenzweig K, Erdi AK et al (2002) Radiotherapy treatment planning for patients with non-small cell lung cancer using positron emission tomography (PET). Radiother Oncol 62(1):51–60

Ford EC, Kinahan PE, Hanlon L et al (2006) Tumor delineation using PET in head and neck cancers: threshold contouring and lesion volumes. Med Phys 33(11):4280–4288

Fox JL, Rengan R et al (2005) Does registration of PET and planning CT images decrease interobserver and intraobserver variation in delineating tumor volumes for non-small-cell lung cancer? Int J Radiat Oncol Biol Phys 62(1):70–75

Gardner M, Halimi P et al (2009) Use of single MRI and 18F-FDG PET-CT scans in both diagnosis and radiotherapy treatment planning in patients with head and neck cancer: advantage on target volume and critical organ delineation. Head Neck 31(4):461–467

Geets X, Daisne JF et al (2006) Impact of the type of imaging modality on target volumes delineation and dose distribution in pharyngo-laryngeal squamous cell carcinoma: comparison between pre- and per-treatment studies. Radiother Oncol 78(3):291–297

Giraud P, Grahek D et al (2001) CT and (18)F-deoxyglucose (FDG) image fusion for optimization of conformal radiotherapy of lung cancers. Int J Radiat Oncol Biol Phys 49(5):1249–1257

Gondi V, Bradley K et al (2007) Impact of hybrid fluorodeoxyglucose positron-emission tomography/computed tomography on radiotherapy planning in esophageal and non-small-cell lung cancer. Int J Radiat Oncol Biol Phys 67(1):187–195

Grills IS, Yan D, Black QC, Wong CY, Martinez AA, Kestin LL (2007) Clinical implications of defining the gross tumor volume with combination of CT and 18FDG-positron emission tomography in non-small-cell lung cancer. Int J Radiat Oncol Biol Phys 67(3):709–719

Guido A, Fuccio L et al (2009) Combined 18F-FDG-PET/CT imaging in radiotherapy target delineation for head-and-neck cancer. Int J Radiat Oncol Biol Phys 73(3):759–63

Hall EJ (2000) Radiobiology for the radiologist, 5th edn. Lippincott Williams and Wilkins, Philadelphia

Hanna GG, McAleese J et al (2009) (18)F-FDG PET-CT simulation for Non-Small-Cell Lung Cancer: Effect in Patients Already Staged by PET-CT. Int J Radiat Oncol Biol Phys

Han D, Yu J et al (2010) Comparison of (18)F-fluorothymidine and (18)F-fluorodeoxyglucose PET/CT in delineating gross tumor volume by optimal threshold in patients with squamous cell carcinoma of thoracic esophagus. Int J Radiat Oncol Biol Phys 76(4):1235–1241

Hebert ME, Lowe VJ et al (1996) Positron emission tomography in the pretreatment evaluation and follow-up of non-small cell lung cancer patients treated with radiotherapy: preliminary findings. Am J Clin Oncol 19(4):416–421

Heron DE, Andrade RS et al (2004) Hybrid PET-CT simulation for radiation treatment planning in head-and-neck cancers: a brief technical report. Int J Radiat Oncol Biol Phys 60(5):1419–1424

Hong TS, Killoran JH et al (2008) Impact of manual and automated interpretation of fused PET/CT data on esophageal target definitions in radiation planning. Int J Radiat Oncol Biol Phys 72(5):1612–1618

Hwang AB, Bacharach SL et al (2009) Can positron emission tomography (PET) or PET/Computed Tomography (CT) acquired in a nontreatment position be accurately registered to a head-and-neck radiotherapy planning CT? Int J Radiat Oncol Biol Phys 73(2):578–584

Igdem S, Alco G et al (2010) The Application of Positron Emission Tomography/Computed Tomography in Radiation Treatment Planning: Effect on Gross Target Volume Definition and Treatment Management. Clin Oncol (R Coll Radiol)

International Commission on Radiation Units and Measurements (1993) Prescribing, recording and reporting Photon Bean Theraphy ICRU Report 50

International Commission on Radiation Units and Measurements (1999) Prescribing, recording and reporting Photon Bean Theraphy ICRU Report 62

Ireland RH, Dyker KE et al (2007) Nonrigid image registration for head and neck cancer radiotherapy treatment planning with PET/CT. Int J Radiat Oncol Biol Phys 68(3):952–957

Ishikita T, Oriuchi N et al (2010) Additional value of integrated PET/CT over PET alone in the initial staging and follow up of head and neck malignancy. Ann Nucl Med 24:77–82

Kalff V, Hicks RJ, Mac Manus MP et al (2001) Clinical impact of (18)F fluorodeoxyglucose positron emission tomography in patients with non-small-cell lung cancer: a prospective study. J Clin Oncol 19(1):111–118

Kiffer JD, Berlangieri SU et al (1998) The contribution of 18F-fluoro-2-deoxy-glucose positron emission tomographic imaging to radiotherapy planning in lung cancer. Lung Cancer 19(3):167–177

Konski A, Doss M et al (2005) The integration of 18-fluoro-deoxy-glucose positron emission tomography and endoscopic ultrasound in the treatment-planning process for esophageal carcinoma. Int J Radiat Oncol Biol Phys 61(4):1123–1128

Krengli M, Milia ME et al (2010) FDG-PET/CT imaging for staging and target volume delineation in conformal radiotherapy of anal carcinoma. Radiat Oncol 5(1):10

Koshy M, Paulino AC et al (2005) F-18 FDG PET-CT fusion in radiotherapy treatment planning for head and neck cancer. Head Neck 27(6):494–502

Kruser TJ, Bradley KA et al (2009) The impact of hybrid PET-CT scan on overall oncologic management, with a focus on radiotherapy planning: a prospective, blinded study. Technol Cancer Res Treat 8(2):149–158

Larson SM, Nehmeh SA, Erdi YE, Humm JL (2005) PET/CT in non-small-cell lung cancer: value of respiratory-gated PET. Chang Gung Med J 28(5):306–314

Lee NY, Mechalakos JG, Nehmeh S et al (2008) Fluorine-18-labeled fluoromisonidazole positron emission and computed tomography-guided intensity-modulated radiotherapy for head and neck cancer: a feasibility study. Int J Radiat Oncol Biol Phys 70(1):2–13

Leong T, Everitt C et al (2006) A prospective study to evaluate the impact of FDG-PET on CT-based radiotherapy treatment planning for oesophageal cancer. Radiother Oncol 78(3):254–261

Mac Manus MP, Hicks RJ, Ball DL et al (2001) F-18 fluorodeoxyglucose positron emission tomography staging in radical radiotherapy candidates with nonsmall cell lung carcinoma: powerful correlation with survival and high impact on treatment. Cancer 92(4):886–895

Mac Manus M, D'Costa I et al (2007) Comparison of CT and positron emission tomography/CT coregistered images in planning radical radiotherapy in patients with non-small-cell lung cancer. Australas Radiol 51(4):386–393

Mah K, Caldwell CB, Ung YC et al (2002) The impact of (18)FDG-PET on target and critical organs in CT-based treatment planning of patients with poorly defined non-small-cell lung carcinoma: a prospective study. Int J Radiat Oncol Biol Phys 52(2):339–350

Matsuo M, Miwa K, Shinoda J et al (2009) Target definition by C11-methionine-PET for the radiotherapy of brain metastases. Int J Radiat Oncol Biol Phys 74(3):714–722

Messa C, Ceresoli GL, Rizzo G et al (2005) Feasibility of [18F]FDG-PET and coregistered CT on clinical target volume definition of advanced non-small cell lung cancer. Q J Nucl Med Mol Imaging 49(3):259–266

Moureau-Zabotto L, Touboul E et al (2005) Impact of CT and 18F-deoxyglucose positron emission tomography image fusion for conformal radiotherapy in esophageal carcinoma. Int J Radiat Oncol Biol Phys 63(2):340–345

Muijs CT, Schreurs LM et al (2009) Consequences of additional use of PET information for target volume delineation and radiotherapy dose distribution for esophageal cancer. Radiother Oncol 93(3):447–453

Murakami R, Uozumi H et al (2007) Impact of FDG-PET/CT imaging on nodal staging for head-and-neck squamous cell carcinoma. Int J Radiat Oncol Biol Phys 68(2):377–382

Munley MT, Marks LB et al (1999) Multimodality nuclear medicine imaging in three-dimensional radiation treatment planning for lung cancer: challenges and prospects. Lung Cancer 23(2):105–114

Newbold KL, Partridge M et al (2008) Evaluation of the role of 18FDG-PET/CT in radiotherapy target definition in patients with head and neck cancer. Acta Oncol 47(7):1229–1236

Nestle U, Kremp S et al (2005) Comparison of different methods for delineation of 18F-FDG PET-positive tissue for target volume definition in radiotherapy of patients with non-Small cell lung cancer. J Nucl Med 46(8):1342–1348

Nestle U, Walter K et al (1999) 18F-deoxyglucose positron emission tomography (FDG-PET) for the planning of radiotherapy in lung cancer: high impact in patients with atelectasis. Int J Radiat Oncol Biol Phys 44(3):593–597

Nishioka T, Shiga T et al (2002) Image fusion between 18FDG-PET and MRI/CT for radiotherapy planning of oropharyngeal and nasopharyngeal carcinomas. Int J Radiat Oncol Biol Phys 53(4):1051–1057

Paulino AC, Koshy M et al (2005) Comparison of CT- and FDG-PET-defined gross tumor volume in intensity-modulated radiotherapy for head-and-neck cancer. Int J Radiat Oncol Biol Phys 61(5):1385–1392

Paulsen F, Scheiderbauer J et al (2006) First experiences of radiation treatment planning with PET/CT. Strahlenther Onkol 182(7):369–375

Paskeviciute B, Bolling T et al (2009) Impact of (18)F-FDG-PET/CT on staging and irradiation of patients with locally advanced rectal cancer. Strahlenther Onkol 185(4):260–265

Patel DA, Chang ST et al (2007) Impact of integrated PET/CT on variability of target volume delineation in rectal cancer. Technol Cancer Res Treat 6(1):31–36

Pehlivan B, Topkan E et al (2009) Comparison of CT and integrated PET-CT based radiation therapy planning in patients with malignant pleural mesothelioma. Radiat Oncol 4:35

Pfannenberg AC, Aschoff P et al (2007) Low dose non-enhanced CT versus standard dose contrast-enhanced CT in combined PET/CT protocols for staging and therapy planning in non-small cell lung cancer. Eur J Nucl Med Mol Imaging 34(1):36–44

Pinkawa M, Eble MJ, Mottaghy FM (2011) PET and PET/CT in radiation treatment planning for prostate cancer. Expert Rev Anticancer Ther 11(7):1033–1039

Rahn AN, Baum RP et al (1998) Value of 18F fluorodeoxy-glucose positron emission tomography in radiotherapy planning of head-neck tumors. Strahlenther Onkol 174(7):358–364

Riegel AC, Berson AM et al (2006) Variability of gross tumor volume delineation in head-and-neck cancer using CT and PET/CT fusion. Int J Radiat Oncol Biol Phys 65(3):726–732

Rothschild S, Studer G et al (2007) PET/CT staging followed by Intensity-Modulated Radiotherapy (IMRT) improves treatment outcome of locally advanced pharyngeal carcinoma: a matched-pair comparison. Radiat Oncol 2:22

Scarfone C, Lavely WC et al (2004) Prospective feasibility trial of radiotherapy target definition for head and neck cancer using 3-dimensional PET and CT imaging. J Nucl Med 45(4):543–552

Schinagl DA, Vogel WV et al (2007) Comparison of five segmentation tools for 18F-fluoro-deoxy-glucose-positron emission tomography-based target volume definition in head and neck cancer. Int J Radiat Oncol Biol Phys 69(4):1282–1289

Schreurs LM, Busz DM et al (2010) Impact of 18-fluorodeoxy-glucose positron emission tomography on computed tomography defined target volumes in radiation treatment planning of esophageal cancer: reduction in geographic misses with equal inter-observer variability*. Dis Esophagus

Schwartz DL, Ford E et al (2005a) FDG-PET/CT imaging for preradiotherapy staging of head-and-neck squamous cell carcinoma. Int J Radiat Oncol Biol Phys 61(1):129–136

Schwartz DL, Ford EC et al (2005b) FDG-PET/CT-guided intensity modulated head and neck radiotherapy: a pilot investigation. Head Neck 27(6):478–487

Schmucking M, Baum RP et al (2003) Molecular whole-body cancer staging using positron emission tomography: consequences for therapeutic management and metabolic radiation treatment planning. Recent Results Cancer Res 162:195–202

Shimizu S, Hosokawa M et al (2009) Can hybrid FDG-PET/CT detect subclinical lymph node metastasis of esophageal cancer appropriately and contribute to radiation treatment planning? A comparison of image-based and pathological findings. Int J Clin Oncol 14(5):421–425

Song Y, Chan M et al (2006) Inter-modality variation in gross tumor volume delineation in 18FDG-PET guided IMRT treatment planning for lung cancer. Conf Proc IEEE Eng Med Biol Soc 1:3803–3806

Soto DE, Kessler ML et al (2008) Correlation between pretreatment FDG-PET biological target volume and anatomical location of failure after radiation therapy for head and neck cancers. Radiother Oncol 89(1):13–18

Steffen IG, Wust P et al (2009) Value of Combined PET/CT for Radiation Planning in CT-Guided Percutaneous Interstitial High-Dose-Rate Single-Fraction Brachytherapy for Colorectal Liver Metastases. Int J Radiat Oncol Biol Phys

Steenbakkers RJ, Duppen JC et al (2006) Reduction of observer variation using matched CT-PET for lung cancer delineation: a three-dimensional analysis. Int J Radiat Oncol Biol Phys 64(2):435–448

Subramaniam RM, Truong M, Peller P, Sakai O, Mercier G (2010) Fluorodeoxyglucose-positron-emission tomography imaging of head and neck squamous cell cancer. Am J Neuroradiol 31(4):598–604

Subedi N, Scarsbrook A, et al (2009) The clinical impact of integrated FDG PET-CT on management decisions in patients with lung cancer. Lung Cancer 64(3):301–307

Stroom J, Blaauwgeers H et al (2007) Feasibility of pathology-correlated lung imaging for accurate target definition of lung tumors. Int J Radiat Oncol Biol Phys 69(1): 267–275

Tonkopi E, Chi PC et al (2010) Average CT in PET studies of colorectal cancer patients with metastasis in the liver and esophageal cancer patients. J Appl Clin Med Phys 11(1):3073

Truong MT, Grillone G, Tschoe C, Chin L, Kachnic LA, Jalisi S (2009) Emerging applications of stereotactic radiotherapy in head and neck cancer. Neurosurg Focus 27(6):E11

van Baardwijk A, Bosmans G et al (2007) PET-CT-based auto-contouring in non-small-cell lung cancer correlates with pathology and reduces interobserver variability in the delineation of the primary tumor and involved nodal volumes. Int J Radiat Oncol Biol Phys 68(3):771–778

van Der Wel A, Nijsten S et al (2005) Increased therapeutic ratio by 18FDG-PET CT planning in patients with clinical CT stage N2–N3M0 non-small-cell lung cancer: a modeling study. Int J Radiat Oncol Biol Phys 61(3):649–655

Vanuytsel LJ, Vansteenkiste JF et al (2000) The impact of (18)F-fluoro-2-deoxy-D-glucose positron emission tomography (FDG-PET) lymph node staging on the radiation treatment volumes in patients with non-small cell lung cancer. Radiother Oncol 55(3):317–324

Vernon MR, Maheshwari M et al (2008) Clinical outcomes of patients receiving integrated PET/CT-guided radiotherapy for head and neck carcinoma. Int J Radiat Oncol Biol Phys 70(3):678–684

Vesprini D, Ung Y et al (2008) Improving observer variability in target delineation for gastro-oesophageal cancer–the role of (18F)fluoro-2-deoxy-D-glucose positron emission tomography/computed tomography. Clin Oncol (R Coll Radiol) 20(8):631–638

Vrieze O, Haustermans K et al (2004) Is there a role for FGD-PET in radiotherapy planning in esophageal carcinoma? Radiother Oncol 73(3):269–275

Wang D, Schultz CJ et al (2006) Initial experience of FDG-PET/CT guided IMRT of head-and-neck carcinoma. Int J Radiat Oncol Biol Phys 65(1):143–151

Wong WL, Hussain K et al (1996) Validation and clinical application of computer-combined computed tomography and positron emission tomography with 2-[18F]fluoro-2-deoxy-D-glucose head and neck images. Am J Surg 172(6):628–632

Wong RJ, Lin DT, Schoder H et al (2002) Diagnostic and prognostic value of [18F]Fluorodeoxyglucose positron emission tomography for recurrent head and neck squamous cell carcinoma. J Clin Oncol 20(20):4199–4208

Wu K, Ung YC et al (2009) PET CT Thresholds for Radiotherapy Target Definition in Non-Small-Cell Lung Cancer: How Close Are We to the Pathologic Findings? Int J Radiat Oncol Biol Phys

Xia P, Anols HI, Ling CC (2004) Three-Dimensional conformal radiotherapy and intensity-modulated radiotherapy. In: Leibel SA, Phillips TL (eds) Textbook of radiation oncology, 2nd edn. Elsevier Inc, Philadelphia

Yu J, Li X, Xing L et al (2009a) Comparison of tumor volumes as determined by pathologic examination and FDG-PET/CT images of non-small-cell lung cancer: a pilot study. Int J Radiat Oncol Biol Phys 75(5):1468–1474

Yu W, Fu XL et al (2009b) GTV spatial conformity between different delineation methods by 18FDG PET/CT and pathology in esophageal cancer. Radiother Oncol 93(3):441–446

Yu HM, Liu YF et al (2009c) Evaluation of gross tumor size using CT, 18F-FDG PET, integrated 18F-FDG PET/CT and pathological analysis in non-small cell lung cancer. Eur J Radiol 72(1):104–113

Zasadny KR, Kison PV et al (1998) FDG-PET Determination of Metabolically Active Tumor Volume and Comparison with CT. Clin Positron Imaging 1(2):123–129

Zheng XK, Chen LH et al (2006) Influence of [18F] fluorodeoxyglucose positron emission tomography on salvage treatment decision making for locally persistent nasopharyngeal carcinoma. Int J Radiat Oncol Biol Phys 65(4):1020–1025

Zhong X, Yu J et al (2009) Using 18F-fluorodeoxyglucose positron emission tomography to estimate the length of gross tumor in patients with squamous cell carcinoma of the esophagus. Int J Radiat Oncol Biol Phys 73(1):136–41

Patients with HIV

Rathan M. Subramaniam, J. M. Davison, D. S. Surasi, T. Jackson, and T. Cooley

Contents

Abstract

This chapter discusses FDG normal variant uptake in HIV patients and the role of FDG PET/CT in malignancies in HIV-infected patients, CNS manifestations of HIV, assessing fever of unknown origin in HIV patients, assessing response to highly active antiretroviral therapy, and assessing complications. FDG PET/CT has proven useful in the diagnosis, staging, and detection of metastasis and post treatment monitoring of several malignancies in HIV-infected patients. It also has the ability to make the important distinction between malignancy and infection in the evaluation of CNS lesions, leading to the initiation of the appropriate treatment and precluding the need for invasive biopsy. However, immunosuppression predisposes patients to a number of opportunistic infections, and therefore special care must be taken interpreting FDG PET/CT in HIV patients

1 Introduction

Globally, approximately 30 million people were living with HIV infection in 2007 (UNAIDS 2008). Over 2.7 million individuals became newly infected with HIV, and approximately 2 million AIDS-related deaths occur annually. In the United States in 2007, an estimated 35,000 individuals were diagnosed with AIDS, with a cumulative estimated number of AIDS diagnoses reaching 1 million (Hall et al. 2008). Almost 75% of the HIV/AIDS diagnoses among adolescents and adults were in men, primarily homosexual, followed by

R. M. Subramaniam (✉)
Russell H Morgan Departments of Radiology and Radiological Sciences Institutions,
The Johns Hopkins Medical Institutions,
601 N. Caroline Street/ JHOC 3235,
Baltimore, MD 21287, USA
e-mail: rsubram4@jhmi.edu

J. M. Davison · D. S. Surasi · T. Jackson
Departments of Radiology, Boston, MA, USA

T. Cooley
Departments of Oncology,
Boston University School of Medicine,
Boston, MA, USA

P. Peller et al. (eds.), *PET-CT and PET-MRI in Oncology*, Medical Radiology. Diagnostic Imaging,
DOI: 10.1007/174_2011_459,

persons infected through high-risk heterosexual contact (Hall et al. 2008). Although African Americans made up only 13% of the population in the 33 surveyed states, they accounted for almost half of the estimated number of HIV/AIDS diagnoses made during 2006 (Hall et al. 2008).

Beginning in the mid-to-late 1990s in the United States, advances in HIV treatments slowed the progression of HIV infection to AIDS and led to dramatic decreases in deaths among persons with AIDS. From 2002 to 2005, the estimated numbers of new AIDS cases and deaths remained stable. More effective treatments have also resulted in an increase in the number of people currently living with AIDS.

2 FDG PET/CT and HIV Pathogenesis

HIV gains entry to its human host by crossing mucosal surfaces (Quinn 1996). The virus then rapidly disseminates throughout lymphoid tissues and is detectable in regional lymph nodes within 2 days of mucosal exposure and in plasma within 4–11 days (Niu et al. 1993). Trapping of HIV-positive effector cells in lymphoid tissues establishes inflammatory conditions and the lymph nodes become reservoirs of viral production and storage throughout the course of the disease (Fox et al. 1991; Pantaleo et al. 1994; Tenner-Racz et al. 1988; Pantaleo et al. 1991). Upon infection with the HIV virus, resting lymphocytes are activated and switch to glycolysis, increasing their glucose uptake by around 20-fold over 24 h (Bental and Deutsch 1993; Marjanovic et al. 1991). This increased cellular glucose utilization by HIV-infected activated lymphocytes in affected nodes can result in increased FDG uptake (Bakheet and Powe 1998; Sugawara et al. 1998) which is quantifiable by FDG PET. Lymph node activation in healthy individuals without intercurrent infections is generally insufficient to generate an FDG signal above background (Brust et al. 2006; Kwan et al. 2001).

3 Normal Variant FDG Uptake in HIV Patients

Whole-body FDG PET images from HIV-positive patients have demonstrated an association between patterns of lymphoid tissue activation and HIV progression (Scharko et al. 2003). In the acute phase of disease, FDG uptake increases in the head and neck (Scharko et al. 2003; Iyengar et al. 2003) (Fig. 1). In mid stages, hypermetabolism in cervical, axillary, and inguinal lymph nodes is observed (Scharko et al. 2003; Iyengar et al. 2003) (Fig. 1). During late-stage disease, significant FDG accumulation in the colon along with mesenteric and ileocecal lymph nodes occurs (Scharko et al. 2003; Iyengar et al. 2003) (Figs. 2, 3). FDG uptake in the bowel and mesenteric lymph nodes, which is observed frequently in HIV-positive patients (Fig. 3), may occur as a consequence of viral replication (Scharko et al. 2003; Iyengar et al. 2003). It is also likely that FDG accumulation in this region may represent physiological glucose uptake due to infection and inflammation rather than a focus of viral replication, as invasion of the bowel by opportunistic pathogens is common in individuals with AIDS. Iyengar et al. examined the relationship between plasma viremia and FDG uptake (Iyengar et al. 2003) and found a tight correlation between net lymphoid FDG uptake and plasma viremia during both recent infection and chronic infection in asymptomatic long-term non-progressors with stable viremia (Iyengar et al. 2003).

Although these general patterns of biodistribution are frequently observed as the disease progresses, there is some disagreement in the literature. For example, Brust et al. observed no difference in FDG biodistribution between early- and late-stage individuals (Brust et al. 2006), but did find a correlation between viral load and whole-body SUV (Brust et al. 2006). Thus, awareness that HIV-positive individuals at various stages have patterns of FDG uptake in several anatomic regions that differ from their HIV-negative counterparts is key. A unique phenomenon also observed in HIV-positive patients is splenic FDG uptake greater than hepatic FDG uptake. This finding is observed most often in the earlier stages of the disease and may indicate a normal variant or lymphomatous involvement of the spleen (Liu 2009).

4 HIV-Related Malignancies

Disorders associated with impaired cellular immunity, such as HIV infection, predispose to the development of neoplasms (Mbulaiteye et al. 2003). In HIV-infected patients, the particular types of neoplasms as well as

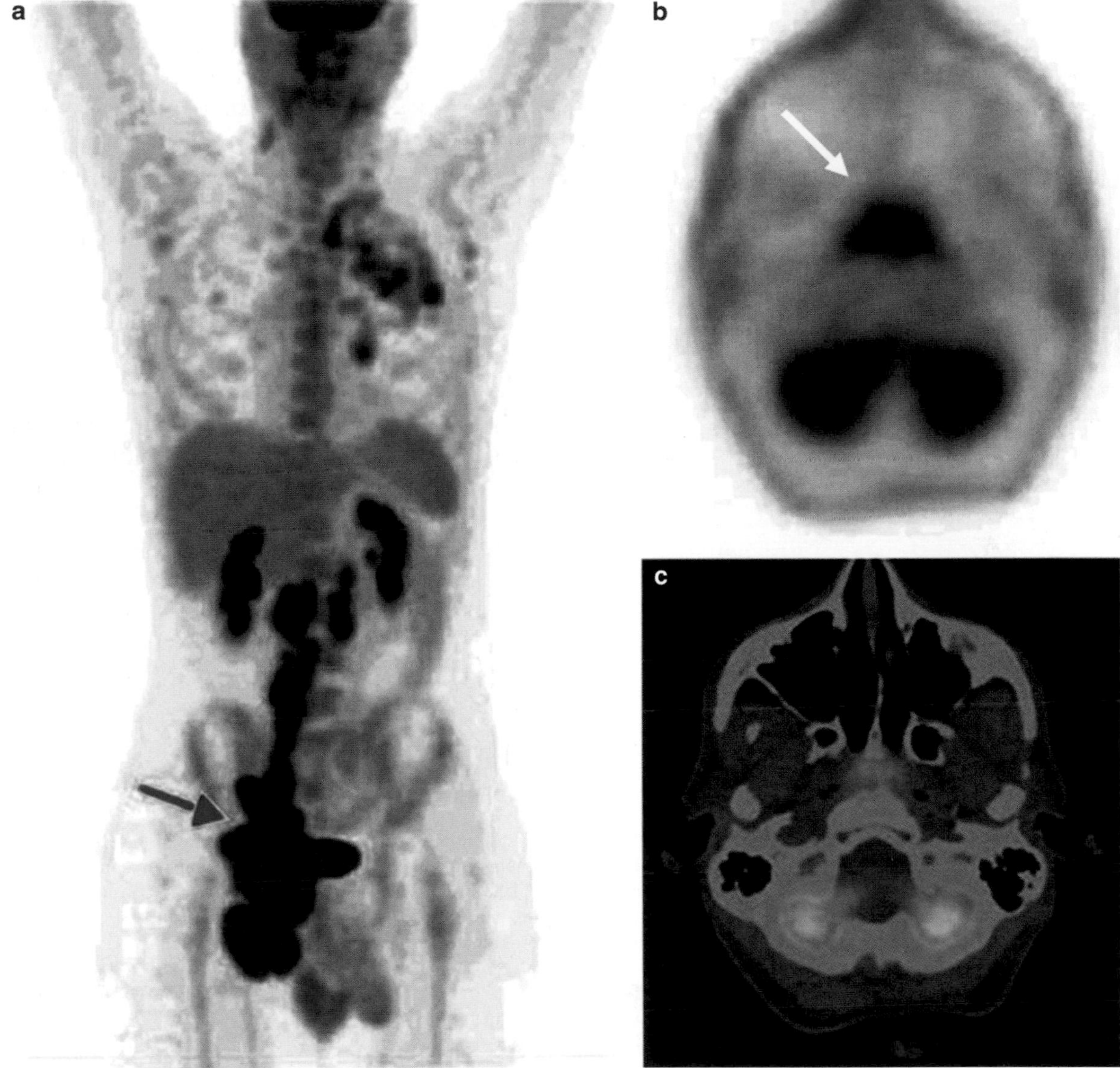

Fig. 1 Variant FDG uptake: a 36-year-old man with history of HIV (CD4 151/viral load 35,000) was referred with a new diagnosis of Hodgkin lymphoma. **a** MIP image demonstrates intense FDG uptake in the (*red arrow*) pelvic and inguinal lymphadenopathy, which was biopsy-proven Hodgkins lymphoma; **b** and **c** axial PET and fused PET/CT demonstrate FDG hypermetabolism in the nasopharynx with an SUV_{max} of 5.9 without a discrete mass. Intense FDG hypermetabolism in the nasopharynx and in the tonsils are common uptake variants in HIV patients

average time for development of these cancers are similar to those observed in solid organ transplant recipients on chronic immunosuppressive therapy as well as in patients with deficiencies of cell-mediated immunity (Euvrard et al. 2003) (Fig. 4). Generally, Kaposi sarcoma will appear within 13–21 months of immune compromise, lymphomas within 32 months, epithelial cancers including skin cancers within 69 months, and anogenital cancers within 84–112 months (Euvrard et al. 2003). In the immunocompromised patient, a common feature of these malignancies is the tendency to occur at a younger age, to involve

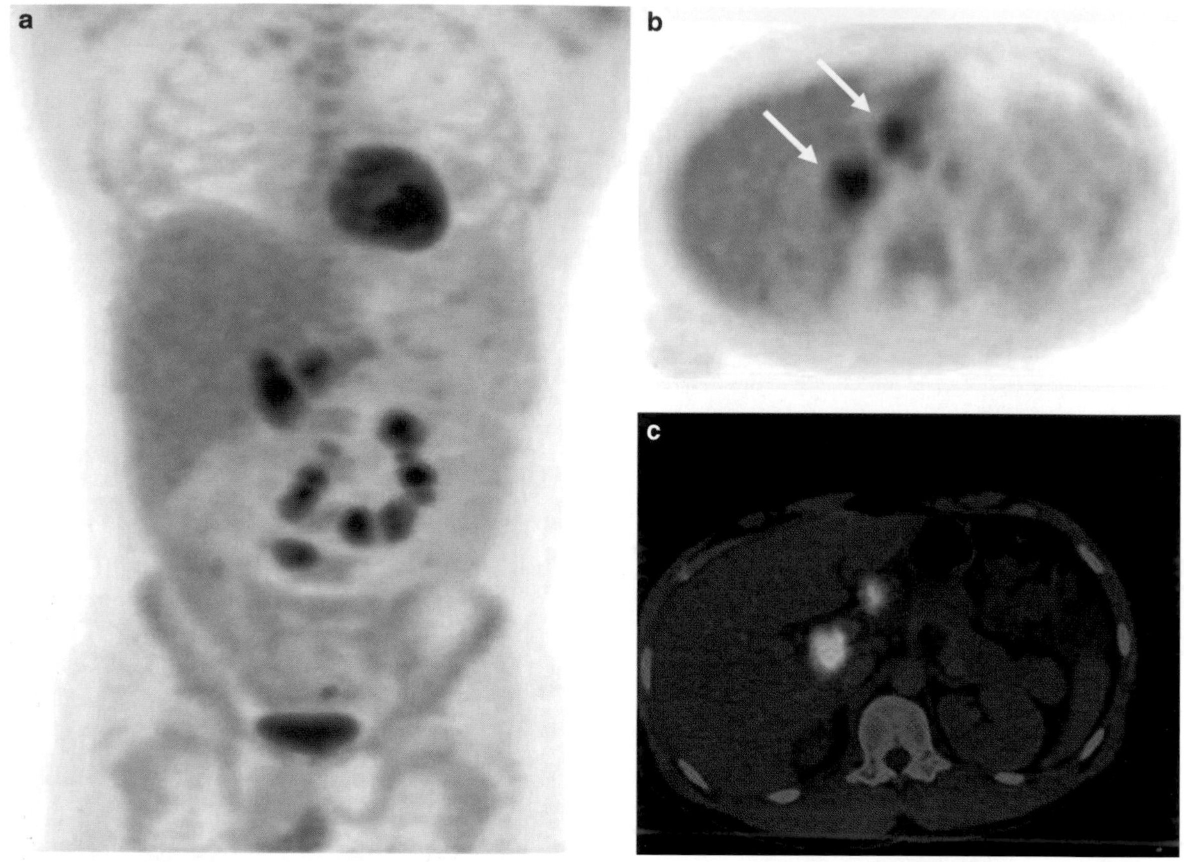

Fig. 2 Variant uptake: a 35-year-old man with AIDS and non-Hodgkin lymphoma underwent two cycles of EPOCH (etoposide, vincristine, adriamycin, cytoxan, and prednisone) before the restaging scan. **a** Restaging PET scan, coronal MIP; **b**, **c** and **d** axial PET. Fused PET/CT demonstrates an interval increase in the size and metabolic activity of the porta hepatic lymph nodes with intense hypermetabolic maximum SUVs of 10.8 and 7.7. The patient underwent EUS and FNA of the peri-hepatic lymph nodes and pathology confirmed non-granulomatous inflammation

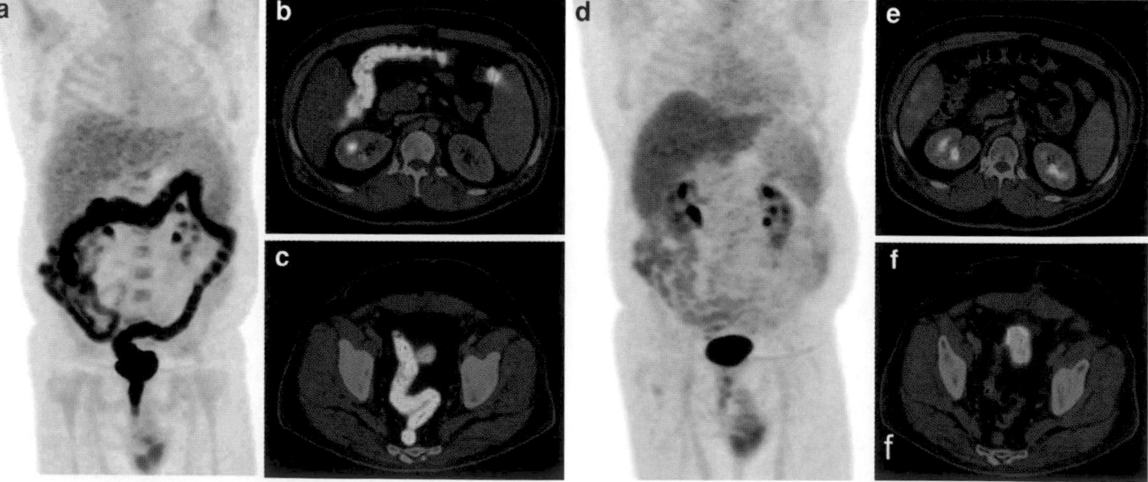

Fig. 3 Variant FDG bowel uptake in an HIV patient: **a** MIP; **b** axial fused PET/CT; **c** axial fused PET/CT of a 42-year-old man with HIV and lymphoma demonstrate increased diffused radio tracer uptake in the colon suggestive of an inflammatory process, likely colitis; **d** MIP; **e** axial fused PET/CT; **f** axial fused PET/CT scan 3 months later demonstrates resolution of hypermetabolic activity within the colon

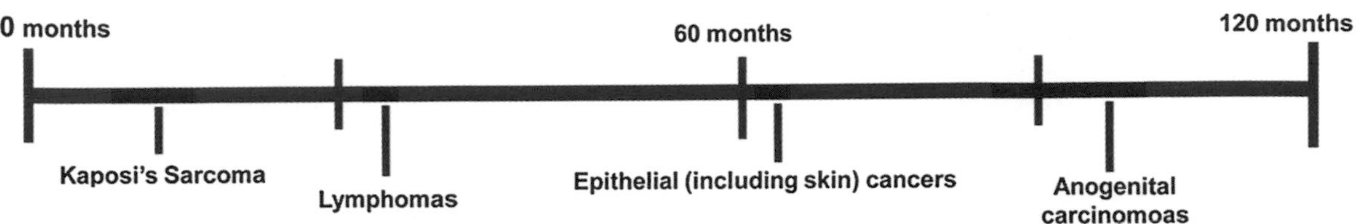

Fig. 4 Average time to development in malignancies with immunosuppression

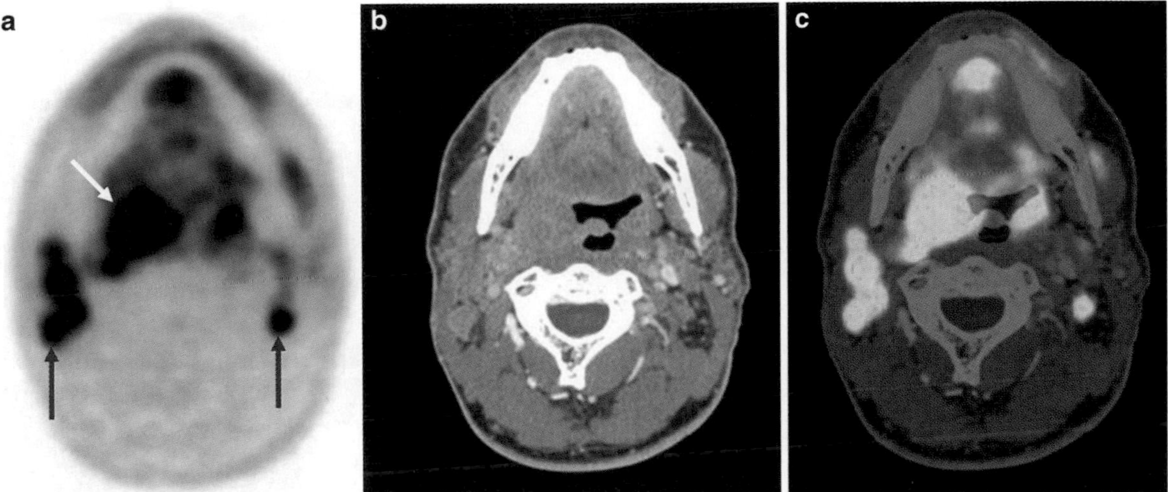

Fig. 5 Squamous cell carcinoma of the right tonsil: **a** Axial PET; **b** axial CT; **c** axial fused PET/CT of a 48-year-old man with AIDS and HPV-related moderately differentiated squamous cell carcinoma of the right tonsil. The lesion SUV_{max} was 14.4, consistent with the patient's known squamous cell carcinoma

unexpected sites, and to follow an aggressive, and often unusual, clinical course when compared to individuals with an intact immune system.

Three cancers are especially prevalent in HIV-positive individuals and are considered AIDS-defining illnesses: Kaposi sarcoma, high-grade B-cell non-Hodgkin lymphoma, and invasive cervical carcinoma (Bower et al. 2006). Most cancers associated with HIV infection are driven by oncogenic viruses such as Epstein-Barr virus (EBV), Kaposi sarcoma-associated herpes virus (KSHV/HHV-8), and human papillomavirus (HPV) (Boshoff and Weiss 2002). However, while these AIDS-defining malignancies are very important in this population, it has become apparent that as patients live significantly longer due to highly active antiretroviral therapy (HAART) they are increasingly more likely to develop non-AIDS-defining cancers (Figs. 5, 6).

4.1 Kaposi Sarcoma

Kaposi sarcoma (KS) is the most common malignancy observed in patients with HIV infection (Frisch et al. 2001; Rabkin and Yellin 1994). Chang et al. first described Kaposi sarcoma-associated herpes virus (KSHV/HHV-8), isolated from cells of an AIDS-KS lesion (Chang et al. 1994) and this virus was subsequently linked to all epidemiological forms of KS (Kedes et al. 1996). KS is characterized by multifocal widespread lesions at the onset of illness followed by rapid progression (Aoki and Tosato 2004). AIDS-KS is more aggressive than non-AIDS-related variants and the lesions often have a different distribution, occupying the nose, mouth, and genitalia (Boshoff and Weiss 2002). Visceral involvement is seen in approximately 50% of AIDS-related KS

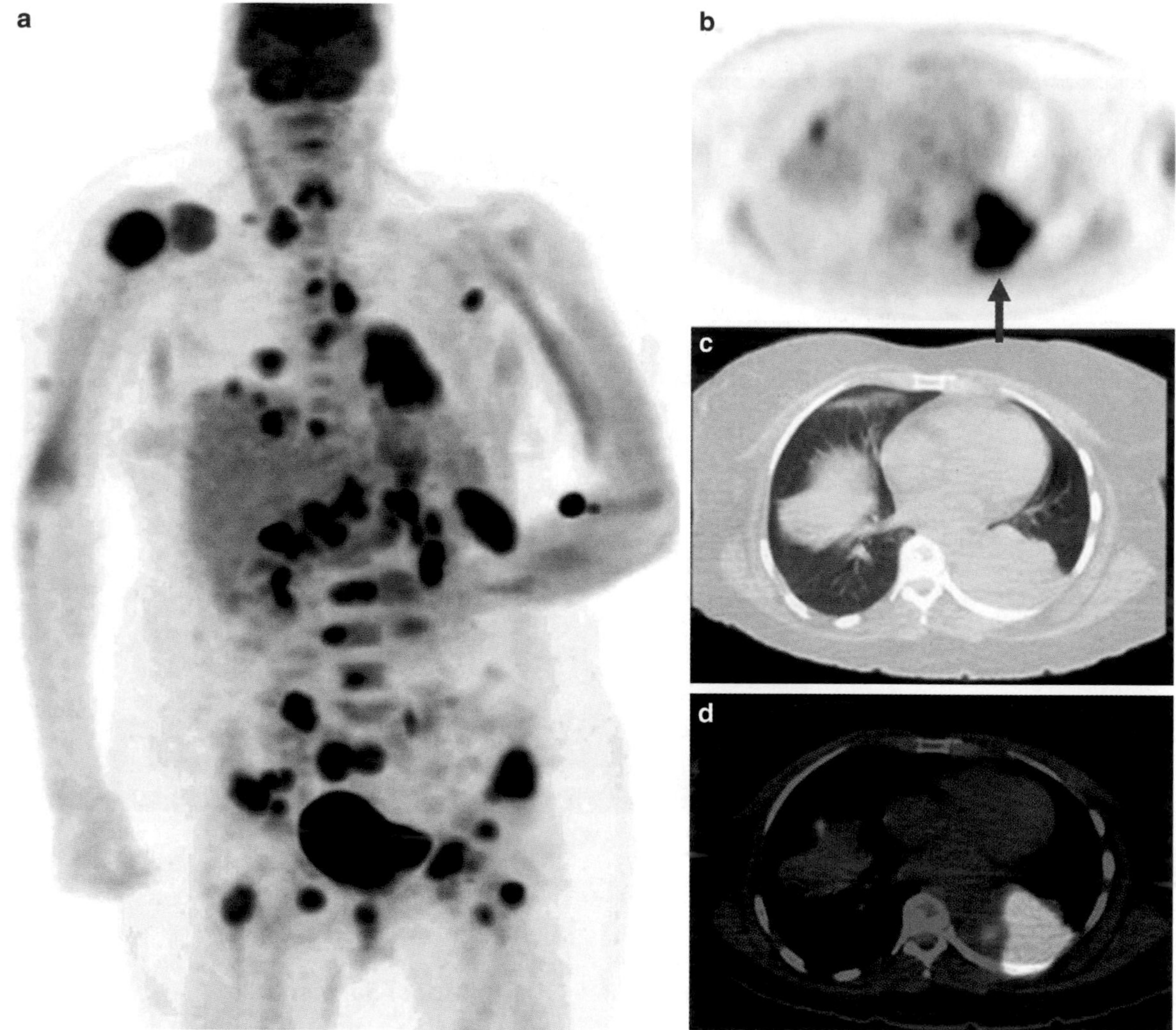

Fig. 6 Squamous cell carcinoma of the lung: **a** MIP; **b** axial PET; **c** axial CT; **d** axial fused PET/CT demonstrating *left lower* lobe mass with an SUV_{max} of 10.2, consistent with squamous cell carcinoma of the lung. **a** Illustrates a diffuse metastatic disease, including adrenal nodal, hepatic nodal, and extensive osseous metastases

patients and is frequently fatal (Aoki and Tosato 2004). The most common site of extra-cutaneous KS is the GI tract (Aoki and Tosato 2004). Pulmonary lesions generally occur at later stages of AIDS-KS and have a poor prognosis (Nasti et al. 2003). The AIDS Clinical Trials Group (ACTG) staging system for AIDS-KS has been used to provide accurate prognostic information on which therapeutic decisions are based (Nasti et al. 2003). This system classifies patients into good- or poor-risk groups based on tumor extent (T), immune system status (I), as measured by CD4 T-lymphocyte count, and evidence for HIV-associated systemic illness (S) (Krown et al. 1989).

Poor-risk tumor extension (T_1) is associated with significantly worse survival and accurate assessment of tumor extent is essential in treatment planning (Krown et al. 1989; Nasti and Tirelli 2005). The role of FDG PET in this evaluation remains to be elucidated (Castaigne et al. 2009; O'Doherty et al. 1997). O'Doherty et al. observed low FDG uptake in two patients with Kaposi sarcoma of the lung and moderate uptake in one (O'Doherty et al. 1997). None of the skin lesions could be visualized with FDG PET (O'Doherty et al. 1997).

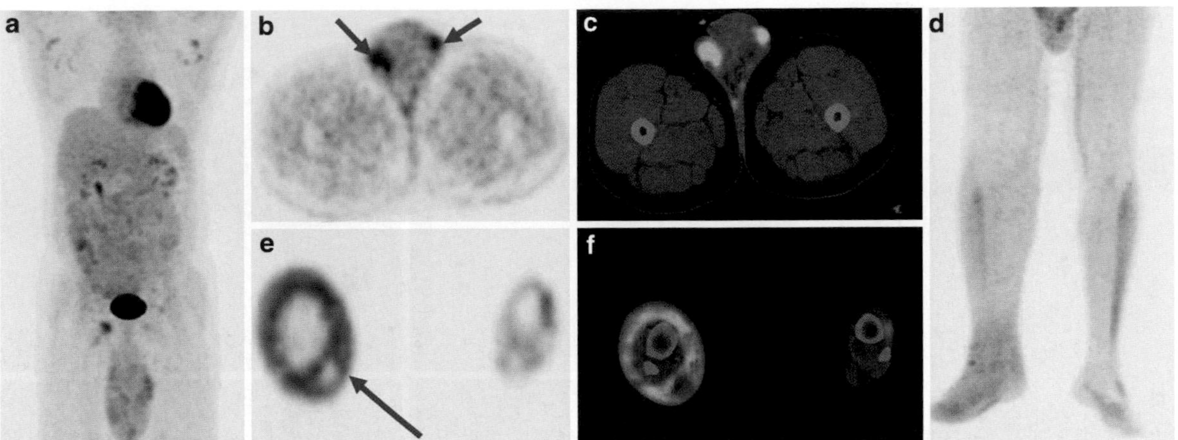

Fig. 7 Kaposi sarcoma: **a** MIP; **b** axial PET; **c** axial fused PET/CT; **d** MIP; **e** axial PET; **f** axial fused PET/CT in a 51-year-old man with Kaposi sarcoma demonstrating mild metabolic activity in the cervical, axillary, mesenteric, and inguinal lymph nodes, likely caused by an inflammatory process due to viral replication. **c**, **f** Multiple nodular lesions found in the scrotum with SUV_{max} ranging from 2.5 to 4.3. Right inguinal node SUV_{max} was 4.6. **d**, **e**, **f** An area of focal hypermetabolism seen in the *right lower* extremity at the level of the foot and ankle with an SUV_{max} of 3.4 and with significant circumferential soft tissue thickening with effacement of subcutaneous fat

In contrast, in a recent retrospective study, FDG PET/CT was useful in distinguishing KS as a malignant lesion and correctly localized the appropriate site for biopsy (Castaigne et al. 2009). With cutaneous Kaposi sarcoma, FDG PET/CT may be an effective modality for localizing and characterizing malignant skin lesions as well as regional nodal involvement (Fig. 7).

In addition to Kaposi sarcoma, KSHV/HHV8 infection is associated with the plasma cell variant of multicentric Castleman disease (MCD), a rare lymphoproliferative disorder. In HIV-infected patients, MCD is highly aggressive and often lethal (Oksenhendler et al. 1996; Dupin et al. 2000). Patients present with non-specific symptoms similar to those observed with opportunistic infections and lymphoma including fevers, anemia, and multifocal lymphadenopathy (Oksenhendler et al. 1996, 2002). The traditional imaging modality for evaluating both HIV-positive and-negative patients with MCD is CT scanning (Hillier et al. 2004). Positive nodes are identified based on size, shape, and enhancement pattern (Hillier et al. 2004). Diagnosis with CT is limited as involvement of normal sized lymph nodes will not be detected and reactive hyperplasia cannot be differentiated from pathological enlargement (Hillier et al. 2004).

Recently, Barker et al. evaluated the efficacy of FDG PET/CT in the diagnosis and monitoring of MCD activity (Barker et al. 2009). Nine patients with histologically confirmed MCD underwent fused FDG PET/CT scans at initial diagnosis, after relapse, or during remission (Barker et al. 2009). FDG PET/CT was able to detect abnormal uptake in lymph nodes more frequently than CT alone detected enlargement (Barker et al. 2009). Scanning with FDG PET/CT may therefore be useful in correctly identifying appropriate sites for biopsy, staging, and monitoring lymphoproliferation due to HIV-associated MCD.

4.2 Human Papillomavirus-Related Malignancies

Human papillomavirus (HPV)-related cancers are frequently encountered in HIV-positive patients. HIV-infected women have an increased risk of developing HPV-associated cervical cancer and both men and women have an increased risk of anal cancer due to HPV (Frisch et al. 2000). FDG PET has been increasingly used in the staging and evaluation of pelvic malignancies, including anal, cervical, ovarian, endometrial, and vaginal carcinoma (Subhas et al. 2005) (Figs. 8, 9). In cervical cancer, FDG PET has been shown to be effective in initial staging, detection of early recurrence, and predicting prognosis (Grigsby et al. 2004; Wong et al. 2004). However, there have

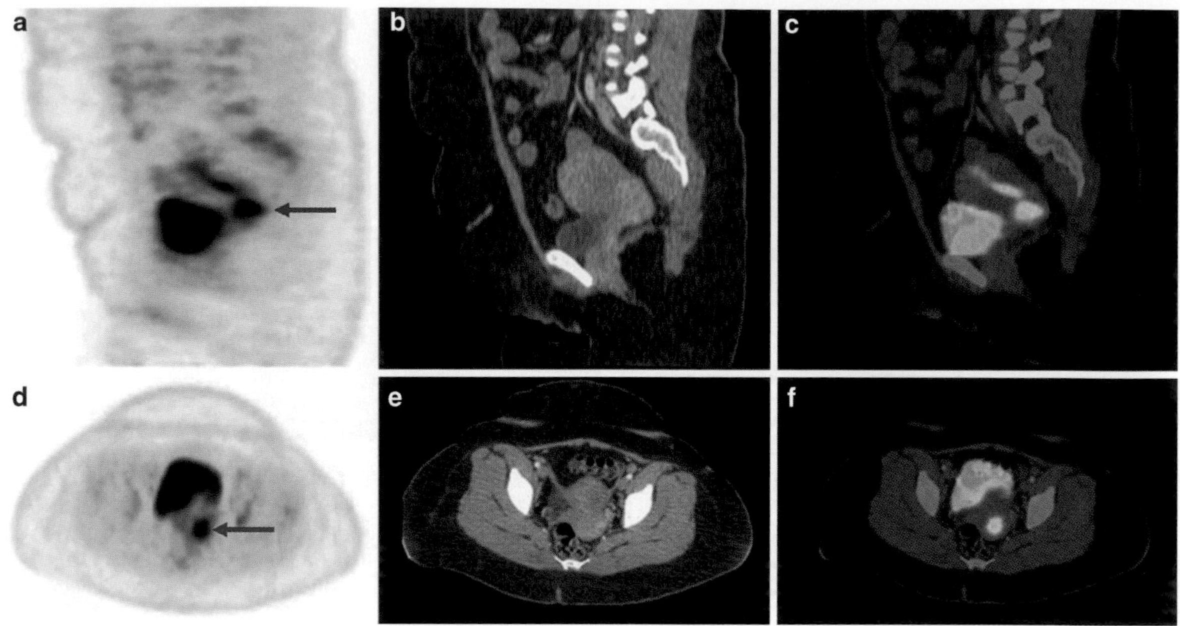

Fig. 8 Cancer of the cervix: **a** Sagittal PET; **b** sagittal CT; **c** sagittal fused PET/CT; **d** axial PET; **e** axial CT; **f** axial fused PET/CT of a 31-year-old woman with AIDS and squamous cell carcinoma of the cervix demonstrating an intense hypermetabolic uptake in the cervix with an SUV_{max} of 8.3

been no studies specifically evaluating the role of FDG PET in managing HIV-positive individuals with cervical cancer. Further analysis of this subgroup of patients is needed as pelvic and extra-pelvic reactive FDG uptake as HIV infection can complicate the evaluation.

One study, which examined the role of FDG PET/CT in the diagnosis and monitoring of patients with anal carcinoma, included a separate evaluation of HIV-positive patients (Hillier et al. 2004). Using FDG PET/CT, 41 patients with anal cancer were assessed, nine of which were HIV-positive (Cotter et al. 2006). In both HIV-negative and HIV-positive individuals FDG PET/CT identified 91% of tumors while CT alone identified only 59% (Cotter et al. 2006). FDG PET/CT also identified significantly more abnormal inguinal lymph nodes than either CT or physical examination (Cotter et al. 2006).

4.3 Lymphoma

As in other immunosuppressive disorders, lymphomas, mainly non-Hodgkin lymphomas (NHL), develop in HIV-infected patients with high frequency (DeMario and Liebowitz 1998; Gallagher et al. 2001). More than 50% of AIDS-related lymphomas are associated with EBV and/or KSHV infection (Boshoff and Weiss 2002). Patients with systemic AIDS-related NHL generally present with advanced-stage disease with an aggressive clinical course (Bower et al. 2006; Boshoff and Weiss 2002). The majority have one of three high-grade B-cell lymphoma histologies: Burkitt lymphoma, diffuse large B-cell lymphoma (DLBCL) with centroblastic features, and DLBCL with immunoblastic features (Aoki and Tosato 2004). Less common types of lymphoma include primary central nervous system lymphoma, primary effusion lymphoma, and plasmablastic lymphoma (Aoki and Tosato 2004; Villringer et al. 1995; Carbone and Gloghini 2005). FDG PET/CT is useful in staging, restaging, and surveillance of HIV-related NHL of various histological subtypes (Figs. 10, 11, 12, 13, 14 and 15). Although it is not considered an AIDS-defining illness, the incidence of Hodgkin lymphoma (HL) is also increased in those infected with HIV (Frisch et al. 2001). AIDS-HL is usually of an aggressive histological subtype, like NHL has a higher incidence of extra-nodal involvement, and is associated with EBV (Boshoff and Weiss 2002).

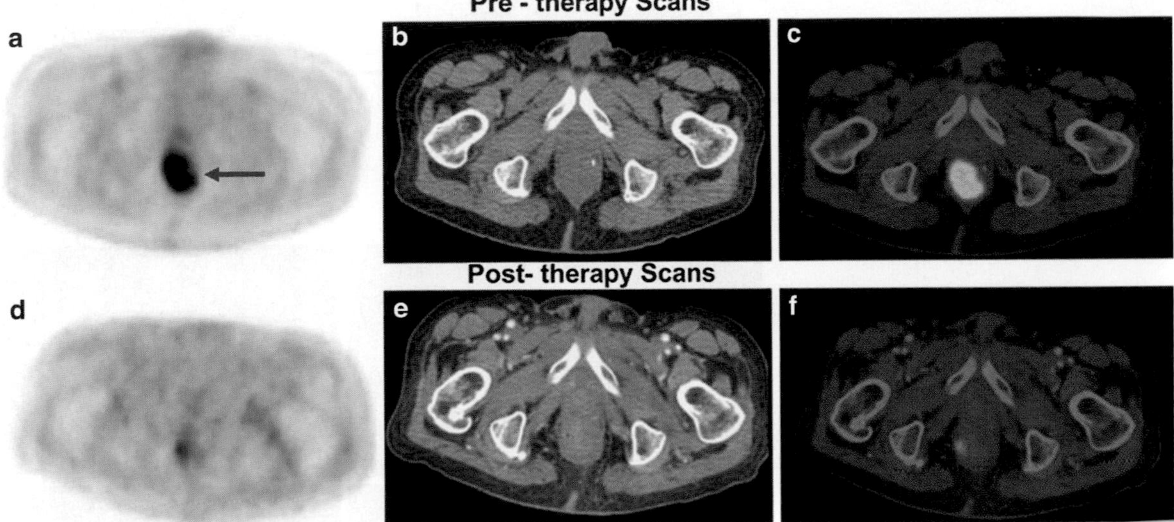

Fig. 9 Adenocarcinoma of the anus and rectum: **a** Axial PET; **b** axial CT; **c** fused PET/CT of a 58-year-old man with AIDS and a hypermetabolic lesion in the *right lateral* aspect of the anus with an SUV_{max} of 10.3; **d** axial PET; **e** axial CT; **f** axial fused PET/CT: Post-therapy scans of a patient treated with chemo radiation (5 Fluorouracil and 50 Gy radiation). Post-treatment scan demonstrates significant improvement of the lesion, with an SUV_{max} of 4.8

One of the most common AIDS-related lymphomas, Burkitt lymphoma, is an aggressive disease best treated with short duration, high-intensity chemotherapy regimens (Blum et al. 2004). Failure to achieve complete remission is a poor prognostic sign associated with relapse and death (Blum et al. 2004). Accordingly, accurate staging and close follow-up is essential in AIDS-related Burkitt lymphoma (Blum et al. 2004). FDG PET/CT has emerged as one of the main imaging modalities for staging, restaging, predicting prognosis, and therapeutic surveillance for patients with Burkitt lymphoma, largely replacing CT or Gallium-67 scans as the modalities of choice (Blum et al. 2004; Jhanwar and Straus 2006). Burkitt lymphoma is an intensely glucose-avid tumor, exhibiting very high FDG uptake and SUVs measured on PET scan (Blum et al. 2004). In the initial staging of AIDS-related Burkitt lymphoma, FDG PET/CT can provide an accurate map of suspected disease and identify unsuspected sites of disease (Just et al. 2008). The high SUVs of lymph nodes involved by Burkitt lymphoma enable differentiation between FDG uptake associated with persistent generalized lymphadenopathy (PGL) (Just et al. 2008). Just et al. also found that a negative FDG PET/CT in HIV-positive patients with Burkitt lymphoma was always associated with a favorable outcome (Just et al. 2008).

5 Central Nervous System HIV Considerations

Neurological complications occur frequently in HIV-positive patients due to opportunistic infection, malignancy, or cytopathic effects of the HIV virus itself (Manzardo et al. 2005). As many as 10% of all AIDS patients initially present with neurologic symptoms and between 40 and 60% will eventually develop CNS complications during the course of their disease (Elder and Sever 1988; Levy et al. 1989). The degree of immunosuppression is the most important factor in establishing a differential diagnosis. Cognitive and motor disorders due to the virus itself are common in patients with CD4 cell counts ranging from 200 to 500/mm^3 (normal 800–1,050/mm^3) and will generally present without focal lesions. Neurologic manifestations due to mass lesions are most common in severely immunosuppressed patients with CD4 cell counts $<200/mm^3$ and are usually a result of opportunistic infections or AIDS-associated tumors such as primary central nervous system lymphoma. The most common cause of neurologic symptoms in AIDS patients is toxoplasmosis (Levy et al. 1989). However, neurosyphilis, cytomegalovirus encephalitis, tuberculosis, cryptococcosis, progressive multifocal leukoencephalopathy (PML), and primary

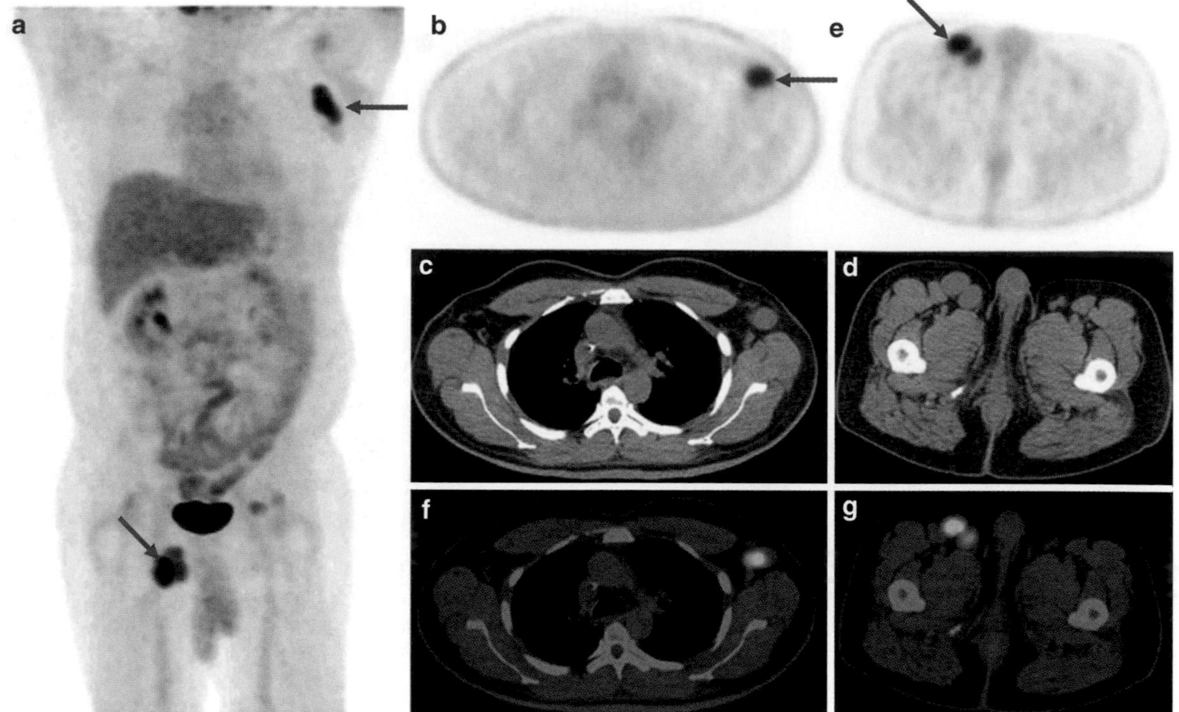

Fig. 10 T-cell lymphoma: **a** MIP; **b** axial PET; **c** axial PET; **d** axial fused PET/CT; **e** axial fused PET/CT; **f** axial PET; **g** axial fused PET/CT of a 58-year-old man with HIV-associated peripheral T-cell lymphoma demonstrate hypermetabolism in the *left axillary* and *right inguinal* areas compatible with malignant lymphoma. *Left axillary* lymph node with an SUV_{max} of 6.5 and right inguinal lymphadenopathy with an SUV_{max} of 7.2, consistent with known malignancy

central nervous system lymphoma are also important causes of neurological dysfunction and should be included in the differential diagnosis (Elder and Sever 1988; Levy et al. 1989).

The evaluation and management of HIV-positive patients presenting with neurologic findings is challenging as the symptoms at initial presentation such as fever, headache, altered mental status, and focal neurologic signs or seizures are not specific. In addition, conventional imaging techniques such as CT or MRI are often not useful in determining the etiologies of mass lesions. For example, both PCL and toxoplasmosis produce similar focal or multifocal ring enhancing lesions with CT and MRI (Offiah and Turnbull 2006). Furthermore, while lesions due to PML do not usually produce edema and are not contrast enhancing, PML occurring in the setting of an immune reconstitution inflammatory syndrome (IRIS) can produce focal edema and a mass effect with contrast enhancement on MRI, resulting in a similar appearance to toxoplasmosis and primary CNS lymphoma. Definitive diagnosis for CNS lesions requires a brain biopsy, an invasive procedure that most physicians avoid when possible in HIV-infected patients (Hoffman et al. 1993). However, establishing the correct diagnosis is essential in directing treatment (Heald et al. 1996). Commonly, antibiotic treatment for toxoplasmosis is administered and confirmation of the diagnosis is made through observation of clinical course after 3–4 weeks (Villringer et al. 1995).

Several studies have evaluated the role of FDG PET in the diagnosis of CNS complications in patients with AIDS, with particular attention paid to the differentiation between toxoplasmosis and lymphoma (Fig. 16). Hoffman et al. performed both a visual and semi-quantitative evaluation of CNS lesions using FDG PET (Hoffman et al. 1993). In every case of lymphoma, FDG uptake was significantly higher than that of nonmalignant lesions (Hoffman et al. 1993). In a similar study, Villringer et al. assessed the ability of FDG PET to differentiate between toxoplasmosis and lymphoma (Villringer et al. 1995). Eleven AIDS patients with CNS lesions

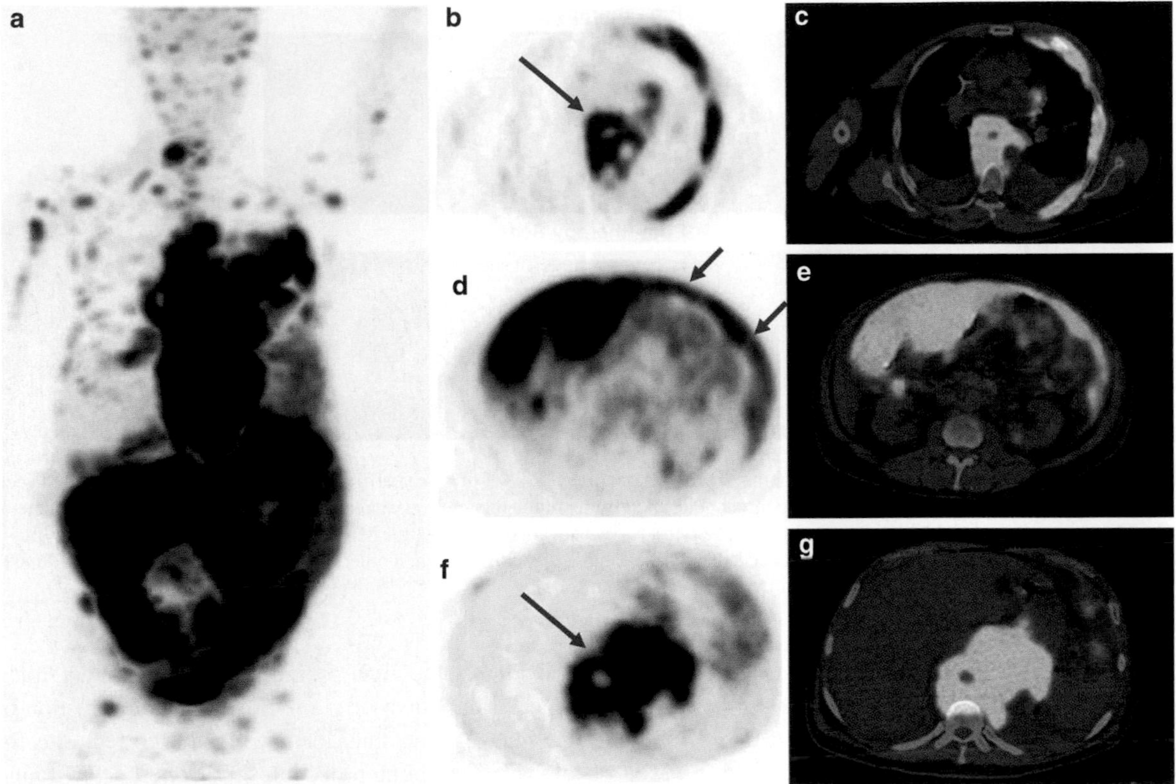

Fig. 11 Burkitt lymphoma: **a** MIP; **b** axial PET; **c** axial fused PET/CT; **d** axial PET of a 50-year-old man with AIDS and Burkitt lymphoma demonstrating a large hypermetabolic retroperitoneal lesion extending from the subcarinal region to the level of the renal arteries. **e** Axial fused PET/CT; **f** axial PET; **g** axial fused PET/CT demonstrating hypermetabolism in the *left pleura* and *left anterior* fourth rib

were examined and the lesion maximum SUVs (SUV_{max}) were compared with that of a contralateral brain area in order to control for differential FDG uptake between lesions in white matter and those in gray matter (Villringer et al. 1995). In all subjects with infections, the SUV_{max} ratio of lesion to contralateral area was significantly lower than the SUV_{max} ratio in patients with lymphoma (Villringer et al. 1995). This study was limited however by the fact that the patients with toxoplasmosis were all being treated at the time of initial PET scan (Villringer et al. 1995). The maximum SUVs of untreated toxoplasmosis lesions may actually be greater. In a prospective study, Heald et al. analyzed FDG PET scans of 18 HIV-positive patients with focal CNS lesions on CT or MRI (Heald et al. 1996). Three groups were compared: patients with infectious lesions, those with biopsy-proven primary CNS lymphoma, and those with presumed primary CNS lymphoma. Lymphoma had a significantly higher FDG uptake than infectious processes in all but two of the 18 cases examined (Heald et al. 1996). High FDG uptake was also observed in two cases of PML and these lesions could not be differentiated from lymphoma (Heald et al. 1996). Consistent with these findings, O'Doherty et al. measured maximum SUVs ranging between 0.14 and 3.7 over cerebral lesions due to toxoplasmosis (O'Doherty et al. 1997), significantly lower than the SUV_{max} of lymphomas which had values between 3.9 and 8.7 (O'Doherty et al. 1997). FDG PET thus has promise as a reliable, non-invasive method of differentiating between primary CNS lymphoma infections. A low SUV_{max} of the lesion adds confidence to a working diagnosis of toxoplasmosis when treated empirically and may avoid a brain biopsy. However definitive diagnosis can only be made by tissue diagnosis.

In some patients a progressive loss of cognitive function accompanied by motor decline will develop due to a condition known as AIDS Dementia Complex

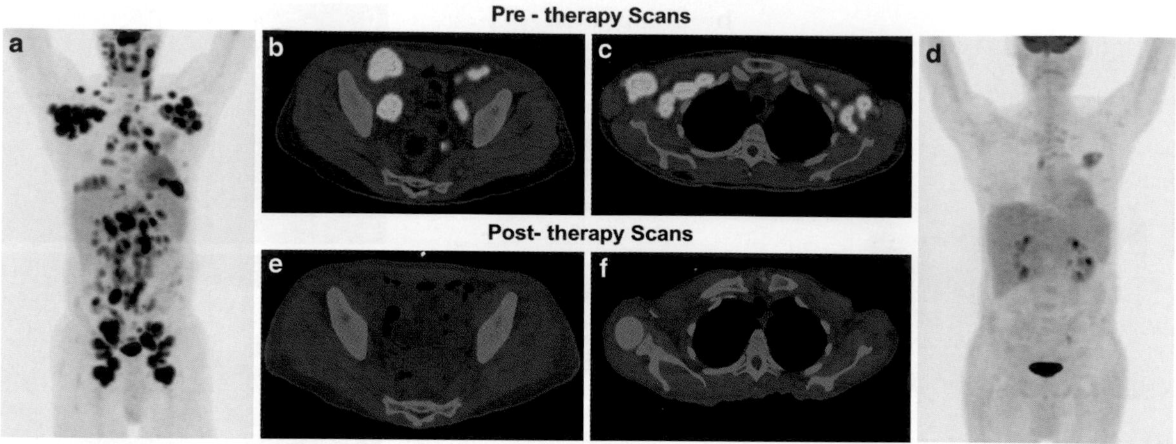

Fig. 12 Therapy assessment of B-cell lymphoma: **a** MIP; **b** axial fused PET/CT of a 54-year-old man with AIDS and diffuse large B-cell lymphoma demonstrating diffuse massive hypermetabolic adenopathy of the bilateral cervical chains, axilla, mediastinum, and bilateral hila. The internal iliac nodule demonstrates hypermetabolic activity with an SUV_{max} of 11. **c** MIP; **d** axial fused PET/CT demonstrating a significant decrease in metabolic activity consistent with a complete response to chemotherapy agents allopurinol and R-EPOCH (Rituximab, etoposide, vincristine, adriamycin, cytoxan, and prednisone)

(ADC) or HIV-Associated Dementia (HAD) (Navia et al. 1986). While ADC generally develops in late-stage AIDS, evidence suggests that a less profound CNS disorder labeled Minor Cognitive Motor Dysfunction (MCMD) may occur even in the systemically asymptomatic stages of infection (Heaton et al. 1995). In HIV-positive patients with subclinical neurologic dysfunction, FDG PET has demonstrated relative hypermetabolism in the basal ganglia, especially in the striatum (Heaton et al. 1995; Rottenberg et al. 1996; von Giesen et al. 2000) followed by late cortical and subcortical hypometabolism or globally reduced cortical FDG uptake (O'Doherty et al. 1997; Rottenberg et al. 1987). Pascal et al. found prominent asymmetries in FDG uptake of the frontal regions in asymptomatic HIV-positive patients, while MRI showed no abnormalities (Pascal et al. 1991). The ability of FDG PET imaging to quantify regional differences in cerebral glucose metabolism may provide a better understanding of the neuroanatomy and activation patterns involved in ADC and MCMD.

6 Fever of Unknown Origin

Immunosuppression due to HIV infection results in a variety of opportunistic infections or tumors, often leading to fever without an obvious cause (Castaigne et al. 2009; O'Doherty et al. 1997). The use of imaging can reduce the time to initiation of treatment for a fever of unknown origin by localizing an infection or malignancy and thus identifying the correct site for biopsy or sampling procedures. O'Doherty et al. found that FDG PET had an overall sensitivity of 92% and specificity of 94% in detecting the cause of unexplained fever, weight loss, or confusion in HIV-positive patients (O'Doherty et al. 1997). FDG PET proved useful in detecting both malignancies and infections (Fig. 17) in HIV-positive patients (O'Doherty et al. 1997). In fact, soft tissue pulmonary infections were observed by FDG PET even before the development of chest radiograph abnormalities (O'Doherty et al. 1997). Castaigne et al. had similar results with FDG PET/CT in successfully diagnosing HIV-related fever of unknown origin (Castaigne et al. 2009).

7 Highly Active Antiretroviral Therapy (HAART)

Treatment with highly active antiretroviral therapy (HAART) has dramatically reduced HIV-associated morbidity and mortality. The ability of HAART to markedly reduce viral load has implications for the evaluation of HIV-positive patients with FDG PET (Brust et al. 2006; Lucignani et al. 2009). Brust et al. demonstrated that, while HAART-na viremic individuals

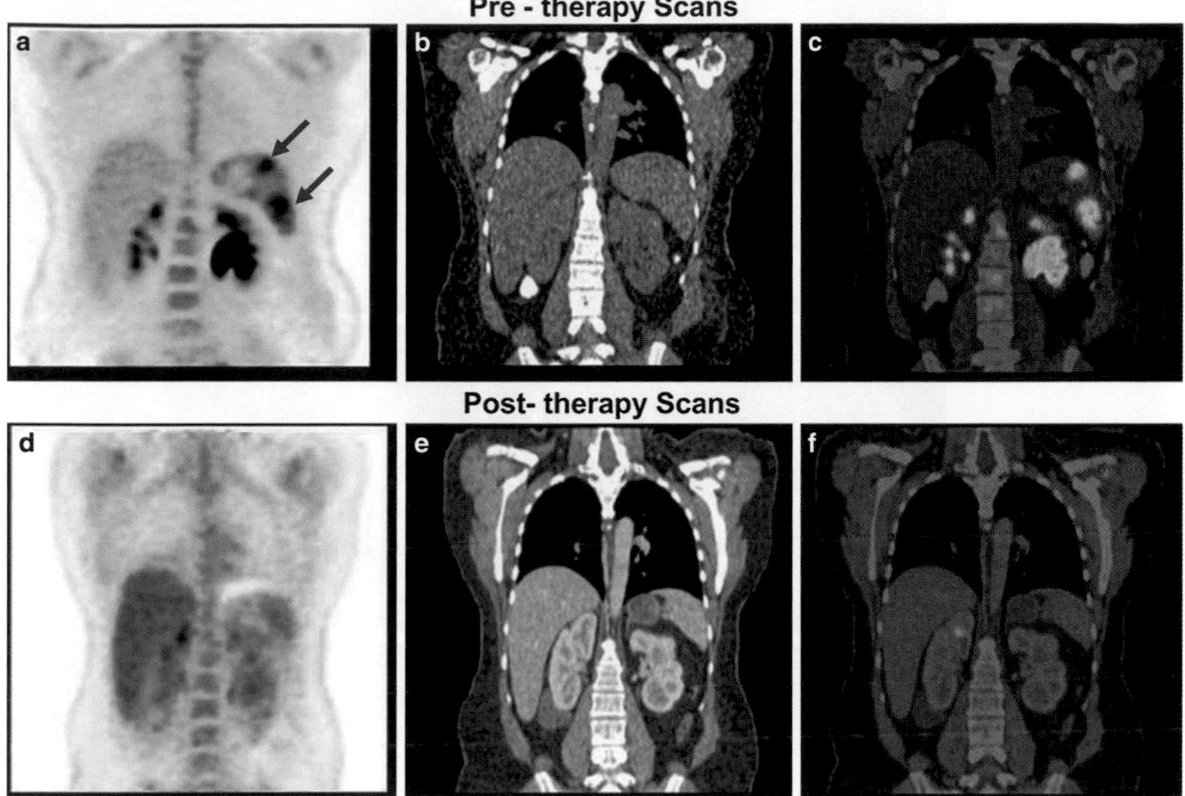

Fig. 13 Therapy assessment of Hodgkin lymphoma: **a** Coronal PET; **b** coronal CT; **c** coronal fused PET/CT, of a 44-year-old woman with HIV and Hodgkin Lymphoma demonstrating multiple abnormal areas of FDG uptake within the spleen prior to chemotherapy. After three cycles of ABVD given with Neulasta, the restaging scans; **d** coronal PET; **e** coronal CT; **f** coronal fused PET/CT demonstrate a complete metabolic response within the spleen with no evidence of abnormal radiotracer activity

with early or advanced HIV had increased FDG uptake in peripheral nodes, patients on HAART demonstrated no significant nodal FDG uptake (Brust et al. 2006). Subsequent interruption of HAART resulted in the appearance of FDG uptake in previously quiescent lymph nodes (Brust et al. 2006).

Current methods used to stage HIV infection and assess response to HAART are based on measurements of variables in the plasma, which may not accurately represent the true level of immune activation and HIV replication in the lymph nodes and other lymphoid tissues. Evaluation of residual immune activation and viral replication in both lymphatic and non-lymphatic organs might allow more accurate staging of HIV infection, and make it possible to design therapeutic approaches based not only immunological variables in the plasma, but also on the state of the immune system target organs of HIV (Lucignani et al. 2009). Lucignani et al. evaluated whether FDG PET could detect specific locations of viral replication in HIV-infected patients, even after an apparent response to HAART (Lucignani et al. 2009). In concordance with Iyengar et al. (Iyengar et al. 2003), they found a significant correlation between plasma viremia and FDG uptake in HAART-na patients (Lucignani et al. 2009). However, in those undergoing treatment with HAART, FDG uptake and plasma viral load were unrelated (Lucignani et al. 2009). FDG PET may be useful in evaluating effectiveness of HAART in suppressing HIV replication in extra-plasmic compartments (Lucignani et al. 2009). Glucose uptake by activated lymphocytes as detected by FDG PET may also be indicative of the efficacy of immune reconstitution by HAART. In HIV-positive patients on HAART, an increase in thymus volume correlates with increased numbers of circulating CD4+ T cells (Rubio et al. 2002). Hardy et al.

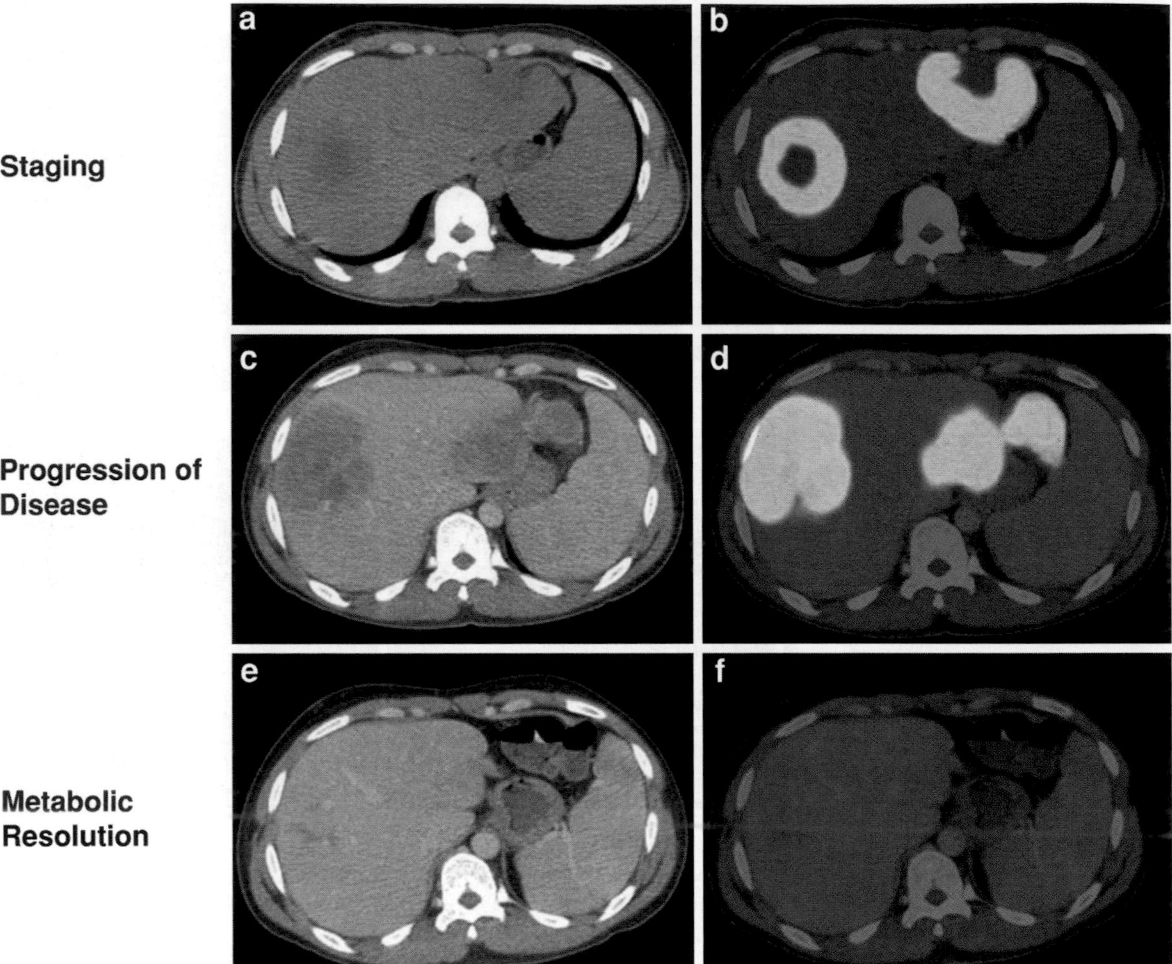

Fig. 14 Stage IV large-cell lymphoma progression: **a** Axial CT; **b** axial fused PET/CT of a 34-year-old man with AIDS and stage IV large-cell lymphoma demonstrating multiple hepatic lesions consistent with biopsy-proven lymphoma. **c** Axial CT; **d** fused PET/CT demonstrates marked progression of the hepatic FDG metabolic uptake consistent with disease progression. **e** Axial CT; **f** fused PET/CT demonstrates significant improvement in the hepatic lesions and interval progression of abdominal and mesenteric lymphadenopathy after a change in chemotherapy instituted after earlier progression

demonstrated increased FDG uptake in the thymus of HIV-positive patients undergoing treatment with HAART, representing thymic reconstitution and possibly correlating with increased numbers of immature T cells in the periphery (Hardy et al. 2004).

While the majority of HIV-positive patients will improve clinically with HAART, a subset of patients will develop a condition known as immune reconstitution inflammatory syndrome (IRIS). Individuals with IRIS demonstrate clinical deterioration with the development of symptoms of opportunistic infections such as tuberculosis, HSV, toxoplasmosis, or bacterial pneumonia (French 2009). This phenomenon is thought to result from the restored ability of the immune system to mount an inflammatory response upon initiation of HAART (French 2009). The response is exaggerated in these patients due to lack of homeostatic regulation (Meintjes and Lynen 2008). IRIS must be considered when evaluating patients with FDG PET/CT undergoing HAART as new, enlarging lymph nodes and multiple inflammatory foci can lead to increased FDG uptake that may be confused with malignancy.

In patients on HAART, an important side effect is lipodystrophy, characterized by peripheral fat wasting and central adiposity, along with metabolic changes such as hyperlipidemia, hyperglycemia, and insulin resistance

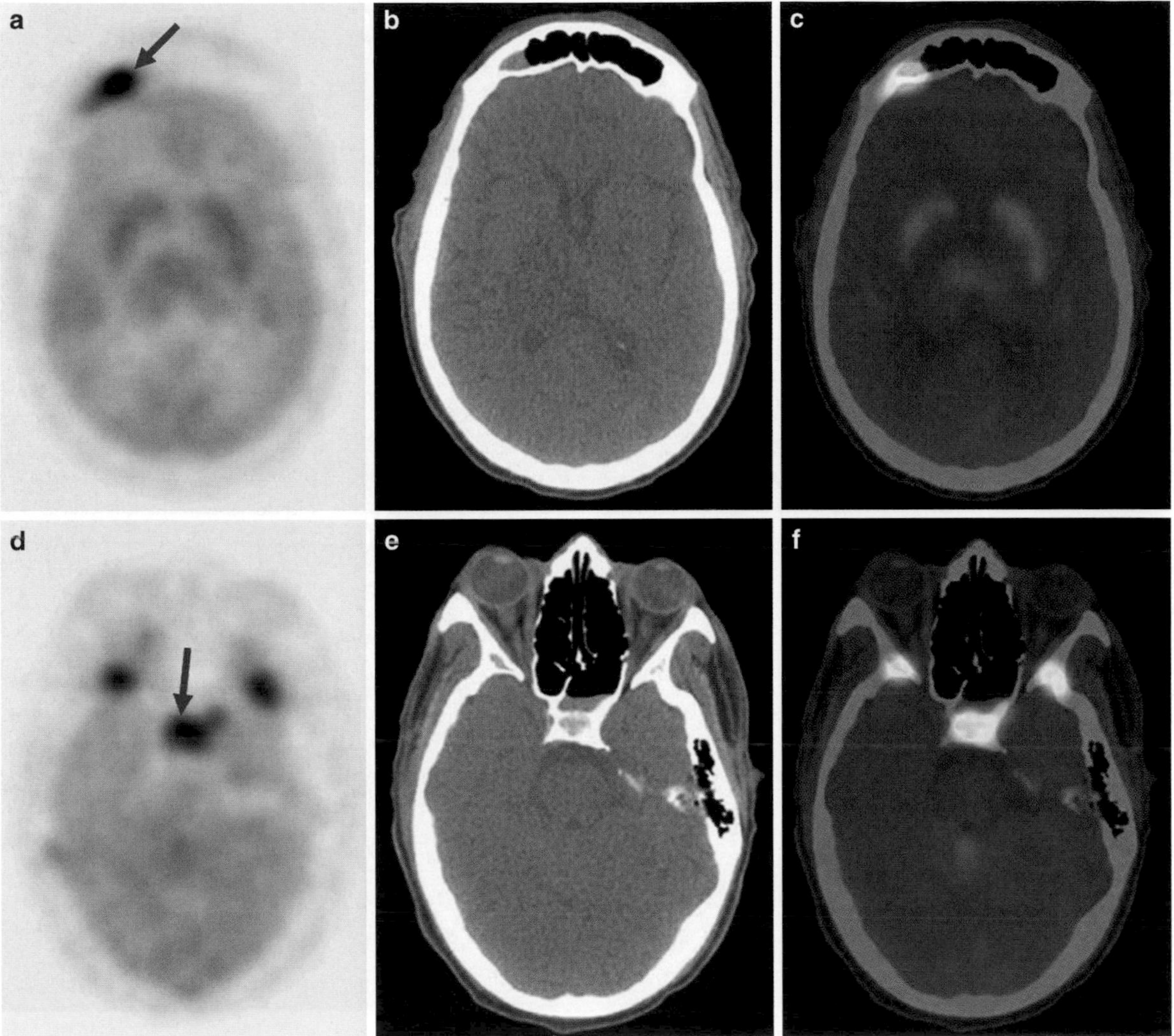

Fig. 15 CNS lymphoma: **a** PET; **b** axial CT; **c** axial fused PET/CT; **d** axial CT; **e** axial fused PET/CT of a 44-year-old man with newly diagnosed HIV and B-cell lymphoma demonstrate increased FDG uptake throughout the cranial cavity and increased proteinaceous fluid in the sphenoid sinus

(Bleeker-Rovers et al. 2004). In a prospective study, Bleeker-Rovers et al. observed increased subcutaneous FDG accumulation in three out of four HIV-infected patients with lipodystrophy on HAART (Bleeker-Rovers et al. 2004) while similar patterns of FDG uptake were absent in HIV-infected controls without lipodystrophy (Bleeker-Rovers et al. 2004). Detecting lipodystrophy with FDG PET may be an effective method for evaluating the adverse effects of HAART. Awareness of this possible variant uptake pattern is important when evaluating FDG PET scans in patients undergoing HAART.

8 Complications in Imaging HIV-positive Patients with FDG PET

Special considerations must be taken into account when evaluating HIV-positive patients with FDG PET. For example, in these individuals, AIDS-related B-cell lymphoma has a propensity to involve unexpected sites (Just et al. 2008). Compared to sporadic variants, AIDS-related B-cell lymphoma has a higher

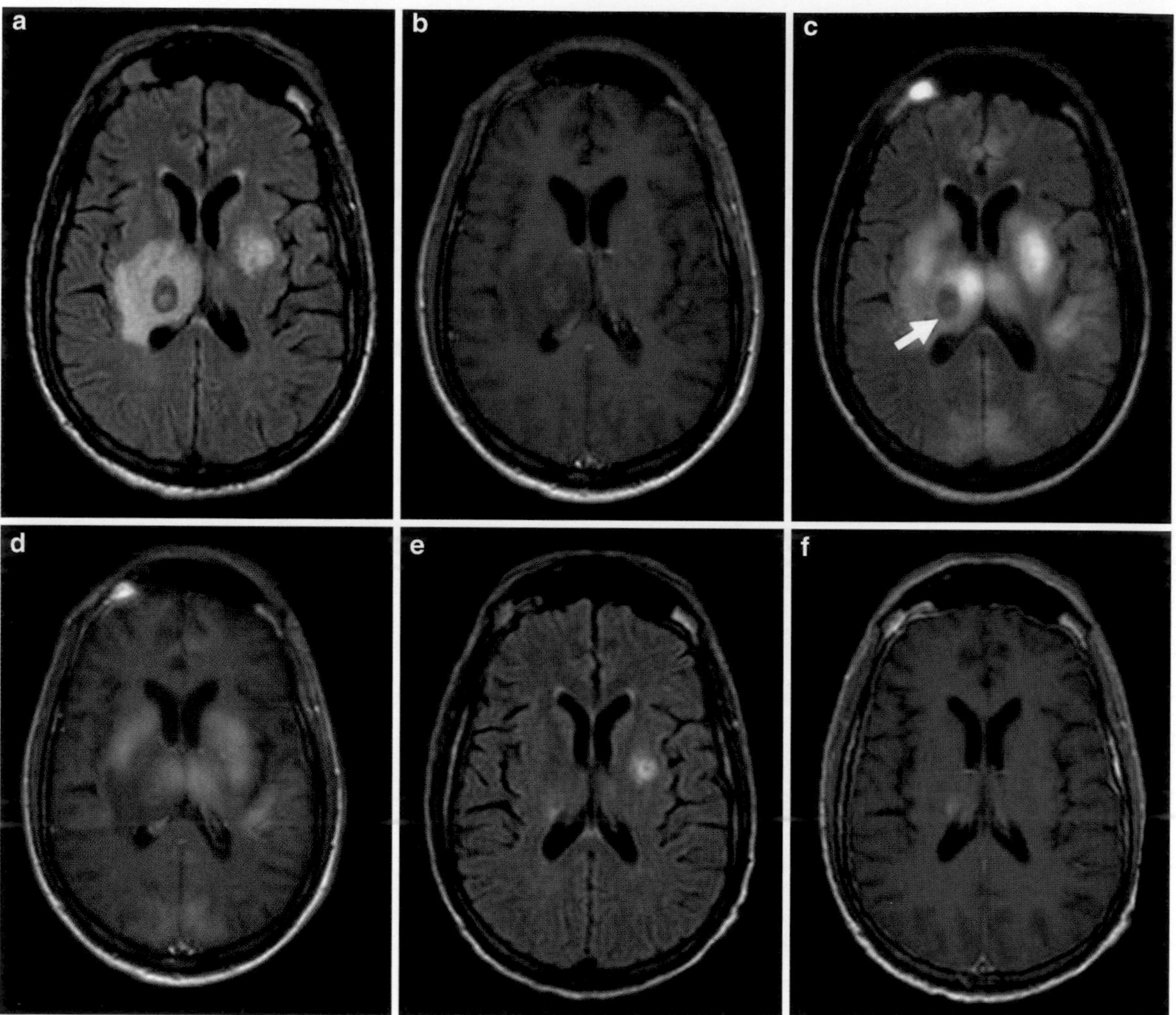

Fig. 16 Cerebral toxoplasmosis: a 44-year-old man with newly diagnosed HIV and large B-cell lymphoma in the pelvis presented with altered mental status. **a** Axial MRI (FLAIR) demonstrates a dominant heterogeneously enhancing lesion in the *right thalamus* measuring 1.8 × 0.7 cm with surrounding vasogenic edema. **b** MRI (T1 with gadolinium) demonstrates a right thalamic lesion with contrast enhancement. **c** Fused PET/MRI (FLAIR) demonstrates a lesion in the *right thalamus* with no FDG hypermetabolism suggesting an infective pathology; toxoplasmosis rather than lymphoma. **d** Fused PET/MRI (post-gadolinium T1) demonstrates enhancement of the lesion without FDG hypermetabolism. Patient was treated for toxoplasmosis with Pyrimethamine and Clindamycin. A follow-up MRI at 26 days of treatment **e** (FLAIR) and **f** (post post-gadolinium T1) demonstrate a decrease in the size, conspicuity, enhancement, and associated edema of the *right* thalamic lesion consistent with toxoplasmosis infection rather than lymphoma (this figure is published with permission from American Journal of Roentgenology Interactive Imaging 2010)

prevalence of bone marrow, cerebrospinal fluid, and lymph node involvement and a lower prevalence of abdominal involvement (Just et al. 2008). Patients with bone marrow and cerebrospinal fluid involvement may not have a distinctive local pattern of FDG uptake (Just et al. 2008).

The predisposition to opportunistic infections associated with immunosuppression also has implications for evaluation with FDG PET. Just et al., evaluated six FDG PET/CT scans from patients with AIDS demonstrating hypermetabolic foci in the lungs. Only one proved to be lymphoma recurrence while increased

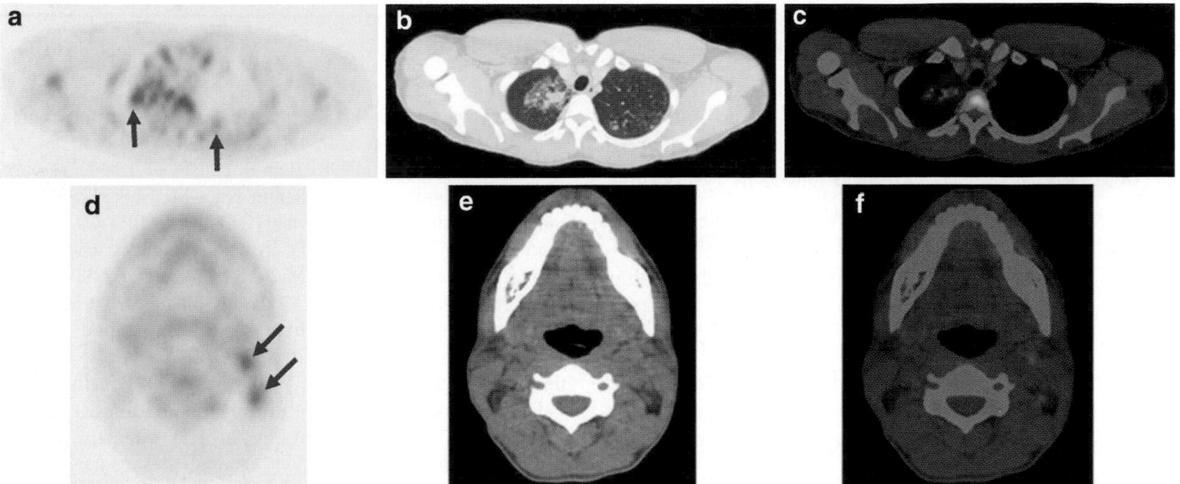

Fig. 17 Opportunistic infections. **a** Axial PET; **b** axial CT; **c** axial fused PET/CT demonstrate a fluffy ground glass pulmonary opacity and scattered pulmonary lymph nodules which may represent infection/inflammatory process, especially in the setting of tuberculosis. Granulomatous inflammation **d** axial PET; **e** axial CT; **f** axial fused PET/CT demonstrate necrotizing granulomas within the lymph nodes which were reported negative on gram stain, AFB smear, PAS stain, PCR for mycobacterium, routine fungal and mycobacterial cultures

FDG uptake in the remaining five scans was due to infections (Just et al. 2008). Inflammatory foci in the lungs are common in immunosuppressed patients and a frequent cause of FDG hypermetabolism. In addition, increased esophageal FDG accumulation observed by Just et al. was always related to infectious or reactive esophagitis (Just et al. 2008). However, low-grade FDG uptake in the oropharynx and distal esophagus observed by O'Doherty et al. proved to be T-cell lymphoma (O'Doherty et al. 1997) suggesting that a malignant etiology cannot immediately be excluded when FDG uptake is observed in these regions.

Generalized lymphadenopathy and distinct patterns of lymphoid tissue activation observed in HIV-positive patients (Brust et al. 2006; Scharko et al. 2003; Iyengar et al. 2003; Lucignani et al. 2009; Goshen et al. 2008) have obvious implications when using FDG PET to detect nodal metastases and disease recurrence. In a study by Goshen et al., seven HIV-positive patients, six with known cases of NHL, were evaluated with FDG PET/CT (Goshen et al. 2008). FDG PET/CT accurately depicted the extent of lymphoma in 12 of 16 scans performed on these patients (Goshen et al. 2008). However, in four scans obtained from two patients, increased FDG uptake was observed in nodes that appeared normal on CT and proved benign after biopsy (Goshen et al. 2008). These patients also had the highest viral loads and lowest CD4 T-cell counts of all patients studied (Goshen et al. 2008). Additionally, when monitoring patients for recurrent anal carcinoma, Cotter et al. found that HIV-positive patients were more likely to have increased FDG uptake in the pelvic lymph nodes and at extra-pelvic sites due to diffuse inflammatory changes (Cotter et al. 2006). Thus, in HIV-infected patients, lymph nodes found to be positive by FDG PET alone may require further study to differentiate malignancy from inflammatory processes, particularly when such findings are encountered in the context of high viral loads and advanced-stage disease.

9 Conclusions

FDG PET has provided valuable insight into the anatomical correlates of HIV progression without the need for biopsy, as the biodistribution of FDG uptake has effectively demonstrated patterns of lymphoid tissue activation in various stages of HIV infection (Brust et al. 2006; Scharko et al. 2003; Iyengar et al. 2003; Lucignani et al. 2009). The observed correlation between FDG accumulation in lymphoid tissues and plasma viremia (Iyengar et al. 2003; Lucignani et al. 2009) supports the key role of

HIV target cell activation and lymphocyte turnover in viral replication and disease pathogenesis.

FDG PET has proved useful in the diagnosis, staging, detection of metastasis, and post-treatment monitoring in the major AIDS-defining malignancies—Kaposi sarcoma, high-grade B-cell non-Hodgkin lymphoma, and invasive cervical carcinoma (Castaigne et al. 2009; O'Doherty et al. 1997; Barker et al. 2009; Cotter et al. 2006). The efficacy of this imaging modality has important implications in treatment planning for HIV-positive patients, particularly in AIDS-related Burkitt lymphoma where a negative PET scan can lead to discontinuation of a chemotherapy regimen that is especially difficult for those with low CD4 counts. It also has the ability to make the important distinction between malignancy and infection in the evaluation of CNS lesions (Villringer et al. 1995; Just et al. 2008; Heald et al. 1996), leading to the initiation of the appropriate treatment and precluding the need for invasive biopsy. When using FDG PET in the initial assessment of cancers in HIV-positive patients, it is important to remember that HIV infection can often lead to phenomena such as persistent generalized lymphadenopathy and that immunosuppression predisposes to a number of opportunistic infections. Special care must therefore be taken in evaluating FDG PET scans from these patients, as benign hypermetabolic foci are common, especially in the context of high viremia, and can lead to false-positive interpretations of malignancy.

The era of highly active antiretroviral therapy has brought about significant changes in the management of HIV-positive patients. When HAART is administered, FDG uptake is unrelated to immunological variables such as plasma viral load (Brust et al. 2006; Lucignani et al. 2009). The complementarity of the information provided by measures of immunological variables and FDG uptake FDG PET may be useful in assessing the extra-plasmic response to HAART (Lucignani et al. 2009). Furthermore, FDG PET may be an important tool not only in monitoring response to therapy, but also in evaluating common side-effects of treatment such as lipodystrophy (Bleeker-Rovers et al. 2004). This will be particularly useful in assessing the lipodystrophy-inducing effect of newly developed antiretroviral regimens.

References

Aoki Y, Tosato G (2004) Neoplastic conditions in the context of HIV-1 infection. Curr HIV Res 2:343–349

Bakheet SM, Powe J (1998) Benign causes of 18-FDG uptake on whole body imaging. Semin Nucl Med 28:352–358

Barker R, Kazmi F, Stebbing J et al (2009) FDG-PET/CT imaging in the management of HIV-associated multicentric Castleman's disease. Eur J Nucl Med Mol Imaging 36:648–652

Bental M, Deutsch C (1993) Metabolic changes in activated T cells: an NMR study of human peripheral blood lymphocytes. Magn Reson Med 29:317–326

Bleeker-Rovers CP, van der Ven AJ, Zomer B et al (2004) F-18-fluorodeoxyglucose positron emission tomography for visualization of lipodystrophy in HIV-infected patients. AIDS 18:2430–2432

Blum KA, Lozanski G, Byrd JC (2004) Adult Burkitt leukemia and lymphoma. Blood 104:3009–3020

Boshoff C, Weiss R (2002) AIDS-related malignancies. Nat Rev Cancer 2:373–382

Bower M, Palmieri C, Dhillon T (2006) AIDS-related malignancies: changing epidemiology and the impact of highly active antiretroviral therapy. Curr Opin Infect Dis 19:14–19

Brust D, Polis M, Davey R et al (2006) Fluorodeoxyglucose imaging in healthy subjects with HIV infection: impact of disease stage and therapy on pattern of nodal activation. AIDS 20:985–993

Carbone A, Gloghini A (2005) AIDS-related lymphomas: from pathogenesis to pathology. Br J Haematol 130:662–670

Castaigne C, Tondeur M, de Wit S, Hildebrand M, Clumeck N, Dusart M (2009) Clinical value of FDG-PET/CT for the diagnosis of human immunodeficiency virus-associated fever of unknown origin: a retrospective study. Nucl Med Commun 30:41–47

Chang Y, Cesarman E, Pessin MS et al (1994) Identification of herpesvirus-like DNA sequences in AIDS-associated Kaposi's sarcoma. Science 266:1865–1869

Cotter SE, Grigsby PW, Siegel BA et al (2006) FDG-PET/CT in the evaluation of anal carcinoma. Int J Radiat Oncol Biol Phys 65:720–725

DeMario MD, Liebowitz DN (1998) Lymphomas in the immunocompromised patient. Semin Oncol 25:492–502

Dupin N, Diss TL, Kellam P et al (2000) HHV-8 is associated with a plasmablastic variant of Castleman disease that is linked to HHV-8-positive plasmablastic lymphoma. Blood 95:1406–1412

Elder GA, Sever JL (1988) Neurologic disorders associated with AIDS retroviral infection. Rev Infect Dis 10:286–302

Euvrard S, Kanitakis J, Claudy A (2003) Skin cancers after organ transplantation. N Engl J Med 348:1681–1691

Fox CH, Tenner-Racz K, Racz P, Firpo A, Pizzo PA, Fauci AS (1991) Lymphoid germinal centers are reservoirs of human immunodeficiency virus type 1 RNA. J Infect Dis 164:1051–1057

French MA (2009) HIV/AIDS: immune reconstitution inflammatory syndrome: a reappraisal. Clin Infect Dis 48:101–107

Frisch M, Biggar RJ, Goedert JJ (2000) Human papillomavirus-associated cancers in patients with human immunodeficiency virus infection and acquired immunodeficiency syndrome. J Natl Cancer Inst 92:1500–1510

Frisch M, Biggar RJ, Engels EA, Goedert JJ (2001) Association of cancer with AIDS-related immunosuppression in adults. JAMA 285:1736–1745

Gallagher B, Wang Z, Schymura MJ, Kahn A, Fordyce EJ (2001) Cancer incidence in New York state acquired immunodeficiency syndrome patients. Am J Epidemiol 154:544–556

Goshen E, Davidson T, Avigdor A, Zwas TS, Levy I (2008) PET/CT in the evaluation of lymphoma in patients with HIV-1 with suppressed viral loads. Clin Nucl Med 33:610–614

Grigsby PW, Siegel BA, Dehdashti F, Rader J, Zoberi I (2004) Posttherapy [18F] fluorodeoxyglucose positron emission tomography in carcinoma of the cervix: response and outcome. J Clin Oncol 22:2167–2171

Hall HI, Song R, Rhodes P et al (2008) Estimation of HIV incidence in the United States. JAMA 300:520–529

Hardy G, Worrell S, Hayes P et al (2004) Evidence of thymic reconstitution after highly active antiretroviral therapy in HIV-1 infection. HIV Med 5:67–73

Heald AE, Hoffman JM, Bartlett JA, Waskin HA (1996) Differentiation of central nervous system lesions in AIDS patients using positron emission tomography (PET). Int J STD AIDS 7:337–346

Heaton RK, Grant I, Butters N et al (1995) The HNRC 500—neuropsychology of HIV infection at different disease stages. J Int Neuropsychol Soc 1:231–251

Hillier JC, Shaw P, Miller RF et al (2004) Imaging features of multicentric Castleman's disease in HIV infection. Clin Radiol 59:596–601

Hoffman JM, Waskin HA, Schifter T et al (1993) FDG-PET in differentiating lymphoma from nonmalignant central nervous system lesions in patients with AIDS. J Nucl Med 34:567–575

Iyengar S, Chin B, Margolick JB, Sabundayo BP, Schwartz DH (2003) Anatomical loci of HIV-associated immune activation and association with viraemia. Lancet 362:945–950

Jhanwar YS, Straus DJ (2006) The role of PET in lymphoma. J Nucl Med 47:1326–1334

Just PA, Fieschi C, Baillet G, Galicier L, Oksenhendler E, Moretti JL (2008) 18F-fluorodeoxyglucose positron emission tomography/computed tomography in AIDS-related Burkitt lymphoma. AIDS Patient Care STDS 22:695–700

Kedes DH, Operskalski E, Busch M, Kohn R, Flood J, Ganem D (1996) The seroepidemiology of human herpesvirus 8 (Kaposi's sarcoma-associated herpesvirus): distribution of infection in KS risk groups and evidence for sexual transmission. Nat Med 2:918–924

Krown SE, Metroka C, Wernz JC (1989) Kaposi's sarcoma in the acquired immune deficiency syndrome: a proposal for uniform evaluation, response, and staging criteria. J Clin Oncol 7:1201–1207

Kwan A, Seltzer M, Czernin J, Chou MJ, Kao CH (2001) Characterization of hilar lymph node by 18F-fluoro-2-deoxyglucose positron emission tomography in healthy subjects. Anticancer Res 21:701–706

Levy RM, Bredesen DE, Rosenblum ML, Davis RL (1989) Central nervous system disorders in AIDS. Immunol Ser 44:371–401

Liu Y (2009) Clinical significance of diffusely increased splenic uptake on FDG-PET. Nucl Med Commun 30:763–769

Lucignani G, Orunesu E, Cesari M et al (2009) FDG-PET imaging in HIV-infected subjects: relation with therapy and immunovirological variables. Eur J Nucl Med Mol Imaging 36:640–647

Manzardo C, Del Mar Ortega M, Sued O, Garcia F, Moreno A, Miro JM (2005) Central nervous system opportunistic infections in developed countries in the highly active antiretroviral therapy era. J Neurovirol 11(Suppl 3):72–82

Marjanovic S, Skog S, Heiden T, Tribukait B, Nelson BD (1991) Expression of glycolytic isoenzymes in activated human peripheral lymphocytes: cell cycle analysis using flow cytometry. Exp Cell Res 193:425–431

Mbulaiteye SM, Parkin DM, Rabkin CS (2003) Epidemiology of AIDS-related malignancies an international perspective. Hematol Oncol Clin North Am 17:673–696

Meintjes G, Lynen L (2008) Prevention and treatment of the immune reconstitution inflammatory syndrome. Curr Opin HIV AIDS 3:468–476

Nasti G, Tirelli U (2005) Highly active antiretroviral therapy in AIDS-associated Kaposi's sarcoma (KS): implications for the design of therapeutic trials in patients with advanced symptomatic KS. J Clin Oncol 23:2433–2434

Nasti G, Talamini R, Antinori A et al (2003) AIDS-related Kaposi's Sarcoma: evaluation of potential new prognostic factors and assessment of the AIDS clinical trial group staging system in the Haart era—the Italian cooperative group on AIDS and tumors and the Italian cohort of patients naive from antiretrovirals. J Clin Oncol 21:2876–2882

Navia BA, Jordan BD, Price RW (1986) The AIDS dementia complex: I. Clinical features. Ann Neurol 19:517–524

Niu MT, Jermano JA, Reichelderfer P, Schnittman SM (1993) Summary of the National Institutes of Health workshop on primary human immunodeficiency virus type 1 infection. AIDS Res Hum Retroviruses 9:913–924

O'Doherty MJ, Barrington SF, Campbell M, Lowe J, Bradbeer CS (1997) PET scanning and the human immunodeficiency virus-positive patient. J Nucl Med 38:1575–1583

Offiah CE, Turnbull IW (2006) The imaging appearances of intracranial CNS infections in adult HIV and AIDS patients. Clin Radiol 61:393–401

Oksenhendler E, Duarte M, Soulier J et al (1996) Multicentric Castleman's disease in HIV infection: a clinical and pathological study of 20 patients. AIDS 10:61–67

Oksenhendler E, Boulanger E, Galicier L et al (2002) High incidence of Kaposi sarcoma-associated herpesvirus-related non-Hodgkin lymphoma in patients with HIV infection and multicentric Castleman disease. Blood 99:2331–2336

Pantaleo G, Graziosi C, Butini L et al (1991) Lymphoid organs function as major reservoirs for human immunodeficiency virus. Proc Natl Acad Sci U S A 88:9838–9842

Pantaleo G, Graziosi C, Demarest JF et al (1994) Role of lymphoid organs in the pathogenesis of human immunodeficiency virus (HIV) infection. Immunol Rev 140:105–130

Pascal S, Resnick L, Barker WW et al (1991) Metabolic asymmetries in asymptomatic HIV-1 seropositive subjects: relationship to disease onset and MRI findings. J Nucl Med 32:1725–1729

Quinn TC (1996) Global burden of the HIV pandemic. Lancet 348:99–106

Rabkin CS, Yellin F (1994) Cancer incidence in a population with a high prevalence of infection with human immunodeficiency virus type 1. J Natl Cancer Inst 86:1711–1716

Rottenberg DA, Moeller JR, Strother SC et al (1987) The metabolic pathology of the AIDS dementia complex. Ann Neurol 22:700–706

Rottenberg DA, Sidtis JJ, Strother SC et al (1996) Abnormal cerebral glucose metabolism in HIV-1 seropositive subjects with and without dementia. J Nucl Med 37:1133–1141

Rubio A, Martinez-Moya M, Leal M et al (2002) Changes in thymus volume in adult HIV-infected patients under HAART: correlation with the T-cell repopulation. Clin Exp Immunol 130:121–126

Scharko AM, Perlman SB, Pyzalski RW, Graziano FM, Sosman J, Pauza CD (2003) Whole-body positron emission tomography in patients with HIV-1 infection. Lancet 362:959–961

Subhas N, Patel PV, Pannu HK, Jacene HA, Fishman EK, Wahl RL (2005) Imaging of pelvic malignancies with in-line FDG PET-CT: case examples and common pitfalls of FDG PET. Radiographics 25:1031–1043

Sugawara Y, Braun DK, Kison PV, Russo JE, Zasadny KR, Wahl RL (1998) Rapid detection of human infections with fluorine-18 fluorodeoxyglucose and positron emission tomography: preliminary results. Eur J Nucl Med 25:1238–1243

Tenner-Racz K, Racz P, Gluckman JC, Popovic M (1988) Cell-free HIV in lymph nodes of patients with AIDS and generalized lymphadenopathy. N Engl J Med 318:49–50

UNAIDS (2008) Report on the global AIDS epidemic. In: JUNPoHA (ed) UNAIDS ,Geneva

Villringer K, Jager H, Dichgans M et al (1995) Differential diagnosis of CNS lesions in AIDS patients by FDG-PET. J Comput Assist Tomogr 19:532–536

von Giesen HJ, Antke C, Hefter H, Wenserski F, Seitz RJ, Arendt G (2000) Potential time course of human immunodeficiency virus type 1-associated minor motor deficits: electrophysiologic and positron emission tomography findings. Arch Neurol 57:1601–1607

Wong TZ, Jones EL, Coleman RE (2004) Positron emission tomography with 2-deoxy-2-[(18)F]fluoro-D-glucose for evaluating local and distant disease in patients with cervical cancer. Mol Imaging Biol 6:55–62

Pitfalls and Artifacts

Geoffrey Bates Johnson and Christopher Harker Hunt

Contents

G. B. Johnson · C. H. Hunt (✉)
Department of Radiology and Immunology,
Mayo Clinic, Rochester, MN, USA
e-mail: johnson.geoffrey@mayo.edu

Abstract

FDG PET is extremely useful in staging and restaging cancer, differentiating malignant from benign processes, and locating otherwise occult sites of malignancy. However, areas of real or apparent FDG activity do not always represent malignancy. In this chapter we will review the more common categories of pitfalls and artifacts and how they can be recognized and avoided. Pitfalls arise when real benign biologic processes result in imaging findings that mimic malignancy. Common pitfalls are seen with abnormal nonmalignant biologic processes, as well as normal physiologic and anatomic variation. Artifacts are imaging findings that arise in the process of patient preparation and imaging. Artifacts can mimic real biologic processes, or can negatively affect the interpretation of real biologic processes. Common artifacts result from errors related to attenuation correction, motion, truncation, glucose and insulin, FDG injection and uptake. When combining PET and CT imaging, some pitfalls and artifacts are avoided, while others may be newly created or multiplied.

1 Pitfalls

1.1 Inflammation

Some of the most common pitfalls in FDG PET/CT are inflammatory and infectious processes. In general, infection and inflammation have abnormally high FDG activity, but usually not as high as most

P. Peller et al. (eds.), *PET-CT and PET-MRI in Oncology*, Medical Radiology. Diagnostic Imaging,
DOI: 10.1007/174_2012_708,

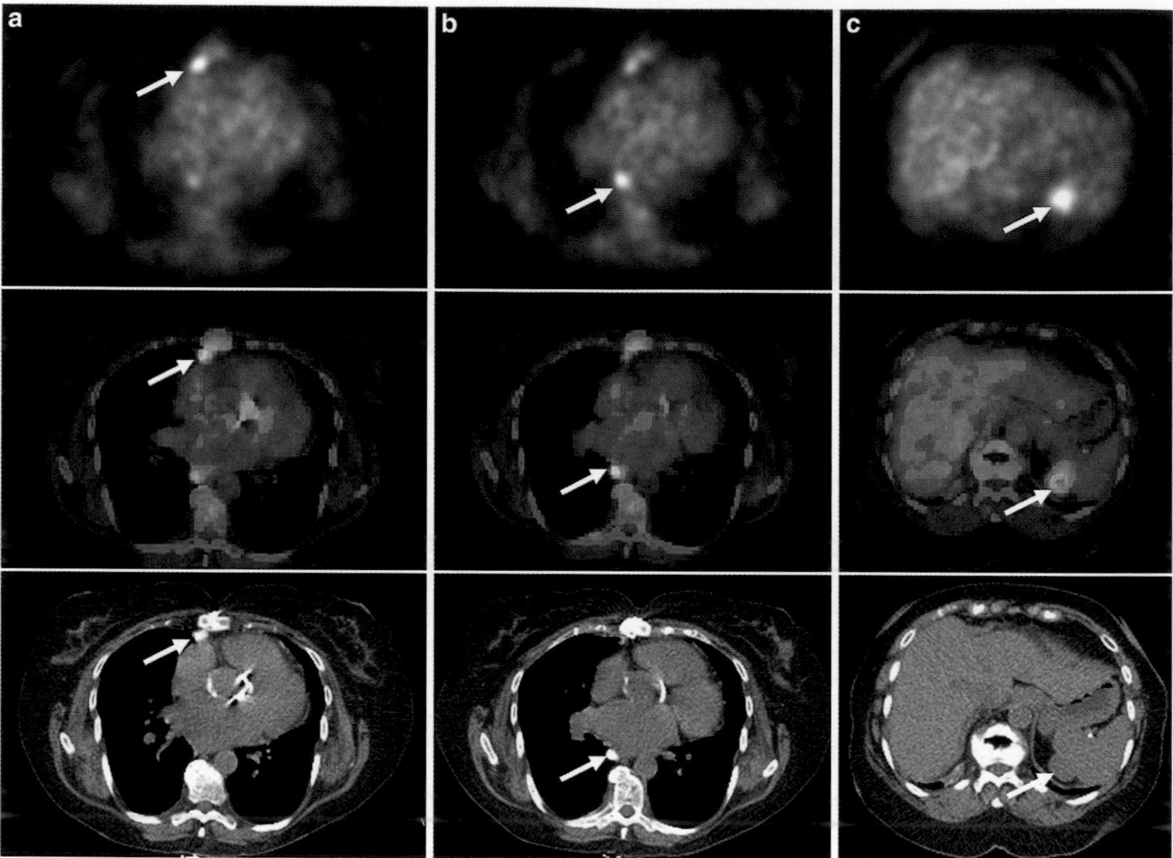

Fig. 1 Talc pleurodesis pitfall. Eighty year-old woman with radiodense FDG-avid right pleural nodules (**a** and **b**), and biopsy proven recurrent noncalcified metastatic ovarian cancer in the left upper abdomen retroperitoneum (**c**). The patient was 9 years post initial surgery and chemotherapy for ovarian cancer. The patient was also 9 years post bedside slurry talc pleurodesis for a benign pneumothorax, which was a complication of port-a-cath placement, and the subsequent inability to remove her chest tube due to large volume pleural effusions. The retroperitoneal mass (**c**) was previously not FDG avid after completion of chemotherapy. The presumed talc deposits with granulomatous foreign body reaction maintained stable high FDG activity on 3 PET-CT scans

malignancies. This general principle requires clinical judgment, and must be applied in a case-by-case basis related to the expected FDG activity in the patient's type of cancer, and the patient's treatment history. For example, a large lymph node with an SUV_{max} of 2.5 in a patient with high-grade metastatic squamous cell cancer is likely reactive. However, a large lymph node with an SUV_{max} of 2.5 could be reactive or represent malignancy in a patient with diffuse low-grade lymphoma. Common situations where it can be particularly difficult to differentiate malignant and nonmalignant processes on PET/CT alone include diverticulitis, mastitis, esophagitis, and pneumonia.

1.1.1 Granulomatous

Granulomatous diseases create findings on CT that mimic malignancy and are often FDG avid. Granulomatous diseases that most commonly result in pitfalls include sarcoidosis (Prabhakar et al. 2008; Chowdhury et al. 2009), tuberculosis, and histoplasmosis (Salhab et al. 2006). Granulomatous diseases are worth considering on a short differential for FDG-avid masses, such as lung nodules or lymphadenopathy (Christensen and Nathan 2006; Lowe and Fletcher 1998). Sarcoidosis can appear as a focal mass or as diffuse disease, such as diffuse splenic activity. When tumors have discordant response to chemotherapy, i.e. some tumors

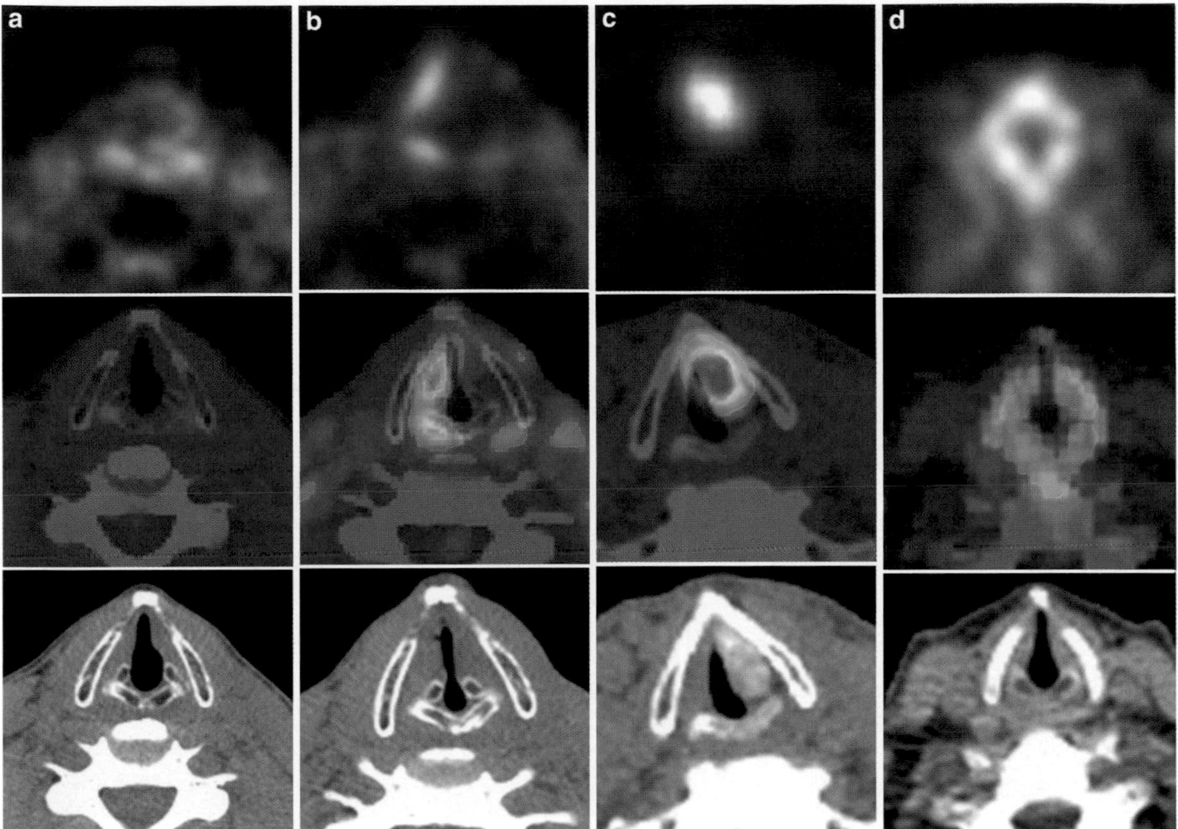

Fig. 2 Vocal cord palsy, teflon granuloma, and normal activity. Forty-six year-old man with a history of history of invasive squamous cell carcinoma of the left tonsil, previously resected, and locally recurred. **a** PET-CT post neoadjuvant chemotherapy shows good response (not shown) with normal vocal cord FDG activity. **b** PET-CT after interval wide left surgical neck resection shows prominent compensatory FDG activity in the muscles of the right vocal cord. This is secondary to left recurrent laryngeal nerve injury during surgery and subsequent left vocal cord paralysis. In patients with history of squamous cell carcinoma of the upper gastrointestinal tract, there is a high risk of secondary cancers, and pitfalls like vocal cord paralysis must be carefully inspected. Flexible nasopharyngolaryngoscopy confirmed left vocal cord paralysis and left pharyngeal paralysis. **c** A different patient who had remote Teflon injection in the left vocal cord to reduce symptoms of left vocal cord paralysis. This injection resulted in chronic granulomatous foreign body reaction, which is seen as a dense mass in the vocal cord on CT and high FDG activity. **d** A different patient who was talking during the FDG uptake phase prior to scanning, showing normal bilateral FDG activity in the muscles of the vocal cords

remain FDG active while others decrease in activity, consider the possibility that some foci of activity may be inflammatory, such as sarcoidosis. Such discordance is not seen when the chemotherapy regimen includes steroids, since sarcoidosis decreases activity in response to steroids.

1.1.2 Foreign Body Reaction

Prolonged and moderate to intense FDG activity can be seen at sites of granulomatous foreign body reactions, even when other imaging modalities show few signs of inflammation. With the proper clinical history, these pitfalls should be easily avoided. Intense and very prolonged FDG activity is seen with talc pleurodesis (Fig. 1) (Nguyen et al. 2009) and Teflon granulomas in vocal cords (Fig. 2) (Truong et al. 2004; Modi et al. 2005; Tessonnier et al. 2008; Ondik et al. 2009). More moderate FDG activity is seen with suture granulomas (Chung et al. 2006), gossypibomas (Tsai et al. 2005; Yu et al. 2008), hernia repair mesh (Aide et al. 2005), synthetic vascular grafts (Wasselius et al. 2008), peritoneal chemotherapy bound to carbon particles

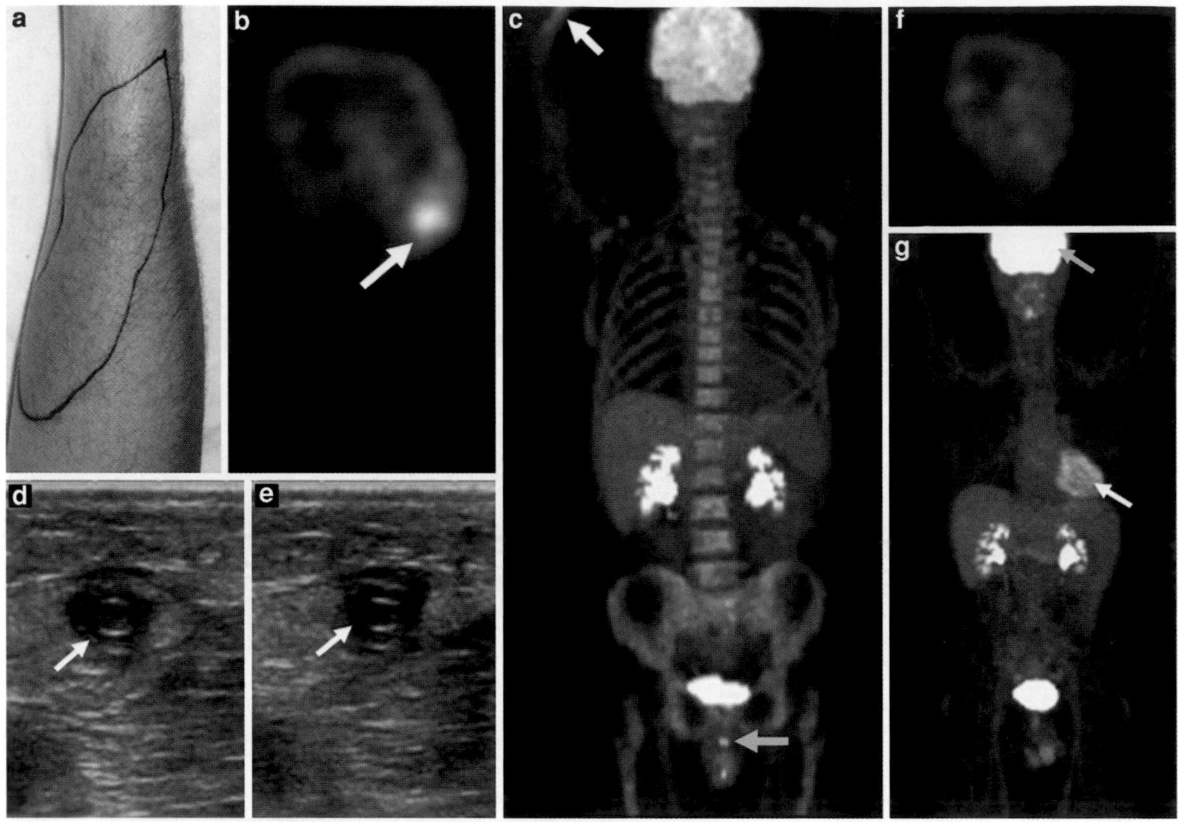

Fig. 3 Acute bland thrombosis. Fifty-four year-old man with history of lymphoma who developed acute thrombophlebitis in his right cephalic vein at a prior IV site. **a** Photo taken 1 day before PET/CT shows erythema. **b**, **c** Moderate linear FDG activity (*arrow*) is seen in the right superficial tissues of the forearm (*white arrows*). **d**, **e** Ultrasound 2 days prior to the PET/CT showed hypoechoic non-compressible acute appearing thrombosis in the right cephalic vein (**d**: without compression, **e**: with compression, *arrows*). In (**c**), also note the diffuse marrow uptake on the PET MIP whole body image in this patient who received a CSF medication (Neulasta) 11 days prior to this PET/CT. This high bone marrow activity acts as a FDG sink, and can reduce FDG activity in the brain and in tumors. This patient also received prednisone for therapy of the forearm pain just prior to the PET/CT, which is known to reduce lymphoma FDG activity. Steroids may artificially reduce FDG activity resulting in falsely negative FDG activity, most pronounced in lymphoma. Therefore, it is generally considered best practice to wait several weeks after steroids before obtaining a PET-CT. For these reasons, the apparent lack of uptake in this patients residual pelvic lymphoma mass is of questionable clinical significance. Also note the urine contamination on the skin below the bladder (*grey arrow*). **f**, **g** Subsequent PET/CT 4 months later shows resolution of thrombophlebitis and bone marrow FDG activity, and the return of normal high brain FDG activity (*grey arrow*). On this PET-CT scan the lack of FDG activity in the residual pelvic lymphoma mass is much more reliable. Also, note the variable cardiac uptake, which is normal (*white arrow*)

(Lim et al. 2008), and prosthetic joints (Kisielinski et al. 2003). In short, virtually any foreign body can result in long-term moderate to intense FDG activity, including reactions to contraceptive devices (Fuechsel et al. 2006) and even rarely to tattoos (Nam et al. 2007). Foreign body pitfalls are further complicated by the fact that the foreign body is not always visible on CT images, the FDG activity can remain high for years or even go up with time, and on occasion the foreign body may also act as a nidus for infection.

1.1.3 Thrombosis

Thrombosis has variable FDG activity, and generally progresses from an acutely inflamed moderately FDG active process to a non-inflamed chronic process that shows little FDG activity (Sopov et al. 2009). In the

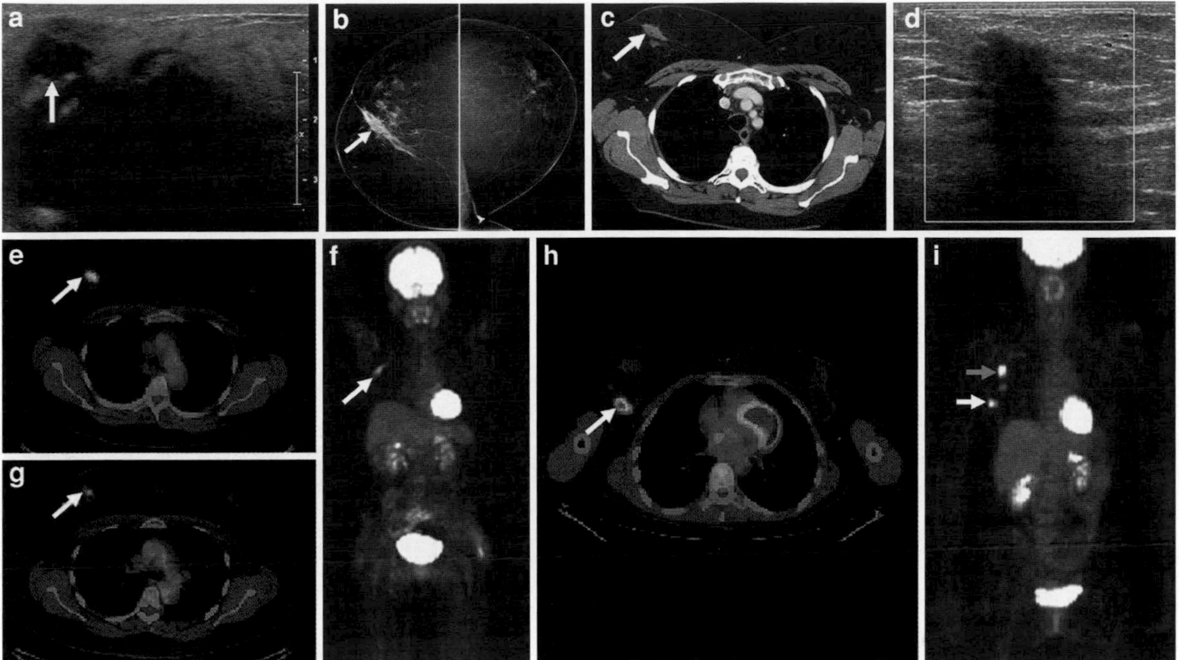

Fig. 4 Resolving hematoma versus malignancy. Sixty-two year-old woman with a history of melanoma who was in a motor vehicle accident and suffered a hematoma in her right breast as seen on outside ultrasound (**a**, *arrow*). One year later there was a new mass seen on screening mammography (**b**, cc views shown), CT (**c**), and ultrasound (**d**). **e**, **f** The breast mass showed moderate FDG activity on PET-CT (*arrows*), SUX max 6.0. Although this was most likely due to healing of a posttraumatic hematoma, biopsy was performed, showing giant cell reaction and fat necrosis. Subsequent PET-CT 2.5 years later showed decrease in FDG activity (**g**, *arrow*). **h**, **i** Comparison case of focal FDG activity in invasive ductal breast cancer (white arrows), SUV max 7.0, with axillary lymph node metastases (**i**, *grey arrow*). Note that normal breast tissue shows widely variable FDG activity in premenopausal women and those on hormone replacement therapy, making careful inspection of breast tissue essential

acute setting, deep venous thrombosis (Fig. 3) (Kikuchi et al. 2004; Do et al. 2006), pericatheter thrombosis (Bhargava et al. 2004), and pulmonary embolus can show moderate FDG activity. Since cancer patients are at increased risk of thrombosis, these pitfalls are common. An acute pulmonary embolus can mimic an FDG-avid pulmonary tumor (Ryan et al. 2007). In addition to FDG activity in the thrombus itself, secondary infarcted lung tissue can appear mass-like on CT and exhibit elevated FDG activity. Thus, pulmonary infarcts are commonly misinterpreted as lung malignancy (Kamel et al. 2005). Peri-catheter thrombosis is more confusing, as FDG activity often remains high even after the thrombus has become chronic (Bhargava et al. 2004a, b). Tumor thrombus and non-malignant, or bland, venous thrombosis are usually easily differentiated on PET/CT, assuming the thrombus is chronic.

1.1.4 Infectious

Infection can be intensely FDG avid in common conditions like bacterial pneumonia, diverticulitis, abscess, and mastitis. Most often it is not difficult to correctly diagnose a bacterial infection with PET, when given the clinical history and CT findings. However, infections are common in cancer patients, and are even more common after surgery and/or chemotherapy, when findings of recurrent or residual malignancy might be subtle. Therefore, differentiating infection from malignancy in some cases can be extremely difficult by PET/CT alone.

A more common pitfall than infections themselves are the secondary immune responses they create in so-called "reactive" lymph nodes. This pitfall is particularly common following head and neck surgery with radiation, bronchoscopy, or endoscopy, and can be associated with aspiration pneumonitis and/or

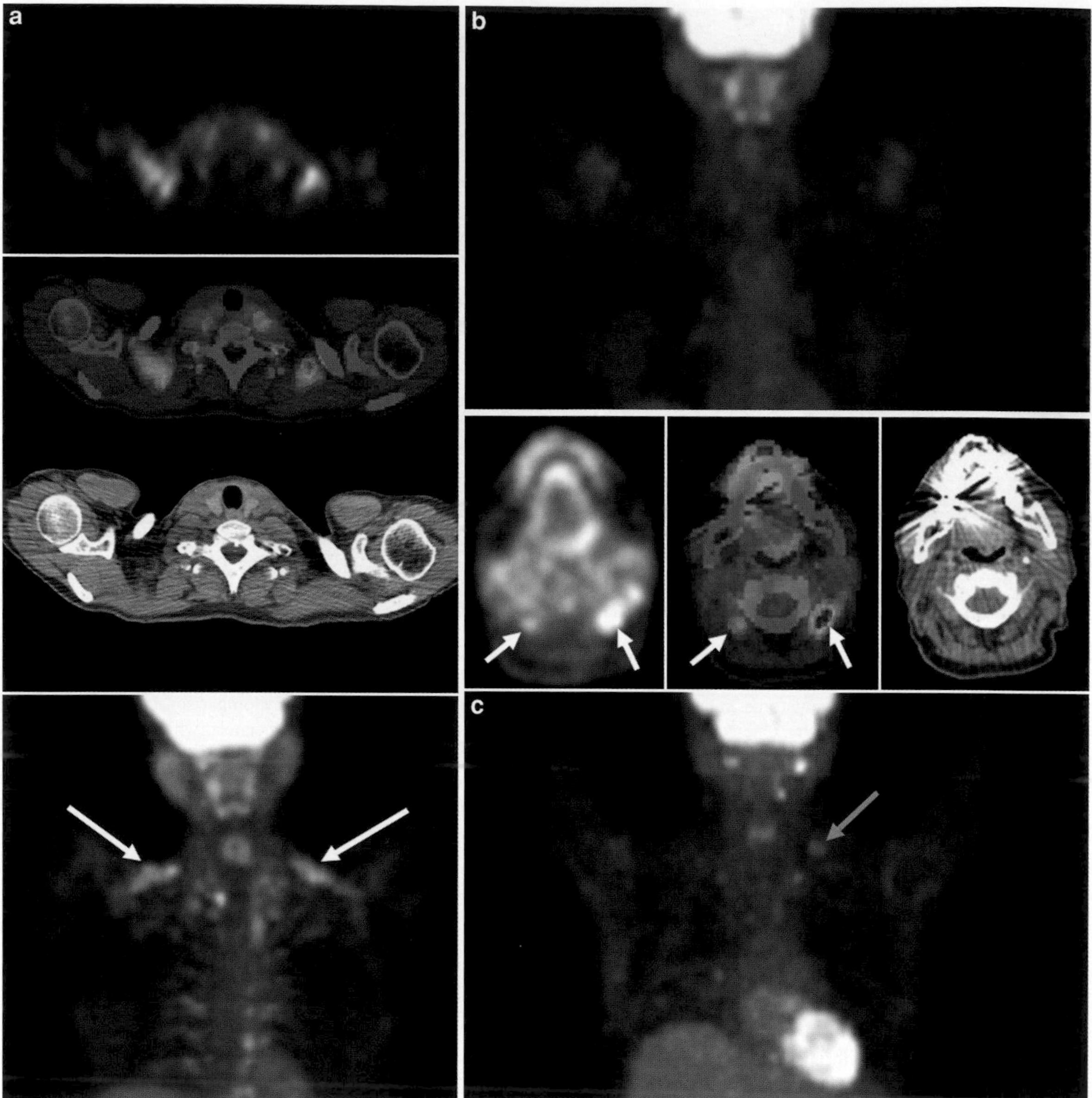

Fig. 5 Physiologic variation-brown fat. **a** Fifty-four year-old female with history of melanoma. Bilateral supraclavicular linear FDG activity (*arrows*) centered on fat, and scattered FDG activity in other fat in the paraaortic and paravertibral mediastinum, consistent with active brown fat. **b** MIP images in the same patient at a later date show resolution without therapy. Usually brown fat is most FDG avid in the bilateral supraclavicular fat, with more distant areas in the neck and mediastinum, and less commonly below the diaphragm. Only rarely is brown fat active in the absence of active brown fat in the bilateral supraclavicular areas. **c** Fifty-nine year-old female with history of metastatic melanoma. Foci of FDG-avid brown fat in the bilateral posterior neck (*white arrows*), and only subtle FDG active left supraclavicular brown fat (*grey arrow*). Active brown fat is most common in young, thin, women, and can be reduced by warming patients

pneumonia (Wang et al. 2010). The FDG activity in these reactive lymph nodes is usually less intense than the primary malignancy. However, in the post-surgical/post-therapy patient, it can be very difficult to differentiate a reactive lymph node from a lymph node with micrometastasis, and biopsy is often performed.

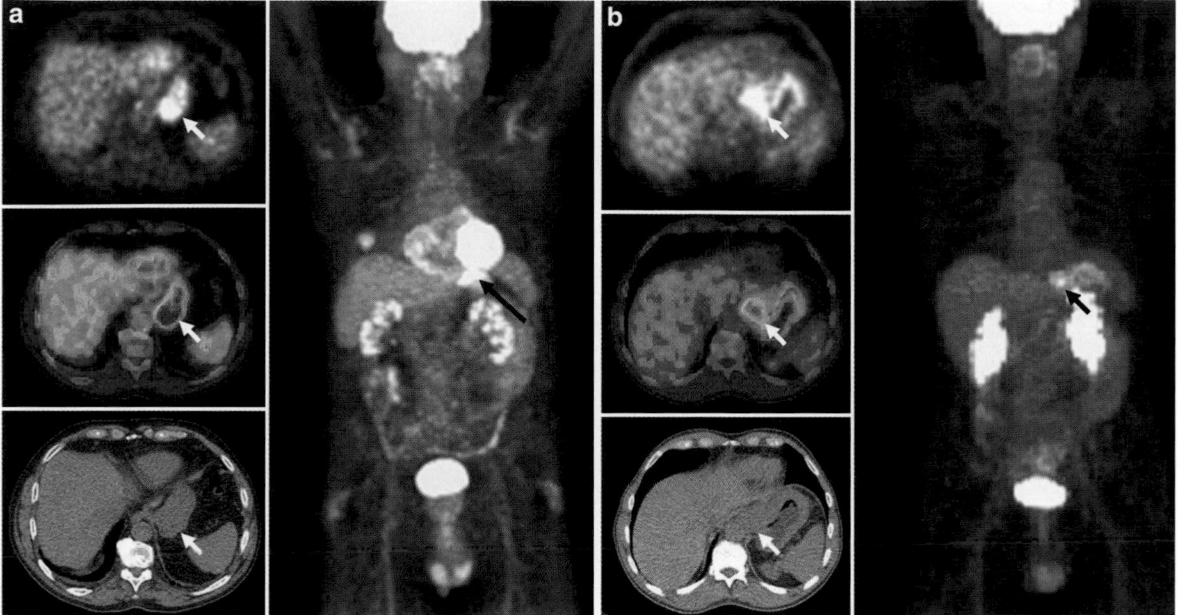

Fig. 6 Physiologic variation-normal esophagogastric activity versus malignancy. **a** Eighty-one year-old man with indeterminate lung mass, and FDG uptake in the esophagogastric (EG) junction and proximal stomach (*white arrows*). Normal FDG activity is commonly seen in the distal esophagus and proximal stomach, as is inflammatory FDG activity related to reflux and chemotherapy. In some cases it can be impossible to tell benign from malignant findings in this location on PET-CT, and EGD should be recommended. **b** Comparison case of 62-year-old man with biopsy-proven grade 4 adenocarcinoma of the distal esophagus through proximal stomach (*white arrows*). Note the normal variability of the cardiac FDG activity between these patients (*black arrows*)

1.1.5 Miscellaneous

Several other presumed inflammatory/infectious processes with unclear etiologies are common pitfalls. Classically, Paget disease results in patchy moderately increased cortical activity with less intense marrow/trabecular bone activity that decreases with the stage of the disease. Paget disease resulting in pathologic fractures and malignant transformation can have intense FDG activity.

Fibrous dysplasia causes intense FDG activity and can be polyostotic, as in McCune-Albright syndrome (Fig. 10), where it mimics diffuse metastatic disease (Kao et al. 2007).

Synovial conditions, such as inflammatory joint diseases (Kubota et al. 2009) and pigmented villonodular synovitis (Nguyen 2007; Yoshida et al. 2007), can have intense FDG activity. Inflammatory joint disease can have associated FDG-avid lytic perarticular findings. In rheumatoid arthritis, nodular disease can be an associated finding and usually has low to moderate FDG activity (Joosen et al. 2000; Gupta et al. 2005), but can rarely have moderate to intense activity, and mimic malignancy (Bakheet and Powe 1998; Strobel et al. 2009). In pigmented villonodular synovitis and its extra-synovial form (called giant-cell tumor of the tendon sheath), there can be a mass in or near the joint space with intense FDG activity (Nguyen 2007).

Atherosclerosis can have mild to moderate FDG activity, and is most commonly patchy and linear in nature with associated easily identifiable irregular wall thickening and calcifications on CT imaging. However, uncommon presentations of this common condition include focal and intense FDG activity, which have been known to mimic malignancy, for example in the mediastinum (Hanif et al. 2004). Giant cell and other diffuse forms of aortitis, can have moderate to intense circumferential FDG activity without calcification, and are not commonly confused with cancer.

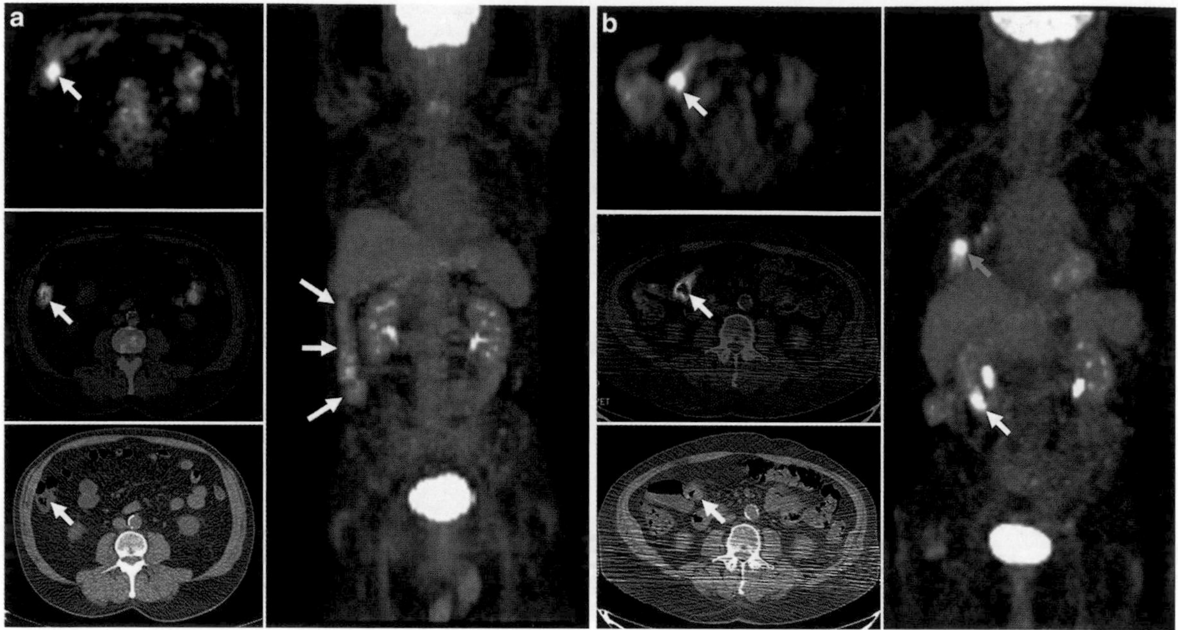

Fig. 7 Physiologic variation-normal cecum activity versus malignancy. **a** Seventy-one year-old man with history of melanoma. PET-CT shows linear uptake in the cecum extending up the ascending colon (*multiple arrows*). This is common and is within the normal variation of FDG activity. Normal FDG uptake can even be more focal than this in the cecum. However, focal uptake in colon cancer can have a similar appearance. **b** Comparison case of a 79-year-old man evaluated for indeterminate lung nodule in the right lower lobe, later surgically proven to be squamous cell cancer (*grey arrow*). This patient also had a focus of intense FDG activity in the ascending colon, and associated circumferential wall thickening on CT, later pathologically confirmed to be adenocarcinoma (*white arrows*)

1.2 Trauma and Healing

1.2.1 Injury

FDG activity is progressively reduced while healing progresses to completion. In some difficult cases, follow-up PET/CT is often helpful. Common etiologies include fractures, muscle and ligament strains, lacerations and hematomas. For example, chronic sterile hematomas can have moderate FDG activity for many months, and in the case of seatbelt injury can mimic breast cancer (Fig. 4) (Hamada et al. 2005). Muscular injuries usually cause FDG activity that is elongated along the course of the muscle fibers, whereas malignancy is often more focal, lobulated, or infiltrative.

1.2.2 Post-Surgical

Post-operative fractures, heterotopic ossification, and infection are common FDG-avid pitfalls (Liu 2009a). Surgical placement of anything through the skin, such as catheters, ports, and stomas cause prolonged moderate FDG activity (Bhargava et al. 2004a, b), until the device is removed and the skin irritation resolves. Stomas to the gastrointestinal tract show moderate FDG activity that does not resolve over time.

Post-surgical altered mechanics, such as vocal cord paralysis, causes intense FDG activity within the muscles of the contralateral vocal cord due to overuse, and hypertrophy (Fig. 2). In addition, as discussed above, direct injection of Teflon into a nonfunctioning and atrophic vocal cord to ameliorate symptoms of vocal cord paralysis, leads to an intensely FDG-avid foreign body reaction (Fig. 2). Teflon is dense on CT, allowing differentiation from paralysis and cancer.

1.2.3 Post-Radiation

When external beam radiation is used, post-radiation changes are classically defined by mild to moderate FDG activity with straight lines at the edges of the irradiated field. FDG activity often peaks within about

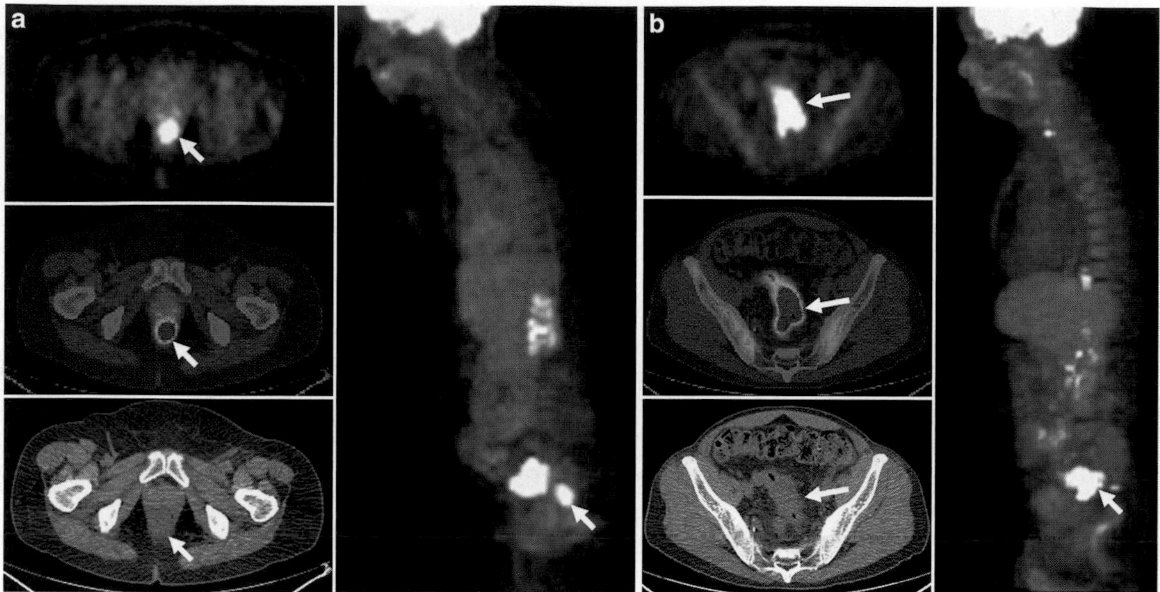

Fig. 8 Physiologic variation-normal rectal activity versus malignancy. Sixty-nine year-old woman with history of melanoma, currently in remission. **a** Intense FDG uptake in the rectum (posterior to normal bladder, *arrows*). FDG activity is commonly seen in the rectum and is most often due to normal physiologic variation, but can also be seen with primary malignancy. MRI was indeterminant (not shown). Physical exam and colonoscopy revealed no malignancy and hemorrhoids. Follow-up PET-CT scans showed no increase in FDG activity. **b** Comparison case of 58-year-old man with metastatic colon cancer to lymph nodes, with the primary site in the sigmoid colon (*arrows*). The sigmoid colon can have a similar appearance on PET-CT with diverticulitis. Note that scan was performed with a dual-lumen flushing bladder catheter in place to remove/reduce FDG activity in the bladder

1 month, then resolves over 4–6 months (Nakahara et al. 2008). It is difficult to confidently diagnose recurrent malignancy in a post-radiation site on a new baseline PET performed shortly after completion of therapy. In this context, malignancy can be best eliminated from the differential diagnosis on subsequent PET exams.

Therapeutic radiation inflammation more commonly becomes a pitfall in patients who have received focused radiation in a type of tissue susceptible to radiation necrosis. Radiation necrosis can appear mass-like and have intense FDG activity (Hung et al. 2005). This issue is particularly common with procedures such as gamma knife therapy for high-grade brain tumors. When inflammation accompanies radiation necrosis, it is not readily distinguishable from recurrent malignancy of high-grade brain tumors by PET (Ricci et al. 1998; Thompson et al. 1999; Chernov et al. 2005). Unfortunately, CT adds little diagnostic benefit in this situation.

1.3 Physiologic Variations

Physiologic FDG activity varies widely in certain normal tissues with respect to time, location, and intensity. The most common pitfalls are seen in cardiac muscle, brown fat, the gastrointestinal tract, the genitals, the uterine lining, breast tissue, skeletal muscle, and the central nervous system.

Cardiac muscle variably shifts between using free fatty acids and glucose as its primary energy source. Therefore, normal cardiac muscle can have focal, heterogeneous, or diffuse FDG activity. Cardiac muscle can also range from background levels to intense activity. Normal variation in myocardial activity can make normal tissue look like focal malignancy, and can make metastatic disease undetectable.

The primary function of brown fat is to generate body heat, and can be activated when physiologically needed. Therefore, brown fat has highly variable FDG activity. The vast majority of patients with active

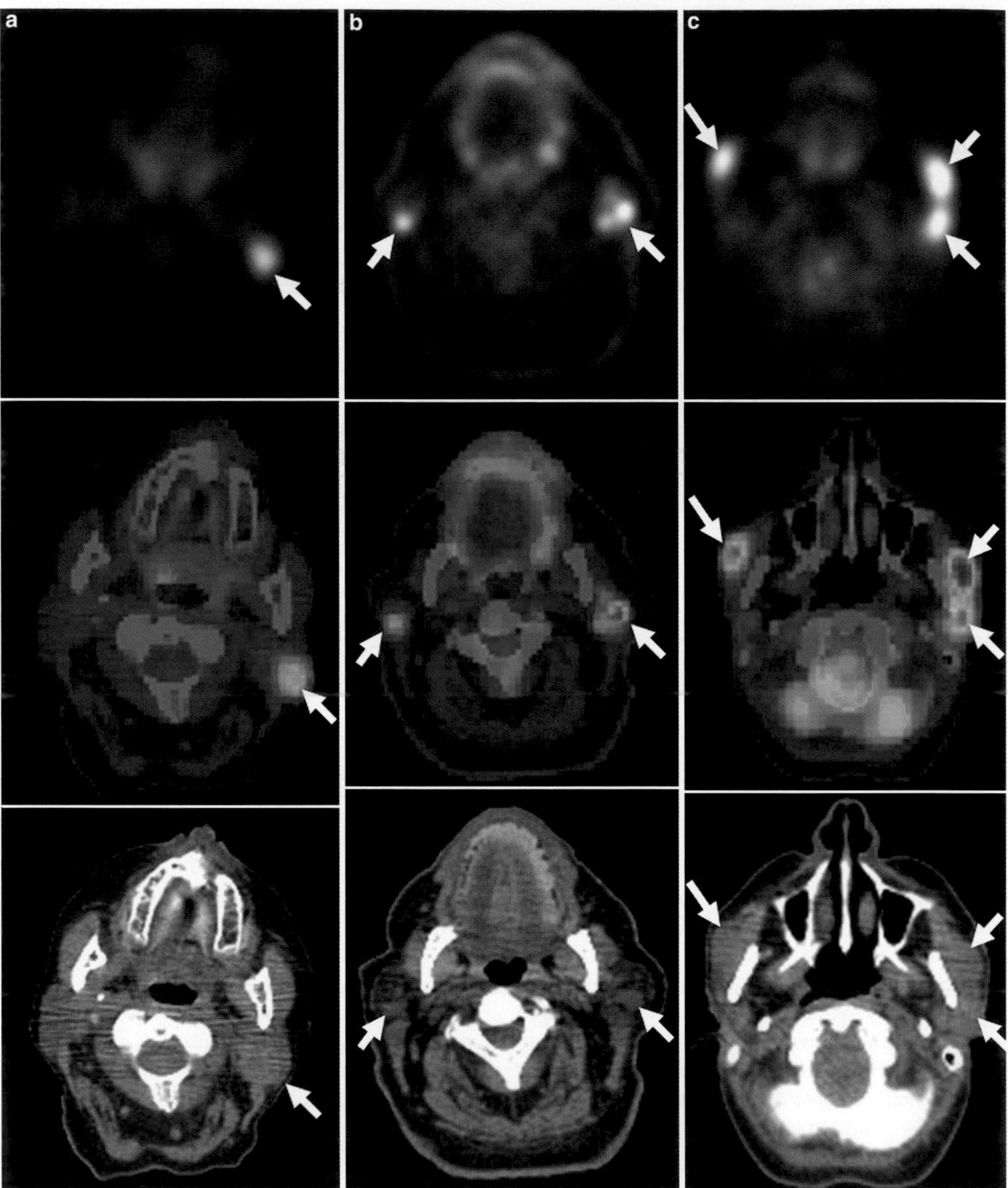

Fig. 9 Benign neoplastic–Warthin's tumors versus malignancy. **a** Seventy-five year-old woman with metastatic lung cancer and a 2 cm FDG avid mass in the superficial left parotid gland on PET-CT (*arrows*). This was resected and found to be a benign Warthin's tumor. **b** 76-year-old man with metastatic lung cancer and multiple bilateral FDG-avid masses in the parotid glands (*arrows*). The largest left intra-parotid mass was biopsied and shown to be benign Warthin's tumor. **c** 78-year-old woman with history of MALT lymphoma and bilateral FDG-avid masses in the parotid glands (*arrows*). Note how the parotids can variably extend anteriorly, which was confirmed on MRI in this patient (not shown). Biopsy showed MALT lymphoma in intra-parotid lymph nodes. There is no reliable way to tell the difference between benign and malignant FDG-avid solid parotid masses on imaging. For clear diagnosis biopsy and often surgical resection is required

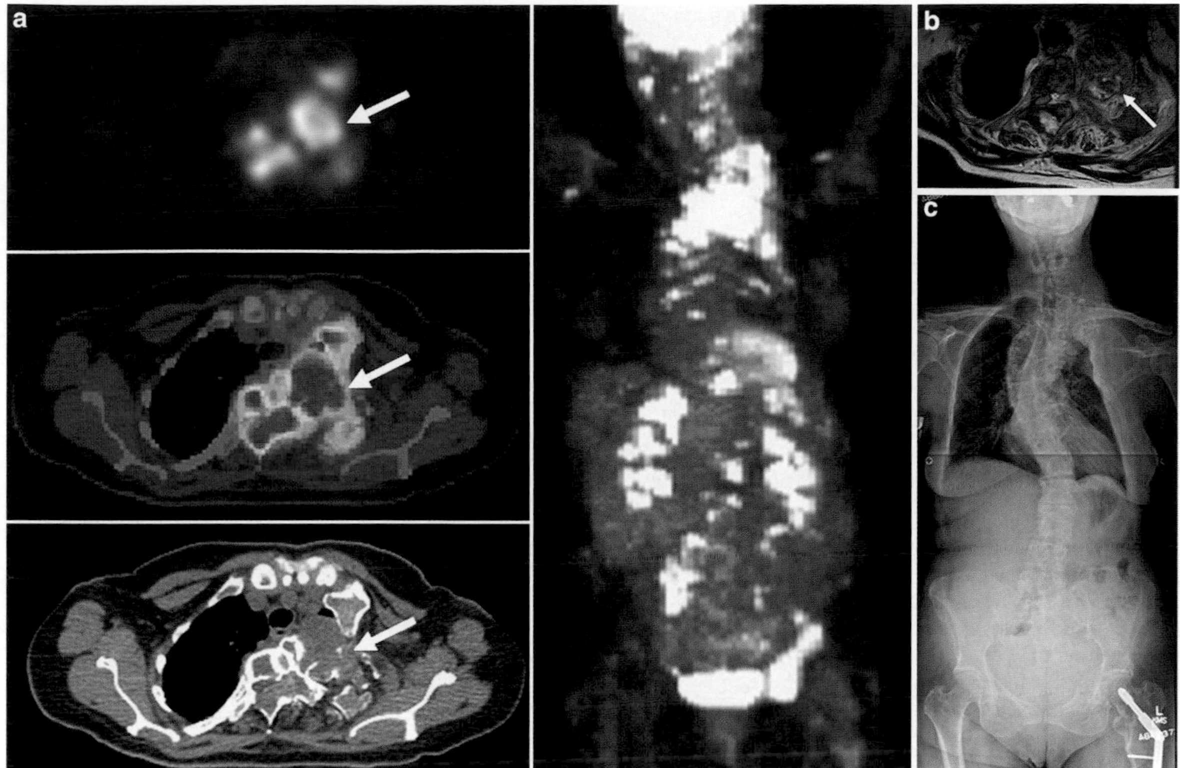

Fig. 10 Benign neoplastic-fibrous displasia pitfall. Fifty-three year-old woman with McCune-Albright syndrome and chronic Polyostotic fibrous dysplasia. **a** PET-CT shows multiple intensely FDG avid partially exophytic expansile skeletal masses (*arrows*). **b** Axial T2-weighted MRI shows the same exophitic tumors with mixed signal characteristics (*arrow*). **c** Whole spine radiograph shows secondary severe scoliosis

brown fat display a pattern of symmetric activity in the bilateral supraclavicular fat elongated along fat plains (Cohade et al. 2003) (Fig. 5) with additional sites of FDG activity in the mediastinal, paraspinal, or even abdominal fat. It is uncommon to see brown fat activity outside of the supraclavicular neck in the absence of bilateral supraclavicular brown fat activity (Fig. 5). Activation of brown fat can be avoided, or at least minimized by proper patient preparation. Brown fat appears FDG active most commonly in young, thin, female patients, and is induced by exposure to cold temperatures prior to and during radiotracer uptake (Ouellet et al. 2010). Keeping patients warm before and during uptake time is the most effective method for reducing brown fat activity. Diazepam also appears to reduce brown fat activity (Garcia et al. 2004).

The gastrointestinal tract has widely variable normal FDG activity (Figs. 6, 7, 8). The true causes of this normal physiologic activity are a subject of debate (Cook et al. 1996). Possible etiologies include peristaltic muscle activity, mucosal cell activity, lymphocyte activity, excretion of FDG into the GI lumen, or activity within bacteria. Methods to reduce GI activity have not been very successful. The most common sites of activity include the distal esophagus through the proximal stomach (Fig. 6) (Koga et al. 2003), cecum (Fig. 7) and rectum (Fig. 8).

Another common pitfall is normal cyclic FDG activity in the ovaries and endometrium in women of childbearing age (Liu 2009a, b). A normal ovarian corpus leutium cyst shows moderate FDG activity. Normal endometrium can show moderate FDG activity during menstruation.

FDG activity in the breast is highly variable, especially in premenopausal women, or women on hormone replacement therapy (Beatty et al. 2009). Lactating breasts are intensely FDG avid and make

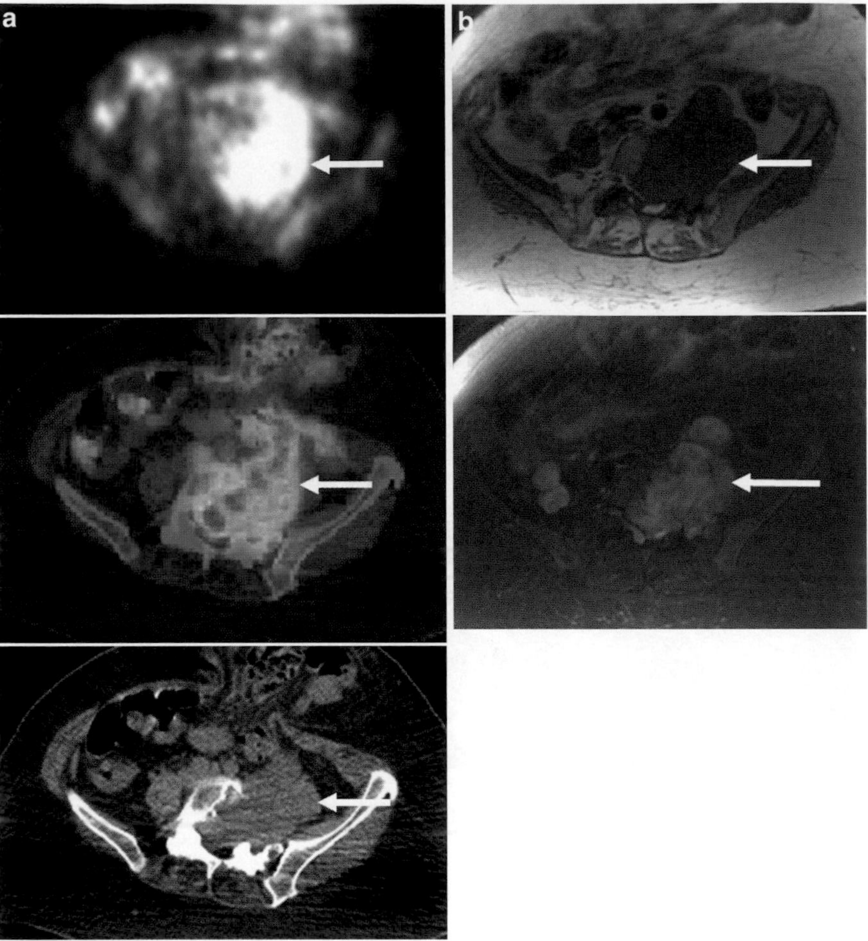

Fig. 11 Benign neoplastic-neurofibroma pitfall. Sixty year-old female with multiple masses along nerves in the sacrum that were stable in size over 5 years in this patient with neurofibromatosis. **a** Note the variable FDG uptake, from mild to intense (*arrows*). Widely variable FDG activity is common in benign neurofibromas. PET-CT alone often cannot differentiate between benign and malignant neurofibromas. Schwannomas by comparison tend to have mild FDG activity. **b** MRI of the same patient: axial T1-weighted (*top*) and T2-weighted images (*bottom*) with fat saturation. The lesion is depicted as hypointensity on T1-weighted and somewhat heterogeneous hyperintensity on T2-weighted image. Incidental ventral hernia is noted

PET/CT very insensitive to malignancy. Normal breast activity is usually diffuse or patchy within the glandular portions of the breasts, as opposed to focal activity within cancer. In post-menopausal women, the tissue immediately subjacent to the areola is normally mildly to moderately FDG avid. However, in the same population hormone replacement will increase the FDG activity, and on sequential PET/CT scans this change can appear to represent the development of bilateral breast cancer.

If a patient has undergone strenuous exercise or must move with altered mechanics in the 24–48 h prior to a PET/CT, FDG activity can be seen in normal muscles (Cook et al. 1996). The activity is often in multiple related muscle groups and is slightly elongated or linear down the muscle fibers as opposed to intense and round. These characteristics are best assessed on the PET rotating MIP images.

Normal moderate FDG activity is variably seen in the conus of the spinal cord, and can be confused with central nervous system drop metastasis or cord malignancy. This pitfall can be even more confusing as the normal conus is often slightly bulbous on CT.

1.4 Anatomic Variations

Anatomic variations, both normal and abnormal, can and do lead to interpretation errors. Several classic examples relate to urine, which is intensely FDG avid. Normal variation in the luminal diameter of the ureters can be mistaken for metastatic lymph nodes. Key to avoiding this pitfall is to note the elongation of activity in the cranial caudal direction on the MIP images. Duplicated collecting systems, bladder diverticula, and transurethral resection of prostate

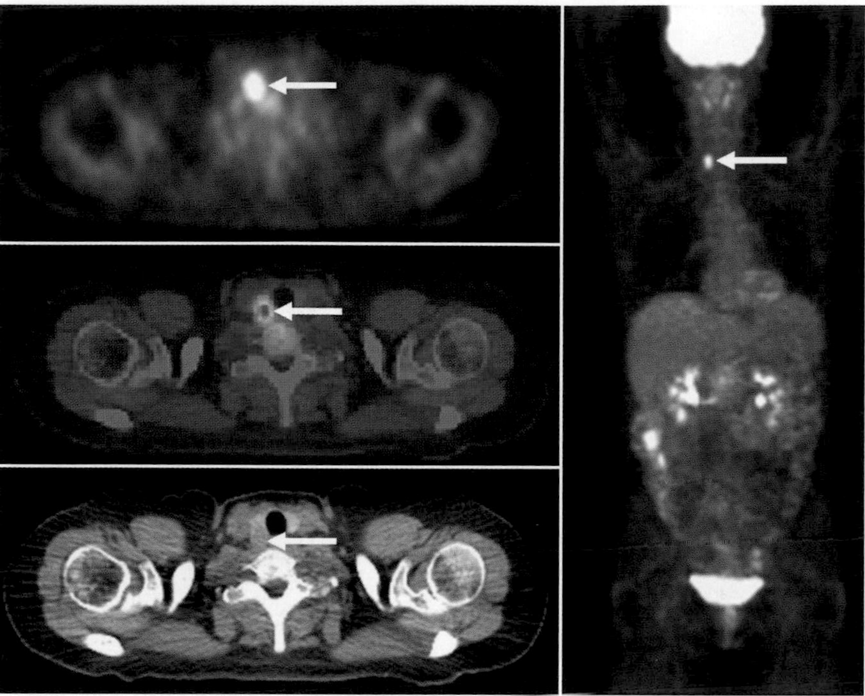

Fig. 12 Benign neoplastic-thyroid adenoma. Thirty-nine year-old woman with history of recurrent pancreatic cancer. Low density mass in left thyroid lobe with intense FDG (*arrows*), stable over several PET-CT scans. Such FDG activity can be seen with adenomas, such as follicular adenoma

(TURP) defects filled with urine are other common pitfalls. Attempts to minimize urine related pitfalls, such as flushing out the urine with furosimide, have not proven very effective at reducing urine activity, and often cause bladder discomfort.

Salivary glands show moderate to intense FDG activity normally. Symmetry cannot be relied on to differentiate a normal salivary gland from a neck lymph node. Not infrequently submandibular glands are markedly asymmetric in size. These glands are also often removed during head and neck surgery.

1.5 Neoplastic

As exemplified by numerous case reports, many nonmalignant neoplasms can have FDG activity, and a handful can occasionally have intense activity. Therefore, the use of PET to evaluate some tumors can actually lower confidence in the benign diagnosis favored on other imaging, perhaps appropriately. Examples of such tumors are Warthin tumors, meningiomas (Lee et al. 2009), uterine leiomyomas (Nishizawa et al. 2008), adenomas of various origins, oncocytomas, fibrous dysplasia, and neurofibromas (Figs. 9, 10, 11, 12).

Warthin tumors of the parotid glands usually have intense FDG activity and therefore can be completely indistinguishable from a malignant parotid mass on imaging (Fig. 9). This is further complicated by the lack of confidence many pathologists have for the diagnosis of parotid tumors based on fine needle aspiration or even core needle biopsy. Some otorhinolaryngologists suggest the only way to accurately diagnose a parotid mass is with surgical resection.

There is wide overlap in FDG activity between benign and malignant thyroid tumors (Fig. 12) (Bogsrud et al. 2007). More diffuse FDG activity in the thyroid is common, and is usually benign, due to conditions such as chronic lymphocytic (Hashimoto) thyroiditis (Karantanis et al. 2007a, b) and Graves disease (Chen et al. 2007).

Meningiomas are common, even in cancer patients, and occasionally even benign meningiomas are intensely FDG active. Follow-up imaging to insure stability, or even surgical biopsy may be needed to confirm the diagnosis.

Renal cell carcinoma and oncocytoma are common and usually cannot be differentiated on anatomic imaging or FDG PET, with both showing low to moderate FDG activity (Blake et al. 2006). Furthermore, renal cell carcinoma and oncocytoma are most

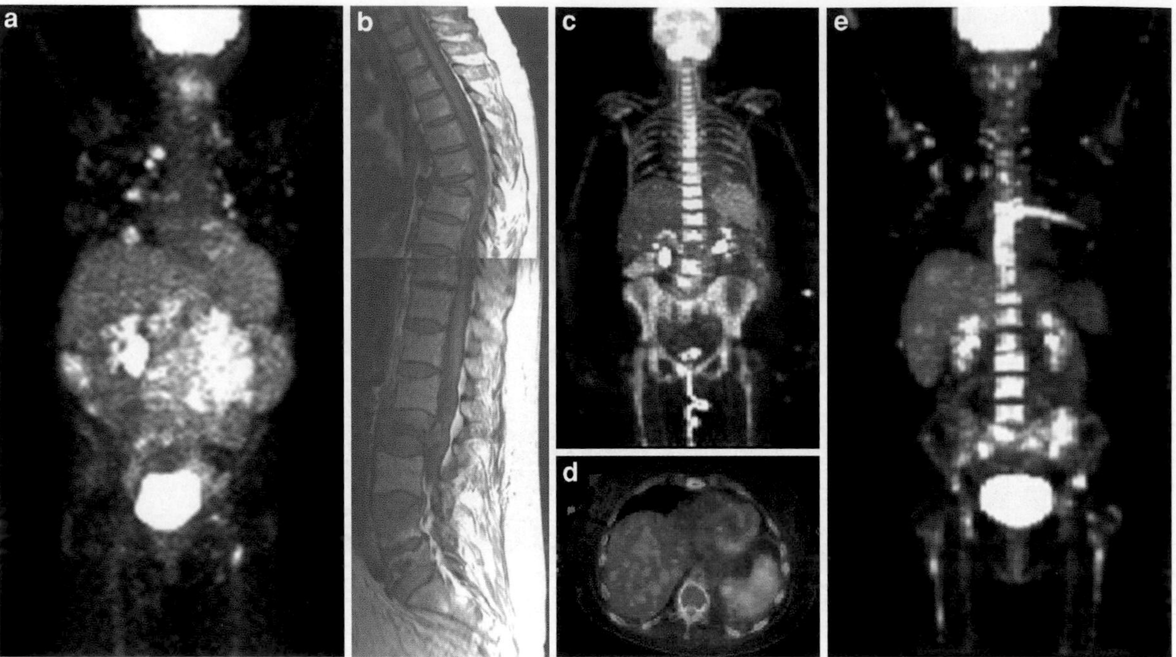

Fig. 13 Neutrophil stimulation therapy versus malignancy. **a** Sixty-six year-old woman with diffuse FDG-avid grade 1 follicular lymphoma in lymph nodes, mesentery, and spleen seen on MIP images of PET data from attenuation-corrected PET-CT, and normal bone marrow FDG activity. Subsequent R-CHOP chemotherapy was complicated by neutropenic fevers after cycle one, resulting in hospitalization. Granulocyte-Colony Stimulating Factor (CSF, Neulasta) was given prophylactically with the second cycle of R-CHOP. **b** Sagittal T1-weighted MRI of the thoracic and lumbar spine confirms lack of bony malignancy. Spinal surgeries for compression fracture and cord compression also resulted in pathologic samples showing osteopenic fractures and lack of marrow malignancy. **b** Sagittal T1 MRI of the thoracic and lumbar spine confirms lack of bony malignancy. Spinal surgeries also resulted in pathologic samples showing osteopenic fractures and lack of marrow malignancy. **c**, **d** Early follow up PET-CT only 8 days after R-CHOP with Neulasta shows apparent dramatic response with reduction in FDG activity of the systemic lymphomatous lymphadenopathy. Also seen is marked diffuse increase in bone marrow and splenic FDG activity (also note Foley catheter, arrow). Dramatic diffuse increase in bone marrow FDG activity, and to a lesser degree splenic FDG activity is common after granulocyte or granulocyte–macrophage colony stimulating factor (CSF) types of medications (such as Neulasta). Generally 4 weeks are required for marrow FDG activity to return to normal. CSF medications are commonly used to boost the neutrophil levels in patients who would otherwise have bone marrow suppression from chemotherapy. Generally bone marrow and splenic activity are considered abnormal if higher than that seen in the liver. When there is high FDG activity diffusely throughout the marrow, it acts as a sink, and tumors present on the scan will have SUV values that are lower then they would be otherwise. Therefore, this scan is non-diagnostic as the patient may be hiding FDG-avid cancer. This diffuse marrow FDG activity also mimics what can be seen with diffuse marrow malignancy and a careful history can be key to the differentiation. **e** For comparison, a 44-year-old female with breast cancer that is diffusely metastatic to the bone marrow. Note there is more heterogeneity in the marrow FDG activity and extension into at least one rib, but these clues for malignancy are not always present

often slow growing. PET/CT is really only helpful for identifying distant metastases.

Uterine leiomyomas, also known as fibroids, are extremely common, and can on occasion have intense FDG activity in pre-menopausal women (Nishizawa et al. 2008). More confusing is the ability of benign leiomyomas to change FDG activity between scans.

Adenomas in general have moderate to intense FDG activity, such as thyroid (Fig. 12; King et al. 2007), parathyroid (Bogsrud et al. 2007; Kim et al. 2009), adrenal (Nunes et al. 2010), and gastrointestinal adenomas (Gollub et al. 2007). Adrenal masses can generally be called benign if less FDG avid than the liver. Focal thyroid FDG activity should lead to ultrasound guided biopsy. Focal FDG activity in the gastrointestinal tract can be normal or represent an adenoma or malignancy, and should prompt either visualization via endoscopy, or repeat PET (Figs. 6, 7, 8).

Hibernomas represent uncommon benign neoplastic tumors of brown fat. Hibernomas are intensely

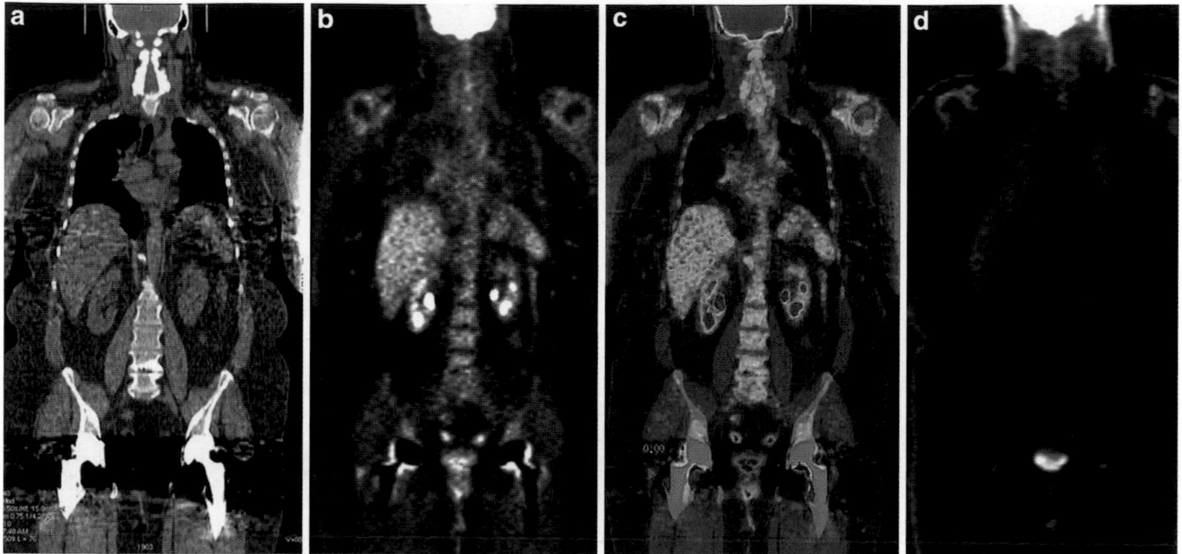

Fig. 14 Misattenuation artifacts-metal misattenuation artifact. Sixty-nine year-old referred to rule out occult malignancy. Coronal CT shows extensive beam hardening artifact from the patients bilateral hip replacements (**a**). On coronal PET and fused PET/CT images (**b**, **c**), increased uptake is noted around the arthroplasties (*arrows*) due to misattenuation artifact. On the non-attenuation correction image (**d**), no significant increased uptake is noted, confirming this artifact

FDG avid (Subramaniam et al. 2007), and are non-responsive to diazepam, warming blankets, or other methods of reducing brown fat activity. Hibernomas tend to have much higher FDG activity than the low grade liposarcomas they resemble on CT and MRI imaging (Tsuchiya et al. 2006).

1.6 Hematopoietic

Chronic severe anemia, such as is seen with thalassemia, can result in expansion of normal bone marrow FDG activity into the appendicular skeleton. Less commonly chronic anemia or systemic conditions that displace bone marrow, such as medullary fibrosis, can result in moderately FDG-avid mass-like extramedullary hematopoiesis.

1.7 Drug Related

Abnormally high diffuse bone marrow FDG activity (greater than liver activity) is commonly seen in patients who have recently received granulocyte or granulocyte–macrophage colony stimulating factors (GCSF, Fig. 13) (Kazama et al. 2005). This appearance closely mimics diffuse marrow malignancy. CSF can also, on occasion, cause increased splenic FDG activity (Sugawara et al. 1999), which mimics lymphoma. CSF is usually given shortly after finishing a cycle of chemotherapy to lower neutrophil counts. Therefore, a delay of 4 weeks between CSF therapy and PET imaging is recommended (Kazama et al. 2005), but 5 days may be sufficient (Hollinger et al. 1998). Rebounding bone marrow in response to the suppressive effects of chemotherapy itself can increase FDG activity, but tends to not be as severe as with CSF therapy. If the marrow activity is more variable with relative hot spots, one should consider marrow malignancy as more likely (Fig. 13).

Anemia is often a side effect of malignancy and/or chemotherapy, and bone marrow ramps up output of erythrocytes in response to this acute anemic state. However, even when severe, anemia as a result of chemotherapy rarely causes intense marrow FDG activity. Even the use of erythropoietin type medications to increase the marrow production of red blood cells does not tend to result in marrow FDG activity levels high enough to be confused with malignancy. However, there are some reports in the literature where erythropoietin has caused a potential pitfall (Blodgett et al. 2004).

Thymic "rebound" is commonly seen after completion of chemotherapy, thought to be the result of

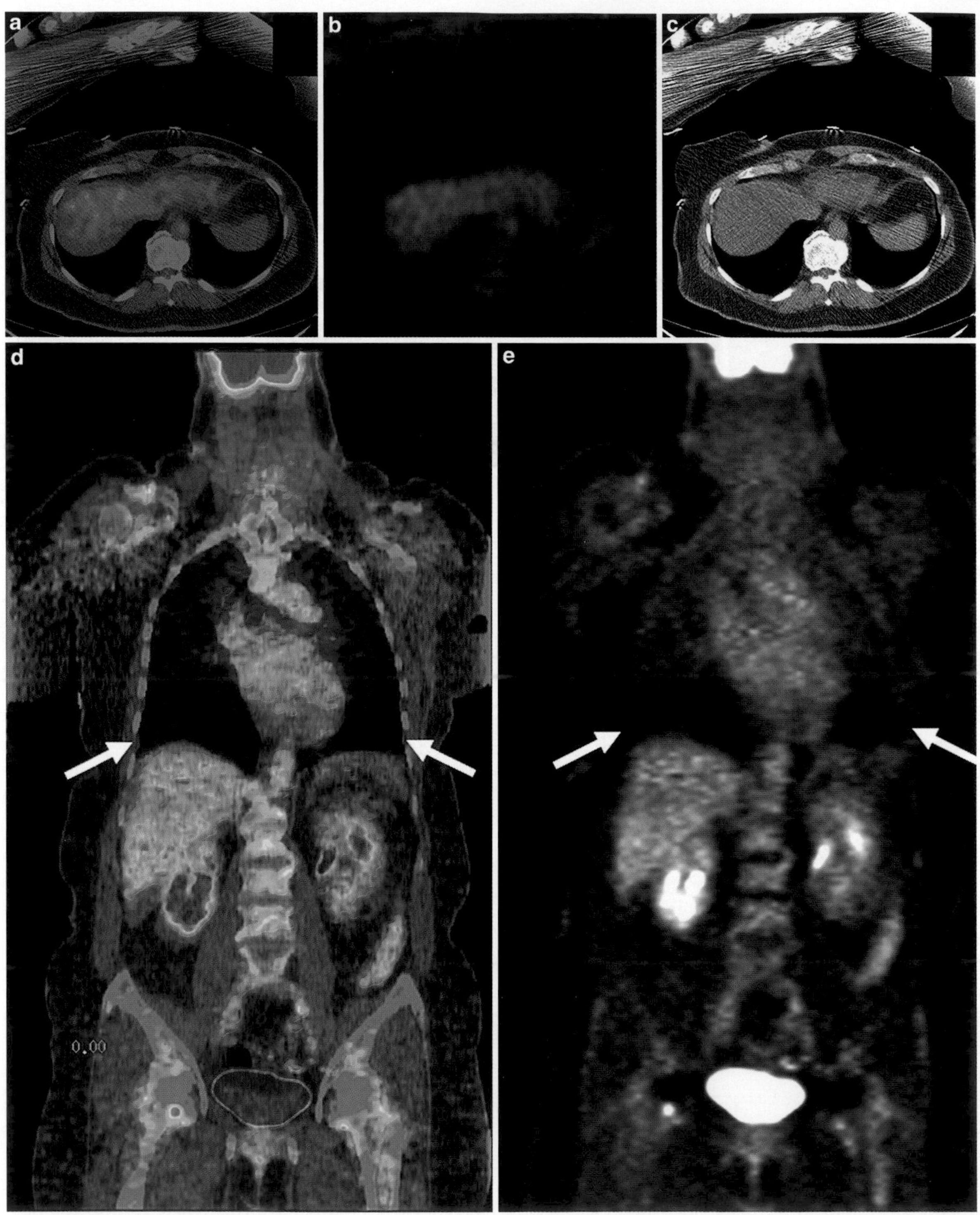

the body's attempt to replenish T cells lost as a result of chemotherapy. In adults, rebounding thymic tissue often forms a round mass and has moderate to intense FDG activity. Hyperplastic thymic tissue can even, on occasion, extend into the superior mediastinum and neck, causing confusion (Smith et al. 2007; Fallanca

◂**Fig. 15** Misattenuation artifacts-arm positioning misattenuation artifact. Sixty-one year-old referred for breast cancer restaging. As this patient was unable to place her arms above her head (**a**–**c**), there is significant misattenuation with relative photopenia involving the upper abdomen and lung bases, best appreciated on the coronal reformatted PET/CT and PET images (*arrows*, **d** and **e**). This example demonstrates the difficulty with misattenuation due to arm position. In this patient, the severity of this artifact could have been lessened by having the patient imaged with the arms straight down at her side rather than laid across the abdomen

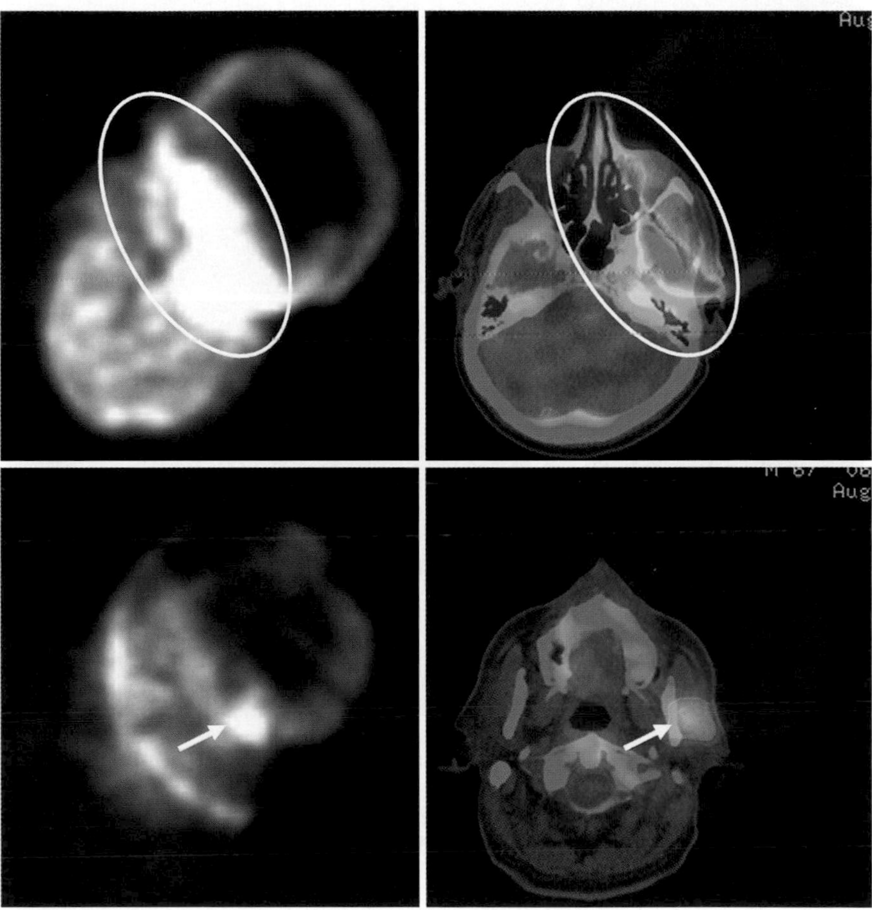

Fig. 16 Motion Artifacts-Gross Patient Motion Artifact. Seventy-two year-old for rectal cancer restaging who moved his head during the PET acquisition. Note that this results in falsely elevated SUV on the left half on the head and neck (circles). Failure to note this motion may result in incorrect identification of a hypermetabolic focus in the left masseter (arrows)

et al. 2008). Some have gone so far as to recommend biopsy confirmation of any possible malignant recurrence in the anterior mediastinum seen on PET (Levine et al. 2006). The general principle of comparison to the initial pretreatment PET scan is helpful, as the vast majority of recurrent malignancies occur in sites of previously FDG-avid malignancy.

In addition to false positive pitfalls related to drugs, there are false negative studies related to the FDG sink effect, where FDG is pulled away from tumors, artificially lowering the tumor activity. This occurs when insulin is active, either after injection or when secreted in response to eating. Insulin pushes FDG into the muscles leaving little FDG available for tumors (Figs. 21, 22, 23). The same sink effect occurs when the bone marrow is diffusely activated by CSF (Chhabra et al. 2006) (Fig. 13). All of these issues should be prevented when possible, and if identified on a study, PET might need to be repeated.

If the patient is scanned too soon after a chemotherapy dose is given, the FDG activity in a malignant tumor can be falsely lowered. In general the best time to image is at least 4–6 weeks after a dose of chemotherapy, or just prior to the next dose of chemotherapy (Glazer et al. 2010), but this may depend on the particular cancer and chemotherapy used. It is not

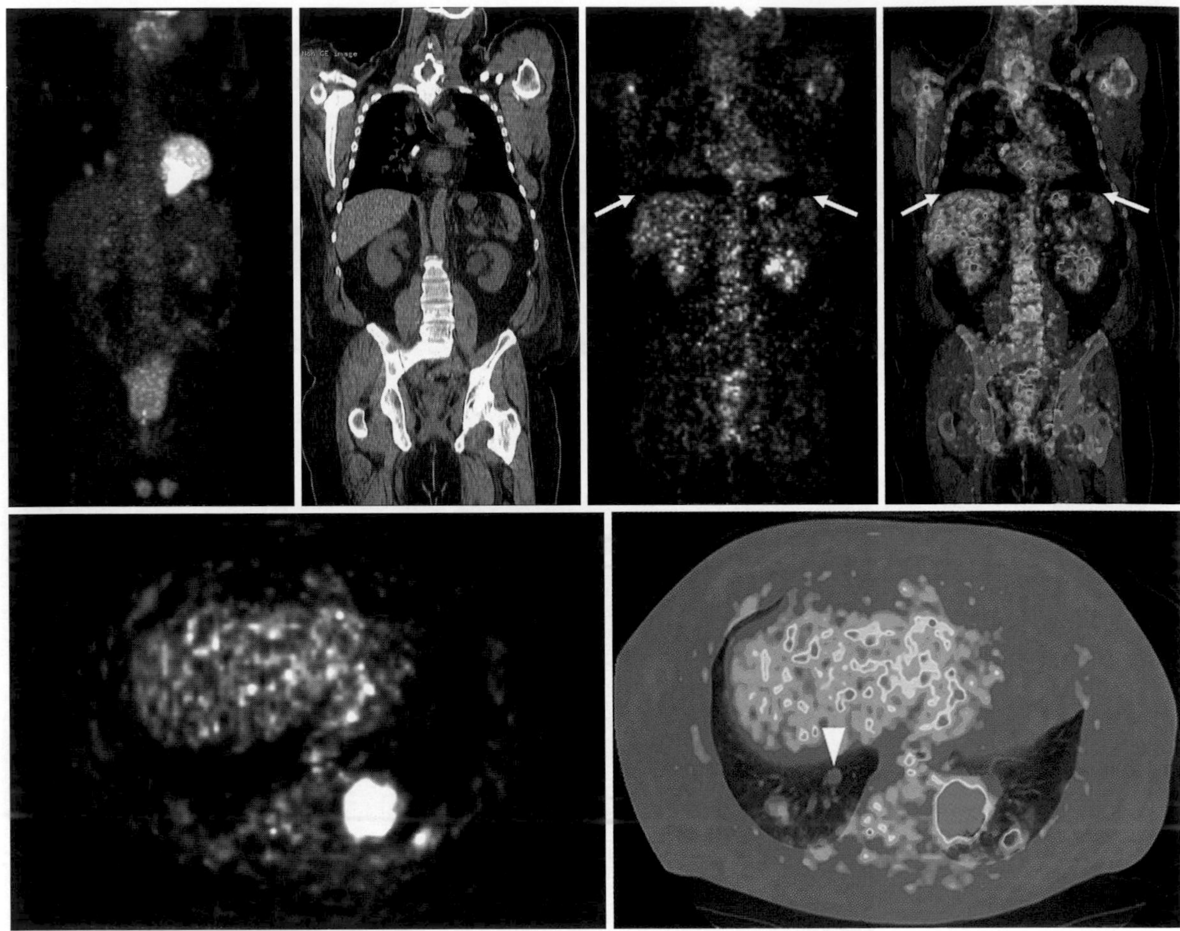

Fig. 17 Motion Artifacts-Respiratory Motion Artifact. Forty - year-old with metastatic colon cancer for restaging. Best noted on the coronal PET and PET/CT images (*arrows*), there is photopenia involving the lung bases from respiratory diaphragm motion artifact ("banana sign"). This artifact can cause falsely lowered SUV in malignant masses of the lung bases. In this patient with multiple pulmonary metastatic nodules, one nodule in the lung base (*arrowhead*) demonstrates no uptake due to this artifact

clear exactly how some tumors can be alive but temporarily FDG inactive immediately after chemotherapy. This concept is referred to as metabolic inhibition (Glazer 2010). Steroids in particular, taken as part of a chemotherapy regimen or for other purposes, can result in complete temporary loss of FDG activity in live tumors.

2 Artifacts

2.1 Attenuation Correction

Without attenuation correction PET images incorrectly show radiotracer activity deep in the body as diminished, and radiotracer near the skin surface as intense (Figs. 14). Using the CT data for the attenuation correction map is advantageous in part because CT is much faster than the older method of using germanium rods, resulting in improved patient comfort (Fanti et al. 2005). This improved speed is achieved because the X-ray tube within the CT can generate far more photons per time than germanium rods. However, attenuation correction artifacts are created by differences in how lower energy X-ray photons from the X-ray tube of the CT scanner and higher energy annihilation photons from radiotracer positron annihilation within the body are attenuated in the tissues. Annihilation photons from PET radiotracers are 511 keV, whereas CT X-ray tubes emit photons over a spectrum of energies with the highest energy often set around 120 keV.

Photons of different energies behave differently in patients, and are attenuated, or stopped, by different tissues and other materials, such as metals in different amounts. One might think that tissue density, which can be estimated by the CT scan, could be mathematically adjusted to calculate the expected attenuation of annihilation photons created by PET radiotracers. Unfortunately, these mathematical adjustments are imperfect, because factors other than density also affect attenuation, leading to inaccurate attenuation correction (Goerres et al. 2002a, b).

Clinically relevant attenuation artifacts are most commonly related to dense material, such as metal. Metal attenuation artifacts are most commonly encountered in dental amalgam, joint prostheses, and pacemakers. The high density metal in these implants almost completely attenuates the CT photons which causes "beam-hardening" artifacts adjacent to the implant on the CT images (Barrett and Keat 2004). Discordance in attenuation between CT and PET photons leads to falsely elevated PET signal adjacent to the implants, which can be confused with pathologic FDG activity mimicking tumor or infection (Figs. 14). Since this artifact is due to the combination of the PET and the CT data, reviewing the non-attenuation-corrected images will often help to make the distinction (Fig. 14).

While attenuation correction artifacts are most commonly encountered adjacent to metallic implants, any high-density material can cause the artifact. This has led some to suggest that intravenous contrast dye should not be used in PET/CT imaging. However, most consider the attenuation artifact from intravenous contrast to be negligible (Yau et al. 2005), and outweighed by the diagnostic benefit of intravenous contrast in many patients. The beam-hardening artifact from intravenous contrast is particularly prominent at the junction of the subclavian veins with the brachiocephalic veins. Therefore, in patients with possible pathology in the upper mediastinum and lower neck, some recommend injecting the arm that is less likely to cause confusing artifacts on a case-by-case basis. Another alternative is to perform the CT without intravenous contrast as part of the PET/CT, and then repeat the CT with contrast after the PET data is collected.

High-density "oral" gastrointestinal contrast causes significant attenuation correction artifacts throughout the abdomen, resulting in much more of a diagnostic problem than intravenous contrast (Prabhakar et al. 2007). The artifact is most marked when barium is used, as opposed to lower density iodinated oral contrast agents. However, some suggest avoiding positive oral contrast altogether when evaluating patients with potential gastrointestinal pathology. In patients who have received oral barium as part of previous imaging studies, it is good practice to delay PET/CT imaging until this contrast has cleared. Negative oral contrast that simply expands the lumen of the gastrointestinal tract but with a density similar to water is an alternative.

In addition to high-density material, such as metal, iodine, and barium, the patient's own tissues can at times result in attenuation correction artifacts. Significant attenuation correction artifacts can occur when the patient's body is too thick and dense to allow CT photons to transmit all the way through (Fig. 15). This is commonly seen when arms are positioned down next to the torso. In addition to poor attenuation correction, the CT itself provides poorer quality images, reducing the benefit of CT for localization and corroboration of PET findings (Bockisch et al. 2004). The vast majority of PET/CT scans are performed with the arms up and out of the field of view, but rarely arms are down to include known or potential tumor sites. When there is a high likelihood of pathology in the head and neck, dedicated imaging of this region with the arms down may be beneficial to reduce artifacts.

2.2 Motion/Anatomic Misregistration

Anatomic misregistration due to patient movement between the CT and PET acquisitions creates artifacts. Motion artifacts can be caused by gross patient movement or movement associated with normal physiologic activities. Patient movement not only causes misregistration of radiotracer activity related to the CT anatomic images, but also results in attenuation correction artifacts leading to incorrect calculated intensity of activity (Fig. 16). This occurs because misregistration of a focus of radiotracer

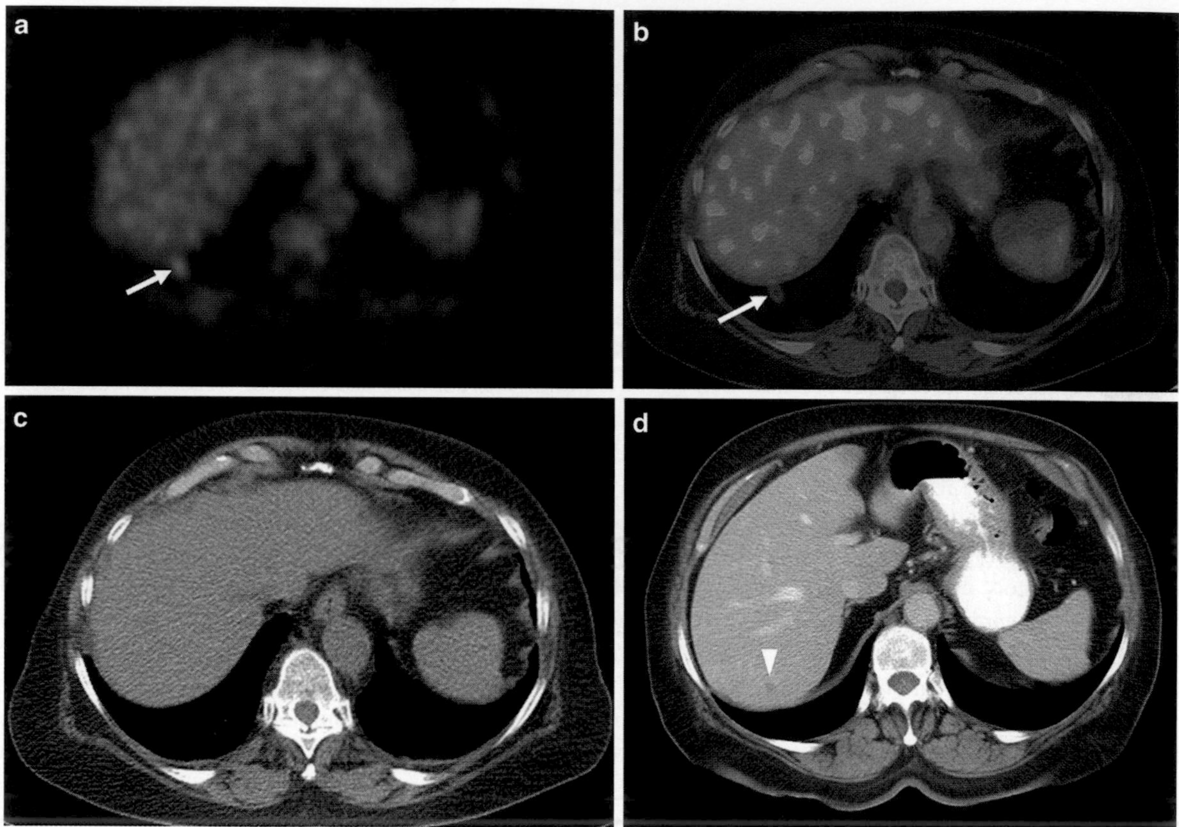

Fig. 18 Motion artifacts-respiratory translation artifact. Sixty-six year-old female for small cell lung cancer restaging has an apparent FDG-avid focus in the right lung base (**a** and **b**, *arrows*). On the non-contrast attenuation correction CT (**c**), no corresponding mass is seen. On the contrast enhanced exam performed the day prior, a metastatic lesion is seen in the hepatic dome (**d**, *arrowhead*). Due to respiratory motion, this mass is falsely translated into the right lung base

activity changes the apparent site of the radiotracer activity on the combined PET/CT images, thus changing the surrounding environment used for attenuation correction by the CT (Goerres et al. 2003; Osman et al. 2003). The end result of motion is that the apparent location and intensity of the radiotracer activity is incorrect, sometimes drastically so.

If motion occurs during the CT acquisition, the CT images may be blurred, and the attenuation map may be affected. If motion occurs during PET acquisition, the resulting images are also blurred, but this may be more difficult to detect. Blurring of PET images as a result of motion effectively reduces the maximum SUV, by spreading the activity over a larger area. Since the SUV_{max} of a tumor can be used to help with diagnosis, prognosis, and evaluation of response to therapy, even subtle motion artifacts during PET scanning can change patient management.

Gross patient motion artifacts can occur when the patient voluntarily or involuntarily moves between the CT and PET acquisitions. This is usually quite easy to recognize, and must be looked for routinely as part of the image quality control prior to every scan interpretation. Many imaging centers require technicians or interpreting physicians to review each PET/CT scan for gross patient motion before the patient leaves. If motion is detected, part or all of the scan may need to be redone. Careful attention to patient comfort and positioning prior to initiating the scan will limit this artifact. Patients are often physically incapable of holding their arms in a given position, and require straps or other fastening devices. Some patients are incapable of cooperating and may require medication for pain, anxiety, or even general anesthesia.

The most common gross patient motion artifacts are caused by movement of the head (Fig. 16). Relaxation

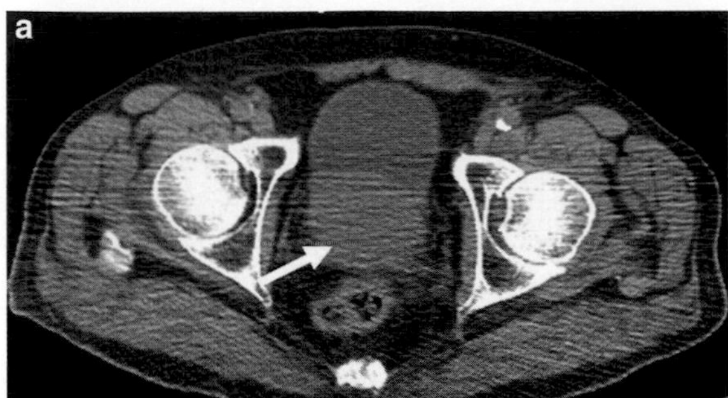

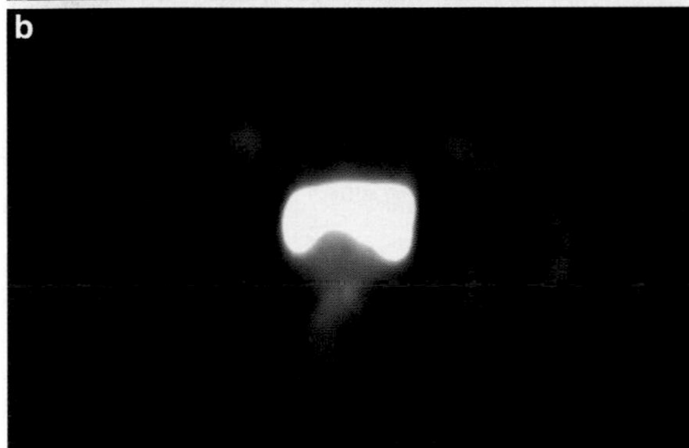

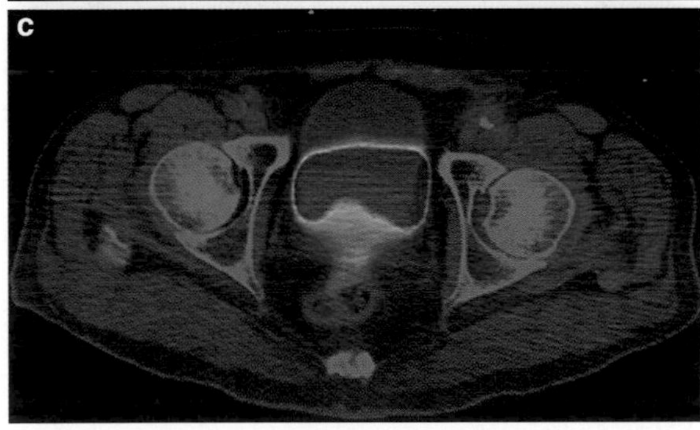

Fig. 19 Motion artifacts-bladder motion artifact. Eighty-two year-old male for lung cancer staging. This patient with marked prostatic enlargement (*arrow*), could not completely empty his bladder prior to CT (**a**) and subsequent PET (**b**) acquisitions. FDG avid urine layers in the posterior portion of an enlarging bladder. Note the disparate bladder size between the two acquisitions which leads to false anatomic coregistration on the fused images (**c**)

of the neck muscles can tilt or rotate the head and neck. This can lead to significant misregistration and attenuation correction artifacts. This type of motion ranges from obvious to very subtle. The resulting artifacts are further complicated by the small size of and short distances between head and neck structures. Unfortunately, head motion can be difficult for the technologist to detect during the course of the exam. Prevention of this artifact with head immobilizers made of foam or vacuum bags is critical, especially when head and neck disease is suspected. One way to check for rotational head motion is by comparing the location of the skin border and mandible on the CT with the radiotracer activity in the belly of the genioglossus muscles (Goerres et al. 2002a, b). The genioglossus muscle bellies almost always have detectable FDG activity and make an upside-down "V" that should reside within the confines of the mandible and skin within the floor of the mouth.

In addition to gross patient movement, normal physiologic motion routinely causes artifacts. Physiologic motion artifacts are always present, but to varying degrees, and are commonly seen with respiration, cardiac contractions, gastrointestinal motility, and bladder filling. Physiologic motion affects the PET acquisition more drastically, since the PET photons must be collected over a much longer period of time. This causes smearing of PET activity over adjacent locations on the CT attenuation correction map. The smeared portions of the PET scan have reduced SUV measurements and also incorrect attenuation correction. Of these types of physiologic motion, respiratory motion most often causes clinically relevant artifacts. Attempts to minimize respiratory motion artifacts have been partially successful, and include shallow breathing during PET acquisition to minimize diaphragmatic excursion, respiratory gating of both PET and CT imaging, and the use of respiration-averaged CT (Pan et al. 2005, 2006).

Respiratory motion artifacts are most pronounced in the lung bases and upper abdomen where the motion covers the greatest distance. This location is also where the relatively dense liver and diaphragm abut the lung, resulting in the greatest secondary attenuation correction artifacts of misregistered radiotracer activity. Respiratory artifacts are often identified as curvilinear photopenic areas on the PET images in the lung bases that parallel the hemi-diaphragms. These photopenic areas have a typical "double banana" appearance on coronal reconstructed images (Osman et al. 2003). If there is a pulmonary nodule within this artifactually photopenic area, it is important to recognize that the SUV will be falsely lowered or even that a malignant nodule may appear to have no radiotracer activity at all (Fig. 17) (Erdi et al. 2004).

In addition to creating artifacts related to lesions in the lung bases, respiratory motion causes artifacts related to lesions in the upper abdomen. Radiotracer-

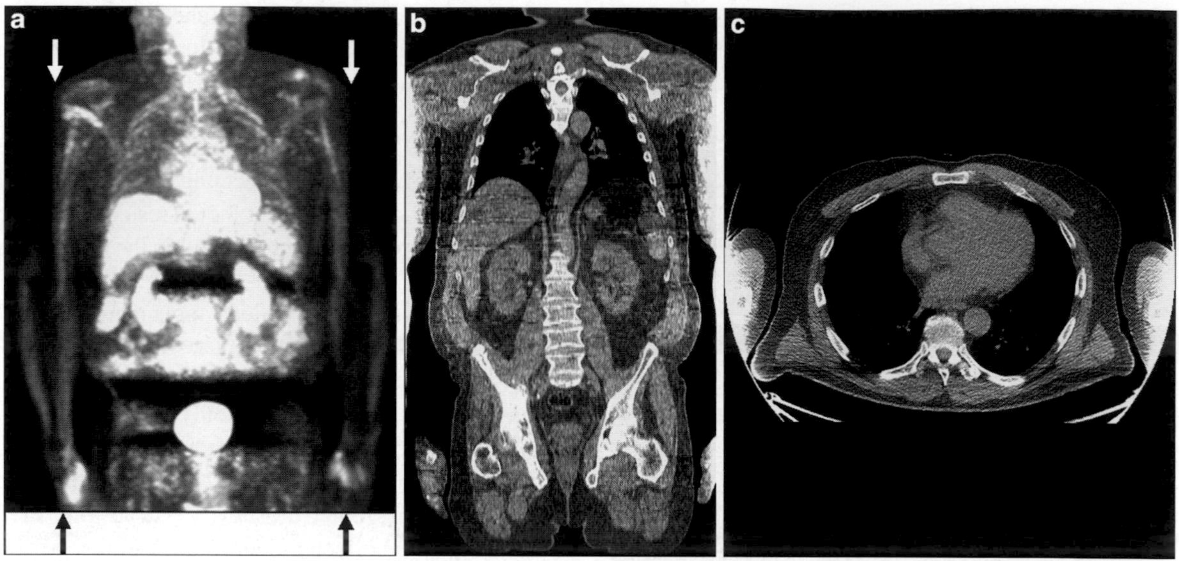

Fig. 20 Truncation artifact. In this larger patient, the CT field of view was set to 50 cm with the PET field of view at 70 cm. The result is truncation artifact on the PET image (**a**) which is seen as linear misattenuation of the lateral aspects of the upper extremities (*arrows*). This is confirmed on the CT images by identifying the "clipping" of the upper extremities which does not allow for any CT information to be available for attenuation correction (**b** and **c**)

avid lesions in the upper abdomen (such as tumors in the dome of the liver) can appear on the combined PET/CT images to be within the lung base, or smeared into the lung base (Fig. 18). If the CT images show a liver lesion and no lung lesion, and the PET images show a focus of radiotracer activity in the lung base just above the liver lesion, one can rightly deduce that the radiotracer activity came from the liver lesion. Adding to the difficulty of interpreting this area of anatomy is that benign lesions in the lung bases are common, and liver radiotracer activity can be misplaced within a benign lung lesion.

The bladder fills with urine during the course of the PET/CT image acquisition. Bladder filling is always present since patients are instructed to come to the exam well hydrated. The bladder should be routinely emptied prior to the initiation of the entire exam, mostly because an overfull bladder leads to patient comfort issues and patient motion. Urine has intense radiotracer activity, because the kidneys excrete FDG rapidly. This intense urine activity makes assessment of activity in surrounding structures very difficult. In addition there are motion artifacts from the significant increase in the size of the bladder between the initial CT acquisition and the subsequent pelvic portion of the PET acquisition, most commonly performed last (Fig. 19). There is no way to accurately measure the activity of low pelvic pathology near the bladder when standard image acquisition is performed, as the intense urine activity is misregistered over the pathology as seen on CT. If pathology is suspected near the bladder, as in patients with a history of prostate or cervical cancer, placement of a bladder catheter to eliminate motion artifact should be considered. Some institutions use a dual lumen catheter with continuous irrigation of the bladder with saline. A flushing catheter not only eliminates motion artifact, but also greatly reduces activity within the bladder. Finally, the image acquisition in patients with pelvic pathology can be done in a caudal to cranial direction to allow for as little bladder expansion and urine radiotracer accumulation as possible (Heiba et al. 2009).

The normal peristaltic activity of the bowel causes motion artifacts. Most of the bowel is also affected by respiratory motion. These two types of physiologic motion can lead to falsely elevated or lowered SUV readings, raising concern for malignancies, or leading to false negative exams (Nakamoto et al. 2004). Bowel paralysis with glucagon can be used to minimize artifacts from peristalsis. However, glucagon is not routinely used, perhaps because peristaltic motion artifact is considered to be minor in comparison to variation in bowel radiotracer activity from other

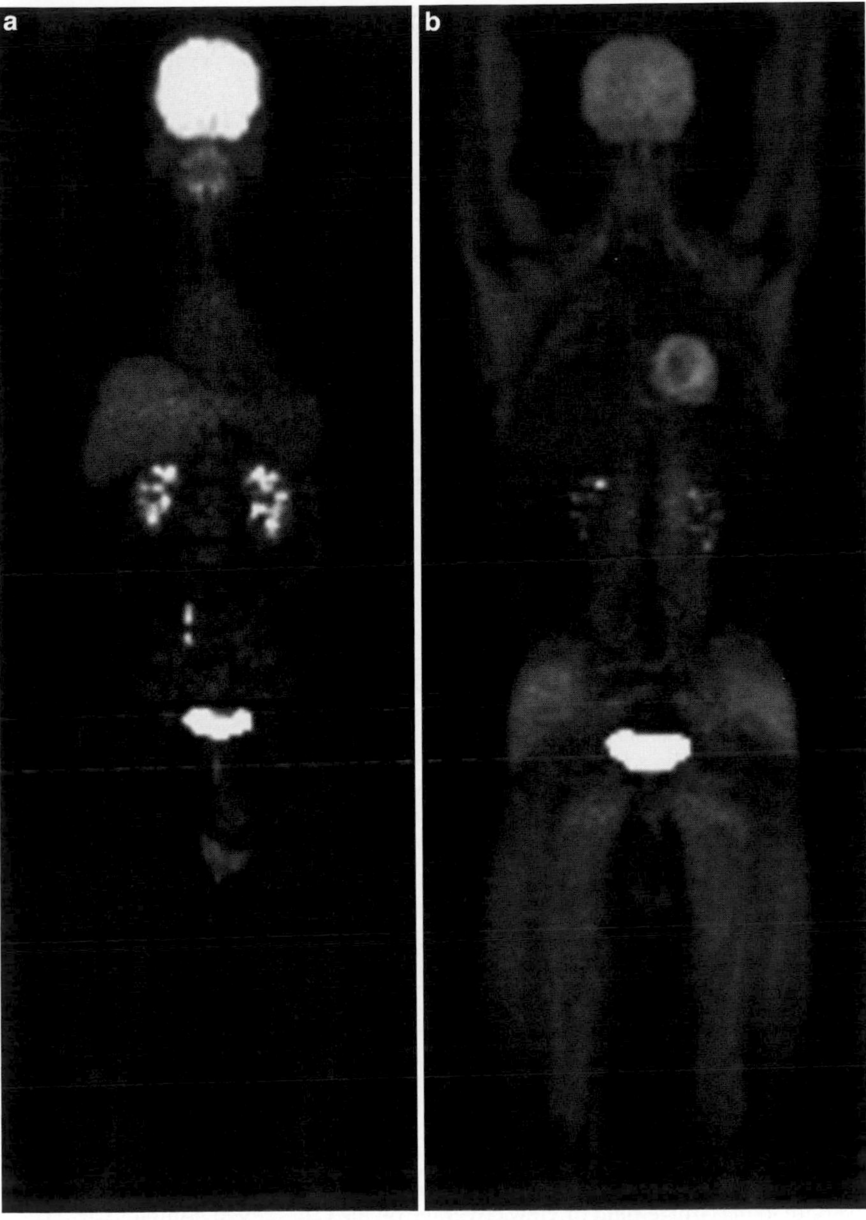

Fig. 21 Glucose related artifacts-non-fasting artifact. Thirty year-old non-diabetic man with a history of metastatic melanoma, currently in remission. **a** PET-CT MIP image showing normal distribution of FDG uptake. **b** PET-CT MIP image showing diffuse intense skeletal muscle FDG activity. Note how the brain, liver, and mediastinal blood pool are markedly lower in FDG activity. One can presume this study would show inaccurately lower FDG activity in any tumor as well, and may even be falsely negative. This patient ate some candy just prior to the exam. When fasting a non-diabetic person can spike their native insulin level in response to sugar, and therefore drive glucose and FDG preferentially into muscle, resulting in a sink effect, even though the measured blood glucose level prior to the exam was normal. Strict fasting for a minimum of 4 h prior to injection is critical (preferably 6 h or more). Note the normal variation of cardiac muscle activity

factors. These other factors derive mainly from respirator motion artifacts in the abdomen and normal physiologic variation in FDG activity in the bowel.

2.3 Truncation

The difference in the diameter of the field of view between the PET (70 cm) and CT (50 cm) exams is an inherent quality of current PET/CT scanner technology. As a result, part of the body can be outside the field of view of the CT, but within the field of view of the PET, causing two types of artifacts, both referred to as truncation artifacts (Fig. 20). One artifact results from no attenuation correction being applied to the portion of the body outside the CT field of view. This causes radiotracer activity to be falsely lowered in the truncated body part outside the CT field of view. The second type of artifact occurs at the edge of, but within, the CT field of view where there can be streak artifacts. Streak artifacts on the CT result in what appears to be extremely dense tissue at the edges of the CT field of

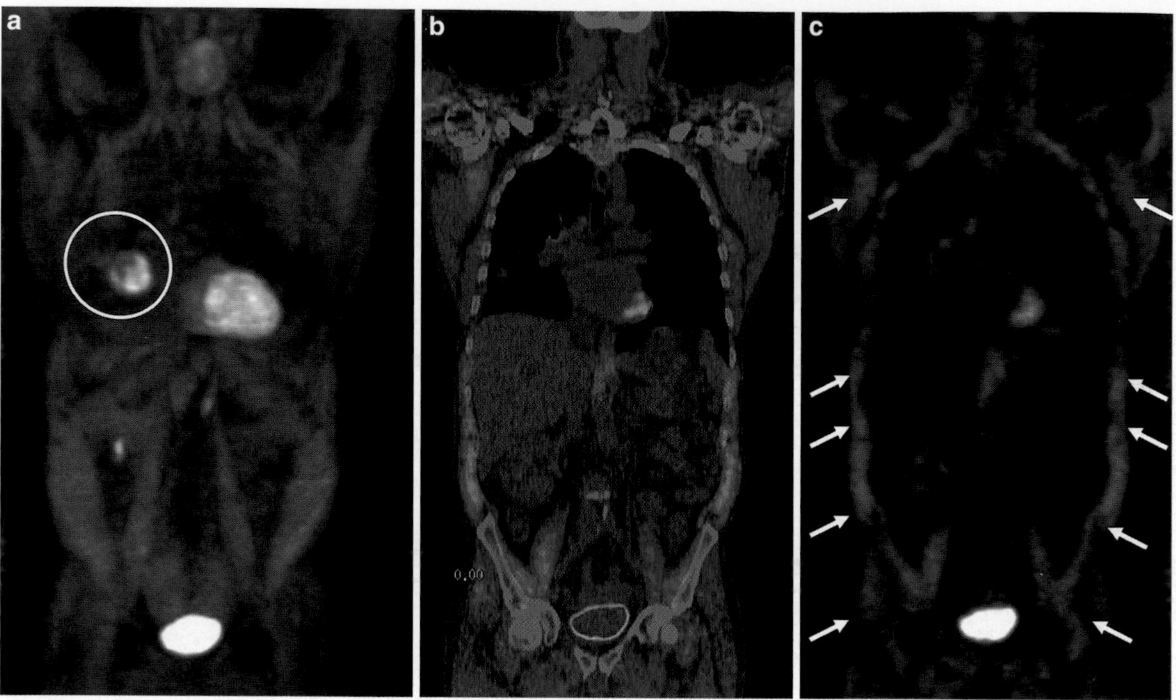

Fig. 22 Glucose related artifacts-hyperinsulinemia artifact. Sixty-six year-old man referred for lung cancer initial staging. This patient, with a history of diabetes, mistakenly took his long acting insulin 2 h prior to this exam. The insulin aggressively drives glucose, and hence the FDG, into the skeletal and cardiac muscle resulting in excessive muscular uptake (*arrows*). While the patient's primary lung neoplasm is still evident (*circle*, **a**), there is essentially no uptake within the mediastinum or hila resulting in a potentially false negative exam (**b** and **c**)

view, which when used for attenuation correction causes falsely elevated radiotracer activity (Sureshbabu and Mawlawi 2005; Mawlawi et al. 2006). Most commonly, truncation artifacts are seen when large patients are scanned with arms down at the side. When possible, the arms should be scanned above the patient's head to minimize this artifact. Careful attention should be made to place the patient in the center of the bore to maximize field of view coverage on the CT. Modern post-processing algorithms can extrapolate the CT to provide attenuation correction for the truncated portion of the PET field of view, which minimizes truncation artifacts (Bockisch et al. 2004).

Another source of artifacts occurs at the cranial and caudal edges of the PET data. Due to the physics of PET photon coincidence detection, the first and the last image in a PET scan are created from very few photons, and have severe quantum model artifacts. As a result, they contain randomly placed false foci of activity, which are not reproducible. Most regard the images as nondiagnostic and ignore any PET findings they contain. However, it remains the convention to include these images in the diagnostic scan.

This same last slice quantum model issue can occasionally result in artifacts in the middle of a series of PET slices due to improper overlap of bed-positions. PET data is collected in multiple bed-positions that overlap. If the PET is performed without proper overlap of the bed-positions, then the same quantum model, or even complete absence of PET data can be seen in the middle of the PET data. This artifact is best detected by looking at the rotating MIP images, as a horizontal line of low or absent PET data can be seen.

2.4 Glucose and Insulin

Severe artifacts can be seen related to glucose intake, insulin activity, hyperglycemia, and diabetes. If not recognized and avoided, these artifacts can render an entire PET/CT nondiagnostic, or falsely negative. Patients are required to fast for at least 4 h, and

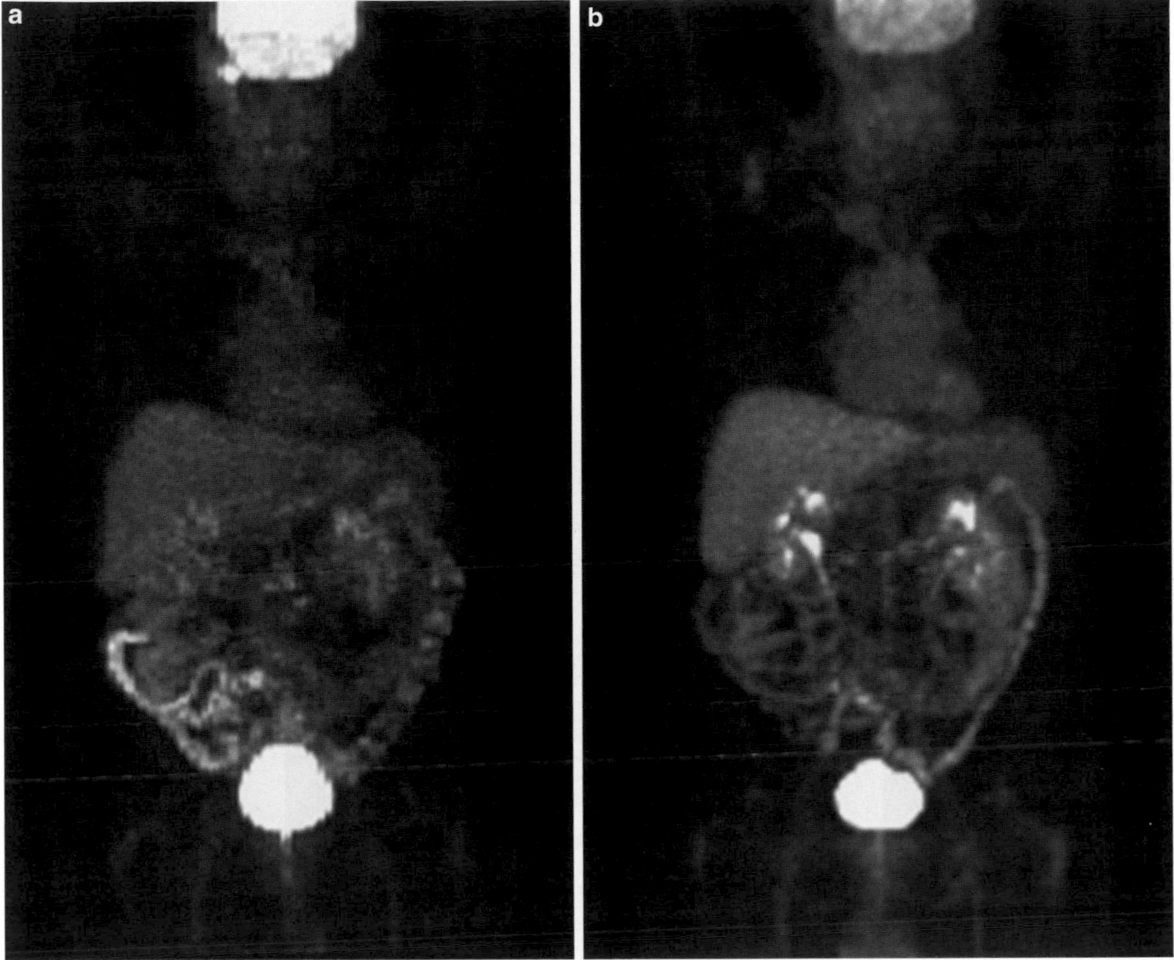

Fig. 23 Glucose related artifacts-hyperglycemia artifact. Sixty-seven year-old diabetic man with a history of metastatic squamous cell cancer. **a** PET-CT MIP image showing normal distribution of FDG uptake, and focal postoperative FDG uptake in the right mastoid bone. **b** PET-CT MIP image showing abnormal distribution of FDG activity, most notably marked decreased activity in the brain, with more normal FDG activity in the mediastinal blood pool and liver. The blood glucose was 100 mg/dl on the first study (**a**) and had jumped to 198 mg/dl on the subsequent follow-up study (**b**). When serum glucose is greater than 150, and especially when greater than 200, it reduces the ability of cells to take up FDG, in part due to competition of glucose with FDG. In non-diabetic patients there is the added complication of driving up insulin and having the muscle behave as an FDG sink (not seen here, presumably because the chronic diabetic patient has muscle tissue that is insulin resistant). Regardless, in the high glucose state a marked decrease in FDG activity is seen in the brain. More critical to the patient, is that tumors also have abnormally low FDG activity, and SUV values are not reliable. In other words, lower than expected brain FDG activity correlates to lower than expected tumor FDG activity and a poor PET scan. Most PET centers test serum glucose in all patients and refuse to do a scan if the serum glucose is greater than 200 mg/dl, and in some cases if it is greater than 150 mg/dl. Some might call this second study (**b**) non-diagnostic

preferably 6 h, prior to PET/CT scanning. This is to make sure that there are low and predictable levels of both glucose and insulin in the blood. Many institutions routinely measure blood glucose just prior to FDG injection. A patient with a serum glucose level above 200 mg/dl typically will not be scanned, as the glucose will significantly reduce FDG activity in any tumor that may be present (Bombardieri et al. 2003) (Fig. 23). Many suggest alerting an interpreting physician if blood glucose is above 150 mg/dl, to decide if the scan should be rescheduled after the glucose level has been reduced. Blood glucose below 150 mg/dl is usually acceptable, and glucose around 100 mg/dl is ideal.

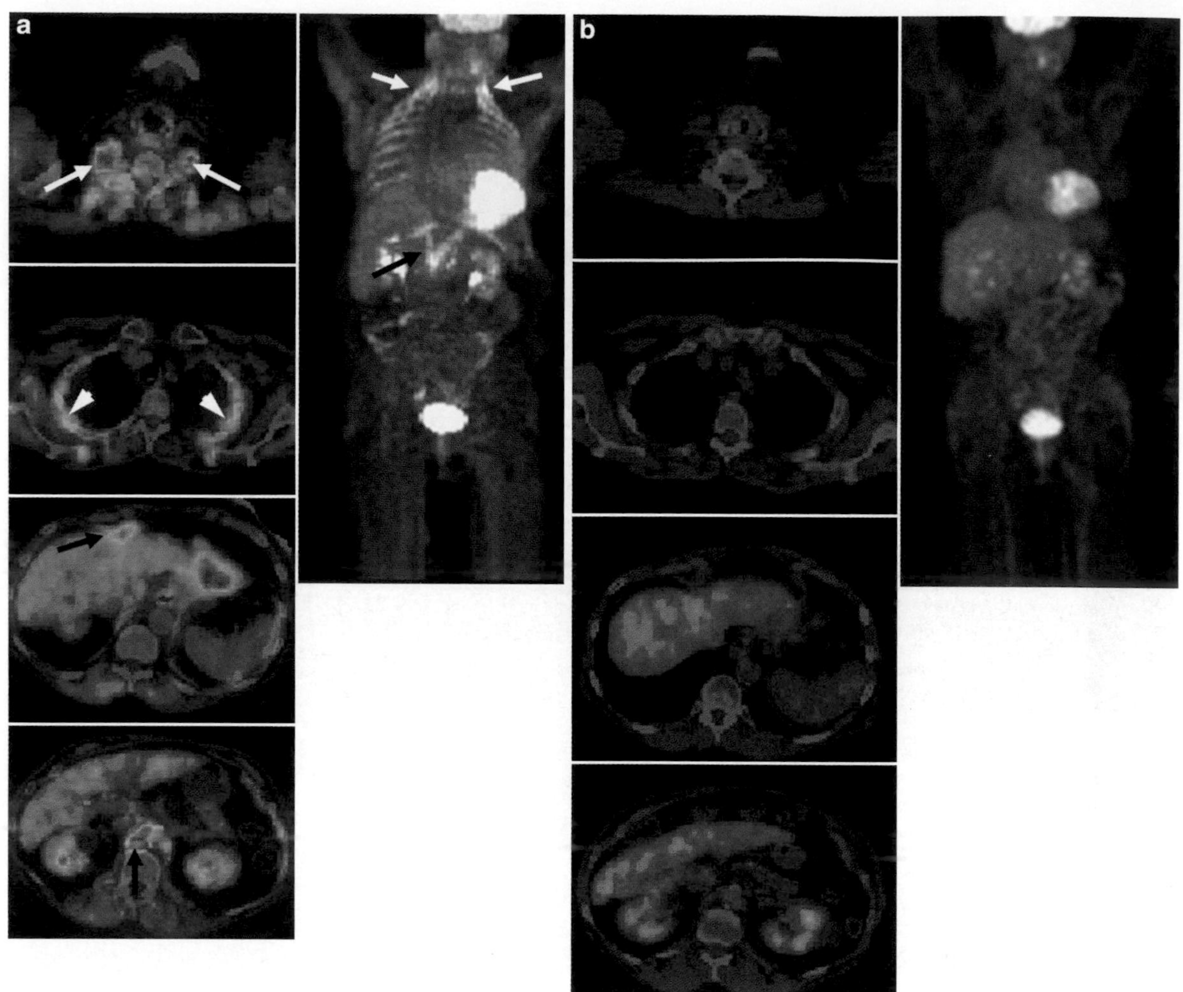

Fig. 24 Uptake phase pitfalls/artifacts-labored breathing pitfall. Seventy-five year-old woman with history of lymphoma, currently in remission, and history of interstitial lung disease, congestive heart failure, and COPD. **a** PET-CT during hypoxemia and new anemia shows intense FDG activity in all of the accessory muscles of breathing, including the middle and anterior scalene (*white arrows*), intercostal (*white arrowheads*), and diaphragm muscles (*black arrows*). Note the scalene, intercostal muscles, and slips of the diaphragm show linear uptake on MIP images. The scalene muscles in the neck, and slips of the diaphragm can be mistaken for masses. The intercostal muscles can be mistaken for bone marrow activity in the ribs. **b** The patient's previous exam, when not actively short of breath, shows normal muscle activity for comparison

Both glucose and insulin dramatically change the biodistribution of FDG in the body. High levels of glucose in the blood directly compete with FDG for entrance into cells through cell membrane glucose transporters (Kapoor et al. 2004). Both FDG and glucose are freely filtered into the renal tubules, but glucose is actively reabsorbed into the blood and FDG is not. Thus FDG is outcompeted by glucose for entry into cells and is preferentially excreted into the urine. The end result of high blood glucose can be very little uptake of FDG within tumors. In addition, when glucose is elevated in non-diabetic patients, there is an expected spike in serum insulin levels. Insulin drives glucose and FDG into the skeletal muscles. This insulin effect causes the muscles to act as an FDG sink, leaving little FDG available for transport into tumor cells. The combination of competition with glucose for transport into tumor cells, preferential urinary excretion of FDG, and systemic muscles acting as a sink, all dramatically reduce tumor FDG activity.

When a non-diabetic fasting patient eats even a small amount of carbohydrate, such as a few cough drops, it

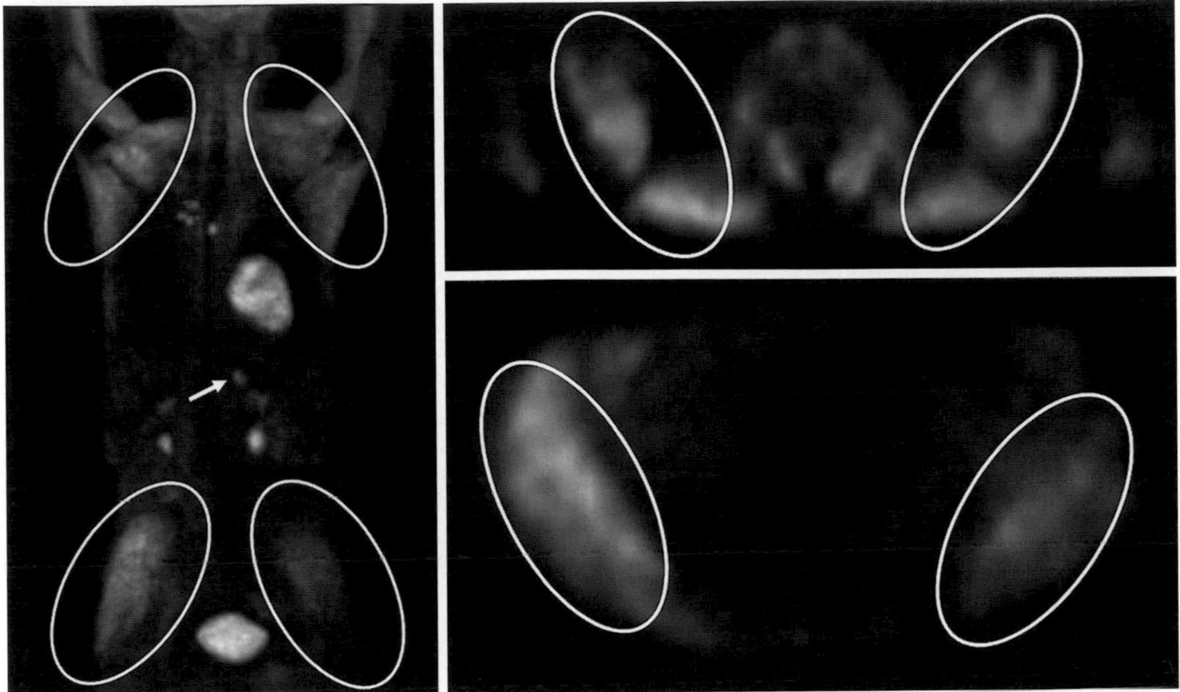

Fig. 25 Uptake phase pitfalls/artifacts-muscle activity artifact. Forty year-old male for non-small cell lung cancer restaging with mediastinal and left adrenal metastases (*arrows*). During the uptake period, prior to imaging, the patient was unable to lay still, resulting in significant diffuse muscular uptake, most prominently around the shoulders and hips (*circles*). This artifact can lead to falsely lowered SUV within the tumor as well as the possibility for missing of other metastatic foci

can cause an insulin spike sufficient to make a PET scan nondiagnostic (Fig. 21). The serum glucose in such a patient may be completely normal, but the insulin is still active, resulting in a PET scan with systemic skeletal muscle activity. Such artifact also results in decreased normal FDG activity in the brain, an obligate glucose user that is not responsive to insulin. The predominant effect is due to insulin, not hyperglycemia in this case. If a non-diabetic patient reports a recent tiny snack, PET scanning should be rescheduled.

If a chronically diabetic patient is hyperglycemic, there may be less insulin effect, as the patient may make little insulin or be resistant to the effects of the insulin present. Therefore, PET may not show significant skeletal muscle uptake, making detection of hyperglycemia artifacts difficult based on subjective interpretation of images alone. Normal brain activity may be reduced, due to competition of FDG with glucose (Fig. 23). Tumor uptake is also reduced or even falsely negative. Hyperglycemia artifacts in diabetic patients are best detected by monitoring serum glucose prior to injection of FDG, and routinely measuring the activity in the brain compared to the liver and mediastinal blood pool. The distribution of FDG in patients with diabetes has been shown to be adequate for accurate diagnosis in patients with blood glucose levels less than 180 mg/ml (Roy et al. 2009).

Controversy continues regarding the administration of insulin prior to FDG injection for patients with hyperglycemia. While the administration of insulin will lower the serum glucose, insulin also will drive FDG into the muscle and away from tumors (Fig. 22). This effect is potentiated by the administration of longer acting insulin preparations. The use of short acting insulin preparations given 2–4 h prior to FDG injection has been suggested to improve overall image quality without resulting in falsely depressed FDG tumor activity in diabetic patients with elevated serum glucose levels.

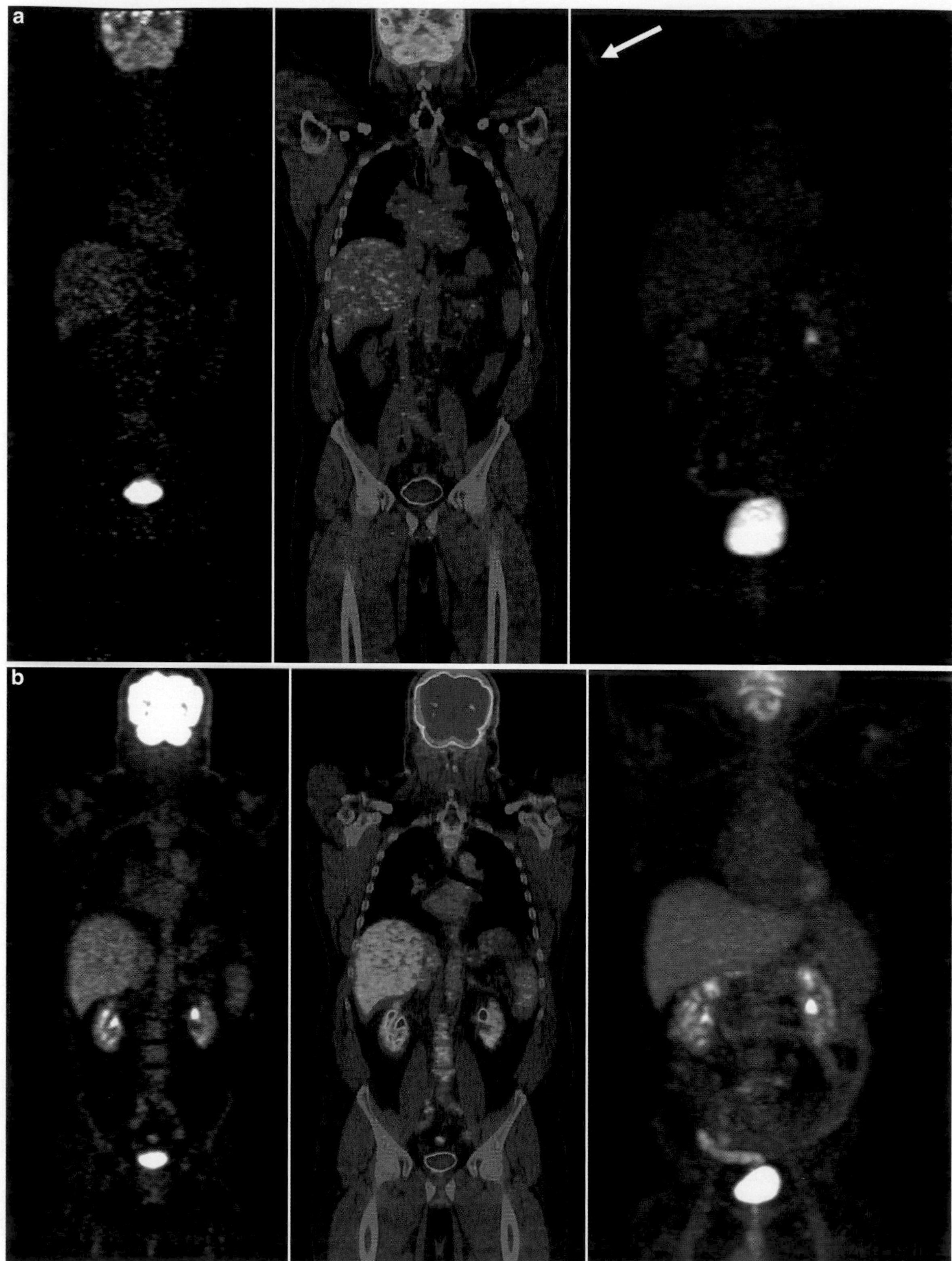
a
b

◀**Fig. 26** Injection artifacts-extravasation Artifact. Fifty-one year-old female for colon cancer restaging who had extravasation of nearly the entire FDG dose in her right antecubital fossa resulting in the markedly "poor count" study on the top row (**a**). Note that while the extravasation site was not imaged, significant uptake in the right upper extremity lymphatic system is seen (*arrow*). On the bottom row (**b**), a repeat exam was performed the next day without extravasation resulting in a normal FDG distribution

2.5 Uptake Phase

There are several key artifacts that can be categorized as related to patient factors during the period of FDG uptake prior to PET scanning. After the patient has arrived at an imaging center, has been interviewed by a nurse or technician, and after serum blood glucose has been tested, the patient is injected with FDG. Then there is a waiting period to allow the FDG to be taken up by the tumors, and also to allow the kidneys to remove excess background FDG activity. The length of the uptake time depends on the PET center's protocol and the type of cancer, and ranges from 45 to 120 min (Fig. 23).

Similar to insulin activity, increased skeletal muscle activity can be seen with movement or increased muscle tension during the FDG uptake period (Figs. 24 and 25). Therefore, it is important to insure that patients remain relaxed, still, and quiet. Excessive muscle activity during the uptake period can result in a sink effect and a potentially non-diagnostic exam. Small repetitive motions can lead to excessive muscle activity artifacts (Fig. 2). Examples include talking (Fig. 2), humming, mouthing silent prayers, posturing to reduce pain, clutching the arms of a chair, or fist pumping to find a vein for injection. Common locations of activity include around the vocal cords, lips, forearm muscles, and neck muscles. Patients are asked not to talk, and to try to relax. Great effort should be made to make the patients comfortable, using towel rolls to prop their head and neck for example. Some institutions give benzodiazepines to many patients to reduce this type of muscular activity (Garcia, et al. 2006). Proper pain control is also critical, and may require narcotics.

COPD, anemia, heart failure, and other problems resulting in shortness of breath are very common in cancer patients. In patients who are short of breath during uptake of FDG, excess activity is seen in the accessory muscles of respiration. The resulting activity can be impressive and involves sternocleidomastoid, scalene, intercostal, and diaphragmatic muscles to varying degrees (Fig. 24). In normal patients the diaphragm does not show significant FDG activity. In patients with labored breathing the slips of the diaphragm, often near the hiatus, can appear like round masses and show intense FDG activity. Intercostal muscle activity is often intense and can be misregistered with CT images due to motion. The pitfall is to misdiagnose the activity as if it were in the ribs. Diffuse rib FDG activity can be a sign of diffuse malignancy in the bone marrow. Patients who are short of breath should be offered supplemental oxygen during uptake, and should minimize exertion and anxiety.

The brain can show variability in activity related to cognition during the uptake phase. These artifacts can have similar appearances to infection, inflammation, and tumors, but are usually recognized and discounted. For example, if the eyes are open the visual cortex of the occipital lobe has about 20 % more activity than the remainder of the cerebral cortex.

Seizures are not uncommon in patients with cancer. Seizures represent pathology, but since they can be avoided or minimized, and since the abnormal brain activity during the uptake period is the key to their appearance on PET imaging, they are discussed here as an artifact. Active seizures can result in marked focal increased FDG activity, often at or near the site of cancer, or previously treated cancer. Seizure related FDG activity often spreads beyond the presumed focus of abnormality. Alternatively, PET imaging performed between seizures can show a focal decrease in FDG activity. Both increased and decreased activity due to seizures can be misinterpreted as malignancy, as many cancers have less FDG activity than the normal brain.

At the end of the FDG uptake phase patients are instructed to empty their bladder, which results in many artifacts. Most often urine contamination artifacts are easily identified in the groin area, on the skin. The potential for bizarre and unexpected appearances of urine contamination are well known to physicians familiar with other nuclear medicine studies such as bone scans. Urine can and does go anywhere you can imagine, and always has high FDG activity. For example, urination onto suspenders can appear like skin malignancy on the shoulders.

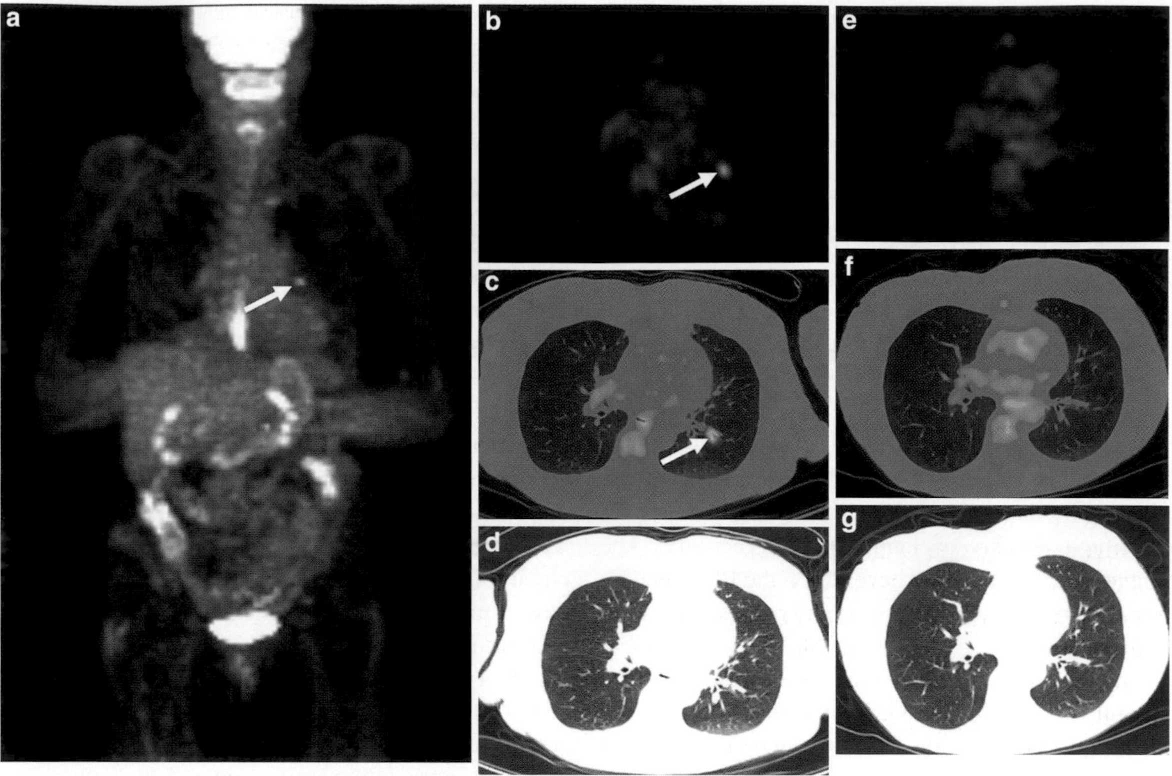

Fig. 27 Injection artifacts-embolization artifact. Sixty-eight year-old female with distal esophageal squamous cell carcinoma with an FDG-avid focus in the left mid lung (*arrows*, **a–c**) without evidence of an underlying mass **d**. This was presumed to be due to inadvertent withdrawal of blood into the FDG syringe prior to injection, resulting in a tiny FDG-avid clot. This was confirmed with repeat imaging 48 h later which demonstrated no abnormal pulmonary uptake (**e**, **f**, and **g**)

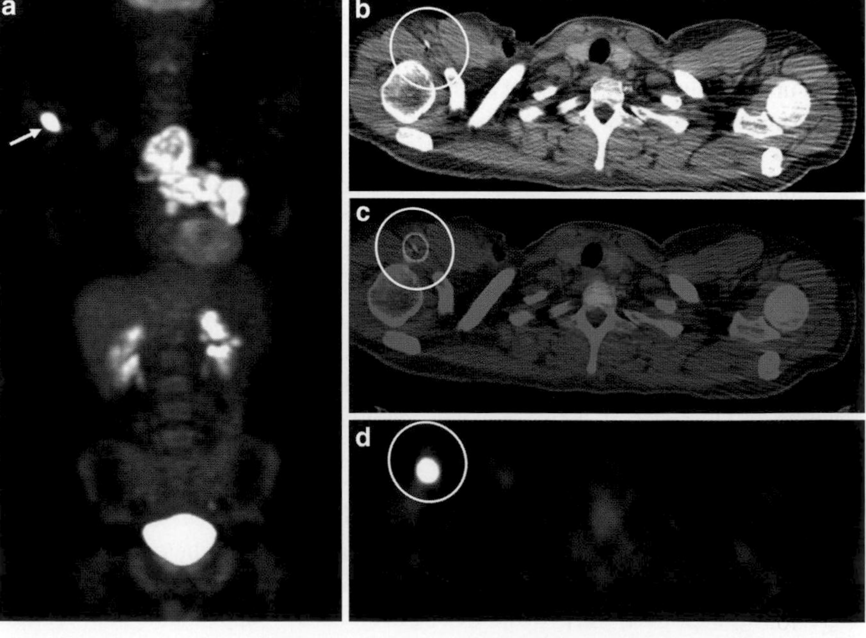

Fig. 28 Injection artifacts-catheter injection artifact. Twenty-one male with large B cell lymphoma. On the MIP image (**a**), the bulk of the patient's disease appears to be mediastinal and hilar with a possible right axillary node (*arrow*). With CT coregistration (**b**, **c**, **d**), this uptake was confirmed to be at the tip of the left upper extremity PICC catheter (*circle*)

2.6 Injection

Meticulous intravenous administration of radiotracer is important to minimize injection-related artifacts. The most common injection-related artifacts are due to extravasation of FDG into the peri-venous soft tissues at the injection site. This results in focal artifactual activity at the injection site, and subsequent drainage of FDG from the injection site through the lymphatic system. This can lead to a lymphoscintigraphy-like appearance with artifactual FDG activity within the lymphatic channels and/or axillary nodes (Fig. 26). Another artifact, especially if the extravasation is large, is the lack of FDG activity in the rest of the patient (Fig. 26). This artifact can cause falsely low activity within tumors or even a completely false negative interpretation of the PET scan.

Peripheral intravenous cannula devices are recommended, as opposed to a direct needle stick (Hamblen and Lowe 2003). Flushing the cannula with saline prior to and immediately after FDG injection is critical. A three-way stopcock adds additional control. In some patients intravenous cannula placement is difficult and a direct needle injection is administered, and should be documented for the interpreting physician. Some advocate routine SUV measurements of the cerebellum, liver, mediastinal blood pool, and injection site as quality control. The development and use of automated radiotracer injectors may also reduce the incidence of injection-related artifacts, with the additional benefit of reducing radiation exposure to the technologist (Covens et al. 2010).

Iatrogenic pulmonary micro-emboli can be intensely FDG avid. Such artifacts are thought to be related to poor injection technique and can be incorrectly interpreted as an FDG-avid tiny pulmonary nodule (Karantanis et al. 2007a, b). One key to detecting pulmonary emboli is the lack of any pulmonary nodule or other mass on the CT images (Fig. 27). In addition, it is also difficult to differentiate artifactual injection-related pulmonary micro-emboli from acute thromboembolic disease, both of which are FDG avid. Several theories exist as the source of iatrogenic FDG-avid micro-emboli, including thrombus formation at the injection site, and clotting in the injection syringe when the technician administering the dose improperly draws back to see a flash of blood prior to injection (Sanchez–Sanchez et al. 2010). The resulting pulmonary micro-embolus can on occasion be shown to be mobile or transient by immediately reimaging the patient, essentially ruling out malignancy.

Injection through indwelling catheters routinely causes artifacts, and should be avoided if at all possible (Ravizzini et al. 2004; Blodgett et al. 2005). FDG is sticky and adheres to deposits on the catheter tip and less so the catheter wall (Fig. 28). If a peripheral vein is used for FDG injection, as is recommended, then activity seen in or around an indwelling catheter is diagnostically helpful, and suggests possible thrombus, infection, or even malignancy. If a central line must be used for FDG injection, the FDG should be diluted (into 5–10 ml) and copious flushing with saline before and after FDG injection is recommended.

References

Aide N, Deux JF et al (2005) Persistent foreign body reaction around inguinal mesh prostheses: a potential pitfall of FDG PET. Am J Roentgenol 184(4):1172–1177

Bakheet SM, Powe J (1998) Fluorine-18-fluorodeoxyglucose uptake in rheumatoid arthritis-associated lung disease in a patient with thyroid cancer. J Nucl Med 39(2):234–236

Barrett JF, Keat N (2004) Artifacts in CT: recognition and avoidance. Radiographics 24(6):1679–1691

Beatty JS, Williams HT et al (2009) The predictive value of incidental PET/CT findings suspicious for breast cancer in women with non-breast malignancies. Am J Surg 198(4):495–499

Bhargava P, Kumar R et al (2004a) Catheter-related focal FDG activity on whole body PET imaging. Clin Nucl Med 29(4):238–242

Bhargava P, Zhuang H et al (2004b) Iatrogenic artifacts on whole-body F-18 FDG PET imaging. Clin Nucl Med 29(7):429–439

Blake MA, McKernan M et al (2006) Renal oncocytoma displaying intense activity on 18F-FDG PET. Am J Roentgenol 186(1):269–270

Blodgett TM, Ames JT et al (2004) Diffuse bone marrow uptake on whole-body F-18 fluorodeoxyglucose positron emission tomography in a patient taking recombinant erythropoietin. Clin Nucl Med 29(3):161–163

Blodgett TM, Fukui MB et al (2005) Combined PET-CT in the head and neck: part 1. Physiologic, altered physiologic, and artifactual FDG uptake. Radiographics 25(4):897–912

Bockisch A, Beyer T et al (2004) Positron emission tomography/computed tomography–imaging protocols, artifacts, and pitfalls. Mol Imaging Biol 6(4):188–199

Bogsrud TV, Karantanis D et al (2007) The value of quantifying 18F-FDG uptake in thyroid nodules found incidentally on whole-body PET-CT. Nucl Med Commun 28(5):373–381

Bombardieri EC, Aktolun et al. (2003) FDG-PET: procedure guidelines for tumour imaging. Eur J Nucl Med Mol Imaging 30(12):BP115–BP124

Chen YK, Wang YF et al (2007) Diagnostic trinity: Graves' disease on F-18 FDG PET. Clin Nucl Med 32(10):816–817

Chernov M, Hayashi M et al (2005) Differentiation of the radiation-induced necrosis and tumor recurrence after gamma knife radiosurgery for brain metastases: importance of multi-voxel proton MRS. Minim Invasive Neurosurg 48(4):228–234

Chhabra A, Batra K et al (2006) Obscured bone metastases after administration of hematopoietic factor on FDG-PET. Clin Nucl Med 31(6):328–330

Chowdhury FU, Sheerin F et al (2009) Sarcoid-like reaction to malignancy on whole-body integrated (18)F-FDG PET/CT: prevalence and disease pattern. Clin Radiol 64(7):675–681

Christensen JA, Nathan MA et al (2006) Characterization of the solitary pulmonary nodule: F-18-FDG PET versus nodule-enhancement CT. Am J Roentgenol 187(5):1361–1367

Chung YE, Kim EK et al (2006) Suture granuloma mimicking recurrent thyroid carcinoma on ultrasonography. Yonsei Med J 47(5):748–751

Cohade C, Mourtzikos KA et al (2003) "USA-Fat": prevalence is related to ambient outdoor temperature-evaluation with 18F-FDG PET/CT. J Nucl Med 44(8):1267–1270

Cook GJR, Fogelman I et al (1996) Normal physiological and benign pathological variants of 18-fluoro-2-deoxyglucose positron-emission tomography scanning: Potential for error in interpretation. Semin Nucl Med 26(4):308–314

Covens P, Berus D et al (2010) The introduction of automated dispensing and injection during PET procedures: a step in the optimisation of extremity doses and whole-body doses of nuclear medicine staff. Radiat Prot Dosimetry 140(3):250–258

Do B, Mari C et al (2006) Diagnosis of aseptic deep venous thrombosis of the upper extremity in a cancer patient using fluorine-18 fluorodeoxyglucose positron emission tomography/computerized tomography (FDG PET/CT). Ann Nucl Med 20(2):151–155

Erdi YE, Nehmeh SA et al (2004) The CT motion quantitation of lung lesions and its impact on PET-measured SUVs. J Nucl Med 45(8):1287–1292

Fallanca F, Giovacchini G et al (2008) Cervical thymic hyperplasia after chemotherapy in an adult patient with Hodgkin lymphoma: a potential cause of false-positivity on [18F]FDG PET/CT scanning. Br J Haematol 140(5):477

Fanti S, Franchi R et al (2005) PET and PET-CT. State of the art and future prospects. Radiol Med 110(1–2):1–15

Fuechsel FG, Weidner S et al (2006) Focal pelvic uptake in 18F-FDG PET due to a contraceptive device; a potential pitfall easily unmasked by PET-CT. Nuklearmedizin 45(4):N42–N43

Garcia CA, Van Nostrand D et al (2006) Reduction of brown fat 2-deoxy-2-[F-18]fluoro-D-glucose uptake by controlling environmental temperature prior to positron emission tomography scan. Mol Imaging Biol 8(1):24–29

Garcia CA, Van Nostrand D et al (2004) Benzodiazepine-resistant "brown fat" pattern in positron emission tomography: two case reports of resolution with temperature control. Mol Imaging Biol 6(6):368–372

Glazer ES, Beaty K et al. (2010) Effectiveness of positron emission tomography for predicting chemotherapy response in colorectal cancer liver metastases. Arch Surg 145(4): 340–345, (discussion 345)

Goerres GW, Burger C et al (2003) Respiration-induced attenuation artifact at PET/CT: technical considerations. Radiology 226(3):906–910

Goerres GW, Hany TF et al (2002a) Head and neck imaging with PET and PET/CT: artefacts from dental metallic implants. Eur J Nucl Med Mol Imaging 29(3):367–370

Goerres GW, Von Schulthess GK et al (2002b) Positron emission tomography and PET CT of the head and neck: FDG uptake in normal anatomy, in benign lesions, and in changes resulting from treatment. Am J Roentgenol 179(5): 1337–1343

Gollub MJ, Akhurst T et al (2007) Combined CT colonography and 18F-FDG PET of colon polyps: potential technique for selective detection of cancer and precancerous lesions. Am J Roentgenol 188(1):130–138

Gupta P, Ponzo F et al (2005) Fluorodeoxyglucose (FDG) uptake in pulmonary rheumatoid nodules. Clin Rheumatol 24(4):402–405

Hamada K, Myoui A et al (2005) FDG-PET imaging for chronic expanding hematoma in pelvis with massive bone destruction. Skelet Radiol 34(12):807–811

Hamblen SM and Lowe VJ (2003) Clinical 18F-FDG oncology patient preparation techniques. J Nucl Med Technol 31(1):3–7, (quiz 8–10)

Hanif MZ, Ghesani M et al (2004) F-18 fluorodeoxyglucose uptake in atherosclerotic plaque in the mediastinum mimicking malignancy: another potential for error. Clin Nucl Med 29(2):93–95

Heiba SI, Raphael B et al (2009) PET/CT image fusion error due to urinary bladder filling changes: consequence and correction. Ann Nucl Med 23(8):739–744

Hollinger EF, Alibazoglu H et al (1998) Hematopoietic cytokine-mediated FDG uptake simulates the appearance of diffuse metastatic disease on whole-body PET imaging. Clin Nucl Med 23(2):93–98

Hung GU, Tsai SC et al (2005) Extraordinarily high F-18 FDG uptake caused by radiation necrosis in a patient with nasopharyngeal carcinoma. Clin Nucl Med 30(8):558–559

Joosen H, Mellaerts B et al (2000) Pulmonary nodule and aggressive tibialis posterior tenosynovitis in early rheumatoid arthritis. Clin Rheumatol 19(5):392–395

Kamel EM, Mckee TA et al (2005) Occult lung infarction may induce false interpretation of F-18-FDG PET in primary staging of pulmonary malignancies. Eur J Nucl Med Mol Imaging 32(6):641–646

Kao CH, Sun SS et al (2007) Misdiagnosis of multiple bone metastases due to increased FDG uptake in polyostotic fibrous dysplasia. Clin Nucl Med 32(5):409–410

Kapoor V, McCook BM et al (2004) An introduction to PET-CT imaging. Radiographics 24(2):523–543

Karantanis D, Bogsrud TV et al (2007a) Clinical significance of diffusely increased 18F-FDG uptake in the thyroid gland. J Nucl Med 48(6):896–901

Karantanis D, Subramaniam RM et al (2007b) Focal F-18 fluoro-deoxy-glucose accumulation in the lung parenchyma in the absence of CT abnormality in PET/CT. J Comput Assist Tomogr 31(5):800–805

Kazama T, Swanston N et al (2005) Effect of colony-stimulating factor and conventional- or high-dose chemotherapy on FDG uptake in bone marrow. Eur J Nucl Med Mol Imaging 32(12):1406–1411

Kikuchi M, Yamamoto E et al (2004) Case report: internal and external jugular vein thrombosis with marked accumulation of FDG. Br J Radiol 77(922):888–890

Kim MK, Kim GS et al (2009) F-18 FDG-avid intrathyroidal parathyroid adenoma mimicking follicular neoplasm. Clin Nucl Med 34(3):178–179

King DL, Stack BC Jr et al (2007) Incidence of thyroid carcinoma in fluorodeoxyglucose positron emission tomography-positive thyroid incidentalomas. Otolaryngol Head Neck Surg 137(3):400–404

Kisielinski K, Cremerius U et al (2003) Fluordeoxyglucose positron emission tomography detection of inflammatory reactions due to polyethylene wear in total hip arthroplasty. J Arthroplasty 18(4):528–532

Koga H, Sasaki M et al (2003) An analysis of the physiological FDG uptake pattern in the stomach. Ann Nucl Med 17(8): 733–738

Kubota K, Ito K et al (2009) Whole-body FDG-PET/CT on rheumatoid arthritis of large joints. Ann Nucl Med 23(9): 783–791

Lee JW, Kang KW et al (2009) 18F-FDG PET in the assessment of tumor grade and prediction of tumor recurrence in intracranial meningioma. Eur J Nucl Med Mol Imaging 36(10):1574–1582

Levine JM, Weiner M et al (2006) Routine use of PET scans after completion of therapy in pediatric Hodgkin disease results in a high false positive rate. J Pediatr Hematol Oncol 28(11):711–714

Lim ST, Jeong HJ et al (2008) F-18 FDG PET-CT findings of intraperitoneal carbon particles-induced granulomas mimicking peritoneal carcinomatosis. Clin Nucl Med 33(5):321–324

Liu Y (2009a) Benign ovarian and endometrial uptake on FDG PET-CT: patterns and pitfalls. Ann Nucl Med 23(2):107–112

Liu Y (2009b) Orthopedic surgery-related benign uptake on FDG-PET: case examples and pitfalls. Ann Nucl Med 23(8):701–708

Lowe VJ, Fletcher JW et al (1998) Prospective investigation of positron emission tomography in lung nodules. J Clin Oncol 16(3):1075–1084

Mawlawi O, Erasmus JJ et al (2006) Truncation artifact on PET/CT: impact on measurements of activity concentration and assessment of a correction algorithm. Am J Roentgenol 186(5):1458–1467

Modi D, Fulham MJ et al (2005) Markedly increased FDG uptake in a vocal cord after medialization with Teflon: PET/CT findings. Clin Nucl Med 30(1):45–47

Nakahara T, Takagi Y et al (2008) Dose-related fluorodeoxyglucose uptake in acute radiation-induced hepatitis. Eur J Gastroenterol Hepatol 20(10):1040–1044

Nakamoto Y, Chin BB et al (2004) PET/CT: artifacts caused by bowel motion. Nucl Med Commun 25(3):221–225

Nam H, Smith S et al (2007) A pitfall of 18-fluorodeoxyglucose-PET in a patient with a tattoo. Lancet Oncol 8(12):1147–1148

Nguyen BD (2007) PET, CT, and MR imaging of extra-articular pigmented villonodular synovitis. Clin Nucl Med 32(6):493–495

Nguyen NC, Tran I et al (2009) F-18 FDG PET/CT characterization of talc pleurodesis-induced pleural changes over time: a retrospective study. Clin Nucl Med 34(12):886–890

Nishizawa S, Inubushi M et al (2008) Incidence and characteristics of uterine leiomyomas with FDG uptake. Ann Nucl Med 22(9):803–810

Nunes ML, Rault A et al (2010) 18F-FDG PET for the identification of adrenocortical carcinomas among indeterminate adrenal tumors at computed tomography scanning. World J Surg 34(7): 1506–1510

Ondik MP, Kang J et al (2009) Teflon laryngeal granuloma presenting as laryngeal cancer on combined positron emission tomography and computed tomography scanning. J Laryngol Otol 123(5):575–578

Osman MM, Cohade C et al (2003) Respiratory motion artifacts on PET emission images obtained using CT attenuation correction on PET-CT. Eur J Nucl Med Mol Imaging 30(4):603–606

Ouellet V, Routhier-Labadie A et al. (2010) Outdoor temperature, age, sex, body mass index, and diabetic status determine the prevalence, mass, and glucose-uptake activity of 18F-FDG-detected BAT in humans. J Clin Endocrinol Metab

Pan T, Mawlawi O et al (2006) Attenuation correction of PET cardiac data with low-dose average CT in PET/CT. Med Phys 33(10):3931–3938

Pan T, Mawlawi O et al (2005) Attenuation correction of PET images with respiration-averaged CT images in PET/CT. J Nucl Med 46(9):1481–1487

Prabhakar HB, Rabinowitz CB et al (2008) Imaging features of sarcoidosis on MDCT, FDG PET, and PET/CT. Am J Roentgenol 190(3 Suppl):S1–S6

Prabhakar HB, Sahani DV et al (2007) Bowel hot spots at PET-CT. Radiographics 27(1):145–159

Ravizzini G, Nguyen M et al (2004) Central line injection artifact simulating paratracheal adenopathy on FDG PET imaging. Clin Nucl Med 29(11):735–737

Ricci PE, Karis JP et al (1998) Differentiating recurrent tumor from radiation necrosis: time for re-evaluation of positron emission tomography? Am J Neuroradiol 19(3):407–413

Roy FN, Beaulieu S et al (2009) Impact of intravenous insulin on 18F-FDG PET in diabetic cancer patients. J Nucl Med 50(2):178–183

Ryan AT, Amesur N et al. (2007) Intense FDG activity on PET/CT in a pulmonary embolus mimicking metastatic disease. Am J Roentgenol 188(5)

Salhab KF, Baram D et al (2006) Growing PET positive nodule in a patient with histoplasmosis: case report. J Cardiothorac Surg 1:23

Sanchez-Sanchez R, Rodriguez-Fernandez A et al (2010) PET/CT: Focal lung uptake of F-18-fluordeoxiglucose on PET but no structural alterations on CT. Revista Espanola De Medicina Nuclear 29(3):131–134

Smith CS, Schoder H et al (2007) Thymic extension in the superior mediastinum in patients with thymic hyperplasia: potential cause of false-positive findings on 18F-FDG PET/CT. Am J Roentgenol 188(6):1716–1721

Sopov V, Bernstine H et al (2009) The metabolic spectrum of venous thrombotic disorders found on PET/CT. Am J Roentgenol 193(6):W530–W539

Strobel K, von Hochstetter AR et al (2009) FDG uptake in a rheumatoid nodule with imaging appearance similar to a malignant soft tissue tumor. Clin Nucl Med 34(10):691–692

Subramaniam RM, Clayton AC et al (2007) Hibernoma: 18F FDG PET/CT imaging. J Thorac Oncol 2(6):569–570

Sugawara Y, Zasadny KR et al (1999) Splenic fluorodeoxyglucose uptake increased by granulocyte colony-stimulating factor therapy: PET imaging results. J Nucl Med 40(9): 1456–1462

Sureshbabu W, Mawlawi O (2005) PET/CT imaging artifacts. J Nucl Med Technol 33(3):156–161, (quiz 163–154)

Tessonnier L, Fakhry N et al (2008) False-positive finding on FDG-PET/CT after injectable elastomere implant (Vox implant) for vocal cord paralysis. Otolaryngol Head Neck Surg 139(5):738–739

Thompson TP, Lunsford LD et al (1999) Distinguishing recurrent tumor and radiation necrosis with positron emission tomography versus stereotactic biopsy. Stereotact Funct Neurosurg 73(1–4):9–14

Truong MT, Erasmus JJ et al (2004) Teflon injection for vocal cord paralysis: False-positive finding on FDG PET-CT in a patient with non-small cell lung cancer. Am J Roentgenol 182(6):1587–1589

Tsai YF, Wu CC et al (2005) FDG PET CT features of an intraabdominal gossypiboma. Clin Nucl Med 30(8):561–563

Tsuchiya T, Osanai T et al (2006) Hibernomas show intense accumulation of FDG positron emission tomography. J Comput Assist Tomogr 30(2):333–336

Wang CH, Sun SS et al (2010) Unexpected left-sided pulmonary aspiration misdiagnosed as malignancy in PET cancer screening following panendoscopy cancer screening under conscious sedation. Clin Nucl Med 35(8):604–606

Wasselius J, Malmstedt J et al (2008) High 18F-FDG Uptake in synthetic aortic vascular grafts on PET/CT in symptomatic and asymptomatic patients. J Nucl Med 49(10):1601–1605

Yau YY, Chan WS et al (2005) Application of intravenous contrast in PET/CT: Does it really introduce significant attenuation correction error? J Nucl Med 46(2):283–291

Yoshida T, Sakamoto A et al (2007) Intramuscular diffuse-type giant cell tumor within the hamstring muscle. Skelet Radiol 36(4):331–333

Yu JQ, Milestone BN et al (2008) Findings of intramediastinal gossypiboma with F-18 FDG PET in a melanoma patient. Clin Nucl Med 33(5):344–345

Index

P. Peller et al. (eds.), *PET-CT and PET-MRI in Oncology*, Medical Radiology. Diagnostic Imaging,
DOI: 10.1007/978-3-642-01139-9,